Biliary Lithiasis

Basic Science, Current Diagnosis and Management

GIUSEPPE BORZELLINO • CLAUDIO CORDIANO

Biliary Lithiasis

Basic Science, Current Diagnosis and Management

Springer

GIUSEPPE BORZELLINO
Department of Surgery
University of Verona
University Hospital O.C.M. Borgo Trento
Verona, Italy

CLAUDIO CORDIANO
Department of Surgery
University of Verona
University Hospital O.C.M. Borgo Trento
Verona, Italy

Library of Congress Control Number: 2008926950

ISBN 978-88-470-0762-8 Springer Milan Berlin Heidelberg New York
e-ISBN 978-88-470-0763-5

Springer is a part of Springer Science+Business Media
springer.com

Cover design: Simona Colombo, Milan, Italy
Typesetting: Graphostudio, Milan, Italy
Printer: Grafiche Porpora Srl, Segrate (Milan), Italy

Printed in Italy
Springer-Verlag Italia S.r.l.,Via Decembrio 28, I-20137 Milan

PREFACE

The first laparoscopic cholecystectomy, performed by Prof. Philippe Mouret in 1987 and described by himself in the first chapter of this book, was an event that revolutionized surgery in the past few decades.

Although the majority of surgeons today are unfamiliar with the history of early minimally invasive surgery developments, it is important to realize that the advent of laparoscopy led not only to new surgical techniques, but also to a change in the doctrine of medical care, by strengthening the concept of minimal invasiveness.

This is particularly the case for biliary lithiasis, for which laparoscopy has provided major benefits in terms of both diagnosis and surgical treatment. However, our understanding of the etiology of this disease, as well as the availability of effective medical therapies, have remained substantially unchanged over time.

The application of the innovative approach has not been, in routine practice, without problems: between 1990 and 2000, the rate of serious complications from laparoscopic cholecystectomy were four times higher than those observed with open surgery. Even initial attempts at laparoscopic treatment of biliary common bile duct stones resulted in excessive complications and associated medico-legal problems. Nonetheless, today, most indications have been stated, techniques have been standardized, and a new aspect to the treatment of biliary lithiasis has appeared.

Such important changes in the field of biliary lithiasis and the extended survey of the new procedures justified an assessment and a setting of the new findings with the aim of establishing a balance among basic medical knowledge, technological possibilities and clinical applications. This revision process represents the collective efforts of surgeons as well as radiologists, gastroenterologists and endoscopists, particularly from the main European groups in the field, most of which have contributed to the present volume. We thank all of our colleagues who accepted our invitation. We also apologize to these authors for the pressure that we sometimes exerted on them in order to harmonize the various contributions to this collective work. Finally, we thank Drs. Barbara Ferrario and Donatella Rizza at Springer-Verlag for expert advice and editorial organization, which were fundamental to the successful publication of this volume in a flawless editorial drafting.

Verona, May 2008

Giuseppe Borzellino
Claudio Cordiano

TABLE OF CONTENTS

CONTRIBUTORS

Francesca Abbatini
Department of Surgery Paride Stefanini
Policlinico Umberto I
University of Rome La Sapienza
Rome, Italy

Stefano Amplatz
Division of Gastroenterology
Central Hospital of Bolzano
Bolzano, Italy

Francesco Ardito
Department of Surgery
Hepatobiliary Surgery Unit
Catholic University of the Sacred Heart
School of Medicine
Rome, Italy

Alberto Arezzo
Department of Surgery
Minimally Invasive Surgery Centre
University of Turin
Turin, Italy

Nicola Basso
Department of Surgery Paride Stefanini
Policlinico Umberto I
University of Rome La Sapienza
Rome, Italy

Consuelo Arnal Bertomeu
ICAD (Instituto de Cirugía General
y Aparato Digestivo)
Quiron Clinic
Valencia, Spain

Luigi Borraccino
Department of Internal Medicine
and Public Medicine
Clinica Medica A. Murri
University of Bari Medical School
Bari, Italy

Giuseppe Borzellino
Department of Surgery
University Hospital O.C.M. Borgo Trento
University of Verona
Verona, Italy

Anne Bouix
Department of General Surgery
Percy Military Hospital
Clamart, France

Christoph E. Broelsch
Clinic for General,
Visceral and Transplantation Surgery
University Hospital of Essen
Essen, Germany

Luigi Brusciano
I Division of General
and Gastrointestinal Surgery
Second University of Naples
Naples, Italy

Jose Bueno Lledó
ICAD (Instituto de Cirugía General
y Aparato Digestivo)
Quiron Clinic
Valencia, Spain

Grant Caddy
Department of Gastroenterology
Ulster Hospital
Belfast, Northern Ireland (G.B.)

Ronan Cahill
IRCAD/EITS Institute
Strasbourg, France

Lorenzo Capussotti
Department of Surgery
Hepato-Pancreato-Biliary Unit
Hospital Mauriziano
Torino, Italy

Miguel Carneiro de Moura
Centre of Gastroenterology
University Hospital of Santa Maria
Lisbon, Portugal

Miguel Carrau Giner
Department of Anaesthesiology
ICAD (Instituto de Cirugía General
y Aparato Digestivo)
Quiron Clinic
Valencia, Spain

Luís Carrilho-Ribeiro
Centre of Gastroenterology
University Hôpitaux de Santa Maria
Lisbon, Portugal

Giovanni Casella
Department of Surgery Paride Stefanini
Policlinico Umberto I
University of Rome La Sapienza
Rome, Italy

Jean-Marc Catheline
Departement of Digestive Surgery
Hospital Avicenne
Assistance Publique-Hôpitaux de Paris
Bobigny, Paris, France

Maria Cervera Delgado
ICAD (Instituto de Cirugía General
y Aparato Digestivo)
Quiron Clinic
Valencia, Spain

Francesco Cetta
Department of Surgery
Interuniversity Center for Research
in Hepatobiliary Disease
University of Siena
Siena, Italy

Olivier Chapuis
Department of General Surgery
Percy Military Hospital
Clamart, France

Fausto Chilovi
Division of Gastroenterology
Central Hospital of Bolzano
Bolzano, Italy

Claudio Cordiano
Department of Surgery
University Hospital O.C.M. Borgo Trento
University of Verona
Verona, Italy

Alberto del Genio
I Division of General
and Gastrointestinal Surgery
Second University of Naples
Naples, Italy

Gianmattia del Genio
I Division of General
and Gastrointestinal Surgery
Second University of Naples
Naples, Italy

Claudia della Corte
Department of Pediatrics
Federico II University
Naples, Italy

Manuela De Luca
Department of Surgery
University Hospital O.C.M. Borgo Trento
University of Verona
Verona, Italy

Giovanni De Manzoni
Department of Surgery
University Hospital O.C.M. Borgo Trento
University of Verona
Verona, Italy

Marianna De Marco
Department of Pediatrics
Federico II University
Naples, Italy

Agostino Di Ciaula
Division of Internal Medicine
Hospital of Bisceglie
Bisceglie (Bari), Italy

Maria Di Martino
I Division of General
and Gastrointestinal Surgery
Second University of Naples
Naples, Italy

Eduardo Escarti Carbonell
Department of Gastroenterology ICAD
(Instituto de Cirugía General
y Aparato Digestivo)
Quiron Clinic
Valencia, Spain

Ciro Esposito
Department of Pediatrics
Federico II University
Naples, Italy

Tiziana Facella
Department of Surgery
University of Palermo
Palermo, Italy

Alessandro Ferrero
Department of Surgery
Hepato-Pancreato-Biliary Unit
Hospital Mauriziano
Torino, Italy

Marco Filauro
Department of Surgery
HPB Unit
Galliera Hospital
Genoa, Italy

Rafael Garcia Espinosa
ICAD (Instituto de Cirugía General
y Aparato Digestivo)
Quiron Clinic
Valencia, Spain

Giacomo Gaverini
Departement of Surgery
Hospital Fatebenefratelli
Milan, Italy

Gian M. Gazzaniga
Department of Surgery
HPB Unit
Galliera Hospital
Genoa, Italy

Girolamo Geraci
Department of Surgery
University of Palermo
Palermo, Italy

Simone Giacopuzzi
Department of Surgery
University Hospital O.C.M. Borgo Trento
University of Verona
Verona, Italy

Jean-François Gigot
Division of Hepatobiliary
and Pancreatic Surgery
Department of Abdominal Surgery
and Transplantation
Saint-Luc University Hospital
Brussels, Belgium

Felice Giuliante
Department of Surgery
Hepatobiliary Surgery Unit
Catholic University of the Sacred Heart
School of Medicine
Rome, Italy

Monica Gualtierotti
IRCAD/EITS Institute
Strasbourg, France

Alfredo Guglielmi
Department of Surgery
and Gastroenterology
G.B. Rossi Hospital
University of Verona
Verona, Italy

Catherine Hubert
Division of Hepatobiliary
and Pancreatic Surgery
Department of Abdominal Surgery
and Transplantation
Saint-Luc University Hospital
Brussels, Belgium

Raffaele Iorio
Department of Pediatrics
Federico II University
Naples, Italy

Anna M. Koivusalo
Department of Anaesthesia
and Intensive Care
Liver Surgery
and Transplantation Clinic
University Hospital
Helsinki, Finland

Hwai-Ding Lam
Department of Abdominal Surgery
Hospital Saint Joseph
Charleroi (Gilly), Belgium

Emilie Lermite
Department of Digestive Surgery
CHU Angers
Angers, France

Emanuele Lezoche
Department of General Surgery
and Organ Transplantation P. Stefanini
Azienda Policlinico Umberto I
University of Rome La Sapienza
Rome, Italy

Francesco Li Volsi
Department of Surgery
University of Palermo
Palermo, Italy

Frauke Löhlein
Department of Visceral
and Transplantation Surgery
University Hospital of Zurich
Zurich, Switzerland

Francesco Lombardo
Department of Surgery
University Hospital O.C.M. Borgo Trento
University of Verona
Verona, Italy

Vincenzo Maffettone
I Division of General
and Gastrointestinal Surgery
Second University of Naples
Naples, Italy

Brice Malgras
Department of General Surgery
Percy Military Hospital
Clamart, France

Riccardo Manfredi
Department of Radiology
University of Verona
G.B. Rossi University Hospital
Verona, Italy

Jacques Marescaux
IRCAD/EITS Institute
Strasbourg, France

David Martin
Department of Upper GI Surgery
Concord and Royal Prince Alfred Hospitals
Sydney, Australia;
Copenhagen Trial Unit
Cochrane Hepato-Biliary Group
Copenhagen, Denmark

Ian Martin
Department of Upper GI Surgery
Princess Alexandra Hospital
Brisbane, Australia

John Meenan
Department of Gastroenterology
Guy's and St. Thomas's Hospital
London, United Kingdom

Sara Mehrabi
Department of Radiology
University of Verona
G.B. Rossi University Hospital
Verona, Italy

Anna M. Minicozzi
Department of Surgery
University Hospital O.C.M. Borgo Trento
University of Verona
Verona, Italy

Giuseppe Modica
Department of Surgery
University of Palermo
Palermo, Italy

Mario Morino
Department of Surgery
Minimally Invasive Surgery Centre
University of Turin
Turin, Italy

Antonio Moschetta
Department of Internal Medicine
and Public Medicine
Clinica Medica A. Murri
University of Bari Medical School
Bari, Italy;
Department of Translational Pharmacology
Consorzio Mario Negri Sud
Santa Maria Imbaro (Chieti), Italy

Massimiliano Motton
Department of Radiology
University of Verona
G.B. Rossi University Hospital
Verona, Italy

Philippe Mouret
Professor of Surgery
Lyon, France

Markus K. Müller
Department of Visceral
and Transplantation Surgery
University Hospital of Zurich
Zurich, Switzerland

Andrea Muratore
Department of Surgery
Hepato-Pancreato-Biliary Unit
Hospital Mauriziano
Torino, Italy

Vincenzo Napolitano
I Division of General
and Gastrointestinal Surgery
Second University of Naples
Naples, Italy

Benoit Navez
Department of Abdominal Surgery
Hospital Saint Joseph
Charleroi (Gilly), Belgium

Yuji Nimura
Department of Digestive Surgery
Aichi Cancer Center
Nagoya, Japan

Gennaro Nuzzo
Department of Surgery
Hepatobiliary Surgery Unit
Catholic University of the Sacred Heart
School of Medicine
Rome, Italy

Alessandro M. Paganini
Department of General Surgery
and Organ Transplantation P. Stefanini
Azienda Policlinico Umberto I
University of Rome La Sapienza
Rome, Italy

Andreas Paul
Clinic for General
Visceral and Transplantation Surgery
University Hospital of Essen
Essen, Germany

Patrick Pessaux
Department of Hepatic Surgery
and Transplantation
Hospital of Hautepierre
Strasbourg, France

Franco Pisello
Department of Surgery
University of Palermo
Palermo, Italy

Francesco Pizza
I Division of General
and Gastrointestinal Surgery
Second University of Naples
Naples, Italy

Manuel Planells Roig
ICAD (Instituto de Cirugía General
y Aparato Digestivo)
Quiron Clinic
Valencia, Spain

Daniela Pontrelli
Department of Internal Medicine
and Public Medicine
Clinica Medica A. Murri
University of Bari Medical School
Bari, Italy

Piero Portincasa
Department of Internal Medicine
and Public Medicine
Clinica Medica A. Murri
University of Bari Medical School
Bari, Italy

Roberto Pozzi Mucelli
Department of Radiology
University of Verona
G.B. Rossi University Hospital
Verona, Italy

Francesco Puglisi
Section of Surgery
Department of Emergency
and Transplant Organs (DETO)
University of Bari Medical School
Bari, Italy

Gabriele Regina
Department of Surgical Sciences
Section of General Surgical Clinics
and Surgical Therapy
Parma University Medical School
Parma, Italy

Mario Rizzello
Department of Surgery P. Stefanini
Policlinico Umberto I
University of Rome La Sapienza
Rome, Italy

Luigi Roncoroni
Department of Surgical Sciences
Section of General Surgical Clinics
and Surgical Therapy
Parma University Medical School
Parma, Italy

Gianluca Rossetti
I Division of General
and Gastrointestinal Surgery
Second University of Naples
Naples, Italy

Adriana Rotundo
Department of General Surgery
and Organ Transplantation P. Stefanini
Azienda Policlinico Umberto I
University of Rome La Sapienza
Rome, Italy

Joël Roussel
Hospital Avicenne
Assistance Publique-Hôpitaux de Paris
Bobigny, Paris, France

Andrea Ruzzenente
Department of Surgery
and Gastroenterology
G.B. Rossi Hospital
University of Verona
Verona, Italy

Edoardo Saladino
Department of Surgery
University Hospital O.C.M. Borgo Trento
University of Verona
Verona, Italy

Angel Sanahuja Santafé
ICAD (Instituto de Cirugía General
y Aparato Digestivo)
Quiron Clinic
Valencia, Spain

Africa Sanchez Salas
ICAD (Instituto de Cirugía General
y Aparato Digestivo)
Quiron Clinic
Valencia, Spain

Leopoldo Sarli
Department of Surgical Sciences
Section of General Surgical Clinics
and Surgical Therapy
Parma University Medical School
Parma, Italy

ROSA C. SASSO
Department of Internal Medicine
and Public Medicine
Clinica Medica A. Murri
University of Bari Medical School
Bari, Italy

STEFAN SAUERLAND
Institute for Research
in Operative Medicine
University of Witten/Herdecke
Cologne, Germany

MARKUS SCHÄFER
Department of Visceral
and Transplantation Surgery
University Hospital of Zurich
Zurich, Switzerland

CARMELO SCIUMÉ
Department of Surgery
University of Palermo
Palermo, Italy

ALESSANDRO SETTIMI
Department of Pediatrics
Federico II University
Naples, Italy

GIANFRANCO SILECCHIA
Department of Surgery Paride Stefanini
Policlinico Umberto I
University of Rome La Sapienza
Rome, Italy

CINTHYA SOLANO
IRCAD/EITS Institute
Strasbourg, France

LUC SOLER
IRCAD/EITS Institute
Strasbourg, France

G. PAOLO SPINA
Department of Surgery
Hospital Fatebenefratelli
Milan, Italy

HORST STEINER
Department of Gynecology
Paracelsus Medical University
Salzburg, Austria

PAUL SUNGLER
Department of Surgery
Paracelsus Medical University
Salzburg, Austria

SALVATORE TOLONE
I Division of General
and Gastrointestinal Surgery
Second University of Naples
Naples, Italy

JÜRGEN TRECKMANN
Clinic for General
Visceral and Transplantation Surgery
University Hospital of Essen
Essen, Germany

PIETRO VAYRO
Department of Pediatrics
Federico II University
Naples, Italy

LUCA VIGANÒ
Department of Surgery
Hepato-Pancreato-Biliary Unit
Hospital Mauriziano
Turin, Italy

HELEN H. WANG
Gastroenterology Division
Beth Israel Deaconess Medical Center
Department of Medicine
Harvard Medical School
Boston, Massachusetts, USA

DAVID Q.-H. WANG
Gastroenterology Division
Beth Israel Deaconess Medical Center
Department of Medicine
Harvard Medical School
Boston, Massachusetts, USA

CHIARA ZUGNI
Department of Surgery
and Gastroenterology
G.B. Rossi Hospital
University of Verona
Verona, Italy

Chapter 1

Reflections on the Birth and on the Concept of Laparoscopic Surgery

Philippe Mouret

Cœlioscopic cholecystectomy turns twenty this year, an age that places it somewhere between the carefree attitude of a child, the follies of an adolescent and the senility and obsoleteness that will arrive when medical therapy will be able to master and control biliary lithogenesis. Until now, there are no signs of any credible harbingers. Even if one day cœlioscopic cholecystectomy disappears into the dustbin of obsolete technologies, I suppose the concept of minimally invasive surgery will nevertheless remain for a long time. More than this, I hope that the concept of reduction in aggressiveness, an approach directly linked to this surgery, will continue and develop even further.

Cœlioscopic cholecystectomy, beyond its existence as a treatment approach for biliary lithiasis, also holds the honor, in the eyes of the international surgical community, of being considered the starting point for cœlioscopic digestive surgery. This is a mistaken notion, or more specifically, an inexact one, from two perspectives. I personally performed my first cœlioscopic cholecystectomy in March of 1987. I shall make a precise report on this operation later. However, somebody else before me, the German Muhe, using a cœlioscope for viewing and lighting, had performed during the years 1985-86, a series of cholecystectomies with a clever piece of equipment resembling an operative anuscope that, within the same operating envelope, allowed room for the optical lens, the insufflation system and the operative tool or tools.

Taking advantage of an unfortunate outcome in one of his patients, the confraternal community of Muhe's country, helped by its repressive justice system, put an end to his series, which at this stage was already well advanced, and did all that was possible to block the spreading of Muhe's new technique. For this reason I didn't know of Muhe in 1987, and I only learned of his trials years later when those bitterly protesting my paternity informed me of Muhe and his work.

The use of a cœlioscope as a viewing device was such an innovation, even if, in terms of technical conception, it was not yet entirely the cœlioscopic surgery of today, that I thought it appropriate to share the honor of the recognition of this first in biliary surgery with Muhe. This did not happen.

Muhe had fully understood the advantages of viewing through the cœlioscope, but not entirely the possibilities of the present-day cœlioscopic technique. He was still limited by the single port access, which permitted only "fleeting glances" of the operative tool, making control difficult or approximate. This technique could be defined as a "micro-laparotomy record", and it therefore faced the same limits as the mini-laparotomy of the time.

I myself contributed the principle of operating by convergent and separate paths via multiple port accesses at a distance from the optic: a technique that had the advantage of being able to be extended to all cœlioscopic interventions. This principle already existed before me. It has become both a rule and a concept.

This ability to become a generalized technique probably explains the enormous success (that I personally find partially unjustified) of this operation, which has become known mythically and symbolically as the birth of operative laparoscopy in digestive surgery.

I had hoped to be able to pay Muhe this homage publicly; this could not be done. Today, I can only do it posthumously.

I would have been even more inclined to share with him the honor of this "première" biliary operation, since it was far from being my first "première". It did not represent my first steps in laparoscopic surgery, but it did mark the completion of a long evolution and experience with laparoscopy both technically and conceptually. I have always thought that cœlioscopy represents the most efficient way of aiding and perfecting digestive surgery, both on tactical and technical levels.

The destiny of a treatise is different from a publication in the specialized press and it strives to be read for a long time to come, without going so far as to evoke eternity. This is why it seemed logical for me to take advantage of the present treatise's vast forum, to report the prehistory of laparoscopic surgery, of which I am a part, and which ran until its historic period for which it has been established it specifically begun in 1987. After this date, I no longer possessed the exclusivity or the mastery of the evolution of laparoscopy: the innovation became a collective one.

I have absolutely no intention of using this occasion to make a personal apology or give self-praise, but the principles that I discovered or, more exactly, applied during this prehistoric phase, still seem essential today for the conception, the evolution and the teaching of laparoscopic surgery. It should be kept in mind that I am by far not the only person to have conceived of this concept. Unfortunately, these facts have been completely obscured by the explosive worldwide diffusion of laparoscopy that surprised the unsuspecting digestive surgical world. Its members admitted this innovation without inspection and almost without reflection.

The explosive character of the diffusion of laparoscopic surgery after the discovery of laparoscopic cholecystectomy brought one and all, including myself, to speak and act in inexact, poorly thought-out ways. It is time to try to get back on track, on this historic and conceptual revisiting occasion of the birth of laparoscopic surgery.

If we must argue over possible paternity of laparoscopic surgery, so be it. But we should remember the enormous advances that came before us. The material was almost entirely created and developed by German industry throughout the first half of the twentieth century. However, it was towards the middle of the twentieth century that a gynecologist, a humanist, a man of conviction and furthermore, of genius, Raoul Palmer, laid both the technical and ethical foundations for modern cœlioscopy.

I say above all a man of conviction, because the idea of systematically replacing exploratory laparotomy with preliminary endoscopy jostled the well-established habits of the time. Effectively, during this period, all women who showed sterility due to tubal obstruction were subjected to pelvic surgical exploration. Most of the time, this exploration resulted only in a report of irreparable post-abortum, or most often post-tubercular, lesions. Revelation of such a misfortune led these young patients not only to feel a loss of any hope, but also, given such weak conclusions, to feel that they had been subjected to uselessly aggressive surgery for no valid reasons. Frankly, no one in the profession really paid heed to it since this behavior was the only and unavoidable option.

Obtaining the same result through endoscopy was a considerable step forward in humanizing surgery. However, convincing the surgical collective of the solidity of this position was not a small task. Nonetheless, at least some gynecologists followed this approach and, thanks to Raoul Palmer, within a few years cœlioscopy became a recognized procedure in their discipline.

The fact that Palmer was a gynecologist caused, however, everyone to pigeonhole cœlioscopy as an exclusively gynecological procedure. The surgeons, of which the well-known adage says that great surgeons can be identified by the great scars they leave, scorned and were even totally unaware of endoscopy and its possibilities. However the real meaning of such an adage was that a clear view of the operating field and lesions was allowed by large incisions, thus permitting everyone, even less talented surgeons, to perform successful interventions. This is still an absolute truth: seeing well is a priority, and paradoxically, cœlioscopy is one of the most developed ways of improving the visibility of the operative field.

However, at that time, the lack of easily accessible and distributable images was an obstacle to understanding the potential and the superiority of endoscopic exploration. I say easily accessible images because Palmer did, in fact, provide images, and this by a most astonishing means: extremely ambidextrous, he could draw with one hand (alternating from one to the other) without looking at his drawing, all the while keeping his eye riveted on the lens he held in his free hand. He also recorded his explorations and his gestures using a heavy 16 mm camera, either directly or through a "spy lens" whose four articulated arms severely encumbered the space of the operative field.

Personally, I discovered cœlioscopy in the 1960s, when image technology was still in its initial stages. It was my gynecological companions, slightly my seniors who, having visited Raoul Palmer, taught me the purely exploratory technique. The fact that it was just an exploratory and not an operative technique is probably the reason why the surgeons of the time paid it little attention. On top of that, investigation had gynecological connotations, so they thought they had nothing to do with it!

However, Palmer had already performed some operative gestures, mainly using a coaxial instrumentation with which he could only perform simple movements because of the limited viewing scope. He had nonetheless initialized the practice of having a complementary operative trocar, separate from the optical one, but he had not yet realized that this would be the basis of the inevitable shift from the classic surgical gesture in cœlioscopy practice.

Finally, all, or almost all, had been imagined by Raoul Palmer, all he needed was to become known and understood. Above all, the universality of this method needed to be understood beyond the domain of gynecology.

Such was my route, and it was accomplished neither easily nor in one quick shot.

The idea that cœlioscopy digestive surgery was born *ex nihilo*, by sudden inspiration, is at the very least a simple, if not entirely unrealistic interpretation. They wrote: "One day, a French gynecologist named Mouret had the idea of removing a gallbladder by laparoscopy". I cannot believe how simplistic and inexact that is! I shall tell the tale because the slow progression was certainly due to the degree of the unknown that I was tackling, and the weakness of the technological means. This however, was fortunate for me because this long learning process allowed me to progressively master the difficulties of spatial vision using the cœlioscope, the interpretation of observed structures, and above all performing the gesture in this so differently dreaded space.

I think it is important to note that digestive cœlioscopy came about in the form of an exploratory procedure, just as it did in gynecology. I recall with pleasure that Raoul Palmer gave his students the following rule: "Do 500 exploratory cœlioscopies before even touching the least little operative tool!" Perhaps I had not done that many, but I was not far off.

The path I followed at that time was the repetition of that of Palmer many years before and the motivations were very similar. At that period, as a young surgeon on duty, I had a real sense of guilt when faced with an urgent abdominal syndrome I was forced to propose an exploratory laparotomy, and the guilt worsened as a matter of course when the laparotomy proved inconclusive.

The cœlioscopic exploration, to which I had been initiated in gynecology, seemed to me, by all evidence, to be adapted for use in contested emergency cases and appendicitis, which, in France was operated upon too frequently – i.e., appendicitis that weren't appendicitis – was the chosen ground for the first intention cœlioscopic procedure.

Today this choice may seem to be painfully obvious, especially to surgeons who systematically practice the cœlioscopic approach for appendectomies. However, at this time, when cœlioscopy appendectomies had not yet been, and were far from being performed, cœlioscopy was diagnostic and therefore followed or not by classic open surgery, depending on the positive or negative discoveries of the diagnostic. In other words, what we call today, in my opinion, very incorrectly a "conversion" (at least a reconversion or a relapse, to keep the vocabulary of religious inspiration!) was a necessary part of the operative protocol.

The principle of the first intention cœlioscopic exploration was not only concerned with appendiceal syndromes. It seemed obvious to me that the lesional diagnostic and topographic precisions brought an improvement in operative tactics by allowing two concepts: first, a better adapted choice for the incision site; and second, a notable diminution in the dimension of the incision because exploration was no longer needed and because simple gestures performed by cœlioscopy for adhesiolysis and mobilization of organs simplified the operative steps of laparotomy.

These surgical gestures of freeing adhesions and mobilizing organs were the key to the birth of laparoscopic surgery. At first they were performed modestly because they allowed structures partially or completely hidden by adherences to be viewed through the cœlioscope.

These gestures are inevitably the basis of all abdominal surgery. They have become so natural that surgeons might almost forget their imperative necessity. Mastering them as thoroughly as possible is the key to surgical expertise. The practice of laparoscopic surgery absolutely requires the same rigor in order to be correctly and safely performed.

In the beginning, these procedures were performed without any intention of creating a new way to perform surgery, but merely a new means of exploring. The rest came about perfectly naturally, by way of the evidence that these procedures could be done and when done by cœlioscopy, they were less aggressive for the patient. Quickly the objective became not only to do the same as in open surgery, but to do better. But moving from idea to reality did not happen overnight.

It should be noted that this adhesiolysis, the key to all surgical acts for liberating or mobilizing organs, had already been performed several years before by pneumologists seeking to recreate pneumothorax in the tubercular pleural symphyses by severing the band of conjunctive tissue. Again, it was Palmer who had initialized this practice once more to offer full vision in cases of cicatricial pelvic peritonitis. The increasingly restrictive pigeonholing of specializations had prevented the surgical world from benefiting from this advance.

The freeing of adhesions in an abdominal cavity implies their pre-existing presence. However, at the end of the 1960s a previous abdominal surgery was a formal and absolute contraindication to cœlioscopic exploration. This taboo had to be removed. I did this in my practice, but I did not formalize this practice. I was taking a great personal risk on a medico-legal level, but experience and reason showed that the prohibition was unjustified, or at the very least excessive. It is true that an operated abdomen presents difficulties and traps; surgery for re-intervention shows this! But not only should such re-interventions be permitted, they are even justifiable. Moreover, surgery is not the unique cause of adhesions, and the frequent appearance of extra-surgical adhesions had shown me that most certainly difficulties existed in these cases, but they did not present impossibilities that justified the imposed taboo. Extreme caution was of course the the imperative compensation for taboo transgression.

This account should help to explain why cœlioscopic surgery was not born of the sudden inspiration that an act such as the cholecystectomy made possible, but from a progressive drift between exploratory and therapeutic action.

This is why the first abdominal surgery performed was the treatment of an occlusion of the small intestine by a single band. In this operation that unwittingly became therapeutic, the objective of the cœlioscopic approach was not to confirm diagnosis (it was radiologically evident), its ambition was to confirm that the treatment would have been feasible by simply revisiting the old McBurney incision that I had myself made in order to perform an appendectomy for a frank acute appendicitis one year earlier.

This exploration exposed the site of the occlusion that was due to a single band of adhesion under the caecum. I knew how to perform the adhesiolysis gestures. Adhesiolysis in this context represented the totality of the operative gestures, and it was done. The conversion (the real one, meaning a change in beliefs!) had just been made for first time in digestive surgery. It was 1972.

But more progress was needed before a gesture that included an exeresis could be taken into account, because the obstacle of keeping the pneumoperitoneum airtight was not immediately overcome. It began first with an appendectomy in 1983, more than ten years later, in such an intervention the cœlioscopic stage prepared the exteriorization of the appendix by a 10 mm trocar at the McBurney point or at any other point justified by an appendix ectopia.

To my mind, the cœlioscopic approach conceptually should be not considered an additional surgery, but an aide. However, this "aide" would become so predominant that it would eventually entirely replace the laparotomy-provided acts. This explains why the appendectomy technique that I used was less exclusively endoscopic (or purely endoscopic, if you will) than the technique that Kurt Semm had initiated three years earlier but at that stage had not yet published.

Maybe less exclusively cœlioscopic, this approach was however immediately capable of treating very acute appendicitis, even peritonitis, in which total cœlioscopic viewing of the abdominal cavity quickly showed that despite the appearances of the reduced-path method, the cœlioscopic approach facilitated a complete treatment of appendicitis and its complications. I had just realized that laparoscopy was equal to the greatest laparotomies (those that made surgeons great!).

The approach to the cholecystectomy was done in an analogous manner and the first cholecystectomy was performed unexpectedly and in the most natural of ways. It was a double operation: one part was gynecological (an ovarian cyst), to be performed by cœlioscopy, and the second was a cholecystectomy. Taking advantage of the cœlioscopic approach that I had performed for the gynecological operation, it seemed to me judicious, still intending to perform a further miniaturization of the mini-laparotomy of the time, to use this approach to make as advanced a preparation as possible for the cholecystectomy.

The gallbladder was thus handled from front to back, as by mini-laparotomy. It was laboriously but precisely removed in a good plane, the cystic arteries' branches were coagulated with a monopolar hook, very close to the gallbladder wall so as to encounter only the small caliber branches that could be easily controlled by coagulation. Once this "preparation" was finished, all that remained was to divide the cystic duct after having blocked it. This seems a simple task today, but back then it was anything but obvious. A traditional clipping device was then introduced directly through the abdominal wall and despite the consequent gas leak, the cystic duct could be quickly clipped. It was out of the question to divide the cystic duct (isolated between two metal clips) with the coagulating hook, the only cutting instrument that I had back then, because in such cases the risk of necrosis is more than evident.

The artifice was to introduce, in the place of the clipping device, long fine thoracic surgery scissors the extremity of which reached the proper depth, while the meeting points of the blades was in the wall, allowing the scissors' blades to open and to obtain a relative air-tightness. This is that it was done.

I distinctly remember having a very negative impression of this operation. First, I had the impression of great difficulty, although I claimed to have a lot of experience in the practice of cœlioscopic gestures (over 6,000 procedures). Above all, I could not see a great advantage of this approach compared to the other very minimally invasive operations that we used to practice until that point.

As we left the operating table I thought, and said to my assisting team: "We have probably accomplished a worldwide first, but I think it will also be the last!" This opinion did not last overnight. During the morning visit, I discovered my patient, who, having not seen a laparotomy scar, was disappointed and rather furious because she believed that we had not performed the planned operation on her gallbladder. She was dressed and ready to leave. Even though we were accustomed to seeing easy recoveries from the operations that were already moving toward minimal aggression, the great value of this new technique became evident.

This was what made me decide to repeat the operation, which I did 15 times in 1987 in selected cases with favorably predicted conditions (no cholecystitis, adequate body weight, etc.). Following this, less favorable and unexpected conditions made me realize that, with increasing experience, I could master difficulties in an absolutely satisfactory and safe manner. In 1987, 15% of cholecystectomies were performed by laparoscopy, such a rate increased to 85% in 1988 and it was in 1991 that I made my last preliminary selection for a case of gangrenous cholecystitis, which on reflection, would have been moreover easily removed by cœlioscopy.

I thus progressively "converted" the open technique to laparoscopy. I have never had to go back, except once, in a far away country, when a biliary pathology known over a 20 years period complicated by recurrent infectious accident, had rendered the region incomprehensible, as it was so for that matter (and may be more) through the opened abdomen.

This historical account seems to me very important because it explains my vision of the cœlioscopic phenomenon; a vision very different from that of the surgical community. For everyone this marked the beginning of the cœlioscopic era, and this opinion prevails in general, but for me it was the end of a long and lonely trek, and the escape from the partial hiding in which I practiced cœlioscopy.

The idea that laparoscopic surgery was born from the first cholecystectomy would not matter to me if it did not bring with it an erroneous (or perverted) vision of the position and meaning of cœlioscopy in surgery.

In 1989 an editorial in a famous North American journal qualified the cœlioscopic cholecystectomy as "the second French Revolution". At the time I took this as an honor and it made me proud. I am certain that the intention was good and I am grateful to its author, but on reflection I began to see the reductive and dangerous side of this kind of vision.

Revolution is a rupture: a breaking with the past, its rules, its practices, its methods, and who knows what else. There are always excesses, and sometimes violence, justified simply by the state of revolution. I understand that the community of digestive surgeons, surprised by the arrival of such an uncommon procedure, could believe in a sudden invention, and in a revolution. Many have vested interests in such an interpretation since the arriving new order offered the industry promoting (and even sponsoring) its diffusion the potential of orienting the choice of surgeons who no longer mastered the techniques employed. The reason is that the very effective tools created at the moment of the diffusion brought with them profit to the industry, a real addiction for surgeons, and therefore a source of a huge market.

I will, however, add that if there was a real rupture (a revolution, if you will), it was not caused by the use of the cœlioscope, but by the act of operating through a monitor, and of no longer using direct vision. I am not responsible for this change and had to accept it and get used to it, just as everyone else did. This was not easy and I found the transition very hard.

Revolution, new order and new leaders of which I am typical example, one would think, but not belonging to any cenacle, I can comment on this revolution completely at my ease.

This new hierarchy in the competency is justified by the fact that the learning process of cœlioscopic vision and gestures demands great effort and it is, I think, difficult to acquire such mastery, especially for the older members of the community.

We have, however, created senseless difficulties by hiding the fact that cœlioscopic technique comes directly from classic operative techniques: this is what my own curriculum shows unquestionably. Within the surgical community, with the help of the revolutionary spirit, the past had to disappear, and laparotomy was doomed. Declared "No Scar Surgery", the incision had to be as invisible as possible, going as far as to claim a victory, even at the price of needless difficulties and safety risks, if one less trocar than the neighbor was used! Childish ambition!

There are still a number of paradoxes. Cœlioscopic surgery is perceived as a new practice that needs to be performed without fault and without accommodations (a real fundamentalism is taking hold), but as soon as any serious difficulty arises, everyone agrees that there should be no hesitation to "convert". We can only approve of this caution, but it implies that traditional surgery is still superior to laparoscopy when difficulties or serious complexities occur. On the other hand, it is more and more apparent that cœlioscopic control brings to the surgical gesture a precision comparable to that of the microscope in other domains. The paradox will disappear one day, most likely when the residual technical problems of the cœlioscopy are mastered.

Another paradox: when surgery is complex, and especially when a voluminous exeresis is expected, it is well accepted (and seen as a distressing and unavoidable necessity by the "cœlioscopy fundamentalists"), that a laparotomy (a mini-laparotomy, usually) called "service entrance access" may be necessary to permit the extraction of the surgical specimen. Such a case refers to the so-called mini-laparotomy aided coelioscopy.

Mini-laparatomy is moreover not so minimal in the minds of the users of the "hand-assisted" laparascopy. However, such a technique can be of help only if it is the assistant who introduces the hand and not the operator. Having operated for years by cœlioscopy with one hand busied with a constant task, I know that it is not comfortable, neither, and most of all, should it be labeled as progress.

If we had not created this artificial split between the two technical methods (the famous revolution), we would have realized that cœlioscopy is a means of assisting and perfecting traditional surgery, this is the way it may be considered even if this assistance may sometimes (and more and more frequently) tend towards a total substitution.

Thus, in my opinion, the diffusion of laparoscopy did not occur as I would have wished. I would have liked the diffusion of the cholecystectomy technique to have been systematically preceded by the acquisition of explorative laparoscopy. This would have prevented the occurrence of most youth sins, which we absolve a little bit too complacently by placing them within the so-called "learning curve".

Despite this, it must be recognized that the cholecystectomy was a pretty fortunate choice. Despite the feeling I had during the first operation, this is an operation with relatively favorable results for a first approach. It is a very frequently performed operation, often carried out for symptomatic but uncomplicated pathologies; that is, when the anatomical conditions are quite close to normal. The surgical site is relatively restricted within the abdominal cavity, so much so that a judicious initial positioning of the trocars can be suitable for the entire duration of the operation.

For these reasons, it has been regardless possible to learn coelioscopy without knowing its basis, as with a "recipe", without knowing the general technique of the cœlioscopic surgery to which it referred. No major insurmountable difficulties arise, but surgeons have found themselves during training in such unexpected, disturbing situations and conditions that, as I mentioned earlier, they believe they are penetrating a totally new technique and environment.

We may, despite all of this, wonder why the cholecystectomy was the trigger for the cœlio-surgical era when all that preceded it, (which, in my opinion, is more interesting for the patient) was, and in essence still remains, misunderstood. As discussed above, the reasons for which this choice has been deemed reasonable provide only a partial explanation. For me, the principal deciding factor was the use of video as a means of demonstration, recording and teaching.

Explaining, describing, writing, even with talents I do not have, is not still enough to spread the global nature of information. Communication always requires a great deal of imagination on the part of the person receiving the information. Not everyone has it, or at least not to the same degree, and above all the differences in personal interpretation are of greatest influence. Image which, by its nature, renders the imagination obsolete possesses a great power to demonstrate and create enormous and universal conviction. Moreover, video is incredibly supple and easy to use, if compared with previous image processing. The strength of video as a vector of information is again increased by the fact that it can be understood (at least in part) even by an uninformed audience. The media destined for the general public have thus taken it over, and in this way have favored and accelerated the public demand for a technique that finally takes into account the limitations aggressiveness of surgery.

Many favorable factors ensured that the spread of laparoscopic cholecystectomy would be achieved in an explosive manner, and without too many accidents. I say this cautiously because I quickly and clearly became aware that the technique I was initially practicing was far from mature enough to be repeatable. Personally I would have waited, but I did not control the wave.

Fortunately, brilliant operators, already experienced in cœlioscopy (François Dubois and Jacques Périssat are foremost in my mind) have provided valuable improvements to a practice that was initially (as one of my first visitors accurately pointed out) very "artisanal".

I have said "with not too many accidents". That is a misuse of language, as any accident is always one too many. The clear advantages of the method (when all goes well) have been so obvious that we made the mistake of tolerating an accident rate superior to that found with the classic techniques. Nothing justified this once, and nothing may justify this today, because the cœlioscopic approach, well mastered and well done (on both the technical and tactical sides) gives a surgeon the means to practically erase lesions on the main bile duct.

I know that this comment will be criticized, but I think that if the "conversion" is presented as a parachute for cœlioscopic surgery, it is, as I have said, the translation of a strategic error in the development, and perhaps even in the conception, of laparoscopic surgery.

Today, we should take into consideration the fact that cœlioscopic surgery, even if it is strictly identical to classic surgery in concept, is technically more difficult to gain in practice than the traditional open surgery. It was popularized before those responsible for its instruction had sufficiently mastered it. I felt, and still feel, personally concerned by this problem, but I have any control on it.

We could imagine that this slightly pessimistic vision is becoming obsolete. This is true, and it is mainly because luck has been on its side, that today the technique of laparoscopy cholecystectomy has reached a certain maturity.

But all further developments in laparoscopy have faced the same problems. Even though more and more Expert Centers have been established and are mastering the techniques, the basic diffusion has not always been so successful. The clear-cut advantages of laparoscopic technique did not justify the errors of youth.

Industry has benefited from the situation, proposing more or less adapted training to surgeons, training always focusing on technological solutions rather than on the technical problems encountered. This was its role. Our own role, however, as surgeons, was to impose our ethic. We have not always done this.

Our industrialized countries' economies will probably support this very high-tech approach, and while I esteem that we have chosen an ill-adapted method to diffuse the cœlioscopic technique, the harmful consequences will be erased little by little. The problem is entirely different in Third World countries where laparoscopic surgery is as frequently required as elsewhere (globalization oblige) and probably particularly necessary because of the economy, healthcare, convalescence, and contamination risks for which cœlioscopy may play a role and thus improve surgical practice.

The eminent technological solutions upon which we are increasingly dependent are, and will be for a long time forbidden to them besides only a few elitist pilot centers, the only existence of which is known and that hide reality.

I think that we do an injustice to these countries by practicing a simple and basic transfer of technology (our technology). If we ourselves did not take the proper approach of acquisition in our own countries, adopting a correct approach in Third World countries, where they do not have the means of compensating for the errors in learning strategy, seems to me a strict necessity. I believe we must stimulate surgeons from these countries to re-invent another approach to the cœlioscopy and to give them the means to do this rather than watching them construct a new parallel surgery to that which they already practice (often with difficulty, because they do not have the means of doing otherwise).

The means to progressively shift from open to cœlioscopic surgery exist. These rely essentially on the suspension of the abdominal wall, for which I believe I created the first device. When one of these devices is watched at work, it is welcomed with enthusiasm. Other suspension devices have been created throughout the world with more or less successful results. But these devices were presented in an incorrect way, and sometimes even stupidly, as if they were substitutes for the pneumoperitoneum. "Gasless laparoscopy" is a ridiculous term, because without gas there is no space and without space, there is no vision!

The objective that I was personally pursuing and that I put into practice daily is to render the surgeon independent, or at least less dependent, on the air-tightness of the pneumoperitoneum. The objective here is not to defend this technological aide, and even less to create my own publicity, because my device is no longer being made! But it allows me to underline the fact that the wall suspension I use in all the cholecystectomies that I perform is not at all a substitute for insufflation. It is in fact and above all a means of lifting the round ligament, exposing the inferior side of the liver. This aide brings an incomparable comfort, an almost absolute security, and thus a feasibility, to the laparoscopic cholecystectomy technique that we currently use. Today I don't know how I'd get along without it.

The argument that suspension necessitates a supplementary path (of 4mm) for its set up is often put forward. I think this argument is unbelievably childish and in bad faith, given the safety that suspension brings. All the while, in the name of safety these same people sing the praises of "conversion" which, in my practice of the cholecystectomy has completely disappeared, largely thanks to the "suspension-lifting of the round ligament". Moreover, this aide frees the operator, quite successfully, of the need for permanent air-tightness. Without conversion, this allows the instruments needed for complementary gestures on the main bile duct to be introduced trans-parietally, at a chosen point determined by the anatomy.

Reticence toward this suspension procedure, for the rigorist vision of integral cœlioscopy practice, is a result of the misconceptualization of cœlioscopic surgery as a new surgery, an idea that I have refuted above. I resolutely challenge this vision, because if I am attributed a paternity, then I am also given the right to think and to say when I do not entirely agree with my descendents! This is not the overblown strictness of the aging "pater familias". I am pleading, as I always have, for adaptable and supple surgery. Contrary to what we so often think, classic and cœlioscopic techniques are not alternatives to each other. The techniques are complementary, but will only truly be so when a (technical) solution for a real "reversibility" between the two techniques is found.

Today we are witnessing a true paradox. On one hand we are aiming to be rigorously cœlioscopic, which leads us toward reduction in the number of trocars, as I mentioned earlier. On the other hand, without hesitation, and to solve any passing difficulty, we do not hesitate to brutally disown everything and perform a laparotomy, as large as before and perhaps larger (because you must have courage of your own opinions!), when a simple gesture by mini-laparotomy (even sometimes micro-) would solve the complication and then allow us to return to the cœlioscopic technique, where we are more comfortable and, above all, safe. This dissociation-opposition of open surgery and cœlioscopic surgery is a sign of immaturity and of a still incomplete integration.

The "reversibility" of the two techniques seems to me a necessity, in both directions. A necessity because it facilitates the training (and we are all very inexperienced in the practice of cœlioscopy as it is, in itself, a very young procedure).

A necessity because it is a means of a less costly development. A necessity so that the two previous reasons can permit cœlioscopic progress to spread throughout Third World countries.

I know that, in saying this, I am going against the grain of current ideas. I know that I am opposing industrial economic interests. But I want to express my convictions. The long solitude that I experienced for some 20-odd years taught me to think and act without needing consenting approval. This allows me to continue my attempt to fully communicate my message; in the haste to diffuse the information, we had forgotten a part of it.

An Asian proverb says "When the wise man points at the moon, the idiot looks at the finger." For years we have been looking at the finger, wondering what it could mean. But by looking at the finger, some thought they were being shown the pathway to the moon! This is the impression that I have today, when seeing the focal points in our meetings. But don't get me wrong, I fervently approve of this high-tech research, and I think that it should be conducted. I am passionate about it and I admire it, and if I only participate as a spectator, it is because I believe I have reached my limits.

As for the rest of this metaphor: Okay! Let us look for a path to the moon, but we should never forget the development of the little car that must transport us on earth. There is still much to do.

For those who want to keep their feet on the ground, I would like to paraphrase Neil Armstrong as he took his first step on the moon: "We have made one small step for technology, but one giant step for humanity."

Chapter 2

Epidemiology of Biliary Lithiasis

Stefan Sauerland

Epidemiology of Biliary Lithiasis in Europe

Biliary lithiasis can be defined as the presence of concrements in the gallbladder, the biliary ducts, or both. These concrements can be stones (>3 mm) or biliary sludge containing particles of smaller size. Biliary lithiasis and gallstone disease are two exchangeable umbrella terms for the same condition. Gallstone disease can be asymptomatic or associated with chronic or acute symptoms. Symptomatic disease is more common when gallstones are present than when biliary sludge alone is present [1].

In Europe, biliary lithiasis has probably been common since antiquity. Egyptian mummies were also found to have suffered from biliary concrements. However, the physicians in the ancient Greek and Roman age often did not recognize gallstones as the cause of biliary symptoms. Galen's writings, for example, fail to mention biliary stones. In pre-Roman cultures, the flow of bile was considered important as a metaphor for nutrition and digestion. Ancient medications, on the other hand, often contained ground gall stones taken from oxen, which were used as a remedy for various conditions. Only after these times was the importance of gallstones understood [2], and it was probably Antonius Benivenius, in his book on hidden causes of death (*De abditis morborum causis*, published 1528), who first described an autopsy-verified case of acute cholecystitis leading to death.

As the prevalence of biliary disease is different in different ethnic groups, it seems worthwhile to summarize epidemiologic data for each continent separately [1–3]. With very few exceptions, sonographic imaging has been used in all epidemiologic studies to detect biliary lithiasis. In spite of some differences in disease definition and observer experience, population-based studies using abdominal sonography as a screening tool allow meaningful comparisons among different subgroups and populations around the world. One study from Siberia found a good correlation between sonography and autopsy as detection methods [4].

One of the largest epidemiologic studies on this topic was the Multicenter Italian Study of Cholelithiasis (M.I.COL.), which sonographically screened nearly 30,000 patients [5]. The main results are shown in Figure 2.1. When these results recorded in the Mediterranean region are compared against results recorded in Central or Northern Europe [6], any differences noted are small, suggesting that the ethnic origin of Europeans is sufficiently similar to justify the expectation of similar prevalences of biliary stones throughout Europe, providing other key risk factors do not differ among the different countries. Nowadays, socioeconomic background, culture, and life expectancy are quite similar in all European countries. The epidemiology of biliary diseases is therefore relatively uniform throughout Europe.

Epidemiology of Biliary Lithiasis Outside Europe

In the Americas, disease prevalence within the population varies with ethnic origin [7]. Northern American whites suffer from gallstone disease with a frequency similar to that observed in Europeans. However, much higher prevalences have been found in different Indian American populations [8], such as the Pima, the Chippewa [9], and the Micmac [10] in North America and the Mapuche in South America [11]. Owing to the American Indian admixture in Mexico, standardized disease prevalence is relatively similar to that in North America or Canada [7, 12]. In each subgroup, ancestry is an important explanatory variable [13] and must be considered when such patients need care.

Epidemiologic data relating to Asian populations are quite contradictory: gallstones are found much more frequently in Chinese [14, 15] than in Japanese [16] populations. Comparison with Europeans indicates that biliary diseases in Asians have slightly different etiology and pathology. A large proportion of biliary calculi in Asians are brown pigment stones, and such stones are often found in the intrahepatic bile ducts (i.e., hepatolithiasis). Since biliary tract infestation with parasites is responsible for some of these stones, the prevalence of biliary lithiasis also depends on the availability of antiparasitic drugs in these countries. This may go some way toward explaining the variations in disease prevalence in Asia. Genetic factors also have to be considered.

Unfortunately, virtually no data are available on the prevalence of biliary lithiasis in Africa. Probably because of their lifestyle, the Bantu and the Masai have one of the lowest prevalences anywhere in the world [17]. In the USA, black Americans still have a slightly lower prevalence of biliary lithiasis [7], which shows that both genetic and environmental factors are responsible for disease development.

Unchangeable Risk Factors

Age is certainly one the most important risk factors for biliary lithiasis [18, 19]. Children under the age of 16 rarely develop gallstones. In adults, prevalence steadily increases (Fig. 2.1). This increase is largely independent of gender, although in women there seems to be a slight decrease in prevalence during the perimenopausal years.

Female gender is an important risk factor for biliary lithiasis [20, 21]. In general, the life-time risk of biliary lithiasis is 2 or 3 times higher for a European woman than for a European man. Owing to relatively lower estrogen levels after menopause, the female predominance is less prominent in older age groups. On the other hand, any estrogen medication before or after the menopause increases the risk of biliary lithiasis. Parity and breastfeeding have also been found to be associated with biliary lithiasis [22].

Although it is evident from epidemiologic data that there is an hereditary component in biliary diseases, little is known about the genetics of gallbladder stones [23–25]. Some studies have assessed the genetic component in biliary lithiasis by analyzing possible target genes [26–28]. These genes may act by indirect metabolic pathways (obesity, cholesterol metabolism, etc.) or have a direct effect on biliary lithogenesis (biliary cholesterol hypersecretion, supersaturation, and crystallization, or bile stasis).

Other risk factors of lesser importance include Crohn's disease [29] and liver cirrhosis [30]. Biliary sludge may also be found after the administration of ceftriaxone or after liver transplantation.

Modifiable Risk Factors and Disease Prevention

Obesity dramatically increases the likelihood of gallstone development [19, 31, 32].

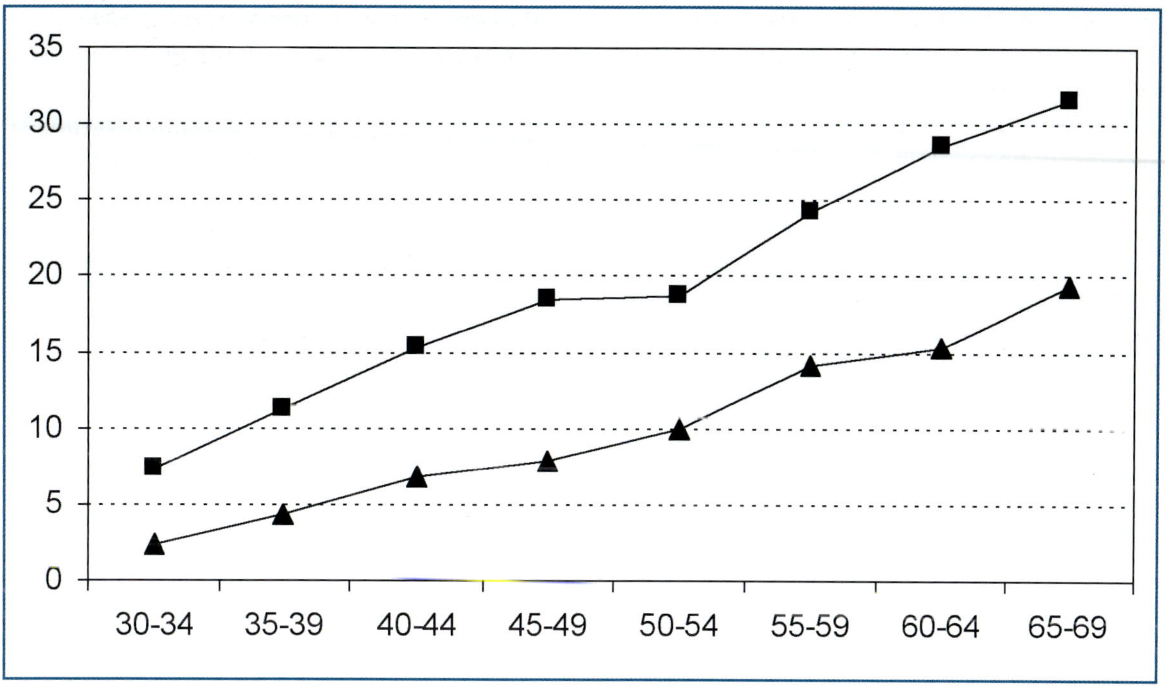

Fig. 2.1 Prevalence of gallstone disease in men (*triangles*) and women (*squares*) with increasing age. Prevalence figures were based on sonographic evidence of biliary lithiasis or cholecystectomy. Years of age are plotted on the *x*-axis and percentages on the *y*-axis

Usually, the body mass index (BMI) is used to define different grades of obesity. A correlation between increasing severity of obesity and gallstone disease has been reliably confirmed especially for female subjects, while in men the association is weaker. For women suffering from overweight (BMI >25), obesity (BMI >30) and morbid obesity (BMI >35) the risk of biliary lithiasis is increased about twofold, fourfold and sevenfold, respectively, relative to that in women with normal body weight [33].

Although weight control and weight loss should be recommended as a possible strategy for disease prevention, initial rapid weight loss can itself cause the formation of gallstones [34]. This side effect of weight loss has been shown most convincingly in bariatric surgery patients, for whom prophylactic cholecystectomy has therefore been proposed [35]. Regardless of whether gastric surgery is carried out for treatment of carcinoma or for weight loss, gastrectomy can cause gallstones [36]. To a lesser extent, a quick succession of episodes of weight loss and weight gain ("weight cycling") can also be a risk factor. It should be noted that even older children can develop gallstones as a consequence of rapid weight loss [37].

Diabetes mellitus and the metabolic syndrome have been examined as potential risk factors [38–40]. However, as diabetes mellitus is strongly associated with obesity and age, sophisticated study designs and analyses are required to assess the specific effect of diabetes on gallstone formation [41]. Similarly, cardiovascular disease is also obviously associated with gallstone disease [42]. However, the direction of causality is uncertain for this association. As some studies have linked biliary lithiasis with decreased levels of physical activity [43], preventive measures should focus primarily on promoting and increasing regular sport activities in the adult population.

As described above, estrogen medication is also a risk factor, with evidence of a dose–response relationship. Accordingly, modern hormonal contraceptives (which are less highly dosed) represent a risk increase of minor importance. Postmenopausal hormone replacement therapy, however, should definitely be avoided.

Drinking coffee has been shown to have a mildly protective effect against biliary lithiasis [44]. Alcohol consumption probably furthers the development of biliary concrements [45, 46]. Other nutritional factors seem to have only minor relevance. The role of fat consumption is generally difficult to evaluate, as obesity may act as a confounding variable. Data on smoking are inconclusive [32, 46].

Economic Impact of Biliary Lithiasis

Owing to its high prevalence, biliary lithiasis is causing enormous expenditures in the health care sector. Once the disease becomes symptomatic, an average patient attends for three outpatient visits before in-hospital treatment (usually with cholecystectomy) follows. Although the advent of laparoscopic cholecystectomy has cut down the length of hospital stay, the overall costs of therapy have remained relatively stable. According to U.S. data from the year 2000 [3], in-hospital treatment for symptomatic cholecystolithiasis costs an average of 11,584 US $. Studies in German hospitals showed much smaller sums of about 2,800 US $ [47, 48].

Assuming an annual cholecystectomy rate of 2.2 per 1,000 population [49], the annual numbers of cholecystectomies can be estimated to be in the range of more than 700,000 for the U.S. population (300 million inhabitants) and more than 1,100,000 for the population of Europe (500 million inhabitants). The associated direct costs, assuming average costs of 2,000 euro per case, amount to more than 2 billion euro annually in Europe. The change from open to laparoscopic cholecystectomy has led to substantial cost reductions owing to shorter hospital stay, but the increase in the total number of procedures, at least in the early years of laparoscopic surgery, has partly cancelled out this effect.

Time Trends

It is evident from historical comparisons that the prevalence of biliary lithiasis has always risen in parallel with socioeconomic progress. Every increase in nutritional intake, obesity prevalence, and life expectancy over time has led to a rise in gallstone prevalence. While the largest improvements in food availability and life expectancy occurred in the nineteenth and early twentieth centuries, obesity is a risk factor that is still growing in importance. Therefore, the number of patients with gallstone disease will most probably continue to increase, although this increase will be slow.

Whether the introduction of laparoscopic cholecystectomy has artificially increased the number of patients with gallstone disease has been the subject of heated debate [49–51]. Certainly, laparoscopic cholecystectomy allows surgeons to lower the threshold and operate on patients with only mild symptoms and those with severe comorbidity. From this viewpoint, the increase in cholecystectomy rates (10–20%) seems generally justifiable. On the other hand, the role of incidental gallbladder surgery still needs further evaluation, both from a medical and from a healthcare perspective.

References

1. Jüngst C, Kullak-Ublick GA, Jüngst D (2006) Gallstone disease: microlithiasis and sludge. Best Pract Res Clin Gastroenterol 20:1053-1062
2. Thudichum JLW (1863) Treatise of gall-stones: their chemistry, pathology, and treatment. John Churchill and Sons, London

3. Shaffer EA (2006) Gallstone disease: epidemiology of gallbladder stone disease. Best Pract Res Clin Gastroenterol 20:981-996
4. Reshetnikov OV, Ryabikov AN, Shakhmatov SG, Malyutina SK (2002) Gallstone disease prevalence in Western Siberia: cross-sectional ultrasound study versus autopsy. J Gastroenterol Hepatol 17:702-707
5. Attili AF, Carulli N, Roda E et al (1995) Epidemiology of gallstone disease in Italy: prevalence data of the Multicenter Italian Study on Cholelithiasis (M.I.C.O.L.). Am J Epidemiol 141: 158-165
6. Muhrbeck O, Ahlberg J (1995) Prevalence of gallstone disease in a Swedish population. Scand J Gastroenterol 30:1125-1128
7. Everhart JE, Khare M, Hill M, Maurer KR (1999) Prevalence and ethnic differences in gallbladder disease in the United States. Gastroenterology 117:632-639
8. Everhart JE, Yeh F, Lee ET et al (2002) Prevalence of gallbladder disease in American Indian populations: findings from the Strong Heart Study. Hepatology 35:1507-1512
9. Thistle JL, Eckhart KL Jr, Nensel RE et al (1971) Prevalence of gallbladder disease among Chippewa Indians. Mayo Clin Proc 46:603-608
10. Williams CN, Johnston JL, Weldon KL (1977) Prevalence of gallstones and gallbladder disease in Canadian Micmac Indian women. Can Med Assoc J 117:758-760
11. Galman C, Miquel JF, Perez RM et al (2004) Bile acid synthesis is increased in Chilean Hispanics with gallstones and in gallstone high-risk Mapuche Indians. Gastroenterology 126:741-748
12. Tseng M, Millikan R, Maurer KR et al (2000) Country of birth and prevalence of gallbladder disease in Mexican Americans. Ethn Dis 10:96-105
13. Miquel JF, Covarrubias C, Villaroel L et al (1998) Genetic epidemiology of cholesterol cholelithiasis among Chilean Hispanics, Amerindians, and Maoris. Gastroenterology 115:937-946
14. Chen CH, Huang MH, Yang JC et al (2006) Prevalence and risk factors of gallstone disease in an adult population of Taiwan: an epidemiological survey. J Gastroenterol Hepatol 21:1737-1743
15. Tung TH, Ho HM, Shih HC et al (2006) A population-based follow-up study on gallstone disease among type 2 diabetics in Kinmen, Taiwan. World J Gastroenterol 12:4536-4540
16. Nomura H, Kashiwagi S, Hayashi J et al (1988) Prevalence of gallstone disease in a general population of Okinawa, Japan. Am J Epidemiol 128:598-605
17. Biss K, Ho KJ, Mikkelson B et al (1971) Some unique biologic characteristics of the Masai of East Africa. N Engl J Med 284:694-699
18. Chen CY, Lu CL, Huang YS et al (1998) Age is one of the risk factors in developing gallstone disease in Taiwan. Age Ageing 27:437-441
19. Maurer KR, Everhart JE, Knowler WC et al (1990) Risk factors for gallstone disease in the Hispanic populations of the United States. Am J Epidemiol 131:836-844
20. Novacek G (2006) Gender and gallstone disease. Wien Med Wochenschr 156:527-533
21. Timmer A, Ahrens W, Stegmaier C et al (2000) Risikofaktoren und Operationsraten des Gallensteinleidens. Ergebnisse einer bevölkerungsbezogenen Studie. Med Klin (Munich) 95:672-677
22. Richardson WS, Carter KM, Helm B et al (2002) Risk factors for gallstone disease in the laparoscopic era. Surg Endosc 16:450-452
23. Attili AF, De Santis A, Attili F et al (2005) Prevalence of gallstone disease in first-degree relatives of patients with cholelithiasis. World J Gastroenterol 11:6508-6511
24. Nürnberg D, Berndt H, Pannwitz H (1989) Familiäre Häufung von Gallensteinen. Dtsch Med Wochenschr 114:1059-1063
25. Grünhage F, Lammert F (2006) Gallstone disease. Pathogenesis of gallstones: a genetic perspective. Best Pract Res Clin Gastroenterol 20:997-1015
26. Bertomeu A, Ros E, Zambon D et al (1996) Apolipoprotein E polymorphism and gallstones. Gastroenterology 111:1603-1610
27. Nakeeb A, Comuzzie AG, Martin L et al (2002) Gallstones: genetics versus environment. Ann Surg 235:842-849
28. Premawardhena A, Fisher CA, Fathiu F et al (2001) Genetic determinants of jaundice and gallstones in haemoglobin E beta thalassaemia. Lancet 357:1945-1946
29. Fraquelli M, Losco A, Visentin S et al (2001) Gallstone disease and related risk factors in patients with Crohn disease: analysis of 330 consecutive cases. Arch Intern Med 161:2201-2204
30. Conte D, Fraquelli M, Fornari F et al (1999) Close relation between cirrhosis and gallstones: cross-sectional and longitudinal survey. Arch Intern Med 159:49-52
31. Rome Group for the Epidemiology and Prevention of Cholelithiasis (GREPCO) (1988) The epidemiology of gallstone disease in Rome, Italy. Part II. Factors associated with the disease. Hepatology 8:907-913
32. Sahi T, Paffenbarger RS Jr, Hsieh CC, Lee IM (1998) Body mass index, cigarette smoking, and other characteristics as predictors of self-reported, physician-diagnosed gallbladder disease in male college alumni. Am J Epidemiol 147:644-651

33. Friedman GD, Kannel WB, Dawber TR (1966) The epidemiology of gallbladder disease: observations in the Framingham Study. J Chron Dis 19:273-292
34. Thijs C, Knipschild P, Leffers P (1992) Is gallstone disease caused by obesity or by dieting? Am J Epidemiol 135:274-280
35. Kiewiet RM, Durian MF, van Leersum M, Hesp FL, van Vliet AC (2006) Gallstone formation after weight loss following gastric banding in morbidly obese Dutch patients. Obes Surg 16:592-596
36. Kobayashi T, Hisanaga M, Kanehiro H et al (2005) Analysis of risk factors for the development of gallstones after gastrectomy. Br J Surg 92:1399-1403
37. Kaechele V, Wabitsch M, Thiere D et al (2006) Prevalence of gallbladder stone disease in obese children and adolescents: influence of the degree of obesity, sex, and pubertal development. J Pediatr Gastroenterol Nutr 42:66-70
38. Mendez-Sanchez N, Chavez-Tapia NC, Motola-Kuba D et al (2005) Metabolic syndrome as a risk factor for gallstone disease. World J Gastroenterol 11:1653-1657
39. Torchio P, Corrao G, Gentile S et al (2004) Prevalence of gallstone disease and related risk factors in 889 diabetic subjects of southern Italy. Dig Liver Dis 36:698-699
40. Chen CY, Lu CL, Lee PC et al (1999) The risk factors for gallstone disease among senior citizens: an Oriental study. Hepatogastroenterology 46:1607-1612
41. Pagliarulo M, Fornari F, Fraquelli M et al (2004) Gallstone disease and related risk factors in a large cohort of diabetic patients. Dig Liver Dis 36:130-134
42. Mendez-Sanchez N, Bahena-Aponte J, Chavez-Tapia NC et al (2005) Strong association between gallstones and cardiovascular disease. Am J Gastroenterol 100:827-830
43. Storti KL, Brach JS, FitzGerald SJ et al (2005) Physical activity and decreased risk of clinical gallstone disease among post-menopausal women. Prev Med 41:772-777
44. Leitzmann MF, Willett WC, Rimm EB et al (1999) A prospective study of coffee consumption and the risk of symptomatic gallstone disease in men. JAMA 281:2106-2112
45. Acalovschi M, Blendea D, Feier C et al (2003) Risk factors for symptomatic gallstones in patients with liver cirrhosis: a case-control study. Am J Gastroenterol 98:1856-1860
46. Volzke H, Baumeister SE, Alte D et al (2005) Independent risk factors for gallstone formation in a region with high cholelithiasis prevalence. Digestion 71:97-105
47. Ure BM, Lefering R, Troidl H (1995) Costs of laparoscopic cholecystectomy. Analysis of potential savings. Surg Endosc 9:401-406
48. Bosch F, Wehrman U, Saeger HD, Kirch W (2002) Laparoscopic or open conventional cholecystectomy: clinical and economic considerations. Eur J Surg 168:270-277
49. Steiner CA, Bass EB, Talamini MA et al (1994) Surgical rates and operative mortality for open and laparoscopic cholecystectomy in Maryland. N Engl J Med 330:403-408
50. Escarce JJ, Chen W, Schwartz JS (1995) Falling cholecystectomy thresholds since the introduction of laparoscopic cholecystectomy. JAMA 273:1581-1585
51. Legorreta AP, Silber JH, Costantino GN et al (1993) Increased cholecystectomy rate after the introduction of laparoscopic cholecystectomy. JAMA 270:1429-1432

Chapter 3

Pathophysiology of Cholesterol Gallstone Disease

Piero Portincasa, Antonio Moschetta, Agostino Di Ciaula, Daniela Pontrelli, Rosa C. Sasso, Helen H. Wang, David Q.-H. Wang

Introduction

Gallstone disease is one of the most costly digestive diseases requiring hospitalization in westernized countries, and its prevalence ranges from 10% to 15% in adults in Europe and the USA [1–4]. The burden of disease is summarized by the prevalence of patients with gallstones, by its incidence (over a million new diagnoses of gallstones a year), and by the number of cholecystectomies performed yearly in the USA (approaching 700,000) [5]. Similar trends in gallstone disease have been confirmed in large epidemiological surveys carried out in Italy [6–10]. In Western societies approximately 80% of gallstones are cholesterol gallstones [11], either pure cholesterol or mixed cholesterol stones (containing more than 50% cholesterol by weight). The formation and growth of cholesterol gallstones implies a major disturbance of cholesterol disposal in the body, and this condition is frequently associated with other metabolic disorders [12]. A complex genetic basis plays also a key role in determining an individual predisposition to developing cholesterol gallstones in response to environmental factors [13, 14]. Pigment stones make up the rest and contain mostly calcium bilirubinate (Fig. 3.1). Black pigment stones (15%) and brown pigment stones (5%) are the two subtypes, the latter type being found mostly in the biliary tract [15].

In this review, the most recent advances and novel insights into the complex pathophysiological mechanisms involved in the formation of cholesterol gallstones will be discussed.

Bile Composition and Secretion

Chemical Composition of Bile

Bile is a complex fluid containing over 95% water [16] and three major lipid components (cholesterol, phospholipids and bile salts), with bile pigments as minor solutes (Table 3.1) [15]. Cholesterol accounts for up to 95% of sterols in both bile and gallstones. Non-cholesterol sterols are found in less than 5% in bile with shellfish free diet, and account for 5-10% of total sterols with shellfish diet. The phospholipids are 15–25% of total lipids in bile, a major compound of which is phosphatidylcholine (lecithin), which is composed of a hydrophilic phosphocholine head group and hydrophobic tails including two long fatty acyl chains. Lecithins are principally synthesized in the endoplasmic reticulum of the liver from diacylglycerol by way of the cytidine diphosphate-choline pathway. The main molecular species of lecithins in human bile are 16:0-18:2 (40–60%), 16:0-18:1 (5–25%), 18:0–18:2 (1–16%), and 16:0-20:4 (1–10%). Bile salts are soluble amphiphiles synthesized from cholesterol in the liver (primary bile salts: in humans the tri-hydroxy cholate, and the dihydroxy chenodeoxycholate) or obtained following intestinal biotransformation from colonic bacteria (secondary bile salts: dihydroxy

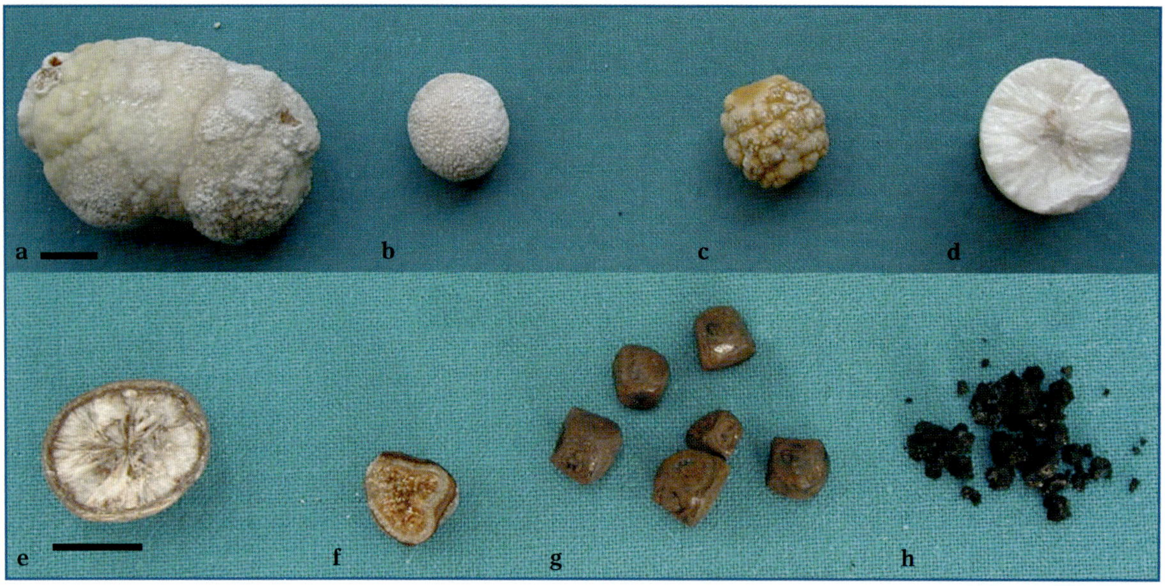

Fig. 3.1 *Upper panel* Morphology of pure cholesterol gallstones: **a** very large stone, probably a conglomeration of several stones; **b** spherical stone with smooth surface; **c** spherical stone with morular surface; **d** cut surface of a spherical stone with smooth surface and typical radial deposition of monohydrate cholesterol crystals. *Horizontal black line* represents 1 cm. *Lower panel* Morphology of mixed cholesterol and pigment gallstones: **e** cut surface of a spherical stone with smooth surface and mixed composition: thick pigment surface and typical radial deposition of monohydrate cholesterol crystals mixed with a brownish pigment core; **f** pigment stone with tiny cholesterol content; **g** group of six small pure pigment stones with multifaceted brownish surface; **h** friable powder of tiny black pigment stones. *Horizontal black line* represents 1 cm

deoxycholate and mono-hydroxy lithocholate, formed from cholate and chenodeoxycholate, respectively). "Tertiary" bile salts are the result of modification of secondary bile salts by intestinal flora or hepatocytes. These are the sulfate ester of lithocholate and ursodeoxycholate, the 7β-epimer of chenodeoxycholate. Bile pigments in bile are minor solutes accounting for approximately 0.5% of total lipids by weight in bile. They are mainly bilirubin conjugates with traces of porphyrins and unconjugated bilirubin. In humans, bile pigments include bilirubin, mono- and diglucuronides predominating: invariably present are other mono- and diconjugates of xylose, glucose, and glucuronic acid as homo- and heteroconjugates. Bile salts are highly soluble, being detergent-like amphiphilic molecules; the hydrophilic (polar) areas of bile salts are the hydroxyl groups and conjugation side chain of either glycine or taurine and their hydrophobic (nonpolar) area is the ringed steroid nucleus. An important feature of bile salts is their high solubility because they tend to self-assemble into micelles when a critical micellar concentration (CMC) is exceeded. The CMC values of common bile salts range from 1 to 20 µM, depending on species, ionic strength, and composition of bile salts, as well as on the types and concentrations of other lipids present in solution. However, because bile is concentrated gradually within the biliary tree, bile salt concentrations steadily exceed their CMCs and bile salts can form simple micelles in bile, which can solubilize cholesterol and phospholipids (mixed micelles in bile). Other bile components include proteins, mainly albumin with some immunoglobulins, and a number of other proteins not yet quantitated, and several ions.

Table 3.1 Major components of human bile

Water	Over 95%	
Lipids		
	Sterols	Cholesterol (95% of sterols)
		Noncholesterol sterols
	Phospholipids	Mainly phosphatidylcholine
	Bile salts	Primary: cholic acid, chenodeoxycholate
		Secondary: deoxycholate, lithocholate
		Tertiary: ursodeoxycholate
Proteins		
	Albumin	
	Immunoglobulins	IgG, IgM
	Apolipoproteins	AI, AII, B, CI, and CII
		Transferrin
		Alpha$_2$ macroglobin
	Other proteins	Epidermal growth factor
		Insulin
		Haptoglobin
		Cholecystokinin
		Lysosomal hydrolase
		Amylase
Ions		
	Sodium	
	Phosphorus	
	Potassium	
	Calcium	
	Copper	
	Zinc	
	Iron	
	Manganese	
	Molybdenum	
	Magnesium	
	Strontium	

Sources of Lipids Secreted in Bile

The metabolic determinants of the supply of hepatic cholesterol that can be recruited for biliary secretion depend on cholesterol input–output balance and its catabolism in the liver. With only low cholesterol or cholesterol free diet, input is related to the amount of cholesterol (both unesterified and esterified) taken up by the liver from plasma lipoproteins plus de novo hepatic cholesterol synthesis. The major sources of preformed cholesterol are hepatic uptake of plasma lipoproteins (mainly HDL, LDL, and VLDL through their receptors on the basolateral membrane of hepatocyte). In keeping with their central role in reverse cholesterol transport, HDL particles are the main lipoprotein source of cholesterol that is targeted for biliary secretion. HDL enters the hepatocyte after specific interaction with the apical plasma membrane transporter scavenger receptor class B type I (SR-BI). Peripheral cells eliminate excess cholesterol through its delivery to HDL, a process mediated by ATP-binding cassette (ABC) transporter protein A1 (ABCA1). The absence of ABCA1 is the cause of Tangier disease, a disorder characterized by very low HDL levels and increased cardiovascular risk. ABCA1 knockout mice with very low circulating HDL levels do not display any appreciable difference in biliary lipid composition, thus proving that metabolic pathways other than HDL-mediated reverse cholesterol transport guarantee biliary cholesterol secretion [17]. An appreciable fraction of cholesterol in bile may also be derived from the diet via apolipoprotein E-dependent delivery of chylomicron remnants to the liver. When there is a high level of cholesterol in the diet, dietary cholesterol reaches the liver through the intestinal lymphatic pathways, such as chylomicrons, and chylomicron remnants after chylomicron hydrolysis by plasma lipoprotein lipase and hepatic lipase.

With high dietary cholesterol, hepatic biosynthesis of cholesterol is reduced, accounting for only approximately 5% of biliary total cholesterol. Overall, the liver can systematically regulate the total amount of cholesterol, and any excess cholesterol is handled efficiently. Conversely, in the fasting state, approximately 20% of the cholesterol in bile comes from de novo hepatic biosynthesis and 80% from pools of preformed cholesterol within the liver. De novo cholesterol synthesis in the liver uses acetate as a substrate and is regulated mainly by a rate-limited enzyme, 3-hydroxy-3-methylglutaryl coenzyme A (HMG-CoA) reductase. This enzyme can be up- or down-regulated, depending on the overall cholesterol balance in the liver. An increase in the activity of this rate-limiting enzyme could lead to excessive cholesterol secretion in bile. Besides biliary secretion, hepatic cholesterol may be converted into cholesterol esters by acyl-coenzyme A:cholesterol acyltransferase (ACAT), either for cytoplasmic storage or for secretion as VLDL and LDL into the bloodstream. In addition, cholesterol can be used for bile salt synthesis by two rate-limited enzymes cholesterol 7α-hydroxylase (CYP7A1) and sterol 27-hydroxylase (CYP27). Bile salts are also secreted in bile, and this represents an additive means of cholesterol disposal (Fig. 3.2).

More than 95% of bile salt molecules secreted into bile are absorbed in the distal ileum via active transport systems and return to the liver, the so-called enterohepatic circulation of bile salts. As a result, the newly synthesized bile salts in the liver account for less than 5% of the total bile salt pool, which compensate for bile salts that escape intestinal absorption and are lost in the feces. The fecal excretion of bile salts is increased in conditions in which the enterohepatic circulation is partially or completely interrupted by surgery, disease states, or drugs (e.g., bile salt-binding resins such as cholestyramine). When enterohepatic circulation is impaired, bile salt synthesis can be up-regulated consistently, in order to restore bile salt secretion rates to approximately 25% of their native values, even in the case of complete interruption. De novo bile salt synthesis employs two sources of cholesterol in the smooth endoplasmic reticulum: cholesterol molecules that are newly synthesized in the smooth endoplasmic reticulum or those that are preformed outside the smooth endoplasmic reticulum. The first step in this process is catalyzed by the enzyme called cholesterol 7α-hydroxylase. It has been found that in the basal state, de novo bile salt synthesis principally utilizes newly synthesized cholesterol as substrate in humans. However, because long-term therapy of competitive HMG-CoA reductase inhibitors (statins) could impair de novo cholesterol biosynthesis to a significantly lesser extent, it is likely that preformed cholesterol from plasma lipoprotein origin could substitute for newly synthesized cholesterol.

Next to cholesterol and bile salts, approximately 11 g of phospholipids are secreted into bile per day in humans. Although biliary phospholipids are derived from the cell membranes of hepatocytes, their compositions differ markedly. The membranes of hepatocytes contain phosphatidylcholine (lecithins), phosphatidylethanolamines, phosphatidylinositols, phosphatidylserines, and

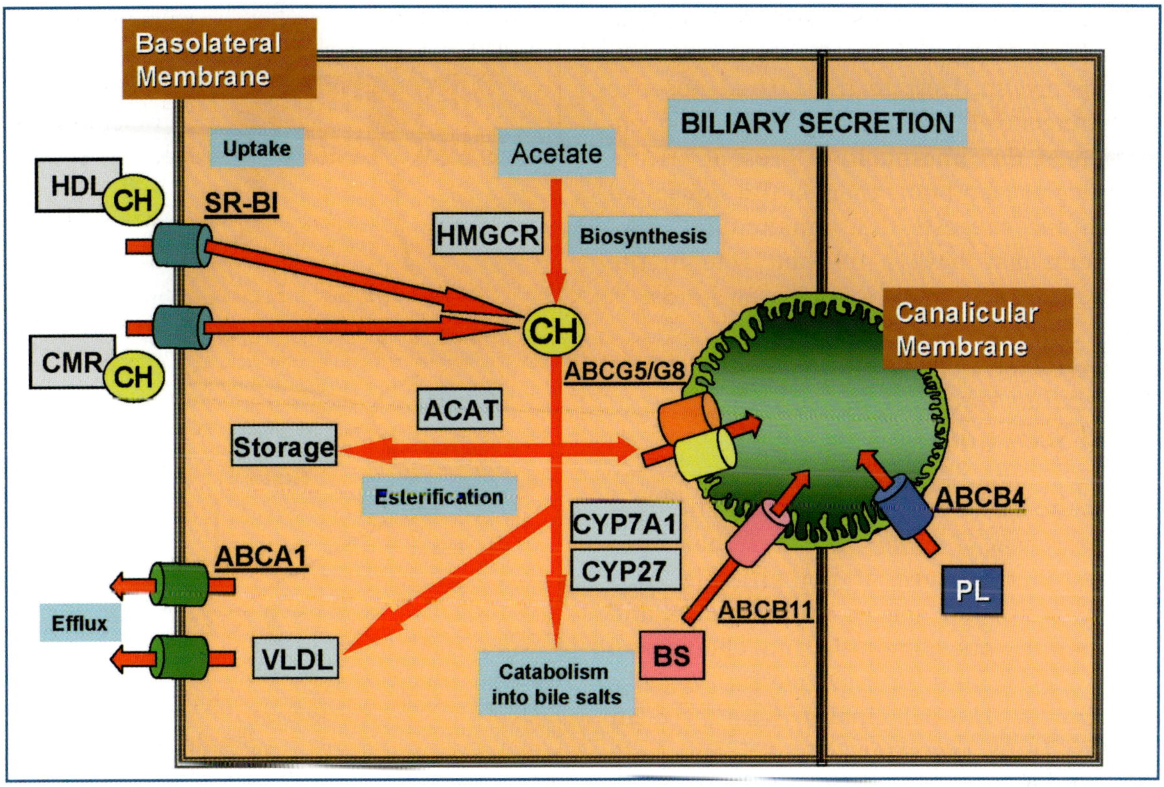

Fig. 3.2 Uptake, biosynthesis, catabolism, and biliary secretion of cholesterol at hepatocyte level. Hepatic uptake of cholesterol is mediated by scavenger receptor class B type I (*SR-BI*) for high-density lipoprotein (*HDL*) and by the chylomicron remnant receptor for chylomicron remnants (*CMR*). Biosynthesis of hepatic cholesterol is regulated by the rate-limiting enzyme 3-hydroxy-3-methylglutaryl-coenzyme A reductase (*HMGCR*). Part of the cholesterol is esterified by acyl-coenzyme A: cholesterol acyltransferase (*ACAT*) for storage in the liver. Some of the cholesterol molecules are used for the formation of very low density lipoprotein (*VLDL*) that is secreted into the circulatory system. The ATP-binding cassette (*ABC*) transporter ABCA1 either directly or indirectly translocates phospholipids and cholesterol to the cell surface, where they appear to form lipid domains that interact with amphipathic α-helices in apolipoproteins. This interaction solubilizes these lipids and generates nascent HDL particles that dissociate from the cell. Binding of apolipoproteins to ABCA1 may also enhance the activity of this lipid-transport pathway. A proportion of cholesterol is used for the synthesis of bile salts via the 'neutral' and the 'acidic' pathways as regulated by two rate-limiting enzymes cholesterol 7α-hydroxylase (*CYP7A1*) and sterol 27-hydroxylase (*CYP27*), respectively. Hepatic secretion of biliary cholesterol (*CH*), phospholipids (*PL*), and bile salts (*BS*) is determined by three ABC transporter proteins, ABCG5/G8, ABCB4, and ABCB11, respectively

sphingomyelins. The major source of phosphatidylcholine molecules destined for secretion into bile is hepatic synthesis. However, a fraction of biliary phosphatidylcholines may also originate in the phospholipid coat of HDL particles. Phosphatidylcholine is by far the most present phospholipid in normal human bile, although the outer leaflet of the hepatocyte canalicular membrane is rich in both phosphatidylcholine and sphingomyelins. The differences between phospholipids present in bile and those in the canalicular membrane are also of interest for the molecular species of both phosphatidylcholine (PC) and sphingomyelin: in contrast to membrane phosphatidylcholine, which is relatively hydrophobic owing to the presence of long acyl chains (mainly 16:0-18:2 PC, 16:0-20:4 PC, 18:0-20:4 PC and 18:0-18:2 PC), biliary phosphatidylcholine is rather hydrophilic (16:0-18:2 PC, 16:0-20:4 PC). Similarly, the tiny percentage of biliary sphingomyelin is more hydrophilic than canalicular membrane sphingomyelin. Despite the virtual absence of sphingomyelin in bile, the higher concentration of this phospholipid present on the canalicular membrane than on the sinusoidal membrane suggests that canalicular sphingomyelin may have a relevant role in the process of canalicular extraction of lipids.

Molecular Mechanisms of Biliary Lipid Secretion

Bile salts exert a stimulatory function for the secretion of biliary lipids. It has been suggested that most, if not all, bile salts enter canalicular spaces as monomers and that biliary phospholipids and cholesterol enter aggregated in unilamellar vesicles (see below). The principal driving force for biliary lipid secretion come from ATP-dependent membrane transporters located on the canalicular membrane of the hepatocyte (Fig. 3.3) [18]. Although the exact mechanisms by which cholesterol is incorporated into biliary vesicles are not yet fully elucidated, recent evidence in molecular genetics points to ABC transporters ABCG5 and ABCG8 as the canalicular transporters responsible for biliary cholesterol efflux. Recently, two groups of scientists [18, 20] independently identified the mutated *ABCG5/G8* genes inducing cytosterolemia (Table 3.2) [19, 21–29], an inherited disorder characterized by plasma accumulation of mainly plant sterols. The role of these two proteins, which work as a functional heterodimer, has been extensively examined in genetically modified mice [30–34]. Overexpression of *Abcg5/g8* in the liver of transgenic mice increases the cholesterol content of gallbladder bile; conversely, ABCG5/ABCG8 knockout mice display drastically reduced biliary cholesterol secretion plus accumulation of high levels of plant sterols in plasma, recapitulating the phenotypes of human cytosterolemia [34]. Despite a reduc-

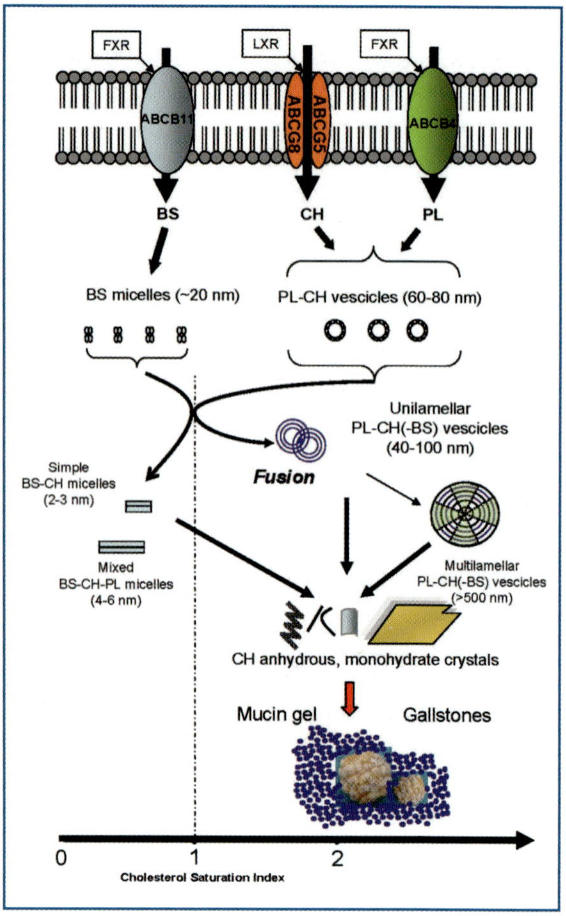

Fig. 3.3 Pathogenesis of cholesterol gallstone formation. Three ATP-binding cassette (*ABC*) transporter proteins (ABCG5/G8, ABCB4, and ABCB11) determining biliary lipid secretion are regulated by farnesoid X receptor (*FXR*) and liver X receptor (*LXR*), respectively. Following biliary secretion, bile salts (*BS*) form simple micelles and phospholipids (*PL*) and cholesterol (*CH*) form meta-stable unilamellar vesicles. During their passage through the biliary tract into the gallbladder, various lipid aggregates are converted into mixed micelles. If bile contains more CH that cannot be solubilized by mixed micelles, it becomes supersaturated with CH so that the cholesterol saturation index (*CSI*) is in excess of 1. These alterations result in the formation and growth of CH-rich multilamellar vesicles, which could fuse larger liquid crystals and are prone to nucleating solid intermediate or monohydrate CH crystals. Thus, conditions that increase the ratio of CH to BS and PC favor the formation of gallstones. The mucous glycoproteins secreted by the gallbladder epithelial cells facilitate the crystallization, precipitation, and aggregation of solid crystals into stone(s) by forming a matrix gel. Adapted from [19]

Table 3.2 Molecular lipid transporters present in the liver and associated human diseases

Transporter	Localization	Function	Disease	References
ABCA1	Apical membrane	Efflux of cholesterol	Tangier disease	[22–24]
ABCB4	Canalicular membrane	Biliary secretion of phospholipids	PFIC type III	[21, 25–27]
ABCB11	Canalicular membrane	Biliary secretion of bile salts	PFIC type II	[28]
ABCG5/G8	Canalicular membrane	Biliary secretion of cholesterol	Cytosterolemia	[18, 29]

tion in the gallstone prevalence rate, gallstone formation is still observed both in Abcg5/g8 double knockout mice and in Abcg5 or Abcg8 single knockout mice challenged with the lithogenic diet, suggesting ABCG5/G8-independent pathways for hepatic secretion of biliary cholesterol, with a role in cholesterol cholelithiasis.

The precise mechanisms responsible for bile salt secretion in bile are not yet fully understood, although consistent data identify the transport protein, ABCB11, as the canalicular bile salt export pump [35–37]. *ABCB11* is the gene mutated in type 2 progressive familial intrahepatic cholestasis (PFIC2), an homozygous disorder characterized by onset in the first years of life, progressive behavior, and a poor prognosis, leading to liver failure before adulthood. Homozygous disruption of the *Abcb11* gene in knockout mice results in severe impairment of bile flow, with total bile acid output as low as one-third of that in wild type mice, with a dramatic reduction of cholic acid secretion and only mild or no change for the remaining bile salts species [36]. Despite the relevant reduction in total output, the persistence of substantial biliary bile salt secretion displayed by *Abcb11* knockouts suggests the existence of as yet unidentified, alternative bile acid transporter(s) on the hepatocyte canalicular membrane. Bile salts are of extreme importance for sustaining biliary secretion, a property termed 'choleretic' activity. Although hepatic secretion of bile salts directly affects cholesterol-phospholipid vesicle secretion, the exact molecular mechanism by which bile salt secretion is coupled to cholesterol and phospholipid secretion remains elusive. The relationship between bile salt secretion and cholesterol secretion is not linear: at low bile salt secretion rates, less than 10 μmol/h/kg, cholesterol secretion per molecule of bile salt is much more than at higher bile secretion rates. Although bile salt secretion rates are not usually low in normal subjects, they diminish during prolonged fasting, during the overnight period, and with substantial bile salt losses, such as in a biliary fistula or ileal resection when the liver cannot compensate sufficiently with increased bile salt synthesis. At high bile salt secretion rates—e.g., during and after eating—biliary saturation is lower than during interprandial periods.

Hepatic secretion of biliary phospholipids is mediated by ABCB4, as shown by the complete lack of biliary phospholipids in mice with deletion of the *Abcb4* gene [21]. ABCB4 is a P-glycoprotein member of the multi-drug resistance gene family, previously known as *Mdr-2* in mice and MDR-3 in men. Mutations of the ABCB4 gene in humans have been identified as the molecular defect underlying type 3 progressive familial intrahepatic cholestasis (PFIC3) [38]. Activation of ABCB4 results in the formation of phosphatidylcholine-rich microdomains within the outer membrane leaflet, supporting the current interpretation of ABCB4 as a transporter responsible for translocation or "flip" of phosphatidylcholines from the endoplasmic (inner) to ectoplasmic (outer) leaflet of the canalicular membrane bilayer. Since detergent-like bile salt molecules within the canalicular space interact with canalicular membrane, it has been suggested that bile salts may partition preferentially into these phosphatidylcholine-rich microdomains in order to destabilize the membrane and release phosphatidylcholine-rich vesicles. A number of diverse observations indicate that bile salts promote vesicular secretion of biliary cholesterol and phosphatidylcholines, although the ectoplasmic leaflet of the canalicular membrane is rich in cholesterol and sphingomyelin and is relatively resistant to penetration by bile salts. Indirect evidence of the importance of bile salts for the process of biliary secretion comes from experiments in laboratory animals in which the rate of organic anions secretion in bile was experimentally increased. Increased concentrations of biliary organic anions do not influence bile salt secretion, but inhibit the secretion of phospholipid and cholesterol into bile as a result of organic anions binding to bile salts within bile canaliculi, thus preventing their interaction with the canalicular membrane.

Lastly, scavenger receptor class B type I (SR-BI) is localized in sinusoidal and, probably, in canalicular membranes of the hepatocyte. Under chow feeding conditions, in transgenic and knockout mice biliary secretion of cholesterol varies in proportion to hepatic expression of SR-BI and the established contribution of SR-BI to sinusoidal uptake of HDL cholesterol that is destined for secretion into bile. Furthermore, cholesterol contents of vesicles may be determined simply by the degree to which cholesterol partitions into phosphatidylcholine-rich microdomains in the canalicular membrane of hepatocyte. Because of the high affinity of sphingomyelin for cholesterol, microdomains form in membranes with sufficient amounts of cholesterol and sphingomyelin on the canalicular membrane [39]. An additional possibility is that bile salts could regulate partitioning of cholesterol into nascent vesicles. Because bile salts reduce the affinity of cholesterol for sphingomyelin, they could induce migration of cholesterol into phosphatidylcholine-rich microdomains.

Regulation of Biliary Secretion by Nuclear Receptors

Bile formation relies on the synchronized function of transport proteins to secrete optimal quantities of each lipid species in order to avoid bile salt detergency and cholesterol precipitation. An important regulatory function is achieved by nuclear receptors, which are ligand-activated transcription factors engaged in the fine tuning of the lipid secretory network. Specifically, the bile acid receptor farnesoid X receptor (FXR) [40–42] and the oxysterol receptor liver X receptors (LXRs) [43, 44] drive gene transcription of lipid canalicular transporters. FXR promotes the expression of bile salt transporter ABCB11 [45] and phospholipid transporter ABCB4 [46]; LXR is responsible for the transcription of cholesterol transporters ABCG5 and ABCG8 [47]. Nuclear receptors share a common molecular structure: the C-terminal ligand-binding domain (LBD) contains an hydrophobic pocket that selectively recognizes and binds the ligand, resulting in a change of the three-dimensional structure of the nuclear receptor, which is now capable of starting gene transcription through the DNA binding domain (DBD). Specific gene transcription starting sites are termed hormone response elements, which are characteristic for each nuclear receptor: FXR binds the chromatin in sites composed of inverted repeated elements of the canonical AGGTCA sequence with one nucleotide separation (IR-1) [48]; LXR, in turn, binds DNA sites consisting of two AGGTCA hexanucleotide repeats separated by four nucleotides (DR4) [49]. Lastly, both FXR and LXR need to form a heterodimer together with retinoid X receptor (RXR) to be operative. The role of FXR and LXR in the liver is not limited to enhancing biliary lipid efflux. Both FXR and LXR are chiefly involved in orchestrating the metabolic pathways responsible for uptake, appraisal, storage, and catabolism of their cognate ligand. FXR keeps bile salt concentration in the physiological range restraining their hepatic synthesis, by means of reduced transcription of rate-limiting enzyme CYP7A1 [50, 51]. LXR, on the other hand, up-regulates CYP7A1 (in rodents but not in man), thus boosting cholesterol catabolism into bile salt [52].

Physical States of Biliary Lipids

Cholesterol is virtually insoluble in aqueous solutions. To be dissolved in bile, cholesterol needs to be solubilized in lipid carriers (Table 3.3). Definite compositions and proportions of biliary lipids result in the formation of micelles and vesicles within the biliary tree and gallbladder, which serve as cholesterol carriers.

Cholesterol Carriers in Bile: Micelles and Vesicles

Bile salts are amphiphilic molecules composed of both hydrophilic and hydrophobic areas. In an aqueous solution, bile salts are present as monomers. As soon as they reach a CMC, bile salt monomers start to aggregate spontaneously. The resulting bile salt aggregates are termed simple micelles: small discoid structures with average diameter of 3 nm. Cholesterol can be solubilized in these simple micelles: the hydrophilic face of bile salts (hydroxyl groups and side chains) are oriented outward, in contact with the water, while the hydrophobic moieties form the core, which dissolves cholesterol molecules. Simple micelles are thermodynamically stable structures, discoid, and formed at bile salt concentrations above the CMC. Although the definition of CMC suggests that micelles rapidly form above a concentration threshold, the bile salt aggregation is a gradual process that starts at concentrations of about 2 mmol/L and proceeds with increasing bile salt concentrations. Phospholipids may also be solubilized and incorporated into simple micelles, resulting in increased cholesterol solubilization capacity: aggregates of bile salts, cholesterol, and phospholipids are termed mixed micelles. On average, mixed micelles solubilize at least three times as much cholesterol as simple micelles can carry out. Mixed micelles are larger, thermodynamically stable structures, with a diameter ranging from 4 to 8 nm. The size of mixed micelles varies depending on the relative proportion of bile salts and phospholipids.

Table 3.3 Lipid carriers responsible for cholesterol solubilization in bile

Structure	Lipid components	Diameter	Localization in the phase diagram	Cholesterol solubilization capacity
Simple micelles	Bile salts	3 nm	One phase	Low
Mixed micelles	Bile salts + phospholipids	4–8 nm	Right two Central three Left two	Intermediate
Vesicles	Cholesterol + phospholipids	40–100 nm	Right two Central three	High

Mixed micelles present a lipid bilayer with the hydrophilic groups of the bile salts and phospholipids aligned outward in contact with the aqueous bile, while the hydrophobic groups are on the "inside". Cholesterol molecules are solubilized inside the bilayer, segregated from the aqueous areas on the outside.

Several clinical observations find different mechanisms than the micellar systems that are also important for cholesterol solubilization in bile. First, in some patients, the presence of supersaturated bile is not associated with solid cholesterol crystals. Second, differences in meta-stability are present both in patients with and without cholesterol gallstones; lastly, some patients still present cholesterol gallstone, despite biliary cholesterol solubility greatly exceeding the limits of meta-stability [53, 54]. Hence, nonmicellar carriers for cholesterol must be present in bile. A more complex mechanism of cholesterol solubilization has been identified by using techniques such as quasi-elastic light-scattering spectroscopy and electron microscopy [55–61]. Gallbladder biles from many healthy individuals are supersaturated with cholesterol, indicating that cholesterol concentrations exceed what can be solubilized by micellar particles. In 1983 the first direct visualization of biliary vesicles was obtained, considerably extending our understanding of cholesterol solubility in bile with respect to cholesterol nucleation and crystallization [62–64], liquid crystal formation [65, 66], and biliary metastability [53, 67].

Vesicles are unilamellar spherical structures and contain phospholipids and cholesterol and only small quantities of bile salts, if any at all. Vesicles are significantly larger than simple or mixed micelles, with diameters between 40 nm and 100 nm, although they are much smaller than liquid crystals, which have diameters exceeding 500 nm and are composed of multilamellar spherical structures. The presence of large quantities of vesicles in hepatic bile suggests the hepatocyte as their likely origin. Unilamellar vesicles are often detected in all freshly collected cholesterol-unsaturated biles as a result of the time-dependent physical chemistry of postcanalicular events during bile formation and because of the very slow disappearance of vesicles by micellar dissolution. Unilamellar vesicles are physically indistinguishable from those present in supersaturated biles. Cholesterol-rich vesicles are remarkably stable in dilute biles, which is consistent with the finding of absent cholesterol crystallization in hepatic biles. Unilamellar vesicles can fuse into larger multilamellar vesicles, which are also termed liposomes or liquid crystals.

When cultured under specified conditions, rat hepatocytes form couplets with isolated "bile canaliculi" at interfaces between adjoining cells, thus providing a valuable tool for in vitro investigation of the physiology of hepatic biliary secretion of lipids. Using laser light-scattering techniques, it has been possible to visualize vesicle formation within these bile canaliculi after exposure to bile salts. Furthermore, with rapid fixation techniques and electronic microscopy, direct morphologic evidence for vesicle formation at the outer surface of the canalicular membrane has been obtained. Unilamellar vesicles have been visualized and their sizes have been determined within canalicular spaces of rat liver by transmission electron microscopy and quasi-elastic light-scattering spectroscopy. The radii of these vesicles by both methods are in general agreement and vary in a range of 60–80 nm. To quantify the changing proportions of micelles to vesicles, the bile formation path in fresh rat bile with unsaturated cholesterol is investigated by dynamic light scattering spectroscopy. These vesicles apparently vary more widely in size, usually being between 40 and 120 nm in radius.

Cholesterol behavior in bile depends strictly on total lipid concentration. In diluted biles with low total lipid concentrations (i.e., less than 3 g/dL), vesicles are extremely stable, not aggregating or fusing, and prevent cholesterol nucleation. Conversely, in concentrated gallbladder biles with high total lipid concentrations (i.e., ~10 g/dL,) vesicles are considerably unstable, resulting in greatly accelerated cholesterol precipitation. Also, the total amount of cholesterol that can be solubilized depends on the relative proportions of bile salts: maximal solubility occurs when the molar ratio of phospholipids to bile salts is between 0.2 and 0.3.

Although vesicles are relatively static structures, the dynamics of vesicles, in terms of size, composition, and interaction with each other and with micelles, is influenced by several factors, such as bile concentrations and the relative ratios of cholesterol, phospholipids, and bile salts in bile. Even though bile is rarely at equilibrium, the physical states of biliary lipids at equilibrium have provided the basis of physical chemistry for describing biliary lipid aggregation in vivo. Because bile is gradually concentrated within the biliary tree, bile salt concentrations approach their CMC values. When this occurs, bile salts begin to modify the structure of phospholipid-rich vesicles that are secreted into bile by the hepatocyte. These interactions indicate the start of a complex series of molecular rearrangements that ultimately form simple and mixed micelles.

The relative ratios of three lipids are influenced by the fasting or feeding state through alterations in bile secretion rates. For example, during fasting, biliary bile salt output is relatively low. Consequently, the ratio of cholesterol to bile salts is increased and more cholesterol is carried in vesicles than in micelles. In contrast, during meals, biliary bile salt output is increased, so that more cholesterol is solubilized in micelles. In addition, when the concentration of bile salts is relatively low, especially in dilute hepatic bile, vesicles are relatively stable and only some vesicles can be converted to micelles. In contrast, vesicles may be transformed or converted completely to mixed micelles because of increased bile salt concentrations in concentrated gallbladder bile. Because relatively more phospholipids may be transferred from vesicles to mixed micelles than cholesterol, the residual vesicles are remodeled, and may be enriched in cholesterol relative to phospholipids. If the remaining vesicles have a relatively low cholesterol-to-phospholipid ratio (less than 1) they are relatively stable. However, if the cholesterol-to-phospholipid ratio in vesicles is greater than 1, vesicles become increasingly unstable. These cholesterol-rich vesicles may transfer some cholesterol to less cholesterol-rich vesicles or to micelles, or may fuse or aggregate to form larger (~500 nm in diameter) multilamellar vesicles (i.e., liposomes or liquid crystals). These liquid crystals are visible by polarizing light microscopy as lipid circular droplets with typical birefringence in the shape of a Maltese cross. Liquid crystals are inherently unstable and could form solid plate-like cholesterol monohydrate crystals, a process termed cholesterol nucleation. As a result, nucleation of cholesterol monohydrate crystals results in a decrease in the amount of cholesterol contained in vesicles but not of cholesterol in micelles, supporting the concept that vesicles could serve as the primary source of cholesterol for nucleation.

Cholesterol Solubility in Bile and the Phase Diagram

Bile salts and phospholipids are the principal agents of solubilization of cholesterol in bile. The relative proportions of these three lipids in bile have a critical role in determining the maximal solubility of cholesterol [53, 68]. In the 1960s, Small et al. defined the maximal solubility (saturation) limits for cholesterol in model bile systems with varying proportions of cholesterol, phospholipids, bile salts, and water together in a quaternary system; three decades later the original description of the phase diagram has been reassessed and improved by Wang and Carey [67–73]. The triangular coordinate diagram is useful to express the solubility of cholesterol for any given solute concentration. The relative proportions (molar percentages) of the three lipids for a fixed total lipid concentration are plotted in a triangular coordinate, which shows the number and type of phases, as determined when the system reaches equilibrium. Hence, the triangular coordinate diagram illustrates the physical phases of cholesterol in bile. For example, the phase diagram shown in Fig. 3.2 is specific for a total lipid concentration of 7.5 g/dL, which is that of human gallbladder biles. For hepatic biles, with a typical total lipid concentration of 3 g/dL, the phase boundaries would be different, with a smaller micellar zone. This effect of total lipid content on cholesterol solubilization in the micellar zone explains why hepatic bile tends to be more highly supersaturated than gallbladder bile in the same patient. Because hepatic bile contains cholesterol-phospholipid vesicles that are relatively stable, solid cholesterol monohydrate crystals are less likely to occur in hepatic bile than in gallbladder bile. In addition, phase diagrams are specific in terms of defining solubility not just for different proportions of lipids but also for different total lipid concentrations. Within the micellar zone, bile is in a visually clear stable solution, which is termed 'unsaturated' because it is capable of solubilizing more cholesterol. At the boundary line of the micellar zone, bile is termed 'saturated' because all the solubilizing capacity for cholesterol is utilized; no further cholesterol can be carried in micelles. Outside the micellar zone, bile is termed "supersaturated" because excess cholesterol cannot be solubilized within micelles. In these circumstances, cholesterol exists in more than one phase (micelles, liquid crystals, and solid monohydrate crystals) and the solution is visually cloudy. Obviously, relatively stable unilamellar cholesterol-phospholipid vesicles solubilize a significant proportion of cholesterol outside the micellar zone. The term meta-"stable zone" refers to the area in the phase diagram (above but near the micellar zone) where bile is supersaturated with cholesterol but may not form solid cholesterol crystals even after many days. The diagram also suggests that when the quantity of cholesterol in bile exceeds that which can be solubilized by the available bile salts and phospholipids the cholesterol crystallizes out of solution. The value of equilibrium phase diagrams relies on their utility to predict the phases in which cholesterol crystals can be found at equilibrium. This model, in fact, reliably predicts cholesterol solubilization or precipitation in bile, providing a pathophysiologic frame to study the prime mover of cholesterol gallstone disease. In the 1970s, these findings were further confirmed in native biles of humans and animals. Consequently, the composition of any bile sample can be represented by a single point on such a triangular coordinate.

Although the equilibration process starts after bile secretion from the hepatocyte and continues in the biliary tree, the evolution to cholesterol monohydrate crystals only occurs in the gallbladder. Cholesterol-unsaturated bile is not at thermodynamic equilibrium, at which all cholesterol can be solubilized with coexisting simple and mixed micelles and therefore relative lipid compositions sited in the micellar zone of the appropriate phase diagram. In contrast, cholesterol supersaturated bile that cannot be completely solubilized by the coexistence of simple and mixed micelles has relative lipid compositions outside the micellar zone of the meta-stable phase diagram. Of note, high degrees of vesicle cholesterol concentrations and high total lipid concentrations are two principal factors that work together in producing the solid crystalline phase. Therefore, with typical physiological lipid ratios, at equilibrium, cholesterol monohydrate crystals are present with saturated simple and mixed micelles, or with saturated micelles plus vesicles that have become multilamellar liquid crystals. The final physical chemical state is also determined by bile salt-to-lecithin ratio and overall hydrophilic–hydrophobic balance of both bile salt and lecithin species.

Pathophysiology of Cholesterol Gallstone Formation

There is now general agreement that hepatic hypersecretion of biliary cholesterol is the prime mover in the pathogenesis of cholesterol gallstone formation. Relative cholesterol hypersecretion into bile may or may not be accompanied by normal, high, or low secretion rates of biliary bile salts and/or phospholipids. Hypersecretion of biliary cholesterol than results in the precipitation of excess cholesterol in the form of solid crystals, the first morphologic evidence of gallstone formation [74, 75]. Besides cholesterol crystals, gallstones contain also glycoproteins, calcium salts and bile pigments.

Classification of Defects Leading to Bile Supersaturation

By definition, bile supersaturated with cholesterol contains cholesterol that cannot be solubilized *at equilibrium* by bile salts and phospholipids. Cholesterol supersaturation could result from (1) hepatic hypersecretion of biliary cholesterol; (2) decreased rates of bile salt or phospholipid secretion into bile; or (3) a combination of cholesterol hypersecretion and hyposecretion of solubilizing lipids. With time and in the presence of a heterogeneous pro-nucleating agent, usually mucin gel, cholesterol supersaturation leads to precipitation of cholesterol monohydrate crystals from a phase-separated liquid-crystalline phase in gallbladder bile, followed by agglomeration and growth of the crystals into mature and macroscopic stones. Many biliary proteins besides mucin gel have been proposed as either pronucleating or antinucleating factors influencing cholesterol nucleation/crystallization in bile; however, their in vivo pathophysiological role, if any, in the pathogenesis of cholesterol gallstone formation remains unclear. Furthermore, proteolysis of soluble biliary glycoproteins does not influence the speed of cholesterol monohydrate crystal detection time in either normal or abnormal gallbladder and hepatic biles, suggesting that soluble biliary proteins may not be an important pathophysiological factor affecting cholesterol crystallization [76].

On the basis of the mechanisms for the saturation of bile with cholesterol, the recognized defects leading to bile supersaturation can be classified into four types.

Type 1: Excessive secretion of biliary cholesterol. Excessive cholesterol is secreted by the hepatocyte into bile, which causes supersaturated bile despite biliary secretion rates and normal pool sizes of bile salts. It is often observed in obese patients with gallstones.

Type 2: Normal secretion of cholesterol in the presence of reduced bile salt pool size, hepatic return, and secretion rate. This defect is often found in nonobese patients with gallstones, possibly because the relatively low rates of recirculating bile salts to the liver are still adequate to depress hepatic bile salt synthesis (i.e., oversensitive hepatic response to feedback of bile salts) but fails to solubilize biliary cholesterol appropriately. During the development of this inappropriate hepatic response to the feedback of bile salts, more bile salts are lost from the enterohepatic circulation than are synthesized, since the rate of synthesis is normal or low. Although some of these patients display a normal bile salt pool, the secretion rate of bile salts is reduced as a consequence of diminished enterohepatic circulations of the pool.

Type 3: Excessive loss of bile salts. Excessive loss of bile salts occurs in patients with ileectomy, diseases of the ileum (e.g., Crohn's disease), or surgical bypass of the ileum. These changes result in significant loss of bile salts, which cannot be recovered even by hepatic bile salt synthesis at the maximal rate. Both the pool and the secretion of hepatic bile salts are decreased, inducing supersaturation of bile despite normal cholesterol secretion.

Type 4: Mixed defect, consisting of excessive secretion of biliary cholesterol, plus reduced bile salt pool size, hepatic return, and secretion rate (combination of types 1 and 2). This condition has been observed in both American Indians and Caucasians with gallstones. In these patients, supersaturated bile results from an oversensitive hepatic response to the feedback of bile salts (causing decreased biliary secretion of bile salts), combined with an increased biliary secretion of cholesterol. The decreased hepatic synthesis of bile salts (when present) and increased biliary secretion of cholesterol may be the result of diminished 7-hydroxylation of cholesterol.

In human bile supersaturated with cholesterol there are two pathways for forming cholesterol-rich vesicles from phospholipid-rich vesicles assembled at the canalicular membrane. Because bile salts solubilize phospholipids more efficiently than cholesterol, cholesterol-rich vesicles may form when bile salts preferentially extract phospholipid molecules directly from phospholipid rich vesicles. The second possibility that has been observed in model bile systems is rapid dissolution of phospholipid-rich vesicles by bile salts. This alteration produces unstable mixed micelles with excess cholesterol. Consequently, structural rearrangements of these unstable micellar particles result in the formation of cholesterol-rich vesicles. Studying the molecular nature of biliary lipid aggregates in bile of typical physiological compositions would help us in understanding the physical state of cholesterol-unsaturated and supersaturated biles in terms of the distribution of biliary lipid aggregates. Unsaturated bile is inferred from the observation that cholesterol is solubilized in thermodynamically stable simple and mixed micelles, whereas 'supersaturated' bile is inferred when cholesterol is solubilized by micellar particles and dispersed in unilamellar vesicles. Concerning relative lipid compositions and physicochemical states of meta-stable model bile plotted on triangular coordinates [53, 67], micellar bile falls within a micellar zone of the phase diagram, whereas supersaturated bile falls outside this zone (Fig. 3.4) [66, 68]. The proportional distance outside the micellar zone directed along an axis joined to the cholesterol apex is often calculated as the cholesterol saturation index (CSI) or lithogenic index [77]. Thus, the degree of saturation of bile with cholesterol can be quantitated. A saturation index for a sample of bile can be estimated directly from the diagram or can be calculated by using a formula. The saturation index is the ratio of the actual amount of cholesterol present in a bile sample to the maximal amount of cholesterol that can be dissolved in it. Bile that has a saturation index of 1 is "saturated"; when the saturation index is less than 1 the bile is "unsaturated"; and when it is greater than 1 the bile is "supersaturated". The degree of saturation can also be expressed as a percentage of saturation by multiplying the saturation index by 100. For example, on the boundary of the micellar zone, bile is saturated and the CSI is 100%. Supersaturated bile has a CSI of over 100% and unsaturated bile has a CSI of less than 100%. The CSI values are also very useful in predicting both the proportions of lipid particles as well as the metastable and equilibrium physical-chemical states of bile.

The degree of cholesterol supersaturation is not a reliable predictor of gallstones: in fact, similar cholesterol supersaturation

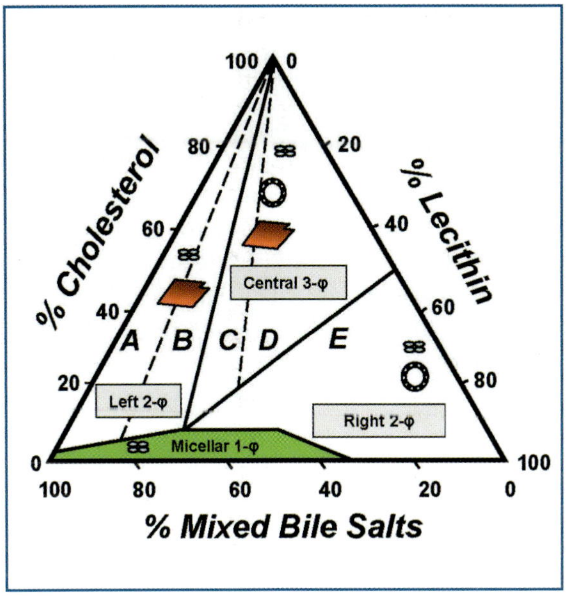

Fig. 3.4 The ternary bile salt–cholesterol–phospholipid phase diagram describes the different pathways of cholesterol solubilization and crystallization in bile. The three axes of the *triangle* represent the concentrations of the three lipids. The diagram is adapted from [67] and [69] for a total lipid concentration at 7.2 g/dl, pH 7 and temperature 37°C. Depicted are a one-phase (φ) (micellar) zone at the *bottom*, a *left* two-phase zone (containing micelles and crystals), a *central* three-phase zone (containing micelles, vesicles and crystals), and a *right* two-phase zone (containing micelles and vesicles). The cholesterol saturation index (*CSI*) has its maximum normal value set at 1 for the micellar-phase boundary. Above this boundary, bile becomes supersaturated and the CSI value is higher than 1. Below this boundary, bile is unsaturated and the CSI value is lower than 1. Based upon the solid and liquid crystallization sequences present in the bile, the left two-phase and the central three-phase regions are divided by *dashed lines* into regions *A* to *D*. The number of phases given represents the equilibrium state

may be present in biles obtained from individuals with or without cholesterol gallstones. In contrast, for identical CSI, there is a clear-cut difference in nucleation times between biles of patients with cholesterol gallstones and of control subjects. Nucleation time is the time until the first appearance of plate-like cholesterol monohydrate crystals in isotropic bile incubated in vitro at 37°C [64]. This measurement provides a reliable means of distinguishing biles from cholesterol gallstone patients and from controls. Moreover, differences in nucleation times suggest that human biles may contain factors that determine gallstone formation by inhibiting or accelerating the appearance of cholesterol crystals. Combined measurements of nucleation and crystal growth (i.e., cholesterol crystal detection time) have been standardized, quantified, and automated. These have proved useful in the search for factors that influence cholesterol crystallization in human bile.

Nucleation/Crystallization of Solid Cholesterol Monohydrate Crystals from Supersaturated Bile

Cholesterol nucleation/crystallization from gallbladder biles in patients with cholesterol gallstones is conventionally defined with reference to the earliest time at which plate-like cholesterol crystals are detected by polarizing light microscopy in a sample of bile previously rendered crystal free (“isotropic”) [64]. Rapid in vitro nucleation/crystallization of cholesterol monohydrate crystals from the ‘isotropic phase’ of gallbladder bile discriminates lithogenic gallbladder biles of cholesterol gallstone patients, from cholesterol-supersaturated biles of controls [78–81]. In understanding the kinetics, characteristics and meta-stable intermediates in the phase transitions of bile, the phase diagram for cholesterol, phospholipids and bile salts has been utilized as a template to study the regions in which different sequences of meta-stable intermediates occur. Recently, five crystallization pathways have been identified in model biles as functions of bile salt to phospholipid ratio, total lipid concentration, bile salt species (hydrophilic-hydrophobic index), temperature, and CSI [67]. These crystallization pathways have been detected and confirmed in fresh human and mouse biles [69, 76, 82, 83]. For cholesterol-phospholipid-mixed bile salt model systems, five distinct crystallization pathways (A-E) have been defined, each illustrating a different sequence of phase transitions, including an anhydrous cholesterol pathway and a liquid crystalline pathway to the formation of solid cholesterol monohydrate crystals [67, 84]. Transient arc-like crystals appear in some pathways, and these are consistent with crystalline 'anhydrous' cholesterol [67, 84–87]. It is not known why anhydrous cholesterol crystals should precipitate in an aqueous environment, but it is characteristic of crystallization pathways that seem to originate from unilamellar as opposed to multilamellar vesicles. It appears that in these pathways the critical nucleus may be a unilamellar vesicle containing liquid anhydrous cholesterol molecules in its core, possibly reflecting internal nucleation. Therefore, these early vesicular 'nuclei' may have already initiated the nucleation cascade by the time bile enters the gallbladder. The current paradigm for nucleation/crystallization, based principally on video-enhanced polarizing light microscopy, suggests that biliary vesicles must fuse or at least aggregate for formation of the crystalline cholesterol monohydrate phase [62, 63]. Since cholesterol nucleation/crystallization is apparently initiated in vesicles, vesicle stability determines the stability of bile. Unstable vesicles can aggregate, fuse, and grow into multilamellar liquid crystalline structures (liposomes) in which cholesterol crystallizes out of solution. Furthermore, evidence from quasi-elastic light-scattering spectroscopy shows that nucleation of solid cholesterol crystals may occur directly from supersaturated micelles in conjugated deoxycholate-rich biles in vitro without an intervening vesicle or liquid crystalline phase. This may occur because of the unusual phase equilibrium relationships of the ternary systems composed with very hydrophobic bile salts.

When phospholipid content is lowest (region A), arc-like crystals with habit and density (d=1.030 g/mL) consistent with anhydrous cholesterol appear first and evolve via helical and tubular crystals to form plate-like cholesterol monohydrate crystals (d=1.045 g/mL). With high phospholipid concentrations (region B), cholesterol monohydrate crystals appear earlier than arc-like and other transitional crystals. With typical physiological phospholipid content (region C), early liquid crystals (d=1.020 g/mL) are followed by cholesterol monohydrate crystals, and arc-like and other intermediate crystals subsequently appear. With still higher phospholipid contents (region D), liquid crystals are followed by cholesterol monohydrate crystals only. At the highest phospholipid mole fractions (region E), liquid crystals are stable and no solid crystals form. Decreases in temperature (37°C→4°C), total lipid concentration (7.5 g/dL→2.5 g/dL), and bile salt hydrophobicity (3α,12α→3α,7α→3α,7α, 12α→3α,7α hydroxylated taurine conjugates) progressively shift all crystallization pathways to lower phospholipid content, also retarding crystallization and reducing micellar cholesterol solubilization. It has been found that cholesterol crystallization pathways and sequences in human gallbladder biles are identical to model biles matched for appropriate physical-chemical conditions. In a physiological state, three of the five crystallization sequences observed in model biles are found in fresh human and mouse gallbladder biles. Most notably, the kinetics of all these phase transitions are faster in lithogenic human biles than in identically patterned model biles, which is most probably due, in part, to the combined influences of increased levels of cholesterol, secondary bile salts, and mucin glycoproteins. In addition, biliary lipid, electrolyte, and protein factors are important in stabilizing supersaturated bile. An example of solid cholesterol crystals, liquid crystals, and gallstones in gallbladder biles is shown in Figure 3.5 [82].

Non-protein factors that retard cholesterol nucleation/crystallization are as follows: (1) total lipid concentrations less than 3 g/dL; (2) reduced hydrophobicity of the

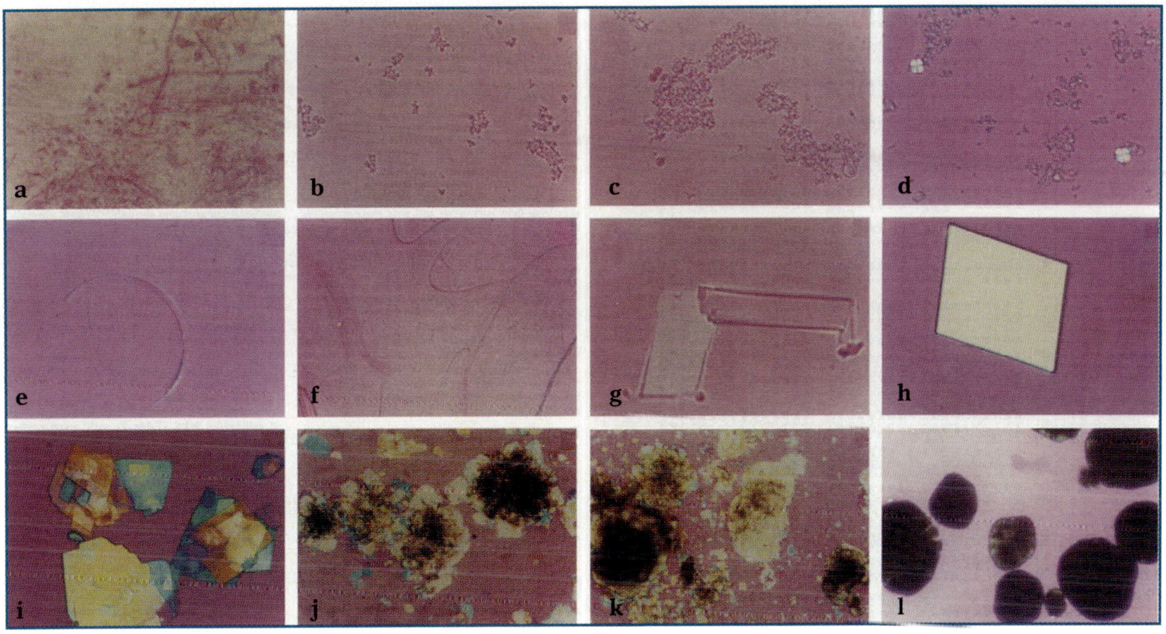

Fig. 3.5 Photomicrographs of mucin gel and habits of solid and liquid crystals, sandy stones, and true gallstones observed in fresh gallbladder biles of gallstone-susceptible mice. **a** Nonbirefringent amorphous mucin gel; **b** Small nonbirefringent liquid crystals; **c** Aggregated nonbirefringent liquid crystals; **d** Fused liquid crystals with Maltese-cross birefringence and focal conic textures; **e** Arc-like (possibly anhydrous cholesterol) crystals; **f** Filamentous crystals; **g** Tubular crystal with fractured extremity to produce plate-like cholesterol monohydrate crystals with notched corners; **h** Typical ChM crystal, with 79.2° and 100.8° angles; **i** Agglomerated cholesterol monohydrate crystals; **j, k** Disintegratable amorphous sandy stones surrounded by mucin gel, with individual cholesterol monohydrate crystals projecting from the edges; **l** Gallstones exhibiting rounded contours and black centers from light scattering/absorption. **a–i** ×1600; **j** ×800; **k, l** ×400, by polarizing light microscopy. Adapted from [82]

bile salt pool; (3) low bile salt-to-lecithin ratios; (4) low cholesterol-to-lecithin ratios in vesicles; and (5) low total calcium ions. The converse of these conditions accelerates nucleation/crystallization. Apart from mucin glycoproteins, the true identity, their quantitative importance, and in vivo roles of putative pro- and anti-nucleating proteins in human biles are much less certain. Mucin glycoproteins are secreted continuously by gallbladders and in great excess during cholesterol lithogenesis . The term 'pro-nucleating factor' has been used to describe a factor that promotes the precipitation of cholesterol crystals from bile and shortens the nucleation time [80, 88, 89]. An 'anti-nucleating factor' has the opposite effect and retards nucleation, increasing the nucleation time. Pro-nucleating and anti-nucleating factors may influence one or several different level of nucleation, in the process of starting the nucleus with cholesterol molecules in bile [90], at the intermediate steps of lipid transfer and vesicle disruption or fusion, and finally the appearance of microscopically detectable cholesterol monohydrate crystals.

Pro-nucleating and Anti-nucleating Factors

Bile may contain both accelerators and inhibitors of crystallization, and the balance between them is essential to determine the physical state of cholesterol in bile. In fact, biles from patients with gallstones display more rapid cholesterol crystallization than those from gallstone-free subjects. This suggests that lithogenic bile may contain components (i.e., pro-nucleating agents) that accelerate crystallization, while normal biles may contain components (i.e., anti-nucleating agents) that inhibit crystallization [75].

Initially, these components were thought to be only biliary proteins. Mucin was the first biliary protein proved to induce rapid crystallization, thereby promoting cholesterol gallstone formation [91]. Mucin or mucin glycoproteins are large molecules consisting of a protein core and many carbohydrate side chains. An important property of mucin is its ability to form a gel phase with higher concentrations; the viscosity of the gel is far higher than that of the sol phase. The epithelial cells of the gallbladder mucosa secrete mucin that normally serves as a protective layer over the mucosa and is considered as a part of the unstirred water layer. Gallbladder mucins, a heterogeneous family of *O*-linked glycoproteins, are divided into two classes: epithelial and gel-forming mucins. It has been proposed that the epithelial mucins produced by mucin genes 1 (*Muc1*), 3 (*Muc3*), and 4 (*Muc4*) do not seem to form aggregates and are integral membrane glycoproteins located on the apical surface of epithelial cells. The gel-forming mucins, *Muc2*, *Muc5ac*, and *Muc5b*, secreted by specialized gallbladder mucin-producing cells provide a protective coating to the underlying mucosa. They form disulfide-stabilized oligo- or polymers, a phenomenon that accounts for their viscoelastic properties. Mucins produced from different organs vary in carbohydrate side chain and protein composition and charge, but generally have similar properties. Mucins have hydrophilic domains to bind water molecules. Mucins have an overall charge and are capable of binding other charged species, such as calcium. Hydrophobic domains of mucin molecule (on the nonglycosylated regions of the polypeptide core) allow binding of lipids such as cholesterol, phospholipids, and bilirubin. Accumulated evidence suggests that gallbladder mucins have an important role in the early stages of cholesterol gallstone formation and are a potent pro-nucleating/crystallizing agent accelerating cholesterol crystallization in native and model biles [76, 91–94]. Indeed, hypersecretion of gallbladder mucins is essential for gallstone formation, and increased amounts of gallbladder mucins are consistently observed in the gallbladder bile in several animal models of gallstones [82, 91]. In addition, mucins are found inside cholesterol gallstones, where they act as a matrix for stone growth, and are a major component of sludge in the gallbladder, and it has been suggested that sludge is a precursor of gallstones [95, 96]. Therefore, two roles in the formation of gallstones have been proposed for mucins: (1) as a pro-nucleating/crystallizing agent for the nucleation/crystallization of cholesterol from saturated bile, and (2) as a scaffolding for the deposition of crystals during growth of stones. The synthesis of mucous glycoproteins secreted by the epithelium of the gallbladder and biliary ducts could be regulated by mucosal prostaglandins that are derived from arachidonic acid-containing biliary phospholipids [97]. It has been proposed that during the formation of gallstones the gallbladder hypersecretes mucins, perhaps stimulated by some component of saturated bile. Then, the carbohydrate groups of the polymers of mucins avidly bind water to form gels. Moreover, the hydrophobic polypeptides in the core of mucous glycoproteins can bind bilirubin and calcium in bile. The resulting water-insoluble complex of mucous glycoproteins and calcium bilirubinate provides a surface for nucleation of cholesterol monohydrate crystals and a framework of matrix for the growth of stones.

Although mucin secretion and accumulation in the gallbladder is determined by multiple mucin genes, it is interesting to explore how individual mucin genes contribute to cholesterol gallstone formation and whether the epithelial mucins influence susceptibility to cholesterol gallstone formation. More recently, it has been found that reduced MUC1 mucin in the gallbladders of mice with a disrupted *Muc1* gene could decrease susceptibility to cholesterol gallstone formation [98]. Also, gene expression of the gallbladder *Muc5ac*, a gel-forming mucin gene, is significantly reduced in *Muc1* knockout mice in response to the lithogenic diet. As a result, cholesterol crystallization and the development of gallstone formation are significantly retarded. This suggests that there may be gene–gene interactions between the *Muc1* and *Muc5ac*, which might affect mucin secretion and its accumulation in the gallbladder. A recent study by QTL mapping in a backcross between SWR/J and AKR/J strains shows that polymorphisms in the *Muc3* gene or its promoter may be linked to gallbladder accumulation of mucin gel and affect cholesterol gallstone formation [99]. Furthermore, increased gallbladder epithelial MUC1 mucin enhances cholelithogenesis mostly by promoting gallbladder cholesterol absorption and impairing gallbladder motility in mice transgenic for the human *MUC1* gene, a lithogenic mechanism that is completely different from the gel-forming mucins [83]. Therefore, these findings support the concept that inhibiting the secretion and accumulation of not only the gel-forming mucins but also the epithelial mucins in the gallbladder may completely prevent the formation of cholesterol gallstones. Taken together, studying *Muc1* knockout and *MUC1* transgenic mice opens avenues to explore whether the epithelial mucins contribute to cholesterol cholelithogenesis and constitutes the basic framework for investigating how other individual mucin genes influence the various cholesterol gallstone phenotypes [83, 98].

Besides mucins, glycoproteins able to bind reversibly concanavalin A-Sepharose have been found to speed up cholesterol crystallization [100]; these include: aminopeptidase N, immunoglobulins, alpha1 acid glycoprotein, phospholipase C, fibronecitin, and haptoglobin. Other pro-nucleating agents include the amphipathic anionic polypeptide fraction/calcium-binding protein, albumin–lipid complexes, and group II phospholipase A_2.

Nonprotein components of bile also expedite cholesterol crystallization. Calcium bound to micelles and vesicles in bile may accelerate cholesterol crystallization by promoting fusion of cholesterol-rich vesicles. The precipitation of calcium salts in biles may lead to rapid crystallization of cholesterol, an effect that is enhanced by the presence of mucins. Rapidity of cholesterol crystal formation also varies in proportion to the deoxycholate content of bile [67, 101]. This effect probably contributes to the influence of this hydrophobic bile salt on the equilibrium phase relationships of biliary lipids. The degree of cholesterol supersaturation of bile may also be a determinant of rapid crystallization of cholesterol [76, 102].

In contrast, identified inhibitors of cholesterol crystallization include apolipoprotein AI, apolipoprotein AII, secretory immunoglobulin A, the hydrophilic bile acid ursodeoxycholic acid (UDCA) [103–105]. Apolipoproteins A-I and A-II have been identified in a sample of human bile that inhibited cholesterol nucleation and later proved to prolong the nucleation time of supersaturated model bile [104]. Since UDCA prolongs the nucleation time in patients with cholesterol gallstones, UDCA has been proposed as anti-nucleating factor [67, 106–108]. UDCA may hinder cholesterol nucleation by increasing vesicle stability. Lastly, a potential anti-nucleating factor has been identified in a slightly acidic glycoprotein with an apparent molecular size of 120 kDa, which has been detected by lectin affinity chromatography and high pressure liquid chromatography (HPLC) ion exchange chromatography. This protein may inhibit crystal growth by attaching to the most rapidly growing microdomains on a crystal face and interfering with further solute attachment. Video-enhanced microscopy studies have suggested that spiral and edge dislocations on cholesterol monohydrate crystals represent areas of rapid growth. Nevertheless, although it is not known whether only one or several anti-nucleating factors exist and how they may inhibit the initiation of cholesterol crystal formation, it has been proposed that unilamellar vesicles may be the key site of action, and further studies are requested. Although evidence supports the significance of various pro- and anti-nucleating proteins for gallstone formation, some of their effects are either nonspecific or unphysiological.

Role of Gallbladder Motility

Under physiological conditions, gallbladder contractions normally occur during both the interprandial and the postprandial periods [109]. In the interprandial period about 25–30 mL (normal fasting volume in lean adults) of bile are stored in the gallbladder [110], which empties out a variable volume of bile following a meal, depending on neurohormonal mechanisms and the meal's composition. Meal-induced cholecystokinin (CCK) release from the duodenum is the principal factor driving gallbladder smooth muscle contraction, accounting for a 70–80% decrease in gallbladder volume from the fasting state. The suppression of postprandial CCK release by somatostatin in acromegalic patients significantly increases the risk of cholesterol gallstone formation by way of a marked decrement in gallbladder contractility [111]. Furthermore, a genetic deletion of the CCK-1 receptor gene in the mouse induces gallbladder stasis, increasing the risk of gallstone formation [112]. In humans at risk of gallstone formation secondary to gallbladder stasis, daily CCK injection during total parenteral nutrition [113] or inclusion of dietary fat to enhance CCK release during rapid weight loss restore gallbladder contractility and may prevent gallstones [114]. The normal pattern of gallbladder motility is frequently altered in subjects with cholesterol gallstones, who show a larger fasting gallbladder volume and incomplete and delayed postprandial gallbladder emptying regardless of gallstone volume [109, 110, 115]. The pattern of gallbladder emptying can be assessed by functional ultrasonography, as shown in Figs. 3.6 [116–118] and 3.7 [110, 116, 117, 119–129]. The gallbladder dysmotility is mainly associated with cholesterol gallstone formation although, to a minor extent (absence of increased fasting gallbladder volume), it has also been described in patients with pigment stones [126]. A subgroup of cholesterol gallstone patients exhibits severely decreased or even absent postprandial gallbladder emptying ("bad contractors"), while gallstone patients with relatively preserved gallbladder emptying ("good contractors") mostly have larger fasting and residual gallbladder volumes than controls [110, 130]. The altered gallbladder motility in gallstone patients does not seem to be linked to the degree of gallbladder wall inflammation, which is usually mild [110]. However, debate continues on whether gallbladder dysmotility is a primary factor in cholesterol gallstone disease or is secondary to inflammation [110, 131]. In gallstone patients, defective postprandial motility is paralleled by defective gallbladder refilling, with lithogenic bile delivered directly from the liver to the small intestine and consequent alterations of the enterohepatic circulation and of the bile salt pool (increased bile salt hydrophobicity). Impaired interprandial motility might thus play a role in cholesterol gallstone pathogenesis [109]. Normally, a 20–30% decrease of gallbladder volume occurs in the fasting state, just before phase III (i.e., intense, regular coordinated contractions) of the intestinal migrating motor complex (MMC), associated

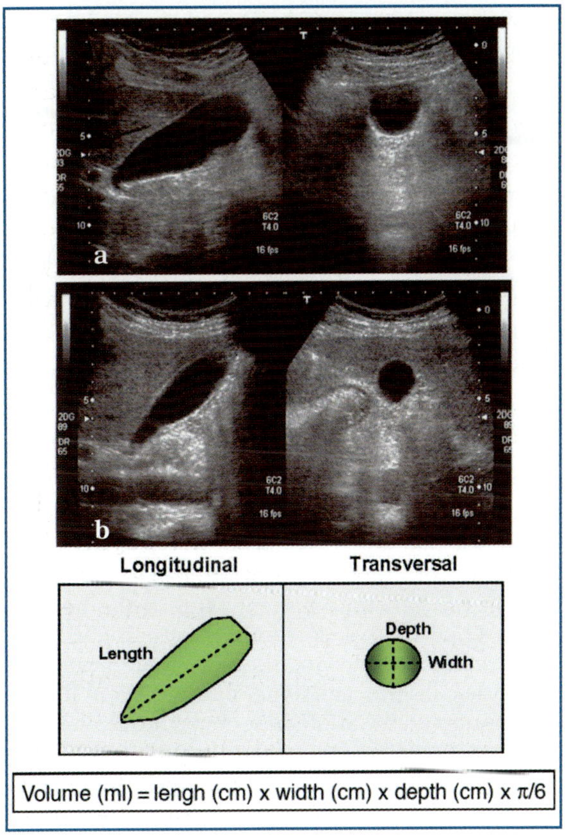

Fig. 3.6 Ultrasound scan of the gallbladder of a healthy subject. The gallbladder image is taken **a** in the fasting state and **b** after ingestion of the standard test meal (see Fig. 3.7 for details). Oblique and sagittal scans are obtained in the right hypochondrium employing a 3.5 MHz probe. The gallbladder content is anechoic and appears as a pear-shaped image (*left panel*) on the longitudinal scan and as a circular image (*right panel*) on the transverse scan. The drawings at the bottom indicate the mathematical algorithm used for the measurement of gallbladder volume according to the ellipsoid formula [116–118]. In this case fasting gallbladder volume was 25.9 mL and postprandial volume was 14.7 mL after 20 min of test meal ingestion

with a rise in plasma motilin concentrations [132-133]. Gallstone patients have less frequent MMC cycles, absent fasting gallbladder emptying, and an abnormal pattern of motilin release compared with controls [134]. Indeed, more frequent food consumption and avoidance of long fasting periods appears to protect against gallstones [9]. The impairment of the gallbladder motor function antedates the appearance of gallstones (as demonstrated in animal models) and has been described in clinical conditions associated with an elevated risk of cholesterol gallstone formation, such as pregnancy, obesity and rapid weight loss in obese patients, diabetes mellitus, and total parenteral nutrition [109, 135]. Furthermore, impaired gallbladder motility persists even after gallstones have disappeared following successful extracorporeal shockwave lithotripsy and oral bile acid dissolution therapy [122, 136].

The concentration of biliary cholesterol is directly related to the degree of gallbladder motility impairment both in gallstone patients and in healthy subjects without gallstones, since cholesterol molecules act as myotoxic agents on the gallbladder smooth muscle. As demonstrated in animals, the direct effect of cholesterol on plasma membranes may cause diminished relaxation of the gallbladder, which is associated with cholesterol gallstone disease [137]. Comparative in vitro studies on gallbladders from cholesterol gallstone patients and controls show that excess accumulation of cholesterol from supersaturated bile in the membranes of gallbladder smooth muscle cells induces a number of alterations in CCK receptors, impaired signal transduction, and reduced contractility of the isolated gallbladder smooth muscle in response to several agonists [109]. Interestingly, it seems these defects can be reversed [138] in an early stage of the disease; this seems to be possible at least until a chronic or an acute-on-chronic gallbladder wall inflammation occurs.

On the other hand, the intracellular mechanisms of muscular contraction seem to be preserved in gallbladders taken from cholesterol gallstone patients. The increased cholesterol absorption from the gallbladder lumen may induce stiffening of sarcoplasma membranes, with a lack of G-protein activation following CCK binding to smooth muscle cell receptors and impairment of gallbladder motor function [139-142].

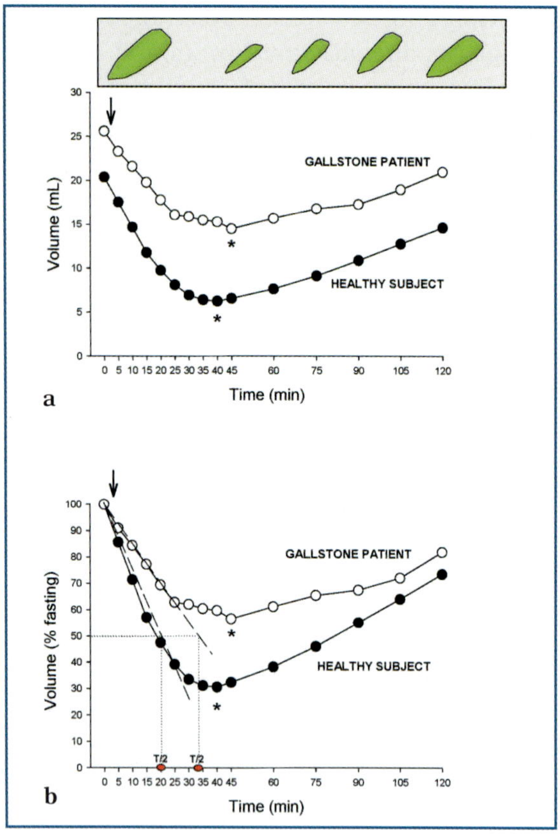

Fig. 3.7 Time-dependent changes in gallbladder volume assessed by real-time "functional" ultrasonography for the study of gallbladder motility function. Curves are obtained with the methodology previously described by our group [110, 116, 117, 119–129]. Overall, indices of gallbladder motility are as follows: fasting volume (mL; mean of 3 measurements at –15, –5 and 0 min before test meal); residual volume (mL and % of fasting volume; minimal volume measured postprandially); $T_{/2}$ (time to achieve decrease by 50% of fasting volume). **a** Gallbladder emptying curves shown as changes in gallbladder volumes (mL). The test meal is 200 mL of a solution of 13 g (39%) fat, 10 g (13%) protein, and 35 g (48%) carbohydrates, for a total of 300 kcal, 1,270 kJ, 365 mosmol/L (*Nutridrink*®, Nutricia, Milan, Italy). The emptying pattern is shown in a healthy subject and in a patient with cholesterol gallstones (in this case one solitary stone with largest diameter of 8 mm). Note that fasting gallbladder volume is larger in the gallstone patient than in the healthy subject (25.6 mL vs 20.4 mL). Postprandial gallbladder volumes following the test meal (*arrow*) are also larger in the gallstone patient than in the healthy subject. **b** Gallbladder emptying curves normalized to the fasting volume (taken as 100%). Note the tri-exponential shape of the emptying curve (meaning rapid emptying, slow emptying, and refilling). An important marker of gallbladder emptying is the half-emptying time ($T_{/2}$), as calculated by regression analysis across points of the rapid emptying. A *horizontal line* is drawn at 50% of gallbladder volume and then interpolated with the regression line and the *x*-axis (time, min). In this case, the half-emptying times are 20 min and 34 min in the healthy subject and the gallstone patient, respectively, meaning that emptying is slightly delayed in the patient. Residual gallbladder volume is indicated by * and is 6.3 mL (30.7%) in the healthy subject and 14.5 mL (56.6%) in the gallstone patient, meaning postprandial gallbladder stasis in the patient

Subsequently, the gallbladder hypomotility provides sufficient time for the nucleation of cholesterol crystals and growth of gallstones in the gallbladder lumen within the mucin gel, which in turn might further worsen motor function by a possible mechanical obstruction of the cystic duct [129, 143].

Role of Gallbladder Concentrating Function

The gallbladder concentrating function may enhance the aggregation of cholesterol crystals [144] and thus be a main contributory factor for cholesterol gallstone formation [67, 144]. Furthermore, the physiological competence of gallbladder in bile acidification seems to be preserved in gallstone patients [145], and this property might induce increased biliary solubility of calcium bilirubinate and calcium carbonate, which in turn may promote nucleation/crystallization of cholesterol molecules. Unlike gallbladder motor function, the gallbladder-concentrating function is preserved in gallstone disease, thus inducing an increment in total lipid concentration that has an effect on the equilibrium phase diagram of the biliary lipids (left shift of all phase boundaries in more diluted biles) [67]. However, a decrement of the gallbladder-concentrating function might be secondary to a reduced expression of some aquaporins (AQP1 and AQP8), since a reduced expression of these water channels could influence gallbladder water transport and, consequently, cholesterol crystallization and gallstone formation in an animal model [146]

In normal subjects, the gallbladder epithelium is able to absorb cholesterol, phospholipids and bile salts in different ways in order to reduce the cholesterol saturation of bile. This is not the case in patients with cholesterol stones, in whom this capacity of selective absorption of cholesterol and phospholipids is lost, with consequent supersaturation of cholesterol in bile during storage [147, 148]. The absorption of cholesterol in the gallbladder wall resembles the events occurring in arterial vessels during atherosclerotic plaque formation. The prolonged exposure of the gallbladder mucosa to a bile supersaturated with cholesterol probably induces continuous absorption of cholesterol by the gallbladder wall [149], allowing unesterified cholesterol molecules to diffuse rapidly towards the muscularis propria. The back-diffusion of unesterified cholesterol molecules into bile is blocked by biliary supersaturation in cholesterol, and, in a lithogenic state, gallbladder mucosal ACAT is able to esterify most, but not all, cholesterol molecules. As a consequence, rather like the atherosclerotic plaque, mucosal and muscle membranes of the gallbladder become markedly saturated with cholesterol and co-exist with stored cholesteryl ester droplets.

The excess absorption of cholesterol molecules from supersaturated, lithogenic bile directly induces proliferative and inflammatory modification in the mucosa and lamina propria of the gallbladder wall, as demonstrated after 2 weeks in prairie dogs fed a 1–2% cholesterol diet [150]. The altered gallbladder absorption function is characterized in vitro in both humans and animal models (cholesterol-fed prairie dogs) by a significant increase in the normal ratio of cholesterol to phospholipid in sarcolemmae. Interestingly, it is possible to restore this level by incubating isolated gallbladder muscle cells with cholesterol-free liposomes [137]. Thus, it is conceivable that unesterified cholesterol molecules become intercalated within the membrane bilayer of muscle cells, which may alter the physical state of phospholipid molecules as reflected by their increased rigidity. As a consequence, this alteration may improve the signal transduction pathway and, therefore, gallbladder motor function.

Role of Intestinal Factors

Recent animal studies suggest that high dietary cholesterol and high efficiency of intestinal cholesterol absorption are independent risk factors for cholesterol gallstone formation [13]. In inbred mice there is a positive correlation between high efficiency of intestinal cholesterol absorption and prevalence of cholesterol gallstones, and gallstone-susceptible C57L mice display higher intestinal cholesterol absorption efficiency than do resistant AKR mice. Furthermore, C57L and AKR mice show a differential metabolism of chylomicron remnant cholesterol that could be used for lithogenic bile formation, because an important resource for biliary cholesterol hypersecretion in mice fed with a lithogenic diet is represented by the cholesterol molecules absorbed from the small intestine [141]. Delayed or impaired intestinal motility might be important in cholesterol gallstone pathogenesis, since it is linked to enhanced intestinal cholesterol absorption, biliary cholesterol secretion, and gallstone prevalence [13].

Impaired intestinal motility and increased deoxycholate seem to be associated with the formation of lithogenic bile in human [151] and in laboratory animal [152, 153] studies. Prolonged large intestinal transit causes a modification of biliary bile salt species by increasing the rate of deoxycholic acid formation. Interestingly, a subgroup of patients with cholesterol gallstones shows both impaired large intestinal motility and increased biliary deoxycholate levels [154-155]. Furthermore, high levels of biliary deoxycholate associated with cholesterol supersaturation in bile and gallstone formation have been found in gallstone-susceptible mice relative to gallstone-resistant mice [13]. Acromegalic patients treated with octreotide (a cholesterol gallstone-inducing agent) also show prolonged large intestine transit times, high levels of deoxycholate in the bile and biliary cholesterol precipitation [156].

Moreover, cecal levels of biliary deoxycholate are higher in cholesterol gallstone patients than in controls, which is associated with increased amounts of Gram-positive anaerobic bacteria and increased activity of 7α-dehydroxylase [157]. Furthermore, an antibiotic treatment that can reduce fecal 7α-dehydroxylation activity also lowers biliary deoxycholate and cholesterol concentrations [158]. An altered enterohepatic circulation of bile salts might also be taken into account in patients with Crohn's disease or in those who have undergone bowel resection or total colectomy. These subgroups of patients usually present a cholesterol-supersaturated bile potentially leading to cholesterol gallstone formation [159], owing to a marked reduction of biliary bile salt secretion and, consequently, to lower cholesterol solubilization in bile. In addition, Crohn's disease induces impaired enterohepatic cycling of bilirubin, increased biliary bilirubin levels, and precipitation of calcium bilirubinate, thus providing a nidus capable of promoting cholesterol nucleation/crystallization in these patients [160].

Animal and human studies have also suggested that a chronic intestinal infection might be considered a potential risk factor in cholesterol gallstone formation. In mouse, distal intestinal infection with various enterohepatic *Helicobacter* species (but not *Helicobacter pylori* [161]) is associated with biliary supersaturation in cholesterol and cholesterol nucleation/crystallization [162]. Interestingly, these *Helicobacter* species have also been identified in the bile and gallbladder tissue from Chilean patients with chronic cholecystitis [163].

Role of the Bile Salt Nuclear Receptor Farnesoid X Receptor

Transcriptional regulation of the biliary secretory network has recently been identified as a central pathophysiologic condition for cholesterol gallstone disease. In detail, it has been proved that the bile salt nuclear receptor FXR is fundamental for correct bile flux and protection against stone formation; LXR, in contrast, enhances the risk of cholelithiasis.

The FXR knockout mice display increased stone formation: after 1 week of an experimental lithogenic diet, cholesterol gallstones occur in FXR knockout mice, but not in wild-type mice. The gallstone phenotype is caused by impaired biliary bile salt and phospholipid secretion associated with decreased expression of ABCB11 and ABCB4, respectively. In parallel, when mice that are genetically susceptible to gallstone formation are treated with synthetic FXR ligands, both cholesterol precipitation and gallstone formation are prevented. The molecular basis for both *loss* and *gain* of functional models, with detrimental and protective effect, respectively, is due to changes in expression levels of biliary transporters; increased expression of ABCB11 and ABCB4 results in the protection against cholelithiasis offered by FXR synthetic agonists [164].

Conversely, owing to increased expression of the cholesterol transporters ABCG5/G8, LXR increases the risk of gallstone formation. In fact, activation of LXR by synthetic ligands results in stone formation even in gallstone-resistant mice, because of ABCG5/G8-dependent increased biliary cholesterol efflux [165]. Although the translational value of these findings has not yet been elucidated, pharmacological manipulation of nuclear receptor activity by synthetic agonists is the most promising therapeutic approach for cholesterol gallstone disease.

Conclusion and Future Perspectives

From the clinical and epidemiological points of view, cholesterol cholelithiasis is a prevalent and costly disease, and the risk of getting it increases with age, obesity, type 2 diabetes, dyslipidemia, hyperinsulinemia, and sedentary lifestyle. All these conditions are also present in the metabolic syndrome, of which cholesterol gallstone disease might be considered, to date, another clinical complication [1, 12, 160]. Cholesterol gallstones derive from the concurrent existence of at least four key factors: biliary supersaturation in cholesterol, accelerated nucleation/crystallization of cholesterol, impaired gallbladder motility, and increased cholesterol availability from the intestine. The development from crystals to gallstones passes from a hypersecretion of mucin by the gallbladder, with gel formation and incomplete gallbladder evacuation, and mechanical factors are also involved. Genetic factors are also conceivable in the light of the epidemiological findings (incidence rates among geographically and ethnically diverse populations, family and twin studies) and results in animal models of inbred mice, which represent a dominant method for the genetic analysis of cholesterol gallstone disease. Several studies have identified some inbred strains of mice susceptible to the formation of gallstones when fed with a lithogenic diet, and other strains resistant to gallstone formation. This gallstone susceptibility in mice, as identified by QTL analysis, has been linked to 25 *Lith* loci on mouse chromosomes so far, and a 'gallstone map' of all known genetic loci determining gallstone susceptibility has lately been drawn for inbred mice. Molecular genetics of cholesterol gallstones in mice will facilitate the identification and positional cloning of *Lith* genes in humans by allowing rapid improvement of techniques for genetic analysis, especially when the nucleotide sequence of the human genome will be available in the near future.

Acknowledgments The authors' experimental work related to the topic of gallstones is supported in part by research grants "Progetti Ateneo 2005-2007" (P.P. and A.M.) from the University of Bari, "COFIN 2005-6" (P.P.), "COFIN 2006-8" (P.P.) by the Ministero Italiano dell'Università e della Ricerca, and DK54012 (D.Q.-H.W.) from the National Institutes of Health (US Public Health Service). P.P. was a recipient of the Short-term Mobility Grant 2005 (Italian National Research Council, CNR) between the University of Bari Medical School and the Harvard Medical School. We thank Paola De Benedictis and Samantha Altini for skillful technical assistance.

References

1. Portincasa P, Moschetta A, Palasciano G (2006) Cholesterol gallstone disease. Lancet 368:230-239
2. Wang DQH, Afdhal NH (2004) Genetic analysis of cholesterol gallstone formation: searching for Lith (gallstone) genes. Curr Gastroenterol Rep 6:140-150
3. Everhart JE, Khare M, Hill M et al (1999) Prevalence and ethnic differences in gallbladder disease in the United States. Gastroenterology 117:632-639
4. Sandler RS, Everhart JE, Donowitz M et al (2002) The burden of selected digestive diseases in the United States. Gastroenterology 122:1500-1511
5. National Institutes of Health (1993) Consensus Development Conference Statement on Gallstones and Laparoscopic Cholecystectomy. Am J Surg 165:390-398
6. Attili AF, De Santis A, Capri R et al (1995) The natural history of gallstones: the GREPCO experience. Hepatology 21:656-660
7. Attili AF, Carulli N, Roda E et al (1995) Epidemiology of gallstone disease in Italy: prevalence da-

ta of the Multicenter Italian Study on Cholelithiasis (M.I.C.O.L.). Am J Epidemiol 141:158-165
8. Attili AF, Capocaccia R, Carulli N et al (1997) Factors associated with gallstone disease in the MICOL experience. Hepatology 26:809-818
9. Attili AF, Scafato E, Marchioli R et al (1998) Diet and gallstones in Italy: the cross-sectional MICOL results. Hepatology 27:1492-1498
10. Festi D, Sottili S, Colecchia A et al (1999) Clinical manifestations of gallstone disease: evidence from the multicenter Italian study on cholelithiasis (MICOL). Hepatology 30:839-846
11. Diehl AK (1991) Epidemiology and natural history of gallstone disease. Gastroenterol Clin North Am 20:1-19
12. Grundy SM (2004) Cholesterol gallstones: a fellow traveler with metabolic syndrome? Am J Clin Nutr 80:1-2
13. Wang DQH, Zhang L, Wang HH (2005) High cholesterol absorption efficiency and rapid biliary secretion of chylomicron remnant cholesterol enhance cholelithogenesis in gallstone-susceptible mice. Biochim Biophys Acta 1733:90-99
14. Lammert F, Sauerbruch T (2005) Mechanisms of disease: the genetic epidemiology of gallbladder stones. Nat Clin Pract Gastroenterol Hepatol 2:423-433
15. Sherlock S, Dooley J (2002) Diseases of the liver and biliary system. Blackwell Science, Oxford
16. Portincasa P, Moschetta A, Mazzone A et al (2003) Water handling and aquaporins in bile formation: recent advances and research trends. J Hepatol 39:864-874
17. Groen AK, Bloks VW, Bandsma RH et al (2001) Hepatobiliary cholesterol transport is not impaired in Abca1-null mice lacking HDL. J Clin Invest 108:843-850
18. Grunhage F, Lammert F (2006) Gallstone disease. Pathogenesis of gallstones: a genetic perspective. Best Pract Res Clin Gastroenterol 20:997-1015
19. Berge KE, Tian H, Graf GA et al (2000) Accumulation of dietary cholesterol in cytosterolemia caused by mutations in adjacent ABC transporters. Science 290:1771-1775
20. Lee MH, Lu K, Hazard S et al (2001) Identification of a gene, ABCG5, important in the regulation of dietary cholesterol absorption. Nat Genet 27:79-83
21. Smit JJM, Schinkel AH, Oude Elferink RPJ et al (1993) Homozygous disruption of the murine mdr2 P-glycoprotein gene leads to a complete absence of phospholipid from bile and to liver disease. Cell 75:451-462
22. Bodzioch M, Orso E, Klucken J et al (1999) The gene encoding ATP-binding cassette transporter 1 is mutated in Tangier disease. Nat Genet 22:347-351
23. Rust S, Rosier M, Funke H et al (1999) Tangier disease is caused by mutations in the gene encoding ATP-binding cassette transporter 1. Nat Genet 22:352-355
24. Brooks-Wilson A, Marcil M, Clee SM et al (1999) Mutations in ABC1 in Tangier disease and familial high-density lipoprotein deficiency. Nat Genet 22:336-345
25. de Vree JM, Jacquemin E, Sturm E et al (1998) Mutations in the MDR3 gene cause progressive familial intrahepatic cholestasis. Proc Natl Acad Sci USA 95:282-287
26. Deleuze JF, Jacquemin E, Dubuisson C et al (1996) Defect of multidrug-resistance 3 gene expression in a subtype of progressive familial intrahepatic cholestasis. Hepatology 23:904-908
27. Dixon PH, Weerasekera N, Linton KJ et al (2000) Heterozygous MDR3 missense mutation associated with intrahepatic cholestasis of pregnancy: evidence for a defect in protein trafficking. Hum Mol Genet 9:1209-1217
28. Strautnieks SS, Bull LN, Knisely AS et al (1998) A gene encoding a liver-specific ABC transporter is mutated in progressive familial intrahepatic cholestasis. Nat Genet 20:233-238
29. Lee MH, Lu K, Hazard S et al (2001) Identification of a gene, ABCG5, important in the regulation of dietary cholesterol absorption. Nat Genet 27:79-83
30. Graf GA, Yu L, Li WP et al (2003) ABCG5 and ABCG8 are obligate heterodimers for protein trafficking and biliary cholesterol excretion. J Biol Chem 278:48275-48282
31. Kosters A, Kunne C, Looije N et al (2006) The mechanism of ABCG5/ABCG8 in biliary cholesterol secretion in mice. J Lipid Res 47:1959-1966
32. Wang HH, Patel SB, Carey MC et al (2007) Quantifying anomalous intestinal sterol uptake, lymphatic transport, and biliary secretion in Abcg8(-/-) mice. Hepatology 45:998-1006
33. Yu L, Li-Hawkins J, Hammer RE et al (2002) Overexpression of ABCG5 and ABCG8 promotes biliary cholesterol secretion and reduces fractional absorption of dietary cholesterol. J Clin Invest 110:671-680
34. Yu L, Hammer RE, Li-Hawkins J et al (2002) Disruption of Abcg5 and Abcg8 in mice reveals their crucial role in biliary cholesterol secretion. Proc Natl Acad Sci USA 99:16237-16242
35. Gerloff T, Stieger B, Hagenbuch B et al (1998) The sister of P-glycoprotein represents the canalicular bile salt export pump of mammalian liver. J Biol Chem 273:10046-10050
36. Wang R, Salem M, Yousef IM et al (2001) Targeted inactivation of sister of P-glycoprotein gene (spgp) in mice results in nonprogressive but persistent intrahepatic cholestasis. Proc Natl Acad Sci USA 98:2011-2016

37. Wang R, Lam P, Liu L et al (2003) Severe cholestasis induced by cholic acid feeding in knockout mice of sister of P-glycoprotein. Hepatology 38:1489-1499
38. de Vree JM, Jacquemin E, Sturm E et al (1998) Mutations in the MDR3 gene cause progressive familial intrahepatic cholestasis. Proc Natl Acad Sci USA 95:282-287
39. van Erpecum KJ, Carey MC (1997) Influence of bile salts on molecular interactions between sphingomyelin and cholesterol: relevance to bile formation and stability. Biochim Biophys Acta 1345:269-282
40. Wang H, Chen J, Hollister K et al (1999) Endogenous bile acids are ligands for the nuclear receptor FXR/BAR. Mol Cell 3:543-553
41. Makishima M, Okamoto AY, Repa JJ et al (1999) Identification of a nuclear receptor for bile acids. Science 284:1362-1365
42. Parks DJ, Blanchard SG, Bledsoe RK et al (1999) Bile acids: natural ligands for an orphan nuclear receptor. Science 284:1365-1368
43. Janowski BA, Willy PJ, Devi TR et al (1996) An oxysterol signalling pathway mediated by the nuclear receptor LXR alpha. Nature 383:728-731
44. Zhang Z, Li D, Blanchard DE et al (2001) Key regulatory oxysterols in liver: analysis as delta4-3-ketone derivatives by HPLC and response to physiological perturbations. J Lipid Res 42:649-658
45. Ananthanarayanan M, Balasubramanian N, Makishima M et al (2001) Human bile salt export pump promoter is transactivated by the farnesoid X receptor/bile acid receptor. J Biol Chem 276:28857-28865
46. Huang L, Zhao A, Lew JL et al (2003) Farnesoid X-receptor activates transcription of the phospholipid pump MDR3. J Biol Chem 278:51085-51090
47. Repa JJ, Berge KE, Pomajzl C et al (2002) Regulation of ATP-binding cassette sterol transporters ABCG5 and ABCG8 by the liver X receptors alpha and beta. J Biol Chem 277:18793-18800
48. Modica S, Moschetta A (2006) Nuclear bile acid receptor FXR as pharmacological target: are we there yet? FEBS Lett 580:5492-5499
49. Willy PJ, Mangelsdorf DJ ()Unique requirements for retinoid-dependent transcriptional activation by the orphan receptor LXR. Genes Dev 11:289-298
50. del Castillo-Olivares A, Gil G (2000) Role of FXR and FTF in bile acid-mediated suppression of cholesterol 7alpha-hydroxylase transcription. Nucl Acids Res 28:3587-3593
51. Lu TT, Makishima M, Repa JJ et al (2000) Molecular basis for feedback regulation of bile acid synthesis by nuclear receptors. Mol Cell 6:507-515
52. Peet DJ, Turley SD, Ma W et al (1998) Cholesterol and bile acid metabolism are impaired in mice lacking the nuclear oxysterol receptor LXR alpha. Cell 93:693-704
53. Carey MC, Small DM (1978) The physical chemistry of cholesterol solubility in bile. Relation to gallstone formation and dissolution in man. J Clin Invest 61:998-1026
54. Holzbach RT, Marsh M, Olszewski M et al (1973) Cholesterol solubility in bile. Evidence that supersaturated bile is frequent in healthy man. J Clin Invest 52:1467-1479
55. Mazer NA, Carey MC, Kwasnick RF et al (1979) Quasielastic light scattering studies of aqueous biliary lipid systems. Size, shape, and thermodynamics of bile salt micelles. Biochemistry 18:3064-3075
56. Mazer NA, Benedek GB, Carey MC (1980) Quasielastic light-scattering studies of aqueous biliary lipid systems. Mixed micelle formation in bile salt-lecithin solutions. Biochemistry 19:601-615
57. Mazer NA, Carey MC (1983) Quasi-elastic light-scattering studies of aqueous biliary lipid systems. Cholesterol solubilization and precipitation in model bile solutions. Biochemistry 22:426-442
58. Mazer NA, Schurtenberg P, Carey MC et al (1984) Quasi-elastic light scattering studies of native hepatic bile from the dog: comparison with aggregative behavior of model biliary lipid systems. Biochemistry 23:1994-2005
59. Somjen GJ, Gilat T (1983)A non-micellar mode of cholesterol transport in human bile. FEBS Lett 156:265-268
60. Somjen GJ, Gilat T (1985) Contribution of vesicular and micellar carriers to cholesterol transport in human bile. J Lipid Res 26:699-704
61. Somjen GJ, Marikovsky Y, Lelkes P et al (1986) Cholesterol-phospholipid vesicles in human bile: an ultrastructural study. Biochim Biophys Acta 879:14-21
62. Halpern Z, Dudley MA, Kibe A et al (1986) Rapid vesicle formation and aggregation in abnormal human biles: a time-lapse video- enhanced contrast microscopy study. Gastroenterology 90:875-885
63. Halpern Z, Dudley MA, Lynn MP et al (1986) Vesicle aggregation in model systems of supersaturated bile: relation to crystal nucleation and lipid composition of the vesicular phase. J Lipid Res 27:295-306
64. Holan KR, Holzbach RT, Hermann RE et al (1979) Nucleation time: a key factor in the pathogenesis of cholesterol gallstone disease. Gastroenterology 77:611-617
65. Holzbach RT, Corbusier C (1978) Liquid crystals and cholesterol nucleation during equilibration

in supersaturated bile analogs. Biochim Biophys Acta 528:436-444
66. Olszewski MF, Holzbach RT, Saupe A et al (1973) Liquid crystals in human bile. Nature 242:336-337
67. Wang DQH, Carey MC (1996) Complete mapping of crystallization pathways during cholesterol precipitation from model bile: influence of physical-chemical variables of pathophysiologic relevance and identification of a stable liquid crystalline state in cold, dilute and hydrophilic bile salt-containing system. J Lipid Res 37:606-630
68. Admirand WH, Small DM (1968) The physicochemical basis of cholesterol gallstone formation in man. J Clin Invest 47:1043-1052
69. Wang DQH, Carey MC (1996) Characterization of crystallization pathways during cholesterol precipitation from human gallbladder biles: identical pathways to corresponding model biles with three predominating sequences. J Lipid Res 37:2539-2549
70. Small DM, Bourges M, Dervichian DG (1966) Ternary and quaternary aqueous systems containing bile salt, lecithin, and cholesterol. Nature 211:816-818
71. Small DM, Bourges MC, Dervichian DG (1966) The biophysics of lipidic associations. I. The ternary systems: lecithin-bile salt-water. Biochim Biophys Acta 125:563-580
72. Small DM (1968) A classification of biologic lipids based upon their interaction in aqueous systems. J Am Oil Chem Soc 45:108-119
73. Small DM, Admirand W (1969) Solubility of bile salts. Nature 221:265-267
74. Hofmann AF, Amelsberg A, Vansonnenberg E (1993) Pathogenesis and treatment of gallstones. N Engl J Med 328:1854-1855
75. LaMont JT, Carey MC (1992) Cholesterol gallstone formation. 2. Pathobiology and pathomechanics. Prog Liver Dis 10:165-191
76. Wang DQH, Cohen DE, Lammert F et al (1999) No pathophysiologic relationship of soluble biliary proteins to cholesterol crystallization in human bile. J Lipid Res 40:415-425
77. Carey MC (1978) Critical tables for calculating the cholesterol saturation of native bile. J Lipid Res 19:945-955
78. Gollish SH, Burnstein MJ, Ilson RG et al (1983) Nucleation of cholesterol monohydrate crystals from hepatic and gallbladder bile of patients with cholesterol gallstones. Gut 24:836-844
79. Harvey PRC, Sömjen G, Lichtenberg MS et al (1987) Nucleation of cholesterol from vesicles isolated from bile of patients with and without cholesterol gallstones. Biochim Biophys Acta 921:198-204
80. Holzbach RT (1990) Current concepts of cholesterol transport and crystal formation in human bile. Hepatology 12:26S-31S
81. Holzbach RT (1990) Nucleation of cholesterol crystals in native bile. Hepatology 12:155S-161S
82. Wang DQH, Paigen B, Carey MC (1997) Phenotypic characterization of Lith genes that determine susceptibility to cholesterol cholelithiasis in inbred mice: physical-chemistry of gallbladder bile. J Lipid Res 38:1395-1411
83. Wang HH, Afdhal NH, Gendler SJ et al (2006) Evidence that gallbladder epithelial mucin enhances cholesterol cholelithogenesis in MUC1 transgenic mice. Gastroenterology 131:210-222
84. Konikoff FM, Chung DS, Donovan JM et al (1992) Filamentous, helical and tubular microstructures during cholesterol crystallization from bile. Evidence that biliary cholesterol does not nucleate classic monohydrate plates. J Clin Invest 90:1156-1161
85. Konikoff FM, Cohen DE, Carey MC (1994) Phospholipid molecular species influence crystal habits and transition sequences of metastable intermediates during cholesterol crystallization from bile salt-rich model bile. J Lipid Res 35:60-70
86. Konikoff FM, Laufer H, Messer G et al (1997) Monitoring cholesterol crystallization from lithogenic model bile by time-lapse density gradient ultracentrifugation. J Hepatol 26:703-710
87. Lammert F, Wang DQH, Hillebrandt S et al (2004) Spontaneous cholecysto- and hepatolithiasis in Mdr2-/- mice: a model for low phospholipid-associated cholelithiasis. Hepatology 39:117-128
88. Holzbach RT (1995) Cholesterol nucleation in bile. Ital J Gastroenterol Hepatol 27:101-105
89. Holzbach RT (1997) Newer pathogenetic concepts in cholesterol gallstone formation: a unitary hypothesis. Digestion 58 Suppl 1:29-32
90. Busch N, Matiuck N, Sahlin S et al (1991) Inhibition and promotion of cholesterol crystallization by protein factors from normal human gallbladder bile. J Lipid Res 32:695-702
91. Lee SM, LaMont JT, Carey MC (1981) Role of gallbladder mucus hypersecretion in the evolution of cholesterol gallstones. Studies in the prairie dog. J Clin Invest 67:1712-1723
92. Afdhal NH, Gong D, Niu N et al (1993) Cholesterol cholelithiasis in the prairie dog: role of mucin and nonmucin glycoproteins. Hepatology 17:693-700
93. LaMont JT (1982) Gallbladder mucin glycoprotein hypersecretion in experimental cholelithiasis: role of mucin gel in nucleation of cholesterol gallstones. Adv Exp Med Biol 144:231-234
94. Levy PF, Smith BF, LaMont JT (1984) Human gallbladder mucin accelerates nucleation of cholesterol in artificial bile. Gastroenterology 87:270-275
95. Lee SP, Nicholls JF (1986) Nature and composition of biliary sludge. Gastroenterology 90:677-686

96. Lee SP, Maher K, Nicholls JF (1988) Origin and fate of biliary sludge. Gastroenterology 94:170-176.
97. Carey MC, Cahalane MJ (1988) Whither biliary sludge? Gastroenterology 95:508-523
98. Wang HH, Afdhal NH, Gendler SJ et al (2004) Targeted disruption of the murine mucin gene 1 decreases susceptibility to cholesterol gallstone formation. J Lipid Res 45:438-447
99. Wittenburg H, Lammert F, Wang DQH et al (2002) Interacting QTLs for cholesterol gallstones and gallbladder mucin in AKR and SWR strains of mice. Physiol Genomics 8:67-77
100. Groen AK, Noordam C, Drapers JAG et al (1990) Isolation of a potent cholesterol nucleation-promoting activity from human gallbladder bile of patients with solitary or multiple cholesterol gallstones. Hepatology 11:525-533
101. Hussaini SH, Pereira SP, Murphy GM et al (1995) Deoxycholic acid influences cholesterol solubilization and microcrystal nucleation time in gallbladder bile. Hepatology 22:1735-1744
102. Miquel JF, Nunez L, Amigo L et al (1998) Cholesterol saturation, not proteins or cholecystitis, is critical for crystal formation in human gallbladder bile. Gastroenterology 114:1016-1023
103. Holzbach RT, Kibe A, Thiel E et al (1984) Biliary proteins: unique inhibitors of cholesterol crystal nucleation in human gallbladder bile. J Clin Invest 73:35-45
104. Kibe A, Holzbach RT (1984) Inhibition of cholesterol crystal formation by apolipoproteins in supersaturated model bile. Science 255:514-516
105. Secknus R, Darby GH, Chernosky A et al (1999) Apolipoprotein A-I in bile inhibits cholesterol crystallization and modifies transcellular lipid transfer through cultured human gall-bladder epithelial cells. J Gastroenterol Hepatol 14:446-456
106. Stolk MFJ, van de Heijning BJM, van Erpecum KJ et al (1994) The effect of bile acid hydrophobicity on nucleation of several types of cholesterol crystals from model bile vesicles. J Hepatol 20:802-810
107. van de Heijning BJM, Stolk MFJ, van Erpecum KJ et al (1994) The effects of bile salt hydrophobicity on model bile vesicle morphology. Biochim Biophys Acta 1212:203-210
108. van Erpecum KJ, Portincasa P, Stolk MFJ et al (1994) Effects of bile salt and phospholipid hydrophobicity on lithogenicity of human gallbladder bile. Eur J Clin Invest 24:744-750
109. Portincasa P, Di Ciaula A, vanBerge Henegouwen GP (2004) Smooth muscle function and dysfunction in gallbladder disease. Curr Gastroenterol Rep 6:151-162
110. Portincasa P, Di Ciaula A, Baldassarre G et al (1994) Gallbladder motor function in gallstone patients: sonographic and in vitro studies on the role of gallstones, smooth muscle function and gallbladder wall inflammation. J Hepatol 21:430-440
111. Moschetta A, Stolk MF, Rehfeld JF et al (2001) Severe impairment of postprandial cholecystokinin release and gall- bladder emptying and high risk of gallstone formation in acromegalic patients during Sandostatin LAR. Aliment Pharmacol Ther 15:181-185
112. Wang DQH, Schmitz F, Kopin AS et al (2004) Targeted disruption of the murine cholecystokinin-1 receptor promotes intestinal cholesterol absorption and susceptibility to cholesterol cholelithiasis. J Clin Invest 114:521-528
113. Sitzmann JV, Pitt HA, Steinborn PA et al (1990) Cholecystokinin prevents parenteral nutrition induced biliary sludge in humans. Surg Gynecol Obstet 170:25-31
114. Gebhard RL, Prigge WF, Ansel HJ et al (1996) The role of gallbladder emptying in gallstone formation during diet-induced rapid weight loss. Hepatology 24:544-548
115. Colecchia A, Sandri L, Bacchi-Reggiani ML et al (2006) Is it possible to predict the clinical course of gallstone disease? Usefulness of gallbladder motility evaluation in a clinical setting. Am J Gastroenterol 101:2576-2581
116. Portincasa P, Moschetta A, Baldassarre G et al (2003) Pan-enteric dysmotility, impaired quality of life and alexithymia in a large group of patients meeting the Rome II criteria for irritable bowel. World J Gastroenterol 9:2293-2299
117. Portincasa P, Moschetta A, Berardino M et al (2004) Impaired gallbladder motility and delayed orocecal transit contribute to pigment gallstone and biliary sludge formation in beta-thalassemia major adults. World J Gastroenterol 10:2383-2390
118. Portincasa P, Moschetta A, Colecchia A et al (2003) Measurement of gallbladder motor function by ultrasonography: towards standardization. Dig Liver Dis (già Ital J Gastroenterol Hepatol) 35 (Suppl 3):S56-S61
119. Portincasa P, Di Ciaula A, Palmieri VO et al (1994) Sonographic evaluation of gallstone burden in humans. Ital J Gastroenterol Hepatol 26:141-144
120. Portincasa P, Di Ciaula A, Palmieri VO et al (1994) Enhancement of gallbladder emptying in gallstone patients after oral cholestyramine. Am J Gastroenterol 89:909-914
121. Portincasa P, Di Ciaula A, Palmieri VO et al (1995) Effects of cholestyramine on gallbladder and gastric emptying in obese and lean subjects. Eur J Clin Invest 25:746-753
122. Portincasa P, van Erpecum KJ, van de Meeberg PC et al (1996) Apolipoprotein (Apo) E4 genotype and gallbladder motility influence speed of gallstone clearance and risk of recurrence after ex-

tracorporeal shock-wave lithotripsy. Hepatology 24:580-587
123. Portincasa P, Di Ciaula A, Palmieri VO et al (1996) Tauroursodeoxycholic acid, ursodeoxycholic acid and gallbladder motility in gallstone patients and healthy subjects. Ital J Gastroenterol Hepatol 28:111-113
124. Portincasa P, Di Ciaula A, Palmieri VO et al (1997) Impaired gallbladder and gastric motility and pathological gastro-esophageal reflux in gallstone patients. Eur J Clin Invest 8:653-661
125. Portincasa P, Altomare DF, Moschetta A et al (2000) The effect of acute oral erythromycin on gallbladder motility and on upper gastrointestinal symptoms in gastrectomized patients with and without gallstones: a randomized, placebo-controlled ultrasonographic study. Am J Gastroenterol 95:3444-3451
126. Portincasa P, Di Ciaula A, Vendemiale G et al (2000) Gallbladder motility and cholesterol crystallization in bile from patients with pigment and cholesterol gallstones. Eur J Clin Invest 30:317-324
127. Portincasa P, Colecchia A, Di Ciaula A et al (2000) Standards for diagnosis of gastrointestinal motility disorders. Section: ultrasonography. A position statement from the Gruppo Italiano di Studio Motilita Apparato Digerente. Dig Liver Dis 32:160-172
128. Portincasa P, Moschetta A, Di Ciaula A et al (2001) Changes of gallbladder and gastric dynamics in patients with acute hepatitis A. Eur J Clin Invest 31:617-622
129. Stolk MFJ, van Erpecum KJ, Renooij W et al (1995) Gallbladder emptying in vivo, bile composition and nucleation of cholesterol crystals in patients with cholesterol gallstones. Gastroenterology 108:1882-1888
130. van Erpecum KJ, vanBerge-Henegouwen GP, Stolk MFJ et al (1992) Fasting gallbladder volume, postprandial emptying and cholecystokinin release in gallstone patients and normal subjects. J Hepatol 14:194-202
131. Xiao ZL, Amaral J, Biancani P et al (2005) Impaired cytoprotective function of muscle in human gallbladders with cholesterol stones. Am. J Physiol Gastrointest Liver Physiol 288:G525-G532
132. DiMagno EP, Hendricks JC, Go VLW et al (1979) (Relationships among canine fasting pancreatic and biliary secretions, pancreatic duct pressure, and duodenal phase III motor activity - Boldireff revisited. Dig Dis Sci 24:689-693
133. Stolk MFJ, van Erpecum KJ, Smout AJPM et al (1993) Motor cycles with phase III in antrum are associated with high motilin levels and prolonged gallbladder emptying. Am J Physiol 264:G596-G600.
134. Stolk MF, van Erpecum KJ, Peeters TL et al (2001) Interdigestive gallbladder emptying, antroduodenal motility, and motilin release patterns are altered in cholesterol gallstone patients. Dig Dis Sci 46:1328-1334
135. van Erpecum KJ, Venneman NG, Portincasa P et al (2000) Agents affecting gall-bladder motility—role in treatment and prevention of gallstones (review). Aliment Pharmacol Ther 14 Suppl 2:66-70
136. Pauletzki JG, Althaus R, Holl J et al (1996) Gallbladder emptying and gallstone formation: a prospective study on gallstone recurrence. Gastroenterology 111:765-771
137. Yu P, Chen Q, Biancani P et al (1996) Membrane cholesterol alters gallbladder muscle contractility in prairie dogs. Am J Physiol 271:G56-61
138. Xiao ZL, Chen Q, Amaral J et al (1999) CCK receptor dysfunction in muscle membranes from human gallbladders with cholesterol stones. Am J Physiol 276:G1401-G1407
139. Yu P, De Petris G, Biancani P et al (1994) Cholecystokinin-coupled intracellular signaling in human gallbladder muscle. Gastroenterology 106:763-770
140. Yu P, Harnett KM, Biancani P et al (1994) Interaction between signal transduction pathways contributing to gallbladder tonic contraction. Am J Physiol 265:1082-1089
141. Yu P, Chen Q, Harnett KM et al (1995) Direct G protein activation reverses impaired CCK signaling in human gallbladders with cholesterol stones. Am J Physiol 269:G659-665
142. Yu P, Chen Q, Xiao Z et al (1998) Signal transduction pathways mediating CCK-induced gallbladder muscle contraction. Am J Physiol 275:G203-211
143. Portincasa P, Stolk MF, van Erpecum KJ et al (1995) Cholesterol gallstone formation in man and potential treatments of the gallbladder motility defect. Scand J Gastroenterol Suppl 212:63-78
144. van Erpecum KJ, Stolk MFJ, van den Broek AMWC et al (1993) Bile concentration promotes nucleation of cholesterol monohydrate crystals by increasing the cholesterol concentration in the vesicles. Eur J Clin Invest 23:283-288
145. Magnuson TH, Lillemoe KD, Zarkin BA et al (1992) Patients with uncomplicated cholelithiasis acidify bile normally. Dig Dis Sci 37:1517-1522
146. Calamita G, Ferri D, Bazzini C et al (2005) Expression and subcellular localization of the AQP8 and AQP1 water channels in the mouse gall-bladder epithelium. Biol Cell 97:415-423
147. Conter RL, Roslyn JJ, Porter-Fink V et al (1986) Gallbladder absorption increases during early cholesterol gallstone formation. Am J Surg 151:184-192

148. Ginanni Corradini S, Elisei W, Giovannelli L et al (2000) Impaired human gallbladder lipid absorption in cholesterol gallstone disease and its effect on cholesterol solubility in bile. Gastroenterology 118:912-920
149. Einarsson C (1999) Lipid absorption by the human gallbladder. Ital J Gastroenterol Hepatol 31:571-573
150. Booker ML, Scott TE, LaMorte WW (1989) Effect of dietary cholesterol on phosphatidylcholines and phosphatidylethanolamines in bile and gallbladder mucosa in the prairie dog. Gastroenterology 97:1261-1267
151. Heaton KW, Emmett PM, Symes CL et al (1993) An explanation for gallstones in normal-weight women: slow intestinal transit. Lancet 341:8-10
152. van Erpecum KJ, vanBerge-Henegouwen GP (1999) Gallstones: an intestinal disease? Gut 44:435-438
153. van Erpecum KJ, Wang DQH, Lammert F et al (2001) Phenotypic characterization of Lith genes that determine susceptibility to cholesterol cholelithiasis in inbred mice: soluble pronucleating proteins in gallbladder and hepatic biles. J Hepatol 35:444-451
154. Portincasa P, van Erpecum KJ, Jansen A et al (1996) Behavior of various cholesterol crystals in bile from gallstone patients. Hepatology 23:738-748
155. Shoda J, He BF, Tanaka N et al (1995) Increase of deoxycholate in supersaturated bile of patients with cholesterol gallstones disease and its correlation with de novo syntheses of cholesterol and bile acids in liver, gallbladder emptying, and small intestinal transit. Hepatology 21:1291-1302
156. Thomas LA, Veysey MJ, Murphy GM et al (2005) Octreotide induced prolongation of colonic transit increases faecal anaerobic bacteria, bile acid metabolising enzymes, and serum deoxycholic acid in patients with acromegaly. Gut 54:630-635
157. Thomas LA, Veysey MJ, Bathgate T et al (2000) Mechanism for the transit-induced increase in colonic deoxycholic acid formation in cholesterol cholelithiasis. Gastroenterology 119:806-815
158. Berr F, Kullak-Ublick GA, Paumgartner G et al (1996) Alpha-dehydroxylating bacteria enhance deoxycholic acid input and cholesterol saturation of bile in patients with gallstones. Gastroenterology 111:1611-1620
159. Pereira SP, Bain IM, Kumar D et al (2003) Bile composition in inflammatory bowel disease: ileal disease and colectomy, but not colitis, induce lithogenic bile. Aliment Pharmacol Ther 17:923-933
160. Brink MA, Slors JF, Keulemans YC et al (1999) Enterohepatic cycling of bilirubin: a putative mechanism for pigment gallstone formation in ileal Crohn's disease. Gastroenterology 116:1420-1427
161. Maurer KJ, Rogers AB, Ge Z et al (2006) Helicobacter pylori and cholesterol gallstone formation in C57L/J mice: a prospective study. Am J Physiol Gastrointest Liver Physiol 290:G175-G182
162. Maurer KJ, Ihrig MM, Rogers AB et al (2005) Identification of cholelithogenic enterohepatic helicobacter species and their role in murine cholesterol gallstone formation. Gastroenterology 128:1023-1033
163. Fox JC, Dewhirst FE, Shen Z et al (1998) Hepatic Helicobacter species identified in bile and gallbladder tissue from Chileans with chronic cholecystitis. Gastroenterology 114:755-763
164. Moschetta A, Bookout AL, Mangelsdorf DJ (2004) Prevention of cholesterol gallstone disease by FXR agonists in a mouse model. Nat Med 10:1352-1358
165. Wang HH, Wang DQH (2004) Overexpression of liver X receptor a (LXRa) enhance cholesterol (Ch) cholelithogenesis in gallstone-resistant AKR mice (abstract). Gastroenterology 126[4, Suppl. 2]: A15-110

Chapter 4

Classification, Composition and Structure of Gallstones. Relevance of these Parameters for Clinical Presentation and Treatment

Francesco Cetta

Classification of Gallstones and Related Clinicopathological and Epidemiological Implications

Gallstones should no longer be considered as a unique entity, but as a heterogenous disease [1–8], which includes at least three different subgroups: cholesterol stones, mixed stones with cholesterol as the main component (for which cholesterol supersaturation of the bile may be of importance) and pigment stones, which are distinguished as black or brown pigment. Supersaturation of the bile with cholesterol is not of prime importance for the formation of pigment stones. In addition to these three main types of gallstone, there are also combination stones and composite gallstones. The former include stones with a central nidus of one type (cholesterol or black pigment) and an outer portion of another type (brown or calcified periphery); the latter occur when pure cholesterol stones are found within the same gallbladder or bile duct together with pure pigment stones, i.e. there are at least two different stone populations in the same subject (Table 4.1).

In epidemiologic studies, the type of detection method used greatly affects the reported prevalence of the various types of gallstones. In fact, studies based on ultrasound can only detect the simple presence or absence of gallstones, with no distinction between cholesterol, mixed, pigment or composite stones. However, this is the most frequently used method in cross-sectional or longitudinal epidemiologic studies. Surgical (or autoptic) series are the only series that give a precise classification of gallstones. However, surgical series are affected by a selection bias for population studies because they mainly include those patients whose stones give rise to severe symptoms

Table 4.1 Classification of gallstones and their composition according to type of stones (2,000 patients)

		Stone composition				
		Cholesterol	Bilirubinate	Carbonate	Palmitate	Phosphate
Cholesterol unique Combination	25%	>70% nucleus	small amounts periphery	5% periphery	- periphery	- -
Cholesterol multiple Mixed faceted	35%	>70% >60%	small amounts 5-10%	- 5%	- small amounts	- -
Black pigmented	8.5%	-	>70%	>5-10%	-	yes
Brown pigmented	6.5%	<15%	>50%	-	>15%	-
Composite stones	21%	variable	-	-	-	-

or complications. In a recent prospective study initially including 1000 [9] and subsequently 2000 consecutive patients who had surgically removed gallstones, stone analysis was performed systematically by infrared spectroscopy and X-ray diffraction analysis [3-9].

Cholesterol Stones

Cholesterol stones, or mixed stones with cholesterol as the main component, were found in 60% of patients in a recent study [3-9]. Less than 5% of patients had "pure" cholesterol stones, which were usually unique and smaller than 0.8 cm. Twenty-five percent of patients had ovoidal cholesterol stones, while 35% had faceted mixed, spherical or mulberry cholesterol stones. Composite calculi were found in 21% of patients in this surgical series. In particular, there were often intraparietal stones of a different type than those present within the main gallbladder lumen. Black pigment stones occurred in 8.5%, whereas brown pigment stones were found in 6.5% of cases (Table 4.1) [9-14].

A precise classification of gallstones based on the stone type, rather than on the total cholesterol amount that may result in a non-homogenous classification [1], is of paramount importance for clinical, pathologic and epidemiologic studies [15]. Such a classification will also give basic information concerning the causes of a particular type of gallstone, as well as the risk factors and pathogenetic mechanisms that led to the formation of stones, whose treatment would therefore be considered during surgery or endoscopy. It has recently been proposed that gallstone-related symptoms are not simply due to "chance" [16], i.e., jaundice occurs in 20% of patients with gallstones and pancreatitis in 10%, regardless of the type of gallstone [16–21]. On the contrary, symptoms greatly depend on the mutual relationships between the content (the type and number of stones), their size, shape and structure, and their container (gallbladder wall, infundibulum, cystic duct, common duct shape, structure and clearing capacity, diameter of the lower portion of the common duct, variable aspect of the cystic duct and of the confluence between the cystic duct and the common duct, etc.) [16, 22–25].

Therefore, small, "young", gallstones of recent onset cause jaundice and pancreatitis more frequently because they migrate more easily through the cystic duct. However, cystic duct diameter, as well as cystic duct insertion, are also independent causative factors. In fact, an increased incidence of pancreatitis has been observed in patients who have a long and tortuous cystic duct, with a medial and low insertion on the common duct within the pancreas [22]. This particular type of cystic duct insertion can be detected by pre- or intraoperative cholangiography, but it can also be suspected intraoperatively, when a cystic artery branch is found antero-inferior to the cystic duct rather than in Calot's triangle.

Brown Pigment Gallstones

Brown pigment stones are completely different from other stones because they are caused by bile stasis and infection; namely by *Escherichia coli*, which produces enzymes, such as betaglucuronidase and phospholipases [9-12]. These enzymes hydrolyze the normal bile components, causing the precipitation of the typical components of brown stones, i.e., calcium bilirubinate and palmitate, whereas cholesterol, if present, accounts for less than 10% of the stone's dry weight (Table 4.1). Brown stones are a "true" infectious disease (not contagious), which is self-maintaining through the vicious cycle of infection-stasis-infection [9–11, 26–63]. Brown stones rarely occur in the gallbladder, but when they do it is normally in patients older than 70 years of age with bile stasis [9]. Brown stones specifically form in the bile ducts, either in the common duct or within the intrahepatic ducts, and usually form in the bile tract after liver transplantation or primary excision of choledochal cysts [54, 56]. Only 60% of all intrahepatic stones are brown [64–69], whereas almost all gallstones entirely formed in the lower common bile duct (CBD) are brown, along with those stones that form cranially to a stricture in the sphincteric portion of the common bile duct after surgical or endoscopic sphincterotomy [13–14]. The same mechanism that is responsible for brown stone formation (bile stasis plus infection) is likely to be responsible for the obstruction of biliary endoprostheses by brown "mud", which has the same composition as brown stones [70–72].

The presence of bacterial microcolonies is the typical finding in brown pigment gallstones. However, bacteria have also been found, to a lesser extent, in the pigment portions of mixed stones and the pigmented centers of certain predominantly cholesterol stones [61–63, 73–94]. Whereas bacteria, namely *E. coli*, are generally responsible for the formation of brown pigment stones, their possible role in the pathogenesis of other types of gallstones remains to be elucidated.

Most bacteria contained in predominantly cholesterol stones produce slime, but not pigment, suggesting that the underlying mechanism is formation of a biofilm nidus that is subsequently covered by cholesterol precipitation. In addition to slime, biliary bacteria can also produce P1-fimbriae [79–94]. A role for adhesion factors in facilitating bacterial colonization and macroscopic stone formation has been suggested. It has also been suggested, namely in elderly people, that the type of bacteria present has an impact on infectious manifestations [88–91]. In particular, patients with *E. coli* and/or *Klebsiella* species commonly show infectious manifestations, patients with *Enterococcus* less so, and those with other species have few infectious manifestations [79].

Black Pigment Gallstones

Black pigment gallstones form exclusively within the gallbladder [9], whereas brown stones occur specifically in the common duct. Black pigment gallstones are not associated with cholesterol supersaturation of the bile. On the contrary, black stones are frequently found in patients with cirrhosis, congenital hemolytic diseases [9], or after heart surgery [26], even if specific risk factors are not detectable in most of cases. Black stones are small or very small and can be found at surgery either as gallstones within the main gallbladder lumen and/or in the CBD, or as intraparietal microstones. These black microstones initially form within the Rokitansky-Aschoff (R-A) sinuses of the gallbladder, subsequently migrate into the main gallbladder lumen and finally into the common duct, through the cystic duct. They can form not only as unique stones, but also in patients with previous stones of other types, namely single ovoidal cholesterol stones. The presumed pathogenetic mechanism is the following: the large cholesterol stone causes repeated episodes of biliary obstruction at the gallbladder infundibulum, facilitating the occurrence of multiple microdiverticula in the gallbladder wall, analogous to the situation in the urinary bladder after prostatic hypertrophy. In these microdiverticula, which behave as microenviroments with sectorial bile stasis, black microstones specifically form, even in patients with previous cholesterol stones and cholesterol supersaturation of the bile in the main gallbladder lumen. The reason for the preferential precipitation of black pigment within the R-A sinuses is not yet well established [23–25]. Black stones are frequently irregular, with a spicular shape in 40% of cases, because they contain large amounts of calcium carbonate and/or phosphate (Table 4.2). Due to these particular features, they frequently cause pancreatitis. However, they never recur after cholecystectomy, indicating that they only form within the gallbladder. Intraparietal black microstones are easily detectable by ultrasound before surgery because they are responsible for a characteristic feature, the so-called comet-tail artifact [25]. This "new" pathophysiologic association is of basic importance in explaining how a patient with ultrasonographic diagnosis of an apparent single ovoidal cholesterol stone can suffer, during the natural history of his/her disease, from multiple episodes of jaundice and/or pancreatitis. In fact, in these cases, a second stone population has formed. These stones are initially black when they precipitate within the R-A sinuses. After migration into the main gallbladder lumen, they may remain as black stones until surgery or may also act as nuclei for the precipitation of cholesterol crystals, resulting in the formation of mulberry or mixed cholesterol stones. The recurrence of symptoms in a patient with a single ovoidal gallstone after a long asymptomatic time lapse is usually due to the occurrence of this new stone population. These microstones can migrate into the CBD and behave as "secondary" common duct stones.

Primary and Secondary Common Bile Duct Stones

Primary CBD stones initially form in the common duct or within the intrahepatic ducts by a mechanism, mainly based on bile stasis and infection, which is different from the mechanism of stone formation in the gallbladder. Primary CBD stones, or recurrent common duct stones, are gallstones that have initially formed, in the CBD, usually after cholecystectomy associated with sphincterotomy or other surgical procedures that alter or by-pass the sphincter of Oddi, facilitating the passage of bacteria from the duodenum into the bile tract. Primary CBD stones have to be distinguished from secondary common duct stones, which initially form in the gallbladder and subsequently migrate into the common duct through the cystic duct and are "missed" at the time of the cholecystectomy (retained stones). Primary or recurrent CBD stones are easily diagnosed at operation because they are brown, earthy, easily crushed with the fingers and on cross-section show alternate light and tan layers, both in the center and in the periphery. They contain bacteria in their central portion (they are "infectious" stones and tell their own history!) and have a characteristic "fecaloid odor". On the other hand, retained stones are purely cholesterol, or mixed faceted stones. They testify their gallbladder origin because they always have a central radiate

Table 4.2 Relationships between types of gallstones and symptoms

	Biliary colic	Jaundice	Pancreatitis	Cholangitis	Biliary fistula	Carcinoma
Cholesterol unique	+	-	-	-	++	+++
Cholesterol multiple	++	++	+	+/-	-	+-
Mixed faceted	++	++	+	+/-	-	+/-
Black pigmented	++	++	+++	-	-	-
Brown pigmented	+	+++	+	+++	-	-
Composite stones	++	++	++	+	+	+++

cholesterol nucleus. A "brown" periphery can sometimes be found, because of secondary precipitations of "infectious" material, due to the long-term stay within the common duct of a cholesterol nucleus initially formed elsewhere [5]. It has recently been suggested that gallstones usually form in the gallbladder in the absence of sectorial bile stasis [67–69], regardless of alterations in bile composition. This statement has important implications for both epidemiologic and clinicopathologic purposes. In fact, metabolic factors, which have systemic effects, cannot be the main cause of precipitation of intrahepatic stones in only one liver lobe or segment, as occurs in most cases; such factors should result in diffuse intrahepatic lithiasis. Local biochemical alterations, such as decreased levels of apolipoprotein A and defects in cholesterol and bile acid formation secondary to sectorial bile stasis, are likely to be found rather than a liver metabolism defect [64, 65]. The pathogenetic hypothesis that a low protein diet causes an increased incidence of brown stones both in the common duct and in the intrahepatic ducts because of a reduced concentrations of glucaric acid (an inhibitor of betaglucuronidase) [36] is far from proven. Our recent findings in a prospective study of patients with previous cholesterol stones and recurrent CBD brown stones after sphincterotomy showed that a low fat-low protein diet was not a basic factor in the occurrence of brown stones in these patients. In fact, for the entire period of postcholecystectomy brown stone formation, these patients had the same diet as in the previous decades when their cholesterol stones had formed [28].

Postcholecystectomy Common Bile Duct Stones

Postcholecystectomy CBD stones can be classified as follows: (1) brown recurrent stones; (2) recurrent stones containing suture material or phytobezoars; or (3) retained or residual stones (Table 4.3) [5–14]. Stones containing foreign bodies can be brown (when the foreign body acts as a co-factor together with bile stasis and infection), cholesterol, mixed or even black pigment stones. The latter never form outside the gallbladder, unless there is a foreign body acting as a nucleus or an obstacle to the free flow of the bile. Retained stones are stones that have been missed at previous cholecystectomy. Therefore, they always show a central cholesterol nucleus with a radiate structure, which is an expression of their gallbladder origin. In addition to these three types, there is another type of postcholecystectomy stone that is always

Table 4.3 Common duct stones

Stones	Pathogenesis	Infection	Risk factors	Treatment
True recurrent or primary	Infection	Yes	Previous SPHT	Repeat SPHT or BE anastomosis
Secondary or retained	Gallbladder origin	Possible	Misdiagnosis	Stone removal
Associated with long cystic remnant	Residual gallbladder mucosa	Rare	Iatrogenic	Stone and cystic remnant removal
Containing foreign bodies	Heterologous nucleation	Possible	Iatrogenic	Stone removal

SPHT, Sphincterotomy; *BE*, Biliary-enteric

cholesterol or mixed, not associated with suture material or metallic clips, and that has certainly formed after cholecystectomy, but not primarily within the common duct: the long cystic remnant postcholecystectomy stone. This stone can become symptomatic from 2 to 30 years after operation. According to the "gallbladder mechanism" it most likely forms in the cystic remnant, which acts as a mini-gallbladder. This is a well-documented finding. A long cystic remnant is responsible for the reformation of cholesterol gallstones after cholecystectomy [29]. The exact pathogenetic mechanism is not well known. There are gallstones which have formed in a cystic remnant of about 1.5 cm, whereas there are patients with cystic remnants larger than 5–7 cm, in whom stones do not reform, even after 27 years [29].

A precise classification of gallstones is easy and can be obtained by the surgeon in the operating room or by the endoscopist after stone removal, simply by cross-sectional examination of the gallstone. A correct classification can help in choosing the method of patient management. In fact, whereas retained stones, cholesterol or mixed stones containing suture material and stones of gallbladder origin can be treated by simple stone removal, with no need for additional sphincterotomy or biliary-enteric anastomosis, in patients with postcholecystectomy stones associated with a long cystic remnant, the removal of the cystic remnant is mandatory. This is not always an easy operation, since it may require intrapancreatic dissection of the lower portion of the common duct, a procedure commonly used for the treatment of congenital choledochal cysts [30]. Finally, if brown stones are found as unique postcholecystectomy CBD stones, stone recurrence is highly probable, irrespective of the treatment strategy. In fact, these stones are caused by a vicious cycle of infection-stasis-infection, simple stone removal leaves therefore the pathogenetic factors responsible for the vicious cycle unchanged [31–36]. In these cases, definitive treatment strongly depends on the age and general condition of the patient, the best policy may be to aim for the disappearance of jaundice and/or clinical cholangitis with the least operative risk and side effects. Therefore, even if previous sphincterotomy, either surgical or endoscopic, was the main cause of the stones, repeat endoscopic sphincterotomy may be a good option, even if restenosis is foreseeable. The patient must be informed that the treatment will be palliative. A biliary-enteric anastomosis could be a more appropriate treatment, but it is associated with a greater operative risk. However, biliary-enteric anastomosis is also a palliative procedure. In fact, the wall of the common duct will be chronically inflamed, colonized by bacteria and will have permanently lost its physiologic properties due to fibrosis. The main advantage of a technically well-performed biliary-enteric anastomosis is the lower incidence of a clinically relevant stricture, as compared with endoscopic sphincterotomy. In fact, brown sludge is going to occur both after sphincterotomy and biliary-enteric anastomosis. However, clinical cholangitis with jaundice and chills is less frequent, because aggregates of brown "mud" less frequently cause sudden intraluminal hyperpressure and secondary passage of bacteria and toxins from the bile into the blood stream.

Gallstone Pancreatitis

Gallstone pancreatitis is thought to be caused by stones that provoke a transient obstruction of the ampulla of Vater and is usually associated with microlithiasis (stones < 3 mm in diameter) [37–43]. Some recent studies gave further insight into possible determinants of gallstone pancreatitis [6, 16–17].

In a study from our institution, systematic stone analysis revealed that 282 of 1421 patients with gallstones had common duct stones [16]. Eighty-two (40 men, 42 women) had pancreatitis that was observed in 4.4% of overall patients with cholesterol stones, 8.1% of those with brown stones, and 13.1% of those with black pigment stones. Some patients with pancreatitis had black microstones in association with large cholesterol stones in the gallbladder. In addition, on the basis of endoscopic retrograde cholangiopancreatography (ERCP) and/or intra-operative cholangiography, it was found that 22 of 51 patients with cholesterol gallstones and pancreatitis had a very low insertion, with a tortuous aspect of the cystic duct, into the common duct close to the papilla of Vater [6, 22].

Acute Cholangitis Associated with Pancreatitis

The incidence of cholangitis associated with gallstone pancreatitis varies greatly according to different authors. In the series of Fan et al. [44], 12% of patients with gallstone pancreatitis treated conservatively developed cholangitis, compared with 0% of patients undergoing emergency ERCP within 24 hours of admission ($p=0.001$). Therefore, these authors recommended urgent ERCP in all patients presenting with acute pancreatitis. On the other hand, Oria et al. [45] reported only a 2% incidence of cholangitis among 110 patients with acute gallstone pancreatitis, whereas Neoptolemos et al. [46] detected a 5% incidence among 229 patients randomized to the non-urgent group. De Virgilio et al. [47], in a retrospective review of 71 subjects with gallstone pancreatitis in whom ERCP was limited to patients demonstrating clinical evidence of biliary sepsis, found that only five patients (7%) had cholangitis. In a prospective study, Chang et al. [38] found that only 3% of patients had cholangitis. This variable incidence of associated cholangitis deserves careful analysis, since it implies different diagnostic and therapeutic attitudes, according to whether the incidence of cholangitis is 3% as opposed to 12% or more in a given population of patients with gallstone pancreatitis. Among other possible explanations, the higher incidence of cholangitis in series from Eastern countries could be due to a greater incidence of pigment gallstones, namely of the brown subtype, which are seen more frequently in the Orient [9–12]. Brown pigment stones are more likely to harbor bacteria, are quite exclusive of elderly patients and have been shown to lead more commonly to infectious complications [9–14].

Original studies from our laboratory have documented that infection precedes, rather than follows, the occurrence of brown stones and is the main cause of their formation [10]. Bacteria not only form the initial nidus, but are also responsible for the precipitation of the various compounds of these stones [9–12]. More recent studies have shown that brown stone formation is a multifactorial phenomenon [11]. Bile infection is a necessary, but not sufficient condition for their formation. Other factors, such as the patient's age (greater than 50), type of bacteria (*Escherichia coli* is more lithogenic than other bacterial strains because it produces greater quantities of β-glucuronidase and phospholipases) [10, 11], grading of associated stricture and bile stasis, concomitant presence of foreign bodies or clots, pancreatobiliary or enterobiliary reflux, host defenses, and immunosuppression all play a role. In particular, old age is a major factor [72]. Old age not only means reduced host defenses, but also hypochlorydria, duodenal or jejunal contamination by coliform bacteria, as well as reduced clearing activity of the bile duct system, among others. All these pathophysiologic aspects must be kept in mind while trying to evaluate the possible risk of cholangitis in a patient with gallstone pancreatitis.

Clinical Predictors of Persistent Common Duct Stones

While acute suppurative cholangitis and severe pancreatitis due to persistent impacted gallstone at the level of the papilla of Vater are obvious indications for emergency endoscopic sphincterotomy and biliary drainage [46–51], which guide-lines can be used to predict persistent CBD stones in patients with an episode of gallstone pancreatitis in the absence of cholangitis?

In one study, in which 12% of patients had gallstone pancreatitis, four clinical variables predicted CBD stones: age > 55 years, admission bilirubin > 30 µmol/ml (1.7 mg/dl), a dilated CBD (> 6 mm) on ultrasonography, and suspected CBD stones on ultrasonography [47]. The presence of all four predictors revealed a 94% probability of CBD stones, but absence of all four predictors was still associated with an 18% probability of CBD stones. In a recent study by Chang et al. [38], who exclusively studied patients with gallstone pancreatitis, the single best independent predictor of CBD stones was total bilirubin greater than 1.35 mg/dl on hospital day two (sensitivity 90.5%, specificity 63%). Urgent ERCP seems to be rarely necessary in Western patients because, as previously stated, cholangitis is uncommon in the course of gallstone pancreatitis and only 21% of these patients usually have persistent CBD stones [38]. Therefore, it should be restricted only to the subgroup showing increased bilirubin after hospital day two.

Endoscopic Sphincterotomy

Endoscopic sphincterotomy is a basic procedure in patients with acute suppurative cholangitis, either alone or in association with acute pancreatitis. However, there is no doubt that unnecessary endoscopic sphincterotomies are sometimes performed [50–53]. This is not only cost ineffective, but also potentially harmful. In fact, the side effects of endoscopic sphincterotomy are well known. They include not only immediate complications, but also long-term side effects, such as recurrent CBD stones. Bergman et al. [53] followed a cohort of 100 patients who had undergone sphincterotomy for gallstones more than 10 years previously. New CBD stones had developed in 24% of patients [53]. Concerns about whether a planned sphincterotomy is really safe and necessary are expressed with increased frequency [50–53]. In particular, a study from our laboratory documented that in subjects with non-brown gallstones at cholecystectomy, brown recurrent stones (i.e., a new disease) were found in 11% of patients who underwent surgical sphincterotomy after a mean follow-up of 6 years (range 3 to 28 years) and in 9% of patients who underwent endoscopic sphincterotomy (mean follow-up 4.3 years; range 3 to 10 years) [13, 14]. Fifty percent of these stones were detected within the first 5 years, whereas the remaining 50% became symptomatic up to 27 years after sphincterotomy [14]. The impairment of the sphincter mechanism is a basic factor or at least a co-factor in the pathogenesis of brown stones. These stones are typical "infectious" stones, the occurrence of which is facilitated by the type of bacteria, old age, grading of associated stricture and bile stasis (see previous chapters). If the duodenum is sterile, as in young healthy subjects, an impaired sphincteric function due to sphincterotomy does not cause the formation of brown stones. Therefore, the incidence of brown stones is very low in young patients, even if they have been followed-up for decades after sphincterotomy, and significantly higher if a given series includes a considerable proportion of old patients. Accordingly, the evaluation of the long-term side effects of sphincterotomy will be affected not only by technical factors, but also by the total number of patients over 60 years of age or under 50, and the types of bacteria colonizing the duodenum in the series of matched patients. Collaborative assessment of patients using a common data base across specialist disciplines [50] will be of help to better define the actual incidence of medium and long-term complications of endoscopic sphincterotomy.

Bacteria and Gallstone Pathogenesis

Bacteria are often found in high concentrations in brown pigment and less frequently in cholesterol gallstones. It is likely that cholesterol stone formation is non-bacterial in nature and principally different from the pathogenesis of "infectious" brown pigment gallstones. However, it is possible that some overlap exists between the two processes [81–83]. Most gallstones are composite in nature. Using molecular-genetic methods, bacteria can be found in most pure cholesterol gallstones (i.e., those whose structure consists of more than 90% cholesterol) [83–86]. The natural history of the gallstone development is unknown. It is likely that brown pigment stones can evolve in their chemical composition after the termination of the infectious process that initiates their formation, and may further develop into either mixed or nearly pure cholesterol stones [81–86]. In a similar fashion, cholesterol-poor or black pigment gallstones may act as foreign bodies to enhance the propensity of bacterial colonization in the presence of pre-existing gallstones or cholangitis, thereby activating pathways of bacterial lithogenesis and resulting in the encasement of cholesterol nuclei with pigment shells and/or in the internal remodeling of existent stones. It is often difficult, if not impossible, to ascertain whether bacterial infection of bile arose before stone formation or vice-versa. The development of gallstones (nucleation, assembly of microcalculi, growth, remodeling) includes the interaction of both bacterial and non-bacterial mechanisms, working discontinuously over years and decades and shaping the structural individuality of each stone. At cholecystectomy, the gallstone removed from the patient represents the end product of a long pathologic process [81–83]. Although the exact temporal contribution of bacteria in lithogenesis is unknown, it is important for the clinician to realize that:

1) There are some gallstones (a minority, i.e., less that 10%), in which infection has been the main, if not the unique determinant of stone formation, if physico-chemical conditions did not change significantly from the beginning of stone formation to the time of stone removal. These stones are "brown pigment stones", which have a definite composition, pathogenesis and clinical behavior [9–12].
2) A greater number of gallstones are colonized by a bacterial biofilm, even though the bile may be culture-negative. In these cases (composite, or even cholesterol or mixed stones), the presence of bacteria likely played a minor role, sometimes a facilitating role for stone nucleation, or may have behaved for some time as "innocent bystanders".
3) For epidemiological, clinical and pathogenetical purposes, it is useful that these two conditions are considered as two separate entities [9–12].

New Pathologic Entities in the Laparoscopic Era

The side effects of sphincterotomy are not the only drawbacks that surgeons must face following the advent of laparoscopic cholecystectomy (LC). In fact, there are some other consequences of LC that may affect common duct stone formation and will be discussed in detail in order to facilitate prevention. CBD stones are a changing entity and, in particular, the incidence and the type of some postcholecystectomy stones could be, at least in part, a side effect or a consequence of the new procedures or therapeutic strategies.

Metallic clips are used in LC instead of traditional ligatures. Time will better define the impact of the use of clips in the reformation of stones in the bile ducts. We have reported a large series of 64 gallstones containing suture material or foreign bodies. Stones containing metallic clips have also been described recently [36]. We have demonstrated that every type of gallstone can form in the common duct in the presence of a non-absorbable foreign object acting as a nucleus [36]. In addition, clips can cause twisting of the cystic stump, temporary or persistent torsion, or obstruction of the common duct. Also, the early slipping of clips or the inappropriate reliance on clips to close an enlarged or swollen cystic duct may cause bile leak. An overlooked injury to the back wall of the cystic duct during catheterization or incidental thermal damage (electrocautery or laser coagulation) to the common duct could also contribute to the increased incidence of bile leakage reported after LC. The consequences of bile leakage need to be evaluated more carefully, not only in terms of immediate postoperative sequeale, but also in terms of long-term local damage, including duct stricture and subsequent stone recurrence [31].

Suggestions for Treatment

A better knowledge of the pathophysiology of CBD stones is of basic importance in the present era of LC in order to select the best therapeutic option for patients with common duct stones found concomitantly with gallbladder stones [31–36]. The best treatment of concomitant common duct stones – endoscopic sphincterotomy before or after cholecystectomy, LC associated with a "wait and see" policy, concomitant treatment of gallbladder and common duct stones by the laparoscopic approach [31–36] – should also be guided by the type of gallstone, taking into consideration the general condition of the patient. In fact, in the presence of one or two small cholesterol or faceted common duct stones, a transcystic or transcholedochal removal through the laparoscopic approach [35] is better than endoscopic sphincterotomy, which is associated with severe long-term side effects, such as the occurrence of brown recurrent stones in a significant percentage of patients [14, 35].

On the contrary, endoscopic sphincterotomy is a more appropriate procedure in the presence of "infectious" brown stones (easily detectable by pre-operative ultrasound), since the biliary-enteric barrier to bile infection is already permanently damaged. Simple LC is an adequate procedure in the presence of black sludge or black microstones, which form exclusively in the gallbladder and never recur after cholecystectomy, without surgical exploration of the common duct, even in patients with previous jaundice and/or pancreatitis. Finally, open surgery is certainly still the best procedure in patients with multiple common duct stones (more than 20–30 gallstones) or the so-called *empierrement du cholédoque* [32]. When CBD stones are associated with intrahepatic stones, the procedure is more complex and may include liver resection and/or cholangiojejunostomy with a Roux-en-Y loop anastomosed to the abdominal wall in order to facilitate postsurgical treatment, including cholangioscopic removal of recurrent or retained stones. In these cases, the use of chemolitholytic drugs, even if effective in stone dissolution in some patients with cholesterol stones, is only a temporary treatment if bile duct stricture is associated. In fact, all gallstones that form cranially to a stricture are invariably going to recur, because of sectorial bile stasis, if the stricture persists [67–69].

In conclusion, new pathophysiologic data that could be of importance for CBD stones include the following:

1) Gallstones are not a unique entity.
2) Gallstones are better classified on the basis of their type, rather than on their cholesterol content.
3) Stone classification is easy and can be achieved by the surgeon or the endoscopist after stone removal, by gross inspection of the stone cross-section.
4) The type of gallstone predetermines its natural history, i.e., different stone types have a different incidence of symptoms and/or complications.
5) A precise classification of gallstones is not only important for epidemiologic and pathogenetic purposes, and to permit a correct comparison of different series, but is also important for clinical and therapeutic purposes. In fact, the type of gallstone could and perhaps should guide the selection of the best therapeutic option for a given disease in a given patient. In particular, biliary pancreatitis and/or cholangitis, which are the most frequent complications of common duct stones, occur in a variable proportion of patients with gallstones. These do not occur by chance, but with specific predisposing factors, concerning either the container or the content, namely the type and consistency of gallstones, the presence or absence of bacteria in the bile, and the type of bacteria.

Acute suppurative cholangitis is a formal indication to ERCP and emergency endoscopic sphincterotomy, but is an infrequent finding in Western countries, particularly in young patients. The different ages of patients and/or the relative incidence of "infectious" brown stones in a given population are possible determinants for differences among various series. Therefore, urgent sphincterotomy should be restricted only to the subgroups of patients with known risk factors for cholangitis (old age, infectious brown stones). Unnecessary sphincterotomy in patients with gallstone pancreatitis is not only useless, but can also be harmful in the long term. In fact, a high incidence (11% and above) of recurrent CBD stones of the brown subtype, causing a self-maintaining vicious cycle and responsible for the occurrence of a "chronic", irreversible disease [9–11], has been observed after both surgical and endoscopic sphincterotomy in patients with previous stones of other types [14]. Therefore, occurrence of brown stones in these subjects can be considered, at least in part, as the result of an iatrogenic lesion, namely the damage of sphincteric function. In the present era of laparoendoscopic surgery, there are a large number of diagnostic and therapeutic options for patients with CBD stones and/or their complications, such as pancreatitis and cholangitis. The range of options is going to become even greater in the future. The proper treatment, in addition to being cost-effective, should be selected on the basis of: (1) a more accurate preoperative diagnosis, including a precise detection of the number, site and type of stones; (2) a better knowledge of the pathogenetic mechanisms determining the occurrence of pancreatitis and cholanitis and/or influencing the post-treatment function of the biliary tree; and (3) awareness of the long-term effects of the various therapeutic options [31]. There is no single treatment suited to all CBD stones. The selected option should be appropriate to the individual, the stones, the type of associated complications, and the aspect of the biliary tract. "Above all, a more accurate knowledge will be required of what is actually minimally invasive, not only in terms of cosmetic results, reduced hospitalization, and early return to work, but also in terms of permanent functional damage and its potential for the occurrence of severe complications in the future" [31].

Acknowledgments
The author wishes to thank Dr. A. Dhamo, Research Doctor, Department of Surgery, University of Siena, Italy, for his cooperation.

References

1. Cetta F, Lombardo F, Giubbolini M et al (1995) Classification of gallstones and epidemiologic studies. Dig Dis Sci 40:2189-2191
2. Cetta F, Bralia A, De Nisi A et al (1984) Physicochemical and microbiological features of recurrent and secondary common duct stones. Gastroenterology 86:1313
3. Cetta F, Tomassini E, Saggese N (1985) Physicochemical analysis of pigment biliary stones. Chir Epatobil 4:173-182
4. Cetta F, Tanzini G, Sianesi M et al (1988) Biliary sludge and microlithiasis: composition, pathogenesis and clinical significance. In: Montorsi M, Granelli P (eds) Proceed 26th World Congr Int Coll Surg VI. Bologna, Monduzzi Publ, pp 345-348
5. Cetta F (1989) Classification, composition and significance of common duct stones after cholecystectomy. In: Gozzetti (ed) Proced Congr Italian Chap HPB Surg. Bologna, Esserre Publ, pp 289-299
6. Cetta F, Lombardo F, Giubbolini M et al (1995) Quantity and location of stone compounds, not the mere presence in small amounts within the stone fabric, are important factors for the correct classification of the gallstones and a better knowledge of their pathogenesis. Hepatology 23:1285-1287
7. Cetta F, Lombardo F (1995) Hypercalcemia. calcium in bile and calcium in gallstones. Gastroenterologv 109:1720-1722
8. Cetta F, Lombardo F, Cappelli A et al (1993) Gallstones: different diseases, not a unique entity. I° Implications for epidemiologic studies. Gastroenterology 104:A354
9. Cetta F (1991) The role of bacteria in pigment gallstone disease. Ann Surg 213:315-326
10. Cetta F (1986) Bile infection documented as initial event in the pathogenesis of brown pigment biliary stones. Hepatology 6:482-489
11. Cetta F (1995) Bacteria and pathogenesis of gallstones. Gastroenterology 109:2050-2052
12. Kaufman HS, Magnuson TH, Lillemoe KD et al (1993) The role of bacteria in gallbladder and common duct stone formation. Ann Surg 104:A369
13. Cetta F (1991) The possible role of sphincteroplasty and surgical sphincterotomy in the pathogenesis of recurrent common duct brown stones. HPB Surg 4:261-270
14. Cetta F (1993) Do surgical and endoscopic sphincterotomy prevent or facilitate recurrent common duct stone formation? Arch Surg 29:336
15. Cetta F, Tanzini G, Civitelli S et al (1993) Relationships among gallstones, carcinoma of the gallbladder and carcinoma of the colon. Gastroenterology 104:A356
16. Cetta F (1996) Biliary sludge: necessity for a better distinction between crushable and not crushable microconcrements. Sludge is responsible for symptoms not by itself, but also in relationship to the variability of the container, i.e., the bile tract wall. Hepatology 23:191-192
17. Lee SP, Hayashi A, Kim YS (1994) Biliary sludge: curiosity or culprit? Hepatology 20:523-525
18. Attili AF, De Santi A, Repice AM et al (1995) The natural history of gallstones. The GREPCO experience. Hepatology 21:656-660
19. Wenckert A, Robertson B (1986) The natural course of gallstone disease: eleven year review of 781 non operated cases. Gastroenterology 50:376-381
20. Cetta F, Calomino N, Malerba M et al (1993) Every type of gallstone can form after total gastrectomy and total parenteral nutrition. Gastroenterology 104:A353
21. Cetta F (1995) The natural history of gallstones. A reappraisal. Gastroenterology 108:A412
22. Cetta F, Lombardo F, Giubbolini M et al (1995) Stone type (black pigment spicular stones) and a low insertion of the cystic duct are important determinants of gallstone pancreatitis. Gastroenterology 108:A411
23. Cetta F, Cariati A, Lombardo F et al (1993) Black microstones form in the fundus of Rokitansky-Aschoff sinuses of patients without increased content of unconjugated bilirubin in the bile. Gastroenterology 104:A353
24. Cetta F, Lombardo F, Malet PF (1995) Black pigment gallstones with cholesterol gallstones in the same gallbladder. Dig Dis Sci 40:534-538
25. Cetta F, Lombardo F, Guidoni E (1992) The comet tail artifact in ultrasound imaging of the gallbladder. Is it a marker of intraparietal black microlithiasis? Gastroenterology 102:A307
26. Cetta F, Montalto G (1997) Gallstone formation after open cardiac surgery. Am J Gastroenterol 92:1-2
27. Matsushiro T, Suzuchi N, Sato T et al (1977) Effects of diet on glucaric acid concentration in bile in the formation of calcium bilirubinate gallstones. Gastroenterology 72:620-623
28. Cetta F, Lombardo F (1992) Epidemiology of brown

pigment gallstones: II Evidence that dietary factors are of low importance, at least in postcholecystectomy stones. Gastoenterology 102:A791
29. Cetta F, Lombardo F, Giubbolini M et al (1995) Cholesterol stone recurrence in the cystic remnant after laparoscopic cholecystectomy. The first case report during a follow-up study of patients with or without postoperative bile acids therapy. Gastroenterology 108:A409
30. Ando H, Kaneko K, Ito T et al (1996) Complete excision of the intrapancreatic portion of choledochal cysts. J Am Coll Surg 183:317-321
31. Cetta F (1994) Common duct stones in the era of laparoscopic cholecystectomy: changing treatments and new pathologic entities. J Laparoendoscopic Surg 4:41-44
32. Pitt HA (1993) Role of open choledochotomy in the treatment of choledocholithiasis. Am J Surg 165:483-486
33. Cotton PB (1993) Endoscopic retrograde cholangiopancreatography and laparoscopic cholecystectomy. Am J Surg 165:474-478
34. Petelin JB (1993) Laparoscopic approach to common duct pathology. Am J Surg 165:487-491
35. Lezoche E, Paganini AM (1995) Single-stage laparoscopic treatment of gallstones and common bile duct stones in 120 unselected, consecutive pattents. Surg Endosc 9:1070-1075
36. Cetta F, Baldi C, Lombardo F et al (1997) Migration of metallic clips used during laparoscopic cholecystectomy and formation of gallstones around them. Surgical implications from a prospective study. J Laparoendosc Surg 7:37-46
37. Cetta F (1998) Gallstone pancreatitis, associated cholangitis, clinical predictors of persistent common duct stones and ERCP or endoscopic sphincterotomy. Editorial Am J Gastroenterol 93
38. Chang L, De Virgilio C, Lo SK et al (1998) Gallstone pancreatitis: a prospective study on the incidence of cholangitis and clinical predictors of retained common bile duct stones. Am J Gastroenterol 93:527-531
39. Acosta JM, Ledesma CL (1974) Gallstone migration as a cause of acute pancreatitis. N Engl J Med 290:484-487
40. Kelly TR (1976) Gallstone pancreatitis pathophysiology. Surgery 80:488-492
41. McMahon MJ, Shefta JR (1980) Physical characteristics of gallstones and the calibre of the cystic duct in patients with acute pancreatitis. Br J Surg 67:6-9
42. Armstrong CP, Taylor TW, Jeacock J et al (1985) The biliary tract in patients with acute gallstone pancreatitis. Br J Surg 72:551-555
43. Farinon AM, Ricci GL, Sianesi M et al (1987) Physiopathologic role of microlithiasis in gallstone pancreatitis. Surg Gynec Obstet 164:252-256
44. Fan ST, Lai EC, Mok FT et al (1993) Early treatment of acute biliary pancreatitis by endoscopic papillotomy. N Engl J Med 328:228-232
45. Oria A, Alvarez J, Chiappetta L et al (1991) Choledocolithiasis in acute gallstone pancreatitis: incidence and clinical significance. Arch Surg 126:566-568
46. Neoptolemos JP, London NJ, James D et al (1988) Controlled trial of urgent endoscopic retrograde cholangio-pancreatography and endoscopic sphincterotomy versus conservative management for acute pancreatitis due to gallstones. Lancet 3:979-983
47. De Virgilio C, Verbin C, Chang L et al (1994) Gallstone pancreatitis: the role of preoperative endoscopic retrograde cholangio-pancreatography. Arch Surg 129:909-913
48. Falsch UR, Nitsche R, Ltidtke R et al (1997) Early ERCP and papillotomy compared with conservative treatment for acute biliary pancreatitis. N Engl J Med 336:237-242
49. Leung JWC, Chung SCS, Sung JJY et al (1989) Urgent endoscopic drainage for acute suppurative cholangitis. Lancet 1:1307-1309
50. Cotton PB (1996) Is your sphincterotomy really safe and necessary? Gastrointest Endosc 44:752-755
51. MacMathuna P, White P, Clarke E et al (1995) Endoscopic balloon sphincteroplasty (papillary dilatation) for bile duct stones: efficacy, safety and follow-up in 100 patients. Gastrointestinal Endosc 42:468-474
52. Flowers L (1996) ERCP versus laparoscopic surgery: the contest over common bile duct stones. Endoscopy 28:438-440
53. Bergman JJ, Van der Mey S, Rauws EA et al (1996) Long-term follow-up after endoscopic sphincterotomy for bile duct stones in patients younger than 60 years of age. Gastrointest Endosc 44:643-649
54. Cetta F, Montalto G, Zuckermann M (1998) Hemobilia, infection, bile stasis, and intrahepatic stones in liver transplant recipients. Surgery 123:115-117
55. Cetta F, Montalto G, Pacchiarotti MC (1997) Gallstone opacification during cholelitholytic treatment. Am J Gastroenterol 92:547-548
56. Cetta F, Montalto G, Nuzzo G (1997) Recurrent hepatolithiasis after primary excision of choledochal cysts. J Am Coll Surg 185:198-200
57. Cetta F, Lombardo F, Baldi C et al (1997) Clip migration within the common duct after laparoscopic cholecystectomy: a case of transient acute pancreatitis in the absence of associated stones. Endoscopy 29:S59-60
58. Figura N, Cetta F, Angelico M et al (1998) Most Helicobacter pylori-infected patients have specific antibodies, and some also have H. pylori antigens and genomic material in bile: is it a risk

factor for gallstone formation? Dig Dis Sci 43:854-862
59. Cetta F, Baldi C, Montalto G et al (1998) Short-term complications after endoscopic sphincterotomy (ES) are not increased in relatively young and healthy patients with small bile ducts, when sphincterotomy for stones is performed by an expert. Ann Surg 228:624-625
60. Cetta F, Rappuoli R, Montalto G et al (1999) New biliary endoprosthesis less liable to block in biliary infections: description and in vitro studies. Eur J Surg 165:782-785
61. Cariati A, Cetta F (2002) Re: Kawai et al. Bacteria are not important in the formation of pure cholesterol stones. Am J Gastroenterol 97:2921-2923
62. Cariati A, Cetta F (2003) Rokitansky-Aschoff sinuses of the gallbladder are associated with black pigment gallstone formation: a scanning electron microscopy study. Ultrastruct Pathol 27:265-270
63. Cariati A, Cetta F (2003) Squamous-cell and non-squamous-cell carcinomas of the gallbladder have different risk factors. Lancet Oncol 4:393-394
64. Ohta T, Nagakawa T, Takeda T et al (1993) Histological evaluation of the intrahepatic biliary tree in intrahepatic cholesterol stones, including immunohistochemical staining against apolipoprotein A-l. Hepatology 17:531-537
65. Shoda J, He B, Tanaka N et al (1995) Primary dual defect of cholesterol and bile acid metabolism in liver of patients with intrahepatic calculi. Gastroenterology 108:1534-1546
66. Kim MH, Sekeijima J, Lee SP (1995) Primary intrahepatic stones. Am J Gastroenterol 90:540-548
67. Cetta F, Lombardo F, Cariati A (1994) The role of the content (decreased level of apolipoprotein Al) and the container (bile duct stricture. sectorial dilatation of the ducts determining bile stasis) in the pathogenesis of hepatolithiasis either pigment or cholesterol. Hepatology 19:1539-1541
68. Cetta F, Lombardo F, Giubbolini M et al (1996) Hepatolithiasis and cholesterol and bile acid metabolism. Gastroenterology 110:963-965
69. Cetta F (1996) Bile stasis, due to bile duct stricture, precedes not follows the formation of primary intrahepatic stones, and plays a basic role in their pathogenesis. Am J Gastroenterol 91:2451-2452
70. Cetta F (1997) Endoscopic stenting for palliation of malignant biliary obstruction and formation of bacterial biofilm resulting in stent clogging. Dig Dis Sci 42:2052-2053
71. Cetta F (1997) Prevention of biliary stent clogging. Am J Gastroenterol 92:542-543
72. Cetta F (1993) Age of gallstones and age of patients at the time of stone formation. Difference among various types of gallstones. Gastroenterology 104:A352
73. Mbongo-Kama E, Harnois F, Mennecier D et al (2007) MDR3 mutations associated with intrahepatic and gallbladder cholesterol cholelithiasis: an update. Ann Hepatol 6:143-149
74. Wu SD, Uchiyama K, Fan Y (2007) The role and mechanism of fatty acids in gallstones. Hepatobiliary Pancreat Dis Int 6:399-401
75. Kawakami H, Kuwatani M, Onodera M et al (2007) Primary cholesterol hepatolithiasis associated with cholangiocellular carcinoma: a case report and literature review. Intern Med 46:1191-1196
76. Grunhage F, Acalovschi M, Tirziu S et al (2007) Increased gallstone risk in humans conferred by common variant of hepatic ATP-binding cassette transporter for cholesterol. Hepatology in press
77. Marschall HU, Einarsson C (2007) Gallstone disease. J Intern Med 261:529-542
78. Castro J, Amigo L, Miquel JF et al (2007) Increased activity of hepatic microsomal triglyceride transfer protein and bile acid synthesis in gallstone disease. Hepatology 45:1261-1266
79. Stewart L, Griffiss JM, Jarvis GA (2007) Gallstones containing bacteria are biofilms: Bacterial slime production and ability to form pigment solids determines infection severity and bacteremia. J Gastrointest Surg 11:977-984
80. Stewart L, Griffiss JM, Jarvis GA (2007) Bacteria entombed in the center of cholesterol gallstones induce fewer infectious manifestations than bacteria in the matrix of pigment stones. J Gastrointest Surg 11:1298-1308
81. Swidsinski A, Lee SP (2001) The role of bacteria in gallstone pathogenesis. Front Biosci 6:E93-103
82. Swidsinski A, Ludwig W, Pahlig H et al (1995) Molecular genetic evidence of bacterial colonization of cholesterol gallstones. Gastroenterology 108:860-864
83. Swidsinski A, Khilkin M, Pahlig H et al (1998) Time dependent changes in the concentration and type of bacterial sequences found in cholesterol gallstones. Hepatology 27:662-665
84. Wu XT, Xiao LJ, Li XQ et al (1998) Detection of bacterial DNA from cholesterol gallstones by nested primers polymerase chain reaction. World J Gastroenterol 4:234-237
85. Lee DK, Tarr PI, Haigh WG et al (1999) Bacterial DNA in mixed cholesterol gallstones. Am J Gastroenterol 94:3502-3506
86. Kawai M, Iwahashi M, Uchiyama K et al (2002) Gram-positive cocci are associated with the formation of completely pure cholesterol stones. Am J Gastroenterol 97:83-88
87. Stewart L, Grifiss JM, Jarvis GA et al (2006) Biliary bacterial factors determine the path of gallstone formation. Am J Surg 192:598-603

88. Stewart L, Griffiss JM, Way LW (2005) Spectrum of gallstone disease in the veterans population. Am J Surg 190:746-751
89. Skar V, Skar AG, Stromme JH (1988) Beta-glucuronidase activity related to bacterial growth in common bile duct bile in gallstone patients. Scand J Gastroenterol 23:83-90
90. Stewart L, Oesterle AL, Erdan I et al (2002) Pathogenesis of pigment gallstones in Western societies: the central role of bacteria. J Gastrointest Surg 6:891-903
91. Stewart L, Oesterle AL, Griffiss JM et al (2002) Gram-negative bacteria killed by complement are associated with more severe biliary infections and produce more tumor necrosis factor-alpha in sera. Surgery 132:408-414
92. Smith AL, Stewart L, Fine R et al (1989) Gallstone disease. The clinical manifestations of infectious stones. Arch Surg 124:629-633
93. Stewart L, Smith AL, Pellegrini CA et al (1987) Pigment gallstones form as a composite of bacterial microcolonies and pigment solids. Ann Surg 206:242-250
94. Stewart L, Griffiss JM, Jarvis GA, Way LW (2007) Bacteria entombed in the center of cholesterol gallstones induce fewer infectious manifestations than bacteria in the matrix of pigment stones. J Gastrointest Surg 11:1298-1308

Chapter 5

Natural History of Biliary Lithiasis

Grant Caddy

Introduction

Biliary lithiasis is a common disease and is present in up to 20–30% of western populations. The prevalence increases with age, being <10% in populations under the age of 30 years and approximately 30% in those over the age of 60 [1]. This prevalence is similar in studies throughout Europe, including the UK. Owing to increasing life expectancy among patients throughout Europe, the prevalence of biliary lithiasis is also likely to increase. This review of the natural history of biliary lithiasis will deal with both choledocholithiasis (bile duct stones) and cholelithiasis (gallbladder stones).

Choledocholithiasis

Bile duct stones can be classified as primary or secondary in their origin. In western populations primary bile duct stones are much less common (5%) than secondary ductal stones (95%), which probably progress from the gallbladder via the cystic duct into the bile duct [2]. Saharia et al. described criteria for the definition of primary bile duct stones, including a 2-year symptom-free interval following cholecystectomy; soft, light brown stones or sludge present in the common duct; and absence of a long cystic duct remnant or a biliary stricture from previous surgery [3]. These primary stones are composed mainly of bilirubinate and are likely to be related to infection and biliary stasis [4–6].

The presence of concomitant secondary bile duct stones at the time of cholecystectomy for gallbladder stones is not uncommon; the prevalence is estimated at approximately 6–30% [7–10]. The prevalence of symptomatic bile duct stones at the time of cholecystectomy has been found to increase with age, ranging from 6% in patients under the age of 80 years up to 33% in patients over 80 [9]. Studies have shown these bile duct stones to be of similar composition to the coexisting gallbladder stones, with cholesterol predominating [11]. In patients with gallstones and concomitant bile duct stones, studies have suggested that an increase in cystic duct diameter is associated with the presence of coexistent bile duct stones [12, 13].

In an early study by Millbourn et al., 38 patients who had retained bile duct stones but were deemed unsuitable for surgery or had refused surgery through personal choice, were followed for up to 13 years. Just over half of these patients developed complications related to retained stones, such as jaundice, sepsis or biliary colic [14]. Wenckert et al. found that approximately 25–50% of patients with retained bile duct stones developed serious complications, mainly jaundice or pancreatitis [15]. Owing to the potential nature of these complications and the high probability of a complication relating to retained bile duct stones in a symptomatic patient, removal of these stones is recommended if this is at all possible.

Conversely, a proportion of symptomatic bile duct stones may migrate spontaneously through the bile duct into the intestine. The size of bile duct stone appears to be the main predictor of spontaneous passage; stones up to 8 mm can be passed spontaneously [16]. In the study by Frossard et al., in which 92 patients had choledocholithiasis identified on endoscopic ultrasound (EUS), 57 patients had endoscopic retrograde cholangiography (ERC) performed between 6 h and 27 days after their EUS procedure. In 12 of these 57 patients (21%) no stones were identified on ERC, which was felt to be the result of spontaneous bile duct stone migration [16]. Given that there is comparable sensitivity and specificity between EUS and ERC, these negative examinations were deemed to be accurate [17]. In the same study only 2 of these 12 patients (17%) with stone migration developed symptoms during the 27 days, the remainder of them remaining asymptomatic (83%).

Similar figures have been reported by Greiner et al. following extracorporeal shock wave lithotripsy of gallbladder stones in 21 patients with stone fragments measuring 0.5–8.0 mm [18]. In this study, 86% of the patients remained asymptomatic during passage of the stone fragments through the biliary tract.

In the study by Frossard, using Cox proportional methods, stone size was the only predictive factor for spontaneous migration, with a stone size of 8 mm or greater having a negative predictive value of 95% for spontaneous migration [16]. Similar spontaneous migration rates have been reported by other authors [19].

Symptomatic Choledocholithiasis

As previously mentioned, up to 50% of patients with symptomatic choledocholithiasis will have recurrent symptoms if left untreated. Commonly these symptoms will include biliary colic, jaundice, sepsis, and pancreatitis, and often patients will have abnormal liver function tests.

Biliary Colic

Biliary colic is typically experienced as pain in the right hypochondrium or epigastrium, or both. The pain can be of variable duration but lasting at least 30 min, and often several hours. Associated symptoms are common and include nausea and/or vomiting, right shoulder tip pain, and fatty food intolerance [20]. Pain is likely to be caused by distension of the bile duct by the offending stone(s) within the bile duct. The probability of stone retention increases with increasing diameter of the stone(s).

Jaundice

When the bile duct becomes obstructed jaundice occurs. This is often the case when the stone(s) become(s) lodged in the distal common bile duct (CBD) as its diameter narrows. Obstruction of the bile duct may be complete or (more often) incomplete, allowing for fluctuating bilirubin levels. Jaundice can occur in isolation, but also occurs less commonly as part of Charcot's triad (pain, jaundice, and cholangitis).

Cholangitis and Pancreatitis

Cholangitis and pancreatitis secondary to choledocholithiasis are discussed in separate chapters and will not be dealt with in detail here.

Abnormal Liver Function Tests

Patients whose liver function tests (LFTs) give abnormal results may or may not have symptoms. Anciaux et al. studied 100 consecutive patients with symptomatic choledocholithiasis and found that the serum levels of gamma glutamyl transpeptidase (GGT) and alkaline phosphatase (ALP) were the most frequent biochemical abnormalities in these patients (increased in 94% and 91%, respectively) [21]. Several studies have used the level of abnormality of LFTs to predict the likelihood of choledocholithiasis and thereby select patients for elective cholangiography. The sensitivity of LFT results alone in detecting choledocholithiasis is approximately 50%, increasing to 98% when LFTs are used in association with other parameters, mainly age, dilatation of the CBD, cholangitis and pancreatitis [22–27].

In those patients with retained bile duct stones at the time of cholecystectomy that are left in place and observed rather than removed, the minority whose stones progress to cause symptoms experience them within 3 years [28, 29].

Asymptomatic Choledocholithiasis

It is likely that the natural history of asymptomatic bile duct stones is associated with fewer complications than that of symptomatic stones. It is known that some bile duct stones pass spontaneously without symptoms. This was demonstrated in an early study by Acosta et al., in which the stools were collected from patients for 10 days during an attack of acute pancreatitis and from a control group of patients with a known history of gallstones but without pancreatitis [30, 31]. Stools were examined using filtration and chemical analysis where appropriate. Gallstones were found in the faeces of 47 (92%) of the 51 patients whose samples were collected during acute pancreatitis and 6 (12%) of the 51 patients who had a history of gallstones but did not have acute pancreatitis (control group). In the patients with acute pancreatitis, the stones detected in the faeces were of a similar chemical composition to those retrieved from the gallbladder following cholecystectomy [31]. This study also reinforces the likelihood that the majority of stones in western populations originally arise in the gallbladder, migrating then into the bile duct before a proportion of them pass into the intestine. In a similar study, gallstones were found in the faeces of 11% of controls—patients with gallstones but without pancreatitis (as against 84% of patients with pancreatitis) [32]. These studies suggest that a proportion of gallstones can pass spontaneously into the intestine without biliary or pancreatic complications.

In historical autopsy studies, Crump et al. found a choledocholithiasis in 24% of patients died from unrelated causes [33]. Again, this study suggests that a proportion of bile duct stones remain asymptomatic.

In these circumstances, do asymptomatic, incidental bile duct stones need to be removed? Currently there is no definitive answer as there is a lack of large controlled studies investigating this issue, but the limited data we do have suggest that a conservative approach may be acceptable. Murison et al. randomly allocated 285 patients undergoing cholecystectomy without a preoperative suspicion of choledocholithiasis to undergo routine intraoperative cholangiogram (IOC) or not [34]. Of those who did undergo IOC, 12% had choledocholithiasis, and it was assumed that the patients who underwent cholecystectomy without IOC would have the same prevalence of choledocholithiasis. Patients were followed up with the aid of a patient questionnaire. Over a median follow up of 4 years, no patients in the observation alone group developed any biliary/pancreatic symptoms or complications. A weakness of this study was that the response rate to the questionnaire survey was only 75%, which means that no information is available for the other 25% of patients. Our data from a retrospective study including follow-up with patients' family practitioners revealed an unsuspected prevalence rate of 6% for choledocholithiasis, but again none of the patients concerned developed any biliary/pancreatic complications over a median follow up of 57 months [35].

In another study, which involved 999 patients with unsuspected choledocholithiasis, IOC was obtained in 962 of them and showed filling defects in 46 (4.8%). No treatment on the CBD was performed but a trans-cystic chatheter was positioned during cholecystectomy and patients were followed-up with trans-cystic cholangiography at 48 hours and 6 weeks. Of these 46 patients, 12 had normal cholangiogram and were considered false positive; in 12 of the remaining 34 patients (35%) with filling defects at 48 hours, bile duct stones were no longer visible on repeat cholangiography at 6 weeks and must therefore have migrated spontaneously [36]. None of these patients developed complications associated with the migration of stones, and 2 of them reported transient pain only. Similar results indicating spontaneous migration of bile duct stones in around one third of patients following laparoscopic cholecystectomy have also been reported from other studies [37, 38]. Routine use of IOC at the time of cholecystectomy will therefore detect bile duct stones more often than the selective use of IOC (12% versus 1–5%), and a significant proportion of the unsuspected stones will remain asymptomatic (50–75%). There are many published studies of IOC in which unsuspected/asymptomatic bile duct stones have been detected [39–42], with an overall detection rate of approximately 4% [43].

Cholelithiasis

Asymptomatic Cholelithiasis

In contrast to choledocholithiasis, the majority of gallbladder stones are asymptomatic. With the widespread use of transabdominal ultrasound, asymptomatic gallstones are commonly detected. Two thirds of patients with gallstones will remain asymptomatic and do not need treatment [44].

In historical studies it was originally thought that asymptomatic gallstones had a relatively high probability of inducing symptoms over a 20-year follow-up, but on reflection these studies included "symptomatic patients" with dyspepsia and the conclusions reached in them are therefore unlikely to be related to gallstones [45–47]. More vigorous follow-up studies suggest that asymptomatic gallstones cause symptoms in approximately 2–4% of cases per year in the first 10 years, perhaps declining to 1–2% per year after that [48–54].

A recent Cochrane review of the literature on the treatment of asymptomatic gallstones found no rigorous studies (randomised or nonrandomised) that adequately justified treating asymptomatic gallstones with cholecystectomy [55]. For the majority of patients, the natural history of asymptomatic gallstones is that they remain silent and do not require treatment. Otherwise there is a small but cumulative risk of developing symptoms over time.

Prophylactic cholecystectomy has however been advocated for certain "high risk" groups of patients (Table 5.1).

Symptomatic Cholelithiasis

If a conservative approach to asymptomatic gallstones is to be recommended, then the consequences of such an approach must be appreciated. By far the most common presenting symptom of symptomatic gallstones is biliary pain, which is reported to occur in approximately 90% of those patients who become symptomatic (Table 5.2) [44, 48, 51, 54, 56].

In the GRPECO study the cumulative probability of developing biliary pain in patients with asymptomatic gallstones at 10 years was 25.8%, as against a 3% probability of their developing a more serious complication, such as cholecystitis or pancreatitis [54]. Approximately 50% of patients who experience biliary pain will have a further episode within 12 months [57]. One third of

Table 5.1 High-risk groups of patients in whom prophylactic cholecystectomy has been advocated

1. Ethnic groups with increased risk of gallbladder carcinoma, e.g. Pima Indians
2. Patients with immune suppression after solid organ transplantation
3. Patients with rapid weight loss, e.g. following bariatric surgery
4. Calcified 'porcelain' gallbladder due to increased risk of gallbladder cancer

Table 5.2 Patients woith gallbladder stones presenting with symptoms of biliary pain. Modified from [58]

First author	No. of patients	No. of years	Percentage presenting with biliary pain as first symptom[a]
Gracie	123	15	90
Attili	118	10	90
Thistle	193	2	100
Cucciaro	125	5	67
Zubler	32	5	83

[a]Mean 86%

these patients will have no further pain or biliary complications. Therefore, the majority of patients who become symptomatic experience biliary pain, rather than developing a more severe complication, such as cholecystitis or pancreatitis. However, in longitudinal studies following patients with symptomatic gallstones, the risk of biliary complications, such as acute pancreatitis, supportive cholangitis, and acute cholecystitis in such patients is 10-fold that in patients with asymptomatic gallstones (1–2% vs 0.1–0.2%) [49, 57]. Previously symptomatic patients who subsequently remain symptom free for 5 years appear to have a reduced future risk of further biliary pain and/or biliary complications and is comparable to that in patients with asymptomatic gallstones [49].

On balance, suitable patients with gallstones who become symptomatic should be offered cholecystectomy in view of the increased risks of potentially serious complications. Complications of symptomatic gallstones left in situ are shown in Table 5.3. These complications are discussed in more detail in other chapters.

Table 5.3 Complications of symptomatic gallstones left in situ

1. Acute cholecystitis
2. Chronic cholecystitis
3. Gangrenous gallbladder
4. Empyema of gallbladder
5. Secondary bile duct stones
6. Calcified 'porcelain' gallbladder due to increased risk of gallbladder cancer
7. Chronic pancreatitis
8. Supportive cholangitis
9. Mirizzi's syndrome
10. Cholecystoenteric fistula with or without gallstone ileus
11. Gallbladder perforation
12. Gallbladder cancer

Summary

In summary, the natural history of biliary lithiasis can be divided into cholelithiasis (asymptomatic and symptomatic) and choledocholithiasis (asymptomatic and symptomatic). The majority of gallstones remain asymptomatic and do not cause symptoms, but approximately 2% of patients per year with gallstones will develop symptoms. Fortunately, the majority of these symptomatic patients will develop biliary pain as their first symptom rather than a more serious biliary complication.

In patients with symptomatic choledocholithiasis, 50% will develop further biliary complications, such as obstructive jaundice or cholangitis.

Asymptomatic choledocholithiasis tends to run a more benign course, but rigorous, high quality studies are lacking in this area. Approximately 6–12% of patients with gallstones will have unsuspected, asymptomatic bile duct stones, and a significant proportion of these will be passed spontaneously with no symptoms found in follow up studies.

References

1. Heaton KW, Braddon FE, Mountford RA et al (1991) Symptomatic and silent gall stones in the community. Gut 32:316-320
2. Johnson AG, Hosking SW (1987) Appraisal of the management of bile duct stones. Br J Surg 74:555-560
3. Saharia PC, Zuidema GD, Cameron JL (1977) Primary common duct stones. Ann Surg 185:598-604
4. Kaufman HS, Magnuson TH, Lillemoe KD et al (1989) The role of bacteria in gallbladder and common duct stone formation. Ann Surg 209:584-591
5. Cetta F (1991) The role of bacteria in pigment gallstone disease. Ann Surg 213:315-326
6. Cetta FM (1986) Bile infection documented as initial event in the pathogenesis of brown pigment biliary stones. Hepatology 6:482-489
7. Denbesten L, Doty JE (1981) Pathogenesis and management of choledocholithiasis. Surg Clin North Am 61:893-907
8. Glenn F, Beil AR Jr (1964) Choledocholithiasis demonstrated at 586 operations. Surg Gynecol Obstet 118:499-506
9. Glenn F, McSherry CK (1975) Calculous biliary tract disease. In: Ravitch MM (ed) Current problems in surgery. Yearbook Publishers, Chicago. pp 1-38
10. Joyce WP, Keane R, Burke GJ et al (1991) Identification of bile duct stones in patients undergoing laparoscopic cholecystectomy. Br J Surg 78:1174-1176
11. Madden JL, Vanderheyden L, Kandalaft S (1968) The nature and surgical significance of common duct stones. Surg Gynecol Obstet 126:3-8
12. Castelain M, Grimaldi C, Harris AG et al (1993) Relationship between cystic duct diameter and the presence of cholelithiasis. Dig Dis Sci 38:2220-2224
13. Taylor TV, Armstrong CP (1987) Migration of gall stones. Br Med J 294:1320-1322
14. Millbourn E (1941) Klinische Studien über die Choledochlithiasis. Acta Chir Scand 86 Suppl 65
15. Wenckert A, Robertson B (1966) The natural course of gallstone disease: eleven-year review of 781 nonoperated cases. Gastroenterology 50:376-381
16. Frossard JL, Hadengue A, Amouyal G et al (2000) Choledocholithiasis: a prospective study of spontaneous common bile duct stone migration. Gastrointest Endosc 51:175-177
17. United States National Institutes of Health (2002) State-of-the-science statement on endoscopic retrograde cholangiopancreatography (ERCP) for diagnosis and therapy. NIH Consens State Sci Statements 19:1-26
18. Greiner L, Munks C, Heil W, Jakobeit C (1990) Gallbladder stone fragments in feces after biliary extracorporeal shock-wave lithotripsy. Gastroenterology 98:1620-1624
19. Oria A, Frider B, Alvarez J et al (1988) Biliary and pancreatic obstruction during gallstone migration. Int J Pancreatol 3:157-164
20. Festi D, Sottili S, Colecchia A et al (1999) Clinical manifestations of gallstone disease: evidence from the Multicenter Italian Study On Cholelithiasis (MICOL). Hepatology 30:839-846
21. Anciaux ML, Pelletier G, Attali P et al (1986) Prospective study of clinical and biochemical features of symptomatic choledocholithiasis. Dig Dis Sci 31:449-453
22. Katz D, Nikfarjam M, Sfakiotaki A Christophi C (2004) Selective endoscopic cholangiography for the detection of common bile duct stones in patients with cholelithiasis. Endoscopy 36:1045-1049
23. Shiozawa S, Tsuchiya A, Kim DH et al (2005) Useful predictive factors of common bile duct

stones prior to laparoscopic cholecystectomy for gallstones. Hepatogastroenterology 52:1662-1665
24. Alponat A, Kum CK, Rajnakova A et al (1997) Predictive factors for synchronous common bile duct stones in patients with cholelithiasis. Surg Endosc 11:928-932
25. Onken JE, Brazer SR, Eisen GM et al (1996) Predicting the presence of choledocholithiasis in patients with symptomatic cholelithiasis. Am J Gastroenterol 91:762-767
26. Rijna H, Borgstein PJ, Meuwissen SG et al (1995) Selective preoperative endoscopic retrograde cholangiopancreatography in laparoscopic biliary surgery. Br J Surg 82:1130-1133
27. Barkun AN, Barkun JS, Fried GM et al (1994) Useful predictors of bile duct stones in patients undergoing laparoscopic cholecystectomy. McGill Gallstone Treatment Group. Ann Surg 220:32-39
28. Hauer-Jensen M, Karesen R, Nygaard K et al (1986) Consequences of routine peroperative cholangiography during cholecystectomy for gallstone disease: a prospective, randomized study. World J Surg 10:996-1002
29. Thurston OG, McDougall RM (1976) The effect of hepatic bile on retained common duct stones. Surg Gynecol Obstet 143:625-627
30. Acosta JM, Ledesma CL (1974) Gallstone migration as a cause of acute pancreatitis. N Engl J Med 290:484-487
31. Acosta MJ, Rossi R, Ledesma CL (1977) The usefulness of stool screening for diagnosing cholelithiasis in acute pancreatitis. A description of the technique. Am J Dig Dis 22:168-172
32. Kelly TR (1976) Gallstone pancreatitis: pathophysiology. Surgery 80:488-492
33. Crump C (1931) The incidence of gallstones and gallbladder disease. Surg Gynecol Obstet 53:447-457
34. Murison MS, Gartell PC, McGinn FP (1993) Does selective peroperative cholangiography result in missed common bile duct stones? J R Coll Surg Edinb 38:220-224
35. Caddy GR, Kirby J, Kirk SJ et al (2005)Natural history of asymptomatic bile duct stones at time of cholecystectomy. Ulster Med J 74:108-112
36. Collins C, Maguire D, Ireland A et al (2004) A prospective study of common bile duct calculi in patients undergoing laparoscopic cholecystectomy: natural history of choledocholithiasis revisited. Ann Surg 239:28-33
37. O'Donovan AN, O'Sullivan G, Ireland A et al (1997) Prospective trial of the role of fine bore intubation of the cystic duct at the time of operative cholangiography. J Am Coll Surg 184:262-264
38. Wilson TG, Jeans PL, Anthony A et al (1993) Laparoscopic cholecystectomy and management of choledocholithiasis. Aust N Z J Surg 63:443-450
39. Jolly PC, Baker JW, Schmidt HM et al (1968) Operative cholangiography: a case for its routine use. Ann Surg 168:551-565
40. Pagana TJ, Stahlgren LH (1980) Indications and accuracy of operative cholangiography. Arch Surg 115:1214-1215
41. Faris I, Thomson JP, Grundy DJ, Le Quesne LP (1975) Operative cholangiography: a reappraisal based on a review of 400 cholangiograms. Br J Surg 62:966-972
42. Adams JD, Haisten AS (1972) Operative cholangiography-its value in the unsuspected choledochal stone. Surg Clin North Am 52:333-340
43. Metcalfe MS, Ong T, Bruening MH et al (2004) Is laparoscopic intraoperative cholangiogram a matter of routine? Am J Surg 187:475-481
44. United States National Institutes Of Health (1992) Gallstones and laparoscopic cholecystectomy. NIH Consens Statement 10:1-28
45. Moynihan BG (1908) An address on inaugural symptoms. Br Med J 2:1597-1601
46. Mayo WJ (1911) "Innocent" gallstones a myth. JAMA 56:1021-1024
47. Comfort MW, Gray HK, Wilson JM (1948) The silent gallstone: a ten to twenty year follow-up study of 112 cases. Ann Surg 128:931-937
48. Gracie WA, Ransohoff DF (1982) The natural history of silent gallstones: the innocent gallstone is not a myth. N Engl J Med 307:798-800
49. Friedman GD, Raviola CA, Fireman B (1989) Prognosis of gallstones with mild or no symptoms: 25 years of follow-up in a health maintenance organization. J Clin Epidemiol 42:127-136
50. Lund J (1960) Surgical indications in cholelithiasis: prophylactic cholecystectomy elucidated on the basis of long-term follow up on 526 nonoperated cases. Ann Surg 151:153-162
51. Newman HF, Northup JD, Rosenblum M, Abrams H (1968) Complications of cholelithiasis. Am J Gastroenterol 50(6):476-496
52. McSherry CK, Ferstenberg H, Calhoun WF et al (1985)The natural history of diagnosed gallstone disease in symptomatic and asymptomatic patients. Ann Surg 202:59-63
53. Ransohoff DF, Gracie WA (1993) Treatment of gallstones. Ann Intern Med 119:606-619
54. Attili AF, De Santis A, Capri R et al (1995) The natural history of gallstones: the Grepco experience. The Grepco Group. Hepatology 21:655-660
55. Gurusamy KS, Samraj K (2007) Cholecystectomy versus no cholecystectomy in patients with

silent gallstones. Cochrane Database Syst Rev Cd006230
56. Zubler J, Markowski G, Yale S et al (1998) Natural history of asymptomatic gallstones in family practice office practices. Arch Fam Med 7:230-233
57. Thistle JL, Cleary PA, Lachin JM et al (1984) The natural history of cholelithiasis: the National Cooperative Gallstone Study. Ann Intern Med 101:171-175
58. Sakorafas GH, Milingos D, Peros G (2007) Asymptomatic cholelithiasis: is cholecystectomy really needed? a critical reappraisal 15 years after the introduction of laparoscopic cholecystectomy. Dig Dis Sci 52:1313-1325

Chapter 6

Preoperative Noninvasive Imaging

Riccardo Manfredi, Sara Mehrabi, Massimiliano Motton, Roberto Pozzi Mucelli

Normal Anatomy Imaging

The liver is divided into the left and right lobes, and each lobe is divided into segments on the basis of its vascular anatomy and biliary drainage. The intrahepatic bile ducts generally follow the internal hepatic segmental anatomy (Figs. 6.1, 6.2). In the left lobe, a left medial segment duct and a left lateral segment duct normally join to form the main left hepatic duct. The right hepatic duct branches near its origin at the common hepatic duct. Frequently, the right hepatic duct has a dorso-caudal branch, draining the posterior segment of the right lobe, and a ventro-cranial branch, draining the anterior segment of the right lobe (Fig. 6.1). Ductal drainage of the caudate lobe is variable and may be related to the left or right ductal system. The left and right hepatic ducts unite just outside the liver to form the common hepatic duct, which is usually 3–4 cm in length (Figs. 6.3, 6.4). The common hepatic duct courses ventrally and inferiorly with the hepatic artery and the portal vein from the porta hepatis into the hepatoduodenal ligament (Fig. 6.4). The common hepatic duct joins the cystic duct to form the common bile duct (CBD) that averages 6–7 cm in length. The

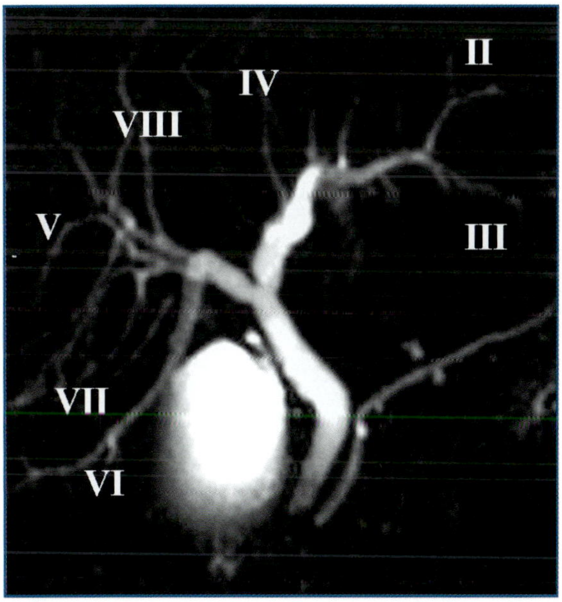

Fig. 6.1 Anatomy of the intrahepatic bile ducts: magnetic resonance cholangiopancreatography (MRCP). Coronal MRCP shows the anatomy of the intrahepatic bile ducts. The hepatic segments are indicated by roman numbers

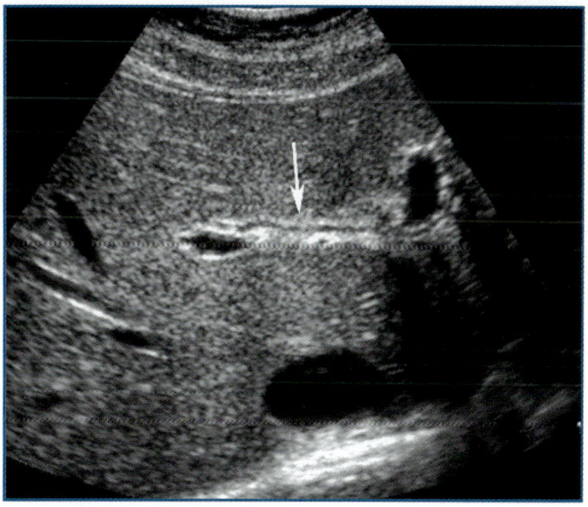

Fig. 6.2 Anatomy of the intrahepatic bile ducts: sonography. The intrahepatic bile ducts appear as hypoechoic structures (*arrow*) within the hepatic parenchyma, surrounded by hyperechoic fat within the portal space

CBD is divided into suprapancreatic, intrapancreatic, and ampullary segments, and enters the posterior-medial aspect of the

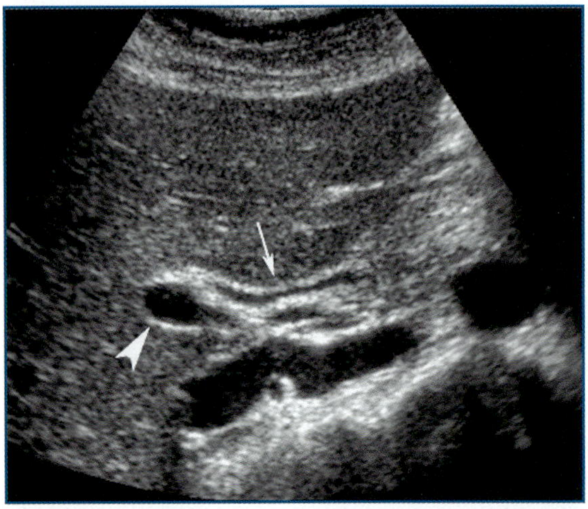

Fig. 6.3 Anatomy of the primary biliary confluence at the hepatic hilum at sonography. The primary biliary confluence appears hypoechoic (*arrow*) in this sonographic scan, located ventrally to the portal vein, at the hepatic hilum (*arrowhead*)

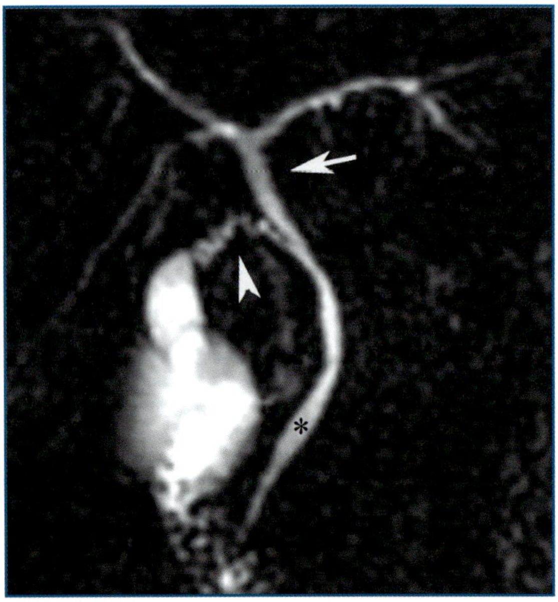

Fig. 6.4 Anatomy of the extrahepatic bile ducts: magnetic resonance cholangiopancreatography (MRCP). The coronal MRCP shows the common bile duct in all its components: common hepatic duct (*arrow*), choledocus (*asterisk*) and cystic duct (*arrowhead*)

second portion of the duodenum through a 1–2 cm long intramural tunnel terminating at the major duodenal papilla (Papilla of Vater) (Fig. 6.4). In many cases, the CBD joins the pancreatic duct in the duodenal wall, and has a short common channel. The sphincter of Oddi surrounds the common channel and the choledochal sphincter surrounds the CBD from its entrance into the duodenal wall to its junction with the pancreatic duct. Microscopically, the extrahepatic ducts are composed mainly of elastic fibers, and are sparse in muscle fibers. This explains their change in size in response to fluctuations in intraductal pressure.

The gallbladder is an elliptical organ that straddles the intersegmental plane between liver segments IV and V (Figs. 6.5 and 6.6). The gallbladder is divided into four parts: the fundus, the body, the infundibulum, and the neck (Fig. 6.5). Usually the organ is attached to the liver by the parietal peritoneum. When relaxed, the normal gallbladder is approximately 10 cm long, 3–5 cm in diameter and has a capacity of approximately 50 ml. The gallbladder wall is usually 2–3 mm thick and composed of columnar epithelium. Lymphatic drainage of the gallbladder descends

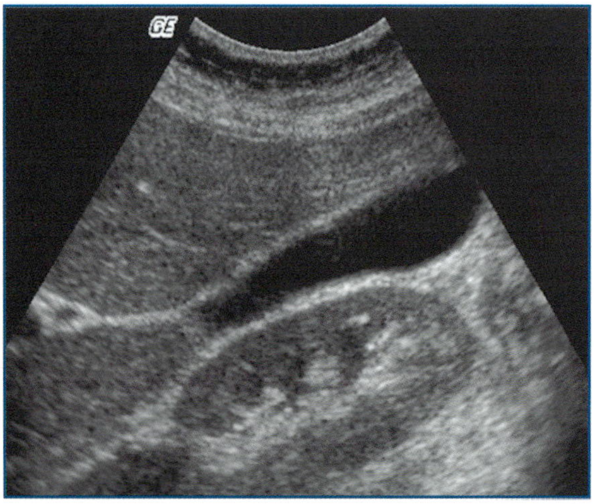

Fig. 6.5 Anatomy of the gallbladder at sonography. The gallbladder appears hypoechoic with thin, hyperechoic walls

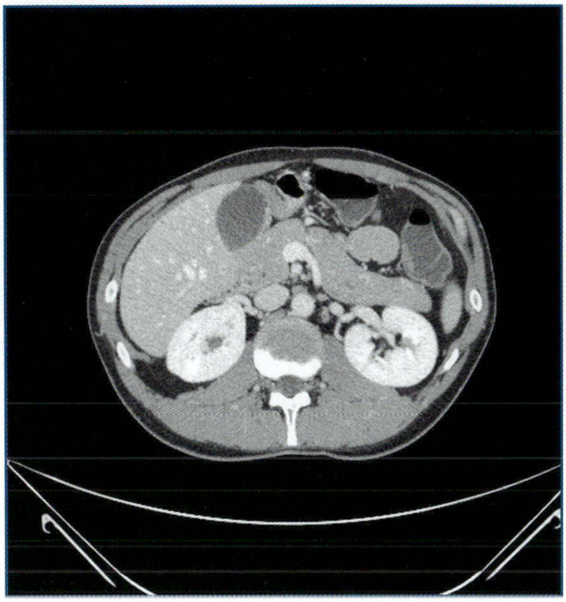

Fig. 6.6 Anatomy of the gallbladder: computed tomography (CT). At CT the gallbladder appears homogenously hypodense, with contrast enhancement of the gallbladder walls

around the bile duct and involves cystic and pericholedochal lymph nodes. From the pericholedochal nodes the drainage continues to nodes found posterior to the pancreas, portal vein, and common hepatic artery and finally reaches the lymphatic flow reaches the lymph nodes of the interaortocaval region, celiac artery, and superior mesenteric artery. The gallbladder communicates with the CBD via the cystic duct, which is 2–4 cm in length, and contains tortuous folds, known as the spiral valves of Heister, near the neck of the gallbladder (Fig. 6.4). The cystic duct usually joins the common hepatic duct approximately halfway between the porta hepatis and the ampulla of Vater to form the CBD.

Variations in ductal plate development can affect any level of the biliary tree, thereby explaining the diversity of anatomical variations congenital bile duct abnormalities.

Biliary tree malformations, with the exception of choledochal cysts, are often asymptomatic. Therefore diagnosis is frequently not made until adulthood.

Gallstones and Imaging Investigations

The most common type of gallstone are cholesterol gallstones, comprising 80% of gallstones in individuals from Europe and the Americas. Whatever the process that promotes the formation of this sort of stones is considered, undissolved cholesterol sticks together and forms particles of cholesterol that grow in size and eventually form larger gallstones [1].

Pigment gallstones are the second most common type of gallstone. They comprise 15% of gallstones in individuals from Europe and the Americas. There are two types of pigment gallstones: black pigment gallstones, and brown pigment gallstones. Calcium bilirubinate is the major component of pigment stones, calcium carbonate being a less common one. However, only 15-20% of stones contains enough calcium to be visible on plain radiographs and, although oral cholecystography has been the main radiographic investigation in the last decades, it has been totally replaced by ultrasonography (US) for the diagnosis of cholelithiasis [1]. Two other characteristics of biliary stones have to be taken into account when deciding imaging investigation: where they are located (gallbladder or biliary tree) and whether associated complications such as cholecystitis or pancreatitis define the clinical picture.

Intrahepatic Biliary Lithiasis

Intrahepatic stones are rare in Western countries, but are seen more frequently in the Far East, where they may be a consequence of parasitic infestation [2].

Conditions predisposing to intrahepatic calculi formation can include congenital abnormalities of the biliary ducts, biliary strictures and choledocholithiasis.

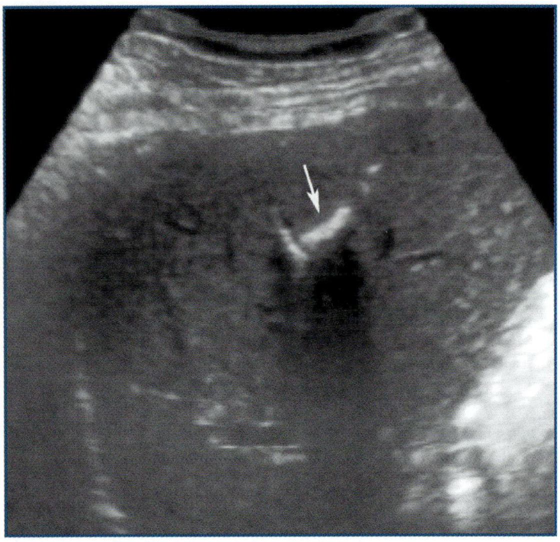

Fig. 6.7 Intrahepatic lithiasis: sonographic signs. At sonography, intrahepatic stones appear as hyperechoic structures (*arrow*) with posterior acoustic shadow

Intrahepatic stones are seen more frequently secondary to CBD stones or to an iatrogenic bile duct stricture or a narrowed biliary-enteric anastomosis.

Ultrasound (US) examination is very accurate in detecting intrahepatic stones, since they appear as echogenic foci centered on the intrahepatic ducts (Fig. 6.7). However, in patients with suspected intrahepatic lithiasis and cholangitis, who have previously undergone to sphincterotomy or biliary-enteric anastomosis, US is less accurate. This is because gas can be present in the lumen of the bile ducts and produce echogenic foci, which may show acoustic shadow or a posterior "comet-tail" artifact, due to reverberation (Fig. 6.7). This may cause a false-positive diagnosis of intrahepatic stones. However, by changing the decubitus of the patient, gas bubbles tend to move within the ducts. On the other hand, extensive pneumobilia may mask the presence of intrahepatic calculi, leading to a false-negative diagnosis [3].

Air within the bile ducts must be distinguished from air in the portal system, which is seen in several pathologic conditions. In both conditions multiple intrahepatic hyperechoic foci are the main ultrasonographic findings. However, they are different in their distribution: gas in the venous system has a peripheral distribution, close to the hepatic capsule, whereas pneumobilia has a more central distribution.

When air is seen in the biliary ducts, it is mandatory to check the patient history for previous sphincterotomy or surgery. If there is nothing relevant in the history, pneumobilia may be suggestive of a spontaneous biliary-enteric fistula: this is the consequence of cholelithiasis with chronic cholecystitis, where inflammation produces migration of the stone into the bowel lumen through erosion of the gallbladder wall [4].

Magnetic Resonance Intrahepatic Biliary Lithiasis

Magnetic resonance cholangiopancreatography (MRCP) is a noninvasive imaging technique that can accurately diagnose the presence and level of biliary stenosis or obstruction [5]. Endoscopic retrograde cholangiopancreatography (ERCP) has long been considered the gold standard for diagnosing bile duct stones, and its easy conversion from a diagnostic imaging technique to a therapeutic interventional procedure is advantageous. However, it is invasive and is associated with a morbidity rate of 1–7% and a mortality rate of 0.1–0.2% [6–8]. It also requires an experienced operator, because technical failure occurs in approximately 4% of patients [7], therefore restricting its accessibility. Based on previous studies [9–14], the diagnostic accuracy of MRCP is comparable to that of ERCP in the evaluation of choledocholithiasis; MRCP has, therefore, gained acceptance as an alternative to ERCP for imaging the biliary tract and the pancreatic duct. Moreover, Kim et al.

[15] recently reported that MRCP was a more effective diagnostic tool than ERCP for the diagnosis of intrahepatic duct stones.

On MRCP, which uses heavily T2-weighted sequences [16], the diagnosis of bile duct stones is based on round, ovoid, or irregularly shaped signal voids being identified within the bile ductal lumen with hyperintensity (Fig. 6.8) [17]. However, it is occasionally difficult to detect bile duct stones based only on the T2-weighted technique of MRCP and on the T2-weighted axial images, especially when the calculi are only partially outlined or they are not outlined at all by the hyperintense bile. In many clinical practices, we have experienced the complementary role of T1-weighted axial images for depicting bile duct stones on MRCP and on axial T2-weighted images. Yet to date, the preliminary studies have focused mainly on the T2-weighted MRCP techniques for the diagnosis of bile duct stones or biliary strictures, except for some studies that have reported on MRCP using mangafodipir as the T1 contrast agent [18–21].

Gallbladder Gallstones

At present, US is the examination of choice for the diagnosis of all gallbladder diseases, including acute and chronic inflammatory disease, benign noninflammatory disease, and malignant tumors. Moreover, it is universally agreed that US should be the first examination for the diagnosis of gallstones, as reported by many authors. Diagnosing gallstones or dilatation of the biliary tree is easy and not operator dependent; however, the subtleties of diagnosis in these areas are still important.

US remains the method of choice for the detection of gallstones, offering several advantages: high sensitivity and accuracy (> 95%), noninvasiveness, the option of performing a bedside examination, lack of ionizing radiation, relatively low cost, and the ability to evaluate adjacent organs [1].

Ultrasonography has been shown to have an accuracy of 96% in the diagnosis of gallstones. However, the measurement of gallstones size on ultrasound scans is accurate when the stones are smaller than 2 cm, but is less so if the stones are larger than 2 cm.

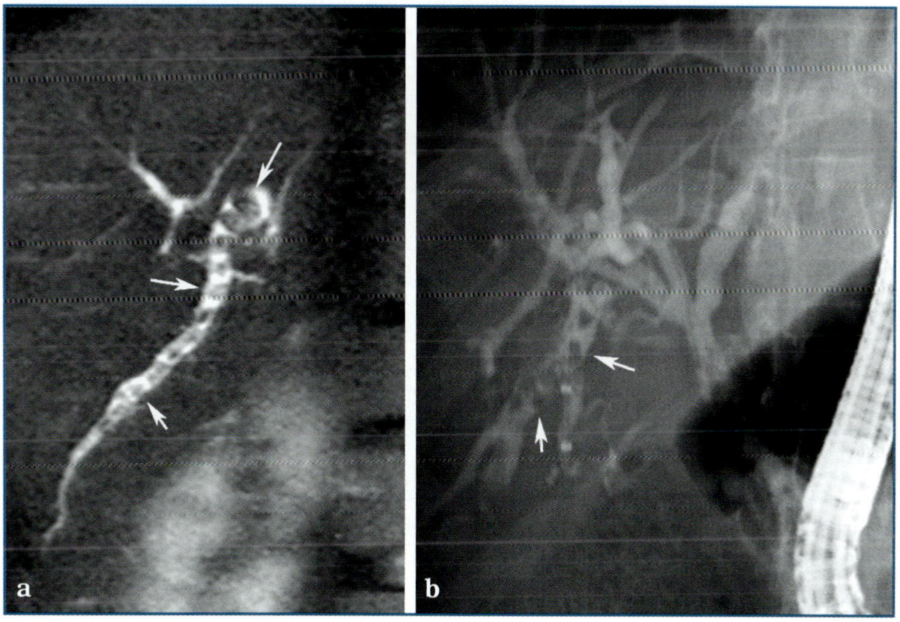

Fig. 6.8 Intrahepatic lithiasis: magnetic resonance cholangiopancreatography (MRCP) and endoscopic retrograde cholangiopancreatography (ERCP). **a** On coronal MRCP images, intrahepatic stones appear as hypointense endoluminal filling defects, within enlarged intrahepatic ducts (*arrows*). **b** The presence of intrahepatic stones is confirmed at ERCP, appearing as endoluminal filling defects (*arrows*)

Furthermore, on ultrasound scans gallstones will often be contiguous or overlap, making their size and number difficult to assess.

US Gallstones

The typical sonographic appearance of a gallbladder stone is an intraluminal echo casting an acoustic shadow, which is important for a high degree of confidence in the diagnosis of cholelithiasis (Fig. 6.9). Small calculi may not produce acoustic shadowing, especially with poor focusing of the ultrasonic beam, as occurs with low-frequency transducers. However, if they can be shown to move when the patient changes position, they can confidently be diagnosed as calculi (the "rolling stone" sign). The presence of the shadow does not depend on the composition of the stones, but rather on their combined ability to both reflect and absorb the majority of the sound energy. Even if the calculi are tiny and a shadow cannot be identified, the rolling stone sign makes the diagnosis convincing [22].

On the other hand, in many cases the gallstones may be fixed in the gallbladder infudibulum or in the cystic duct; this pattern is associated with a hydropic gallbladder and pain in the right upper quadrant of the abdomen. Most gallstones lie in the dependent portion of the gallbladder; very rarely, the stones will have a lower specific gravity than the bile and will float ("buoyancy sign").

It is important to be decisive in diagnosing gallstones. False-negatives and false-positives should be rare. The actual false-negative rate cannot be determined accurately. Most patients who do not have gallstones identified do not undergo surgery. Patients with persistent symptoms do undergo surgery or subsequent studies and are more likely to have had a false-negative diagnosis. The stones may also have formed since the time of the first negative examination.

On the other hand, false-positive diagnoses are easier to prove and can be embarrassing. A surgeon can lose confidence in the radiologist if diagnosed stones are not found. If the calculi are small, they may pass spontaneously. In these cases we recommend a repeat scan if surgery is contemplated later.

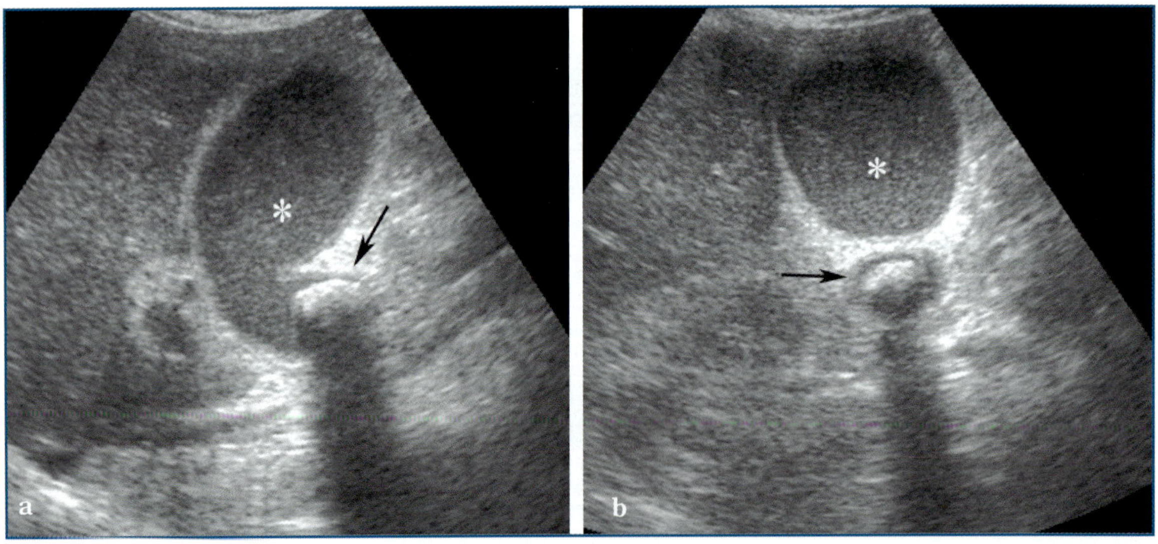

Fig 6.9 Cholelithiasis: sonographic findings. The gallbladder is well distended with endoluminal stone that appears hypoechoic (*arrow*), with posterior acoustic shadow. The bile within the gallbladder shows increased echogenicity (*asterisk*) indicating concentrated bile

A gallstone may be missed if it is impacted in the neck of the gallbladder or cystic duct. Gallstones are also easy to miss if the gallbladder cannot be moved from behind the obscuring costal margin. If the patient has not been fasting, the contracted gallbladder is more difficult to see, but if it is seen, small gallstones can be identified. Sometimes, the gallbladder can be contracted and completely full of calculi, which can make the diagnosis of cholelithiasis more difficult. The most specific sign of a contracted, stone-filled gallbladder is a hypoechoic wall superficial to a curvilinear echo from the stones and an acoustic shadow: the WES triad (Wall, Echo, Shadow) or the "double arc-shadow sign" [23].

False-positive diagnosis of gallstones is rare but can occur if pills in the stomach are mistaken for gallstones or a loop of bowel indenting the gallbladder can mimic a large gallstone.

Emphysematous cholecystitis [24] or a cholecystoduodenal fistula (as with a gallstone ileus) can cause air to obscure the gallbladder. If the gallbladder wall is calcified ("porcelain gallbladder") the appearance is similar [25]. Usually, there is enough suspicion during the scan to suggest performing a confirmatory plain film of the abdomen.

Computed Tomography Gallstones

It is well known that computed tomography (CT) is inferior to US for the detection of (noncalcified) gallstones. The appearance of gallstones on CT images is variable and depends on their composition (cholesterol versus calcium bilirubinate). In a study of 39 patients, Bova et al. [26] found that the information obtained from CT can be used to predict the cholesterol content of gallstones and consequently their solubility. They identified six different CT patterns as follows: pattern 1: negative defect within the bile (2.5%); pattern 2: gallstone invisible (56.5%); pattern 3: faint homogeneous central calcification (10%); pattern 4: thin rim of calcification (21%); pattern 5: thick rim of calcification (7%); pattern 6: dense homogeneous central calcification (2.5%) (Fig. 6.10).

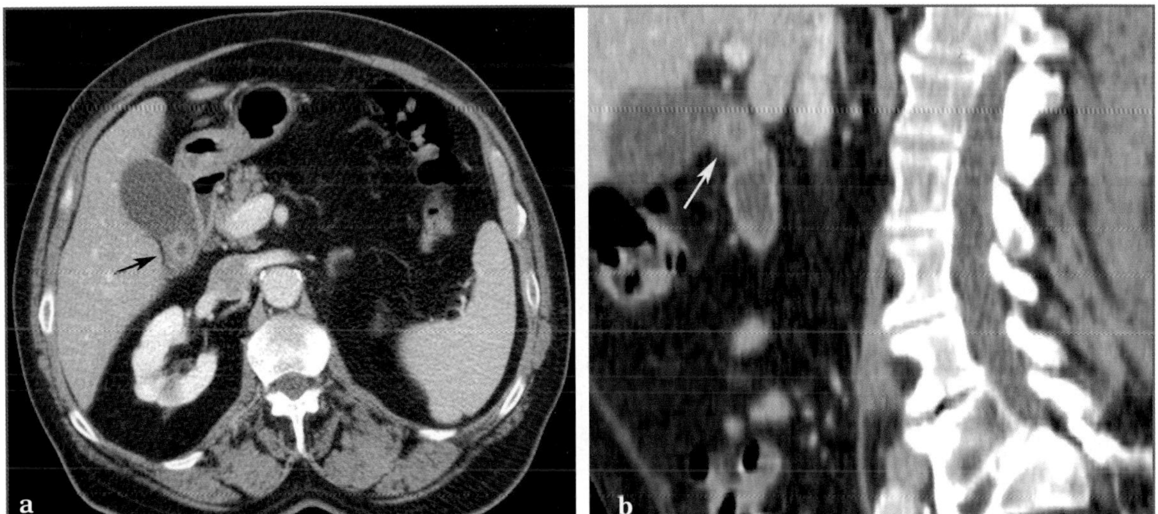

Fig. 6.10 Cholelithiasis: axial computed tomography (CT) and multiplanar reconstruction along the sagittal oblique plane. **a** On axial, contrast enhanced CT image, the gallbladder is well distended with a hypodense endoluminal stone with a thin peripheral hyperdense rim (*arrow*). **b** The stone is located at the gallbladder neck, as shown in the reformatted sagittal oblique image (*arrow*)

MR Gallstones

The accuracy of magnetic resonance imaging (MRI) in the detection of cholelithiasis is not known, the reason being that MRI plays no role in the diagnosis of gallstones, since US is usually used to diagnose cholelithiasis with a high degree of accuracy.

With a high field-strength magnet, the majority of gallstones appear as areas of signal void of both T1- and T2-weighted spin-echo images. In the heavily T2-weighted sequences used to obtain MR cholangiography, even small gallstones are depicted in a background of hyperintense bile. Occasionally areas of high signal are present in the center of the stones on T1- and T2-weighted sequences, and less commonly, the stones are entirely hyperintense on T1-weighted sequences. Since the advent of laparoscopic cholecystectomy, the need to characterize gallstone composition with imaging has substantially decreased, since the therapeutic indications are no longer based on the composition of the stones present.

The ability of MRI to image the entire biliary tree allows evaluation of the gallbladder and cystic duct as well as the intra- and extrahepatic bile ducts for the presence of lithiasis [16].

Cholecystoses

Acalculous gallbladder disease does not draw too much attention from researchers because of its low incidence of malignancy, no symptoms, and good prognosis, and therefore there is not any unanimous terminology. Emerging in 1960, the term "hyperplastic cholecystoses" refers to gallbladder adenoma, adenomyomatosis, and cholesterolosis [27].

Cholecystoses are a group of noninflammatory conditions of the gallbladder wall. The prevalence of the disease varies from 2 to 40% in autopsy studies [28].

Cholecystoses can be divided into hyperplastic and "thesaurismotic" (accumulating forms). The hyperplastic forms are characterized by normal growth of the wall components, while the thesaurismotic forms accumulate deposits of organic and inorganic materials in the gallbladder wall.

Adenomyomatosis, cholesterolosis, and porcelain gallbladder are the most common forms of cholecystosis [27].

Adenomyomatosis is the most frequently seen condition. It is characterized by segmental or diffuse thickening of mucosa and muscular wall (Fig. 6.11) [29]. In the thickened wall, more specifically, small cystic spaces are present, representing the dilated Rokitansky-Aschoff sinuses [30]. The most frequent site of the segmental form of adenomyomatosis is the gallbladder fundus. The sonographic signs are an irregular profile of the internal mucosa and wall thickening, in which may be seen hypoechoic cyst-like zones corresponding to Rokitansky-Aschoff sinuses. These cystic zones may contain debris or little stones, have an acoustic shadow or, more frequently, a "comet tail artefact", which is considered a specific finding [31].

Cholesterolosis can be diffuse and micronodular (nodules less than 1 mm) or focal (nodules larger than 3 mm). The focal type has a characteristic US appearance and is called the polypoid form, which accounts for 90% of all gallbladders polyps. Rarely, the cholesterol pseudopolyp has a diameter larger than 1 cm [32]. These pseudopolyps are usually discovered incidentally and can be distinguished from gallstones by their fixed position, the absence of acoustic shadow, and their attachment to a nondependent portion of the gallbladder wall [22].

Porcelain gallbladder consists of calcifications of the gallbladder wall; the calcified wall produces shadowing of the acoustic signal.

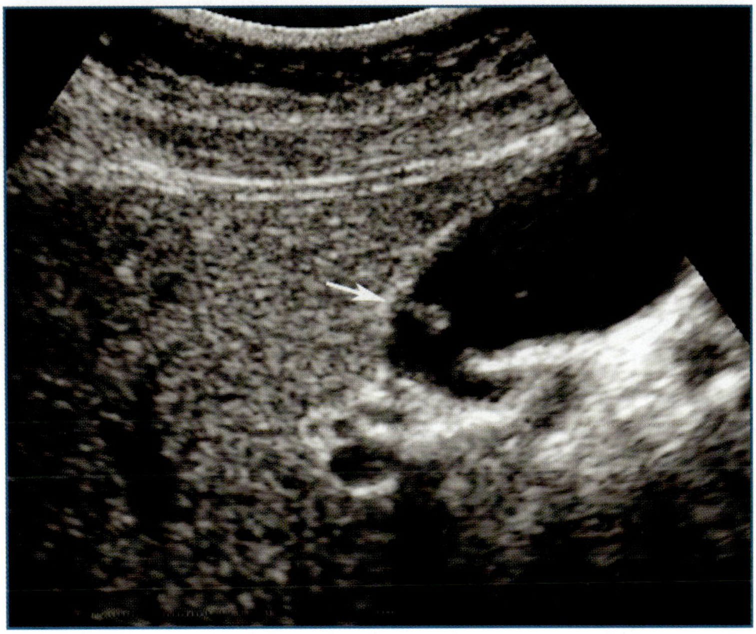

Fig. 6.11 Adenomyomatosis of the gallbladder: sonography. A polypoid thickening of the gallbladder wall adjacent to the non-dependant wall of the gallbladder body (*arrow*), representing adenomyomatosis

Acute Cholecystitis

US Acute Cholecystitis

In cases of acute right upper quadrant pain and tenderness with fever and an elevated white blood cells (WBC) count, imaging plays a central role in the differential diagnosis of acute cholecystitis. US is complementary to clinical and laboratory data, and it is particularly helpful when the clinical pattern is ambiguous. Diagnostic difficulties consist of differentiating acute calculous from acute acalculous cholecystitis and in identifying the evolution of acute cholecystitis into empyema, ischemic necrosis, or perforation.

The main sonographic signs of acute cholecystitis are [33]: the presence of gallstones or sludge and debris, the gallbladder size and its wall thickness.

Gallstones can be detected in 85–90% of cases. They may be impacted in the neck or the cystic duct. Stones in this location can frequently be missed since they are not surrounded by bile and may be situated as far as 1–2 cm from the bile-filled gallbladder [34]. If the gallstone appears to be impacted in the neck of the gallbladder, the patient should be rolled over to see if the stone will roll out. Sometimes the patient has to be turned almost prone to get the stone to roll out.

Acalculous acute cholecystitis most commonly occurs in critically ill patients, especially following surgery, trauma, or burns, or in association with hyperalimentation.

In 25% of uncomplicated cases and 85% of complicated cases of acute cholecystitis it is possible to detect the presence of sludge and debris inside the gallbladder lumen (Fig. 6.12). This is a nonshadowing echogenic material caused by biliary stasis, which may be due to prolonged fasting, extrahepatic biliary obstruction, or, rarely, the chronic situation of cystic duct obstruction. Biliary sludge is composed of calcium bilirubinate granules and cholesterol crystals [35]. Typically, sludge appears as homogeneous low-amplitude-dependent echoes that tend to form a fluid-fluid level that moves very slowly when the patient changes position. If the echogenic material completely fills the gallbladder lumen, the gallbladder becomes similar in appearance to the adjacent liver ("hepatization of the bile") or even more echogenic than the liver. Occasionally the sludge forms round, echogenic masses ("sludge balls"), which can resemble gallbladder tumors. In the complicated forms of acute cholecystitis it is possible to see echogenic material without a level, which does not move or moves reluctantly. This finding is caused by pus, debris, and fibrinous exudate. In gangrenous cholecystitis one may see the sloughed gallbladder mucosa as a thin membranous echo parallel to the wall of the gallbladder.

In 58% of uncomplicated and in 76% of complicated cases of acute cholecystitis an increase in gallbladder size is also reported. The gallbladder may become distended with a short-axis diameter greater than 4 cm; the majority of normal gallbladders are smaller than 4 cm across the short axis. Unfortunately this finding lacks specificity.

Another finding in acute cholecystitis is represented by wall thickening that usually is uniform in uncomplicated cases, and not uniform in complicated cases (64%) (Fig. 6.12). In the fasting patient the gallbladder wall usually measures less than 3 mm thick, but it may appear thicker when contracted. In acute cholecystitis, but also in many other conditions, the gallbladder wall may be thickened and may contain a hypoechoic band. This sign of acute cholecystitis is related to the edema and cellular infiltration of the subserosa and submucosa. In the complicated forms (empyema, gangrenous cholecystitis) the thickened gallbladder wall shows discontinuous, irregularly margined hypoechoic and echogenic intramural bands and foci due to hemorrhage and intramural abscesses [33]. In cases of perforation a fluid collection may be seen in the gallbladder bed or in the intraperitoneal cavity (pericholecystic abscesses). Distinguishing between the two is important to determine the proper treatment: elective surgery in cases of abscess of the gallbladder bed, and emergency surgery or ultrasound-guided drainage followed by surgery in cases of abscess of the intraperitoneal cavity.

The presence of gas in the gallbladder wall and/or lumen may be seen in emphysematous cholecystitis ("effervescent gallbladder") [36]. Adenomyomatosis can also cause segmental gallbladder wall thickening.

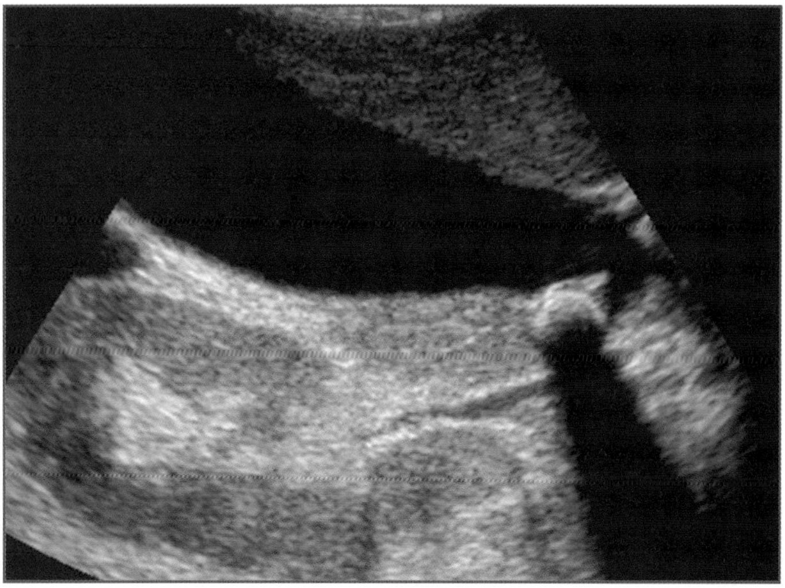

Fig. 6.12 Cholecystitis: sonographic signs. The gallbladder is well distended with thickened walls and gallstones, sludge and debris within the lumen

In patients with acquired immune deficiency syndrome (AIDS), thickening of the wall of the gallbladder is particularly evident, varying from 4 to 15 mm [37]. This finding in AIDS may indicate opportunistic infection of the biliary tract [37].

Many conditions unrelated to gallbladder disease may thicken the wall of the gallbladder, especially hepatitis, hypoalbuminemia, ascites and dilatation of the cystic veins in portal hypertension. These conditions are associated with a single hypoechoic zone between two relatively echogenic layers. Nonetheless, the combined finding of gallstones with thickening of the gallbladder wall in a patient with the appropriate clinical presentation has a high positive predictive value, in excess of 90%, for the diagnosis of acute cholecystitis.

Color and power Doppler may demonstrate hypervascularization of the gallbladder wall in acute cholecystitis.

A pericholecystic abscess can be a complication and definitive evidence of acute cholecystitis. However, other fluid collections can mimic a pericholecystic abscess. Ascites can form in a pocket around a normal or inflamed gallbladder. Veins on the surface of the liver with or without portal hypertension can mimic fluid. Rarely, a large choledochal cyst or a gallbladder duplication is seen, which may mimic a pericholecystic abscess.

Sonographic Murphy's sign has been reported as having a high positive predictive value for acute cholecystitis, greater than 90%. The sonographic Murphy's sign is defined as the presence of pain elicited by direct pressure of the transducer over a sonographically located gallbladder.

CT Acute Cholecystitis

The diagnosis of acute cholecystitis is usually made by clinical examination or US. The major disadvantage of CT is that the presence or absence of Murphy's sign cannot be assessed. Typical CT signs of acute cholecystitis are: focal or diffuse thickening of the wall of the gallbladder, fluid in the gallbladder fossa, enlargement of the gallbladder, and infiltration of the surrounding fat (Fig. 6.13). Hyperdense areas may be seen in the liver parenchyma adjacent to the gallbladder on images obtained early after

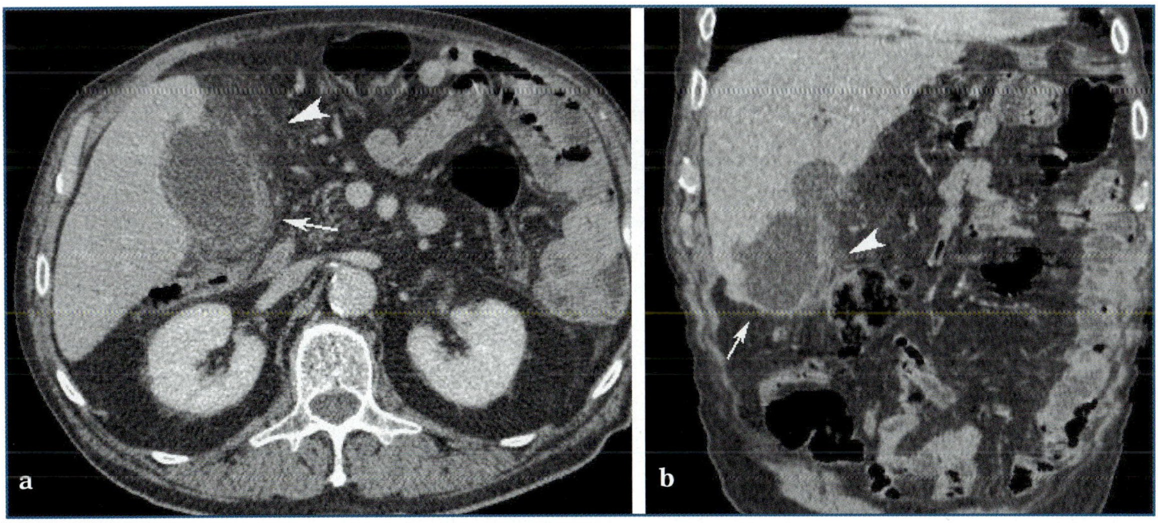

Fig. 6.13 Cholecystitis: axial computed tomography (CT) and multiplanar reconstruction along the coronal plane. **a** On axial contrast-enhanced CT image, the gallbladder is well distended with contrast-enhancing, thickened walls (*arrows*). Fluid can be depicted in the gallbladder fossa (*arrowhead*) as depicted both on axial (**a**) and multiplanar coronal reconstruction image (**b**)

contrast injection [38]. These areas are caused by hyperemia secondary to cholecystitis. It is important to differentiate fluid in the gallbladder fossa from marked hypodense thickening of the gallbladder wall since the latter condition may be secondary to other disease processes such as hepatitis, malignancy, and hypoalbuminemia and thus unrelated to inflammation of the gallbladder. Typical CT findings in cases of concentric gallbladder wall thickening are: two concentric enhancing rims with intervening low-density material; small enhancing punctuate structures within the apparent fluid, corresponding to vessels in the gallbladder wall and a diffusely thickened gallbladder wall.

While the diagnosis of acute cholecystitis can usually be made by clinical examination or US, CT may be useful in the diagnosis of acalculous cholecystitis by showing pericholecystic fluid collections, perforation of the gallbladder wall, or inflammation of pericholecystic fat [39].

Gallbladder perforation is a common complication of acute cholecystitis. Common signs are a pericholecystic fluid collection, streaky omentum or mesentery, and a gallbladder wall defect on CT [40]. While US is well suited to the diagnosis of acute cholecystitis, CT is superior to US for diagnosis of gallbladder perforation [40].

Emphysematous cholecystitis is a complication of acute cholecystitis. In this condition gas is present in the gallbladder lumen or wall or in the pericholecystic space. The diagnosis can be made by CT in the clinical setting of acute cholecystitis. The differential diagnosis includes biliary-antral anastomosis from previous surgery, fistula secondary to gallstone erosion into bowel, and reflux of air through an incompetent sphincter of Oddi or following ERCP.

MR Acute Cholecystitis

The presence of gallstones and thickening of the gallbladder wall, associated with an ultrasound Murphy's sign, are typical signs of acute cholecystitis. However, these signs lack both sensitivity and specificity, and the diagnosis, especially of acalculous acute cholecystitis, remains difficult. MRI can demonstrate the presence of gallstones and gallbladder wall thickening sometimes associated with intramural abscesses or pericholecystic fluid (Fig. 6.14) [41]. However, in addition to this morphological information, MRI can provide data on the chemical composition of the bile and the vascularization of the gallbladder wall.

Pathophysiologically, in acute cholecystitis the water content of the gallbladder bile is higher than in either chronic cholecystitis or normal states [42]. This results in a decrease in signal intensity of the gallbladder bile on T1-weighted sequences.

In summary, although US has the advantage over all other imaging techniques in that it can accurately localize the patient's pain with the ultrasound transducer (ultrasound Murphy's sign), and is the most sensitive technique in gallstone detection, MRI can also demonstrate classic morphological features of acute cholecystitis. In addition, the relative liver/gallbladder bile signal

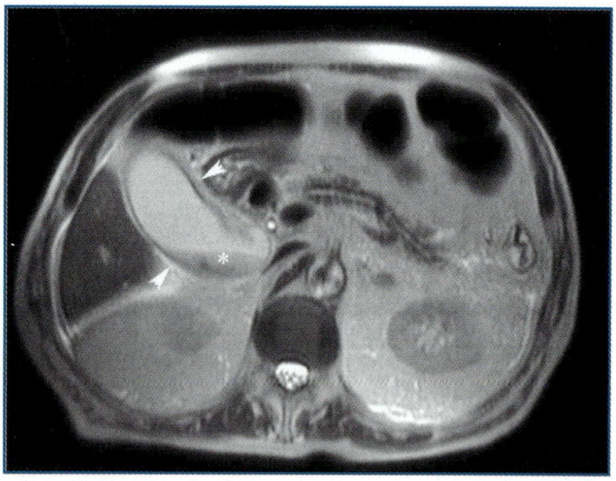

Fig. 6.14 Cholecystitis: magnetic resonance (MR) image. On an axial T2-weighted image, the gallbladder is well distended with endoluminal sludge and debris (*asterisk*) and thickened walls (*arrowheads*)

intensity ratio may be significantly decreased on T1-weighted sequences in patients with acute cholecystitis, compared to that of patients with chronic cholecystitis or normal gallbladders. The percentage of contrast enhancement of the gallbladder wall is also higher in patients with acute cholecystitis.

Mirizzi Syndrome

Mirizzi syndrome is a rare benign cause of obstructive jaundice that results from a stone impacted in either Hartmann's pouch or the cystic duct, thereby causing obstruction of the common hepatic duct (Fig. 6.15) [43, 44].

The Mirizzi syndrome subclassification [45] is based on the results and data from ERCP that indicates that constant pressure from within could create a fistulous communication between the gallbladder and the bile duct. Mirizzi syndrome is consequently divided into two groups: Type I is characterized by simple compression of the common hepatic duct, whereas Type II is defined by the presence of a cholecystocholedochal fistula.

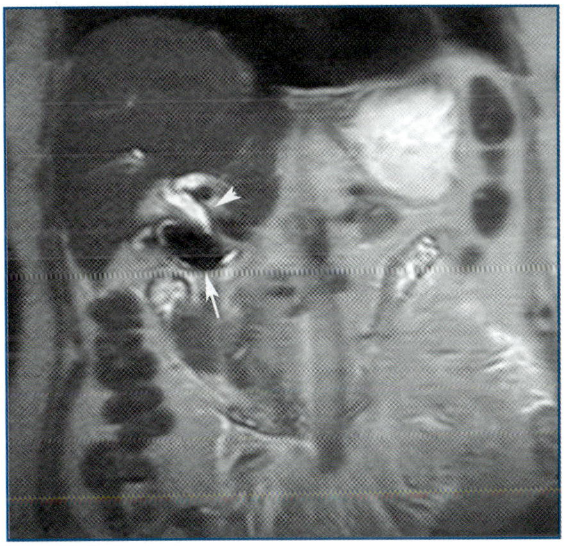

Fig. 6.15 Mirizzi syndrome: magnetic resonance (MR) imaging and magnetic resonance cholangiopancreatography (MRCP). On coronal T2-weighted MR image a hypointense stone can be observed within the gallbladder lumen, impacted in the gallbladder neck (*arrow*), responsible for stenosis of the common bile duct, as shown on the coronal T2-weighted and MRCP images (*arrowhead*)

The ultrasonographic findings of bile duct dilation associated with a contracted gallbladder and stone in the CBD may indicate the presence of the second type of Mirizzi syndrome.

Choledocholithiasis

Choledocholithiasis is a common complication of cholelithiasis. The reported incidence of CBD stones in patients undergoing cholecystectomy varies between 4 and 7% but may be as high as 33% in high-risk groups, such as patients over 80 years of age. CBD stones are far more difficult to detect and result in greater morbidity and mortality than stones within the gallbladder. Multiple imaging tests have been used to diagnose stones in the CBD. In patients with suspected biliary tract disease and jaundice, sonography is typically the initial imaging technique used. The reported sensitivity of sonography for detecting choledocholithiasis varies between approximately 20% [46] and 80% [47]. Traditionally, ERCP was the gold standard for investigation for bile duct diseases, but its role is now limited to therapeutic use. Improved safety profiles means that MR cholangiography [48, 49] and endoscopic sonography have replaced ERCP for the diagnosis of bile duct stones.

Although CT is not the imaging technique of choice for patients with clinical suspicion of choledocholithiasis, it is commonly used in patients with jaundice, abnormal liver function test results, or other symptoms possibly related to the biliary tract. Previous studies have reported the performance of CT using different techniques for showing CBD stones.

These include incremental [50] and helical CT [51–53] acquired both with [51] and without the addition of an intravenous contrast agent [53]. Reported sensitivities have ranged from 20% [54] to as high as 88% [52].

US Choledocholithiasis

Common bile duct stones are identified by the presence of echogenic material within the duct. Stones may be a few millimeters to 2–3 cm in size (Fig. 6.16). They may be obstructive, nonobstructive, or cause only intermittent obstruction. They can be located anywhere in the common duct, but are most often found in the intrapancreatic duct, where they may be associated with dilation of Wirsung's duct [34].

In most series the lowest values are reported for detecting stones in the intrapancreatic bile duct and stones in nondilated ducts. Air in the duodenal lumen, lack of bile surrounding the stone within the duct, absence of distal acoustic shadowing, calcifications in the pancreatic head and undilated common duct containing stones, are conditions that increase difficulties in CBD stone detections. Air in the duodenal lumen may impede ultrasonographic demonstration of stones in the more distal portion of the common duct [34]. Air can be displaced by a water load. Air in the CBD after sphincterotomy or biliaryenteric anastomosis can obstruct visualization of the main bile duct or mimic the presence of stones. This artifact can be eliminated by changing the decubitus of the patient.

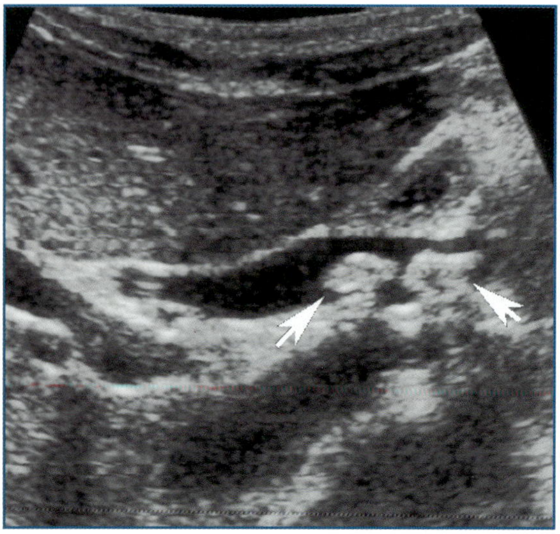

Fig. 6.16 Choledocholithiasis: sonography. On sonographic scan the common bile duct is slightly dilated with endoluminal stones (*arrows*)

There is a natural contrast between echo-free bile and hyperechoic stones in the intrapancreatic duct, and if bile is lacking, the stone is more difficult to perceive, because it is surrounded by glandular parenchyma and tissue-stone contrast is less than bile-stone contrast. Sometimes the common duct, if filled by a large number of stones, may produce a highly reflective image with a distal acoustic shadow that can be misdiagnosed as gas in the duodenum.

Absence of distal acoustic shadowing can occur in about 10% of cases, especially when stones are in the distal portion of the common duct. It maybe due to the stone content (most CBD stones are cholesterol and pigment stones, with little or no calcium) or to technical factors such as transducer frequency gain setting and reflection/refraction of the ultrasound by the duct walls [3]. It is extremely difficult to distinguish a stone without a distal acoustic shadow from blood clots, neoplasms, or sludge.

Calcifications in the pancreatic head, due to chronic pancreatitis or calcified arterial vessels, if located along the course of the bile duct, may simulate stones.

Undilated common duct-containing stones are reported to be present in about 25% of cases of acute biliary obstruction [34], and are considered to be due to the so-called "ball-valve effect", where the intermittent nature of the obstruction prevents the bile duct from becoming dilated. Another reason that ductal dilation may be absent in choledocholithiasis is that the examination is performed early after the acute onset of symptoms, in the "temporal lag" between obstruction and dilation.

CT Choledocholithiasis

Identification of bile duct stones by CT depends more on chemical composition than does identification by sonography. Calcium bilirubinate stones are fairly easily seen as dense white filling defects ringed with bile (Fig. 6.17) [55, 56]. Most other pigment and cholesterol stones with calcium rims are also seen by CT. Small stones, pigment stones with little calcification, and pure cholesterol bile duct stones may be impossible to differentiate from bile, especially if no bile duct dilatation is present. About 75% of biliary stones can be identified by CT using narrow collimation and contiguous sections [50].

Identification of bile duct stones by CT requires direct visualization of the stone. The stone is seen as a calcified filling defect, usually surrounded by bile at the upper curved edge of the stone. The cross-sectional appearance has been called the target sign [57]. More distally the stone may fill the entire duct. Patients with bile duct stones are more likely to have gradual tapering of the CBD than abrupt termination. Abrupt termination of the bile duct is more common in malignancy, with some overlap. Enhancement of the wall of the CBD can be seen in many inflammatory and neoplastic conditions. This wall enhancement should not be confused with calcification of an impacted duct stone [57].

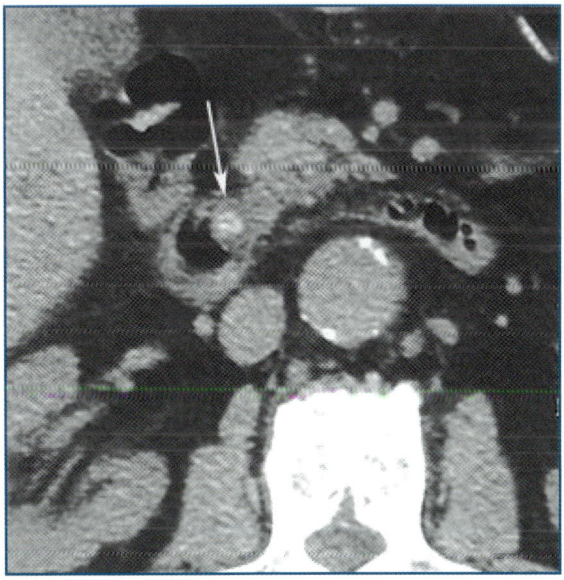

Fig. 6.17 Choledocholithiasis: computed tomography. Axial computed tomography shows a hyperdense stone within the lumen of the common bile duct, impacted in the papilla (*arrow*)

MR Choledocholithiasis

Although sonography and CT are often used in the initial evaluation of patients with suspected choledocholithiasis, neither has a high sensitivity for the detection of CBD stones. Specifically, the sensitivity of sonography for detecting common duct stones ranges from 18 to 70% [46]. This variability in sensitivity is due in part to the operator-dependent nature of sonography and obscuration of the bile duct by bowel gas. The sensitivity of CT for detecting common duct stones ranges from 76 to 87% [46, 50]. Until the advent of MRCP, many patients with suspected choledocholithiasis and a negative sonogram or CT underwent diagnostic ERCP. Although ERCP yields high-resolution images of the biliary tract and provides access for therapeutic intervention, it is invasive and consequently is associated with complications such as pancreatitis, hemorrhage, gastrointestinal tract perforation, and sepsis in approximately 5% of patients [58]. In fact, pancreatitis occurs in up to 1.8–5% of all attempts, and may range in severity from subclinical to life threatening [58, 59]. MRCP provides a noninvasive means of detecting CBD stones. For MRCP to be accepted as an alternative to diagnostic ERCP, however, its sensitivity and specificity in the setting of suspected choledocholithiasis must at least equal to those of ERCP. The determination of the sensitivity and specificity of ERCP in the diagnosis of choledocholithiasis is difficult because ERCP is considered the standard of reference for CBD stone detection. In an analysis of 72 patients studied with intraoperative cholangiography and ERCP, Frey et al. [59] found a sensitivity of 90% and a specificity of 98% for ERCP in the setting of choledocholithiasis. Early studies focusing on the role of MRCP in the detection of CBD stones yielded sensitivities ranging from 81 to 92% and specificities ranging from 91 to 100% [9, 11]. Technical advances resulting in improvements in signal-to-noise and spatial resolution and in minimization of motion artefacts have further enhanced the MRCP diagnosis of choledocholithiasis. Recent studies note sensitivities of 90–100% and specificities of 92–100%, matching and, in most cases, exceeding those of ERCP [10, 12, 48]. Positive predictive values range from 96–100% [10, 12, 48]. Equally important as the sensitivity, specificity, and positive predictive value of MRCP is its negative predictive value, which ranges from 96 to 100% [11, 13, 49]. Therefore, if an MRCP is interpreted as negative for common duct stones then one can avoid the performance of a diagnostic ERCP in most cases. At MRCP, CBD stones are seen as low signal intensity filling defects in the high signal intensity bile

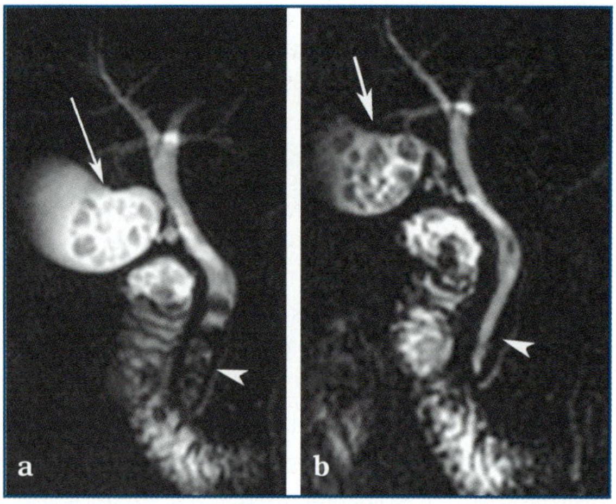

Fig. 6.19 Choledocholithiasis: magnetic resonance cholangiopancreatography (MRCP). **a** Coronal MRCP shows endoluminal filling defects within the lumen of the gallbladder (*arrow*). Multiple stones are present also within the lumen of the distal third of the common bile duct (*arrowhead*). **b** After sphincterotomy, the choledocholithiasis is removed (*arrowhead*)

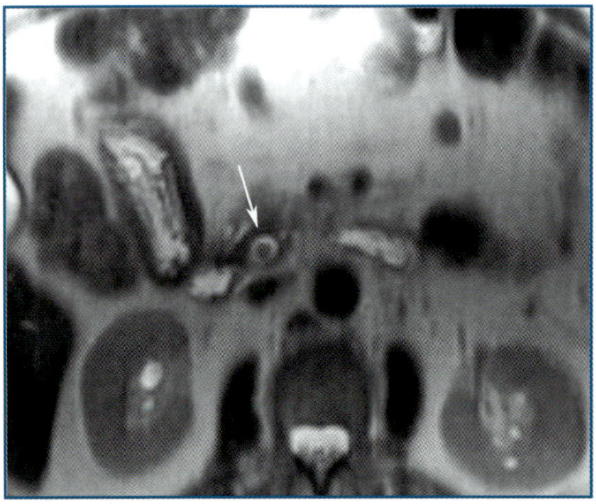

Fig. 6.18 Choledocholithiasis: magnetic resonance imaging. On axial T2-weighted image there is an endoluminal filling defect within the center of the lumen of the common bile duct: the "target sign"

(Figs. 6.18, 6.19). MCRP is accurate not only in the detection and exclusion of common duct stones but also in determining their number, size, and location. With current techniques, common duct stones as small as 2 mm can be detected with MRCP [9, 10]. At times, it is necessary to alter the angle of acquisition to optimize detection of small stones. MRCP is able to detect stones in dilated ducts and in nondilated ducts. Although MRCP provides an accurate, noninvasive means of detecting and excluding choledocholithiasis, one must be aware of mimickers of ductal calculi. These include pneumobilia, compression of the duct by an adjacent vessel, and en face visualization of the cystic duct as it enters the extrahepatic bile duct [60].

References

1. Bortoff GA, Chen MY, Ott DJ et al (2000) Gallbladder stones: imaging and intervention. Radiographics 20:751-766

2. Nakayama F (1982) Intrahepatic calculi. A special problem in East Asia. World J Surg 6:802
3. Irving HC, Bates L (1993) Bile duct pathology. In: Cosgrave D, Meire H, Dewbury K (eds) Abdominal and general ultrasound, vol 1. Edinburgh, Churchill Livingstone, pp 172-184
4. Sauerbrei EE, Nguyen KT, Nolan RL (eds) (1992) Abdominal sonography. New York, Raven, pp 51-72
5. Kim YK, Kim CS, Lee JM et al (2006) Value of adding T1-weighted image to MR cholangiopancreatography for detecting intrahepatic biliary stones. AJR Am J Roentgenol 187:267-274
6. Teplick SK, Flick P, Brandon JC (1991) Transhepatic cholangiography in patients with suspected biliary disease and non-dilated intrahepatic bile ducts. Gastrointest Radiol 16:193-197
7. Bilbao MK, Dotter CT, Lee TG, Katon RM (1976) Complications of endoscopic retrograde cholangiopancreatography (ERCP): a study of 10,000 cases. Gastroenterology 70:314-320
8. Lenriot JP, Le Neel JC, Hay JM et al (1993) Retrograde cholangiopancreatography and endoscopic sphincterotomy for biliary lithiasis. Prospective evaluation in surgical circle. Gastroenterol Clin Biol 17:244-250
9. Guibaud L, Bret PM, Reinhold C et al (1995) Bile duct obstruction and choledocholithiasis: diagnosis with MR cholangiography. Radiology 197:109-115
10. Fulcher AS, Turner MA, Capps GW et al (1998) Half-Fourier RARE MR cholangiopancreatography: experience in 300 subjects. Radiology 207:21-32
11. Becker CD, Grossholz M, Becker M et al (1997) Choledocholithiasis and bile duct stenosis: accuracy of MR cholangiopancreatography. Radiology 205:523-530
12. Reinhold C, Taourel P, Bret PM et al (1998) Choledocholithiasis: evaluation of MR cholangiography for diagnosis. Radiology 209:435-442
13. Chan YL, Chan AC, Lam WW et al (1996) Choledocholithiasis: comparison of MR cholangiography and endoscopic retrograde cholangiography. Radiology 200:85-89
14. Soto JA, Barish MA, Yucel EK et al (1996) Magnetic resonance cholangiography: comparison with endoscopic retrograde cholangiopancreatography. Gastroenterology 110:589-597
15. Kim TK, Kim BS, Kim JH et al (2002) Diagnosis of intrahepatic stones: superiority of MR cholangiopancreatography over endoscopic retrograde cholangiopancreatography. AJR Am J Roentgenol 179:429-434
16. Motohara T, Semelka RC, Bader TR (2003) MR cholangiopancreatography. Radiol Clin North Am 41:89-96
17. Barish MA, Yucel EK, Ferrucci JT (1999) Magnetic resonance cholangiopancreatography. N Engl J Med 341:258-264
18. Mitchell DG, Alam F (1999) Mangafodipir trisodium: effects on T2- and T1-weighted MR cholangiography. J Magn Reson Imaging 9:366-368
19. Vitellas KM, El-Dieb A, Vaswani KK et al (2002) Using contrast-enhanced MR cholangiography with IV mangafodipir trisodium (Teslascan) to evaluate bile duct leaks after cholecystectomy: a prospective study of 11 patients. AJR Am J Roentgenol 179:409-416
20. Marchal G, Ni Y, Zhang X et al (1993) Mn-DPDP enhanced MRI in experimental bile duct obstruction. J Comput Assist Tomogr 17:290-296
21. Sheppard D, Allan L, Martin P et al (2004) Contrast-enhanced magnetic resonance cholangiography using mangafodipir compared with standard T2W MRC sequences: a pictorial essay. J Magn Reson Imaging 20:256-263
22. Cooperberg PL, Gibney RC (1987) Imaging of the gallbladder. Radiology 163:605-613
23. MacDonald FR, Cooperberg PL, Cohen MM (1981) The WES Triad: a specific sonographic sign of gallstones in the contracted gallbladder. Gastrointest Radiol 6:39-41
24. Nemcek AA, Gore RM, Vogelzang R et al (1988) The effervescent gallbladder: a sonographic sign of emphysematous cholecystitis. AJR Am J Roentgenol 150:575-577
25. Kane RA, Jacobs R, Katz J et al (1985) Porcelain gallbladder: ultrasound and CT appearance. Radiology 154:769-770
26. Bova JG, Schwesinger WH, Kurtin WE (1992) In vivo analysis of gallstone composition by computed tomography. Gastrointest Radiol 17:253-256
27. Liu YL, Wang JT (2006) Hyperplastic cholecystoses: efforts should be made to recognize and treat them. Hepatobiliary Pancreat Dis Int 5:334-336
28. Rapaccini GL, Pompili M, Caturelli E (1993) Colecisti e vie biliari. In: Poletto F (ed) Trattato italiano di ecografia, vol 1. Milan, Società Italiana di Ultrasonologia in Medicina e Biologia, pp 271-295
29. Berk RN, Van Der Vegt JH, Lichtenstein JE (1983) The hyperplastic cholecystoses: cholesterolosis and adenomyomatosis. Radiology 146:593-601
30. Kidney MR, Goiney R, Cooperberg PL (1986) Adenomyomatosis of the gallbladder: a pictorial exhibit. J Ultrasound Med 5:331-333
31. Fowler RC, Reid WW (1988) Ultrasound diagnosis of adenomyomatosis of the gallbladder: ultrasonic and pathological correlation. Clin Radiol 39:402-406
32. De Albertis P, Quadri D, Serafini G, Cajano A (1995) Le lesioni benigne e maligne delta parete

delta colecisti. In: Gnocchi G (ed) Colecisti. Naples, Liviana Medicina, pp 57-72
33. Bazzocchi M, Pozzi-Mucelli RS, Brizzi F et al (1984) Aspects echographiques des maladies infiammatories de la vesicule biliarie. J Fr Echo 1:23-28
34. Laing FC, Jeffrey RB Jr (1983) Choledocholithiasis and cystic duct obstruction: difficult ultrasonographic diagnosis. Radiology 146:475-479
35. Filly RA, Allen B, Minton MJ (1980) In vitro investigation of the origin of echoes within biliary sludge. J Clin Ultrasound 8:193-200
36. Nemcek A, Gore RM, Vogelzang RL, Grant M (1988) The effervescent gallbladder: a sonographic sign of emphysematous cholecystitis. AJR Am J Roentgenol 150:575-577
37. Romano Al, Van Sonnenberg E, Casola G et al (1988) Gallbladder and bile duct abnormalities in AIDS: sonographic findings in eight patients. AJR Am J Roentgenol 150:123-127
38. Gryspeerdt S, Van Hoe L, Marchal G, Baert AL (1995) Imaging of hepatic perfusion disorders with double phase spiral CT. Radiology 193:511
39. Blankenberg F, Wirth R, Brooke Jeffrey R (1991) Computed tomography as an adjunct to ultrasound in the diagnosis of acute acalculous cholecystitis. Gastrointest Radiol 16:149-153
40. Kim PN, Lee KS, Bae WK, Lee BH (1994) Gallbladder perforation: comparison of US findings with CT. Abdom Imaging 19:239-242
41. Weissleder R, Stark DD, Compton CC et al (1988) Cholecystitis: diagnosis by MR imaging. Magn Reson Imaging 6:345-348
42. Svanik J, Thornell E, Zettergren L (1981) Gallbladder function in experimental cholecystitis. Surgery 89:500-506
43. Johnson LW, Sehon JK, Lee WC et al (2001) Mirizzi's syndrome: experience from a multi-institutional review. Am Surg 67:11-4
44. Haritopoulos KN, Labruzzo C, Tayar AR et al (2002) Mirizzi syndrome: a case report and review of the literature. Int Surg 87:65-68
45. McSherry CK, Fertenberg H, Virshup M (1982) The Mirizzi syndrome: suggested classification and surgical therapy. Surg Gastroenterol 1:219-225
46. Mitchell S, Clark R (1984) A comparison of computed tomography and sonography in choledocholithiasis. AJR Am J Roentgenol 142:729-733
47. Wermke W, Schulz HJ (1987) Sonographic diagnosis of bile duct calculi: results of a prospective study of 222 cases of choledocholithiasis [in German]. Ultraschall Med 8:116-120
48. Soto JA, Alvarez O, Munera F et al (2000) Diagnosing bile duct stones: comparison of unenhanced helical CT, oral contrast-enhanced CT cholangiography and MR cholangiography. AJR Am J Roentgenol 175:1127-1134
49. Griffin N, Wastle ML, Dunn WK et al (2003) Magnetic resonance cholangiopancreatography versus endoscopic retrograde cholangiopancreatography in the diagnosis of choledocholithiasis. Eur J Gastroenterol Hepatol 15:809-813
50. Baron RL (1987) Common bile duct stones: reassessment of criteria for CT diagnosis. Radiology 162:419-424
51. Miller FH, Hwang CM, Gabriel H et al (2003) Contrast-enhanced helical CT of choledocholithiasis. AJR Am J Roentgenol 181:125-130
52. Neitlich J, Topazian M, Smith RC et al (1997) Detection of choledocholithiasis: comparison of unenhanced helical CT and endoscopic retrograde cholangiopancreatography. Radiology 203:753-757
53. Jimenez CI, del Olmo LM, Perez HM (2001) Helical CT without contrast in choledocholithiasis. Eur Radiol 11:197-201
54. Pasanen P, Partanen K, Pikkarainen P et al (1992) Ultrasonography, CT and ERCP in the diagnosis of choledochal stones. Acta Radiol 33:53-56
55. Baron RL, Stanley RJ, Lee JKT et al (1982) A prospective comparison of the evaluation of biliary obstruction using computed tomography and ultrasonography. Radiology 145:91-98
56. Jeffrey RB Jr, Federle MP, Laing FC et al (1983) Computed tomography of choledocholithiasis. AJR Am J Roentgenol 140:1179-1183
57. Baron RL, Tublin ME, Peterson MS (2002) Imaging the spectrum of biliary tract disease. Radiol Clin N Am 40:1325-1354
58. Masci E, Toti G, Mariani A et al (2001) Complications of diagnostic and therapeutic ERCP: a prospective multicenter study. Am J Gastroentrol 96:417- 23
59. Frey CF, Burbige EJ, Meinke WB et al (1982) Endoscopic retrograde cholangiopancreatography. Am J Surg 144:109-114
60. Watanabe Y, Dohke M, Ishimori T et al (2000) Pseudo-obstruction of the extrahepatic bile duct due to artefact from arterial pulsatile compression: a diagnostic pitfall of MR cholangiopancreatography. Radiology 214:856-860

Chapter 7

Three-dimensional Imaging

Luc Soler, Ronan Cahill, Jacques Marescaux

Introduction

Modern medical imaging provides essential preoperative knowledge of patient anatomy and pathology. This imaging is composed of many kinds of techniques and protocols, the choice of which is fully dependent on the targeted structures that practitioners want to see and analyse. Virtual reality can then be used to facilitate interpretation. Virtual reality is based on three main concepts: immersion, navigation and interaction (Fig. 7.1). Immersion is a mental concept consisting of the feeling of being inside a virtual world visualized on a screen or using immersive devices such as a realistic environment or a head mounted display. Navigation is a concept that allows the virtual world to be traversed. Finally, interaction is a physical concept that allows modification of the properties of the virtual world. These concepts were initially developed for aeronautic simulators and have more recently been extended to computer games, which represent their main market. Applied to medicine, they allow an easier and more extensive visualization and exploitation of medical images. Such an improvement is essentially based on the three dimensional (3D) visualization of patient anatomy from medical images. We will describe how it is possible to use these concepts on the basis of medical images and especially in biliary lithiasis images through a virtual 3D cholangioscopy.

Current 2D-3D Medical Imaging of Biliary Lithiasis

Diagnosis and management algorithms for choledocholithiasis remain controversial.

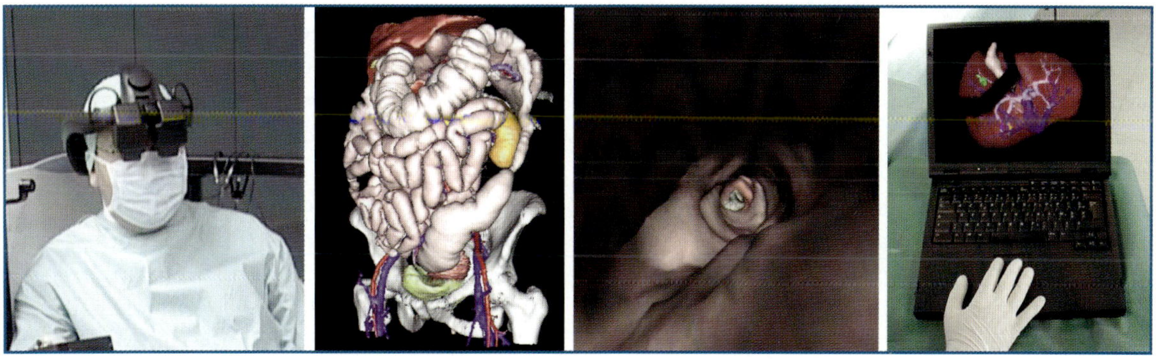

Fig. 7.1 Virtual reality concepts used in medicine (ULIS and 3D VSP ©ircad). Immersion (*left*) is the feeling of being surrounded by a virtual world; navigation (*center*) is being able to go anywhere inside the virtual world; interaction (*right*) is the ability to interactively modify the virtual world

The main medical imaging systems are ultrasound, endoscopic retrograde cholangiopancreatography (ERCP), intra-operative cholangiography (IOC), cholangiocomputerized tomography (CCT), and magnetic resonance cholangiopancreatography (MRCP) [1–3]. These medical image protocols have all been proposed by different teams but without any evidence-based proof owing to accept a definitive strategy for diagnosis. However, it currently seems that MRCP and CCT are more accurate only in staging malignant stenosis [4], with CCT providing a better accuracy, sensitivity and specificity in the diagnosis of lithiasis [4]. Furthermore, preoperative performing of these imaging techniques does not allow to consider spontaneous migration of stones, as it can clearly be demonstrated with intra-operative cholangiography leading then to perform useless procedures which have own risk of morbidity and mortality [5]. These limits stress the need for newer tools and/or strategies that ensure both high diagnostic accuracy and reduced invasiveness. Therefore, there is an objective clinical interest in virtual cholangioscopy due to its potential to obtain high diagnostic accuracy without being invasive.

Currently, efforts to define precise predictive criteria for the presence of common bile duct (CBD) stones are frequently hampered by methodological pitfalls. Preoperatively, surgeons have to choose between transabdominal ultrasonography, endoscopic ultrasonography, computerized tomography (CT) and MRCP, all of which carry a failure rate between 5 and 10% [6]. Performing systematic preoperative ERCP has not gained wide acceptance as it is associated with a morbidity and mortality rate from 3 to 6.4% and 0.2 to 0.8%, respectively [7], with specific severe complications including pancreatitis and perforation. Additionally, ultrasound, CT and magnetic resonance imaging (MRI) are purely diagnostic, whereas ERCP offers the opportunity of therapeutic intervention if needed. Many teams perform routine IOC, but since the advent of laparoscopy, IOCs have been associated with errors in performance [8] or interpretation, and up to 30% of films were not able to render a diagnosis, leading to a mean false positive rate between 2 and 19%, and a false negative rate of 2–3% [7–9]. Therefore, systematic IOC still remains controversial. Its major benefit seems to lie in the identification of CBD injury rather than the 5–10% incidence of identification of unsuspected CBD stones [10].

Many authors have proposed preoperative MRCP as an alternative strategy for detecting the presence of choledocholithiasis. The sensitivity and specificity of MRI have been reported to be 88.9% and 100%, respectively [7]; however, much of the potential of MRI is lost because of limited interpretation of the greyscale. Theoretically, more than 2000 different shades of grey from pure white to pure black are generated with MRI, each corresponding to a specific digital value [11, 12]. In practice, however, the number of shades of grey that the human eye can distinguish on a monitor or a radiographic film does not exceed 256 [11, 13–15], thus a radiologist's basis of interpretation is limited by the biology of human vision. Hence, a large amount of potentially useful information is not considered. The software developed at our institute is able to incorporate all of the digital 'greys' generated by MRI to automatically detect polyps, stones or abnormalities of the duct. The data are analyzed to distinguish noise or artifacts from usable data using a filtering system called anisotropic diffusion [16]. The software performs automatic thresholding, which in turn allows for a completely automated reconstruction of the biliary tree and hepatic structures [17]. From this perspective, 3D reconstructions seem to have an advantage over conventional imaging, and indeed, our prospective results support this idea as evidenced by the higher sensitivity we found with the 3D reconstructions. Virtual reality reconstructions admittedly have some limitations. The most important disadvantage is that they are based on the original MRI data and therefore, despite improvements in data analysis performed by the software, the limitations of MRCP in detecting stones less than 5 mm or stones present in the last portion of the CBD over the papillary sphincter remain, even with 3D reconstruction. A stone located in the terminal 5 mm of the CBD is the most difficult to identify [18, 19]. Likewise, a CBD less than 3 mm in diameter and the presence of a short stenosis or aerobilia may lead to difficult identification. In this study [17], in three cases of false negative results from MRCP, 3D cholangioscopy suggested the presence of a choledocholithiasis. In all these patients, stones were located at the third inferior part of the CBD; in all three patients also, IOC and/or ERCP confirmed the findings of the 3D imaging, leading to successful stone extraction. The size varied from 1.5 cm in two of the cases to less than 0.5 mm in the other case. These findings confirm the reported higher incidence of failure in detecting stones in the most inferior part of the CBD when using MRCP; a lower efficacy in the last third of the CMD is also a possible drawback of our 3D cholangioscopy, as the reconstruction depends on data acquired through the MRCP. This is also suggested by the findings that all false negatives in 3D virtual cholangioscopy occurred in patients with stones in the inferior third of the CBD. Moreover, the 3D cholangioscopy had less false negatives than MRCP and even detected stones smaller than 0.5 mm (which were missed at the MRCP), thus suggesting that the virtual cholangioscopy may improve outcomes of MRCP, and approach the accuracy of more invasive methods. Furthermore, the need for a routine MRI could be criticized as being both expensive and an over-utilization of available resources. In fact, hospital charges for an MRI have been reported as $361,000 in France [20], where this study was conducted, and $1,145,000 in the United States [21]. Although routine MRI may be too expensive to justify, selected performance of MRI with biliary tree reconstruction may gain legitimacy when weighed against the relative cost of a biliary tree injury during a cholecystectomy, which has been reported to have a mean value of $51,411 [22], with mean legal costs at $507,000 [23]. If using 3D reconstruction could prevent even a small number of biliary tract injuries by preoperative identification of anatomic variations, it may actually turn out to be cost-effective. The rationale advocated by centers that practice routine IOC is often that IOC provides information regarding potential anatomic hazards that may subsequently prevent a biliary tract injury, which has been reported to affect around 2,000 patients annually in the United States [24]. Centers that do not practice routine IOC may argue that these injuries are often associated with the performance of the IOC itself, and the study therefore only serves to identify the injury [10]. If a virtual cholangioscopy based on MRI could eliminate the need for routine use of an invasive procedure, and thereby decrease the incidence of biliary tract injuries, one may see a very large decrease in costs. Indeed, the problem of costs related to the implementation of all new technologies may seem discouraging at first glance, but a more comprehensive evaluation of the possible clinical advantages may reveal them to be an opportunity for cost-saving. Moreover, virtual reality is today more and more compatible with standard low-cost personal computers thanks to the development of 3D games. The extra cost of this new technology will then be reduced to a minimum.

From Medical Image to Virtual Patient

The most standard 3D visualization method is direct volumetric rendering [25]. This technique, available on all current imaging systems (MRI or CT scans), can be sufficient for a good 3D visualization of anatomical and pathological structures (Fig. 7.2). It consists of replacing the standard slice view by the visualization of all slices together in 3D. In order to see internal structures, the initial grey level is replaced by an associated colour and transparency. This transparency gives the impression of delineated organs that in reality are not delineated. Indeed, with this technique organ and pathology volume are not available and it is not possible to perform a virtual resection of an organ without cutting the entire surrounding structure. To overcome this limit, each anatomical and pathological structure in the medical image has to be delineated. From the delineated structure a 3D mesh can be created and exported for its visualization in conventional 3D formats such as X3D or VRML. Such a delineation is a long and difficult manual task for radiologists using standard software. Therefore, several research teams have developed automated 3D patient modeling softwares that can interactively or automatically provide the main visible organs from CT scans or MRI [26–30]. We have developed several 3D patient modeling softwares that automatically or interactively provide the main visible organs from CT scans or MRI for the digestive area [31, 32]. Our latest software, 3D Virtual Patient Modelling (*3D VPM ©IRCAD 2006*), also allows 3D modeling of the thoracic or pelvis area to be performed thanks to an improved management of medical knowledge combined with an interactive process [33–35] (Fig. 7.2). The main interest of such modeling is to obtain a surface rendering that will work on all current low-cost computers using an Open GL graphic card.

Several companies propose today such 3D modeling as an online remote service by delivering a DICOM image mainly for dental pathologies, but also more recently for the digestive area (MeVis Distant Services AG, PolyDimensions GmbH). These services are currently not adapted to biliary lithiasis pathologies and provide in the best case a 3D modeling of liver and gallbladder.

Since 2001 we have set up several collaborations with distant university hospitals (Geneva, Montreal and Strasbourg) in order to offer a similar experimental 3D modeling service named MEDIC@, which is not limited to a specific area. A total of 623 clinical cases have been modelled in 3D for the thoraco-abdominal area (Fig. 7.2), 64% being reconstructed for liver pathologies, among which 80 were specifically dedicated to biliary lithiasis for virtual cholangioscopy. Using this distant service, the radiological department can send their anonymous images in a DICOM format through a secured FTP connection to the 3D modeling department. This can be done manually or using the automated MEDIC@ consol that

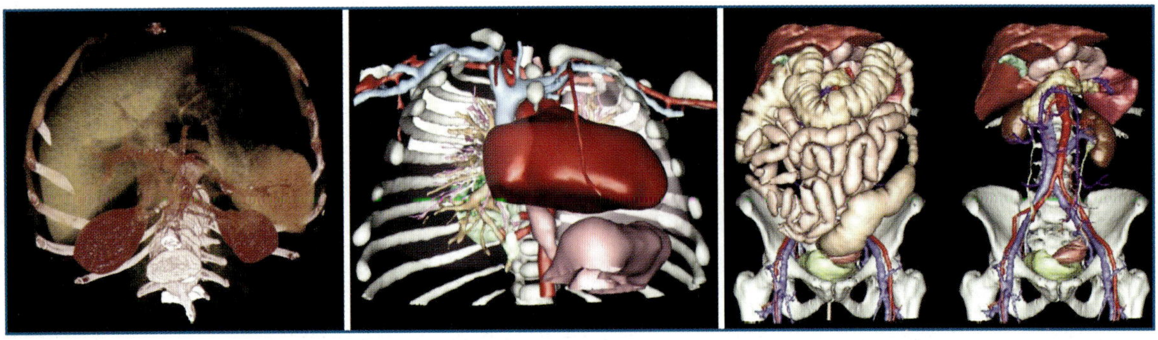

Fig. 7.2 From patient CT scans, samples of volume rendering (*left*) and 3D modeling of thorax (*center*) and abdomen (*right*) performed with 3D VPM © IRCAD 2006

can be installed in the radiological department and linked to the hospital network. In this last case, images are anonymized, encrypted and compressed in order to improve security and transfer speed. Once the IRCAD 3D modeling department has performed the 3D modeling, the hospital downloads the result on their own network. Like the MeVis Distant Services, this distant 3D modeling service efficiently provides an accurate 3D model of patient anatomy and pathology within a short time (between one and three days). In the case of biliary lithiasis, the 3D modeling is performed in only 7.5 minutes on average [32], the result being sent the same day to the distant user.

The results varied according to the initial protocol. From MRCP, the software provides a 3D model of the biliary tract, choledoc and gallbladder, thus allowing a virtual cholangioscopy. From CCT, the software provides a more complete 3D model, integrating the biliary tract, choledoc, gallbladder and also all surrounding anatomical structures such as liver, pancreas and duodenum (Fig. 7.3). From CCT, the different hepatic networks (arteries, portal veins, hepatic veins and biliary tract) are obtained in different acquisition times. It is then necessary to make a registration of these different times in order to obtain a complete 3D view of all networks, which is currently a complex and imprecise task that is not yet totally automated.

From 3D Visualization to Surgical Planning

3D modeling becomes more interesting if surface rendering can be accomplished on all current low-cost computers using an Open GL graphic card. For instance, an export of the surface through a VRML format allows an efficient visualization with any Internet Explorer software combined with a free VRML plug-in. Most of these can be freely installed for non-commercial use (FreeWRL, OpenVRML, CosmoPlayer, Cortona® © Parallel Graphics 2001-2007, Flux Player™ 2.0 © Media Machine 2007, Octaga player © Octaga AS 2001-2007). However, such visualization remains limited to a simple 3D visualization. The major teams developing 3D modeling software have developed specific surgical planning tools [36–38], but they remain specialized to liver segmentectomy and are not adapted for biliary lithiasis analysis. We have developed a specific software dedicated to all surgical applications [39]. 3D Virtual Surgical Planning (*3D VSP ©IRCAD 2003*) allows an optimal surgical strategy to be defined using the 3D-modelled patient. Furthermore, this system allows all structures to be made in transparency, to interact and navigate everywhere, thus allowing any kind of simulation (such as laparoscopy, colonoscopy, cholangioscopy, fibroscopy). It also allows virtual resections to be defined

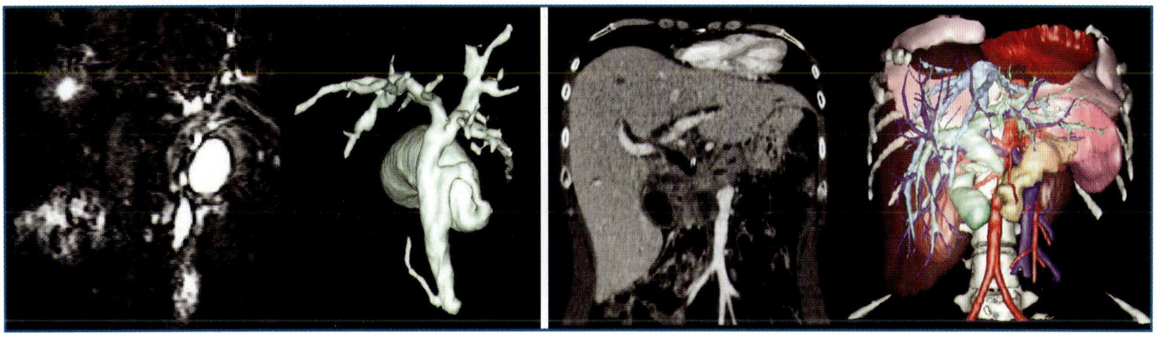

Fig. 7.3 3D modeling from MRCP (*left*) and CCT (*right*) show the biliary tract in green

by interactively positioned cutting planes, and provides the volume of all visualized structures (Fig. 7.4). Due to its compatibility with current standards, this system can be used on a laptop fitted with a 3D graphic card and can thus be used during the intervention to improve gesture control.

Used for biliary pathologies, this software creates a virtual reality environment where interactivity and navigation inside the lumen are feasible, allowing the user to perform a 3D virtual cholangioscopy [32]. It thus permits a virtual navigation in the biliary lumen, the visualization of internal structures such as stones, and an interactive distance and size computation (Fig. 7.5). The virtual navigation mode is composed of two windows providing the endoluminal view and a global external view of the biliary tract in transparency, allowing the position of the virtual endoscope in the lumen to be seen.

As shown in 65 clinical cases from MRCP imaging, an important feature of virtual reality technology is that the software generates a very accurate 3D reconstruction and avoids subjective human interpretation [32]. The software can make stone detection easier by making the differences in shape of the distal duct in normal versus abnormal situations more apparent. Furthermore, the combination and superimposition of conventional MR images on the 3D reconstruction with transparency views can also facilitate visualization during stone detection and virtual navigation.

An inherent advantage of using virtual reality is that the reconstruction is not just a better image, but a real 3D virtual representation. This means that one can be immersed

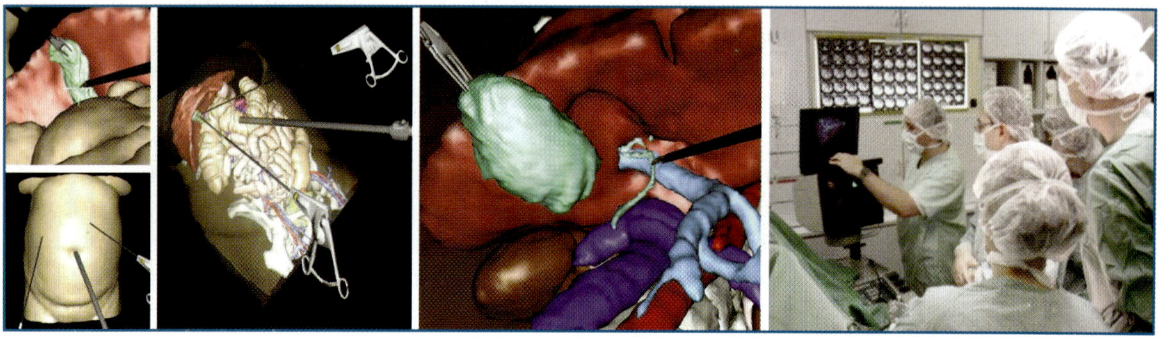

Fig. 7.4 Virtual laparoscopic tool positioning for cholecystectomy (*left*), virtual resection of a 3D reconstructed gallbladder from medical images (*center*) and intra-operative clinical use of the planning software on a laptop (*right*)

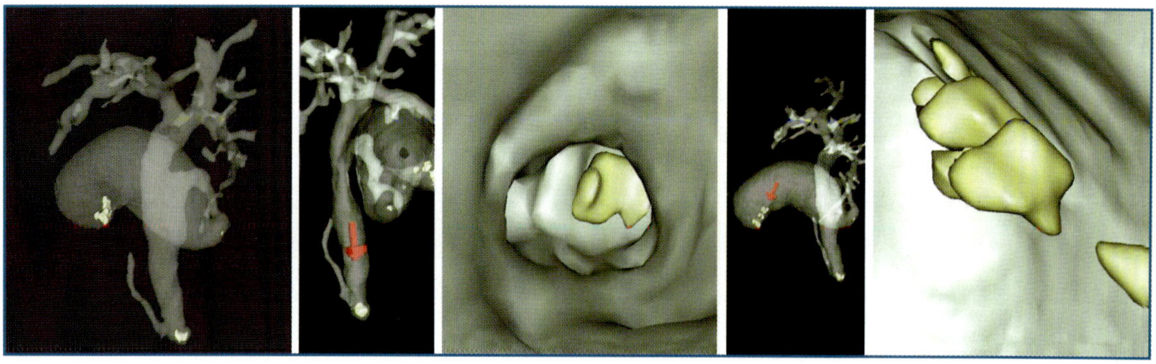

Fig. 7.5 Virtual cholangioscopy from MRCP. The virtual navigation provides two views allowing internal structures such as stones and the virtual endoscope position to be seen (*red arrow* in a transparent biliary tract)

in the image, navigate through the system and interact with the image. In the near future, interaction with the image will likely enable performance of virtual common bile duct surgery using actual patient data. The software is able to generate images much faster than conventional interpretation without concerns about the quality of the radiologist's interpretation. An image that is reconstructed with a high-speed computer can be accomplished in a few minutes and transmitted to the operating team. Although the generation of reconstructions requires a high-speed computer, reconstructions themselves can be displayed and manipulated on a standard laptop, which can also be brought to the operating room. Abnormalities should be easily identified by the operating surgeon, thus potentially reducing or eliminating the need for IOC, as well as facilitating the management of choledocholithiasis. An additional advantage is the ease of transmission of digital data to the operating room team or any other team in any location for consultation or collaboration almost immediately via the Internet. Finally, this preoperative tool can be used to plan the surgical procedure and thus to define the best operative strategy.

A further benefit would appear if these techniques could also provide preoperative training, an ability to evaluate surgeons through surgical simulators, and intra-operative computer-assistance to the surgical gesture. As we will now see, these future revolutions, currently developed and tested in research protocols, will soon be available.

Perspectives of 3D Imaging: from Patient-Specific Simulation to Augmented Reality

As we have seen, surgical planning allows the best operative strategy to be defined, but it does not provide the possibility of evaluating the surgeon's ability. This is the objective of realistic surgical simulators. To be efficient, these simulators have to reproduce sensations linked to operative gestures: realistic visual perception and realistic haptic rendering through force feedback. The most simulated surgeries are abdominal surgery, urology, gynecologic and arthroscopic procedures. Several companies propose virtual laparoscopic cholecytectomy: Surgical Science (www.surgical-science.com), Simbionix™ (www.simbionix.com), SimSurgery (www.simsurgery.no) and Haptica (www.haptica.com). The increasing realism of visual rendering, due to the use of textures obtained from real images, and progress in force feedback mechanisms have increased the quality of these products. All these simulators propose training exercises to learn basic gestures. Pedagogy follows a step-by-step training logic allowing the ultimate realization of more complex gestures, including a grading. Though they are attractive, these simulators are limited to the simulation of restricted and determined virtual models in a set database. Thus, they do not exploit the 3D modeling of patients that can be derived from the medical images, and do not allow a surgical intervention on a copy of the patient to be prepared.

The main idea of a patient-specific simulator is to offer surgeons the opportunity to carry out preclinical training on a virtual copy of the patient. There are thus two main steps: 3D modeling of the patient and patient-specific simulation. As previously seen, a 3D model of a patient can be locally reconstructed from the medical image of the patient, or through a web-based service. Furthermore, there is currently no preoperative patient-specific laparoscopic simulator. To overcome this limit, we are currently developing a simulator called ULIS (Unlimited Laparoscopic Immersive Simulator), in partnership with the Karl Storz Company. The objective of the first version is to be the first patient-specific laparoscopic basic skill training simulator using the Karl Storz Force Feedback System. This Force Feedback system is composed of two Force Feedback entry ports, allowing the introduction of Karl Storz instruments that are real surgical tools (Fig. 7.6).

This simulator uses 3D-modelled patients extracted from CT scan reconstructions that can be deformed locally with force feedback rendering when a virtual instrument is in contact with tissues. A photo-realistic texturing of tissues is performed interactively. ULIS includes camera and surgical instrument manipulation, and simulation of suction and coagulation procedures. Finally, the main advantage of this simulator is that it proposes a new vision of basic skills that are much closer to real laparoscopic surgery than existing ones, thanks to the use of real surgical instrumentation, patient-specific 3D models, photo-realistic rendering and realistic physical rendering including gravity (Fig. 7.7). The next step of this work will consist of developing a preoperative version, i.e, an automatic texturing of 3D modelled organs and the integration of the complete simulator engine SOFA [40], allowing multiple interactions for laparoscopic liver surgery including cholecystectomy.

Preoperative surgical planning and simulation will mainly improve the efficiency of Minimally Invasive Surgery (MIS) procedures thanks to preoperative familiarity with the patient's anatomy and real preoperative training. However, preoperative use of virtual reality is not sufficient to ensure safety during surgical procedures. Such an improvement can be provided by an intraoperative use of virtual reality through Augmented Reality (AR). Indeed, AR consists of superimposing the preoperative 3D patient model onto the real intraoperative patient view (Fig. 7.8). AR provides a transparent

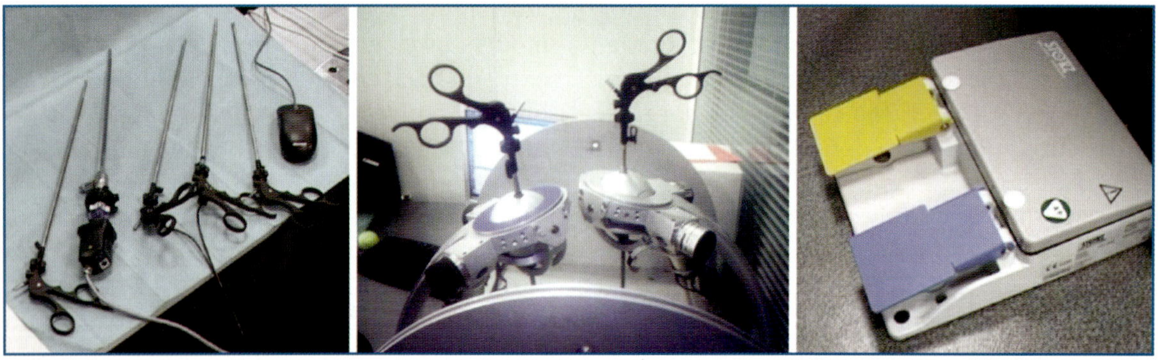

Fig. 7.6 The Karl Storz Force Feedback System for laparoscopic surgical simulation includes all surgical instruments

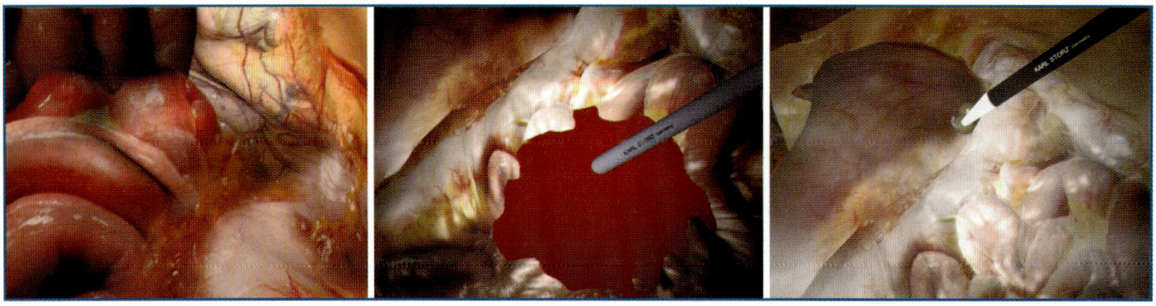

Fig. 7.7 Several screenshots of the ULIS simulator illustrating the laparoscope manipulation (*left*), a virtual blood injury in the bowel area (*center*) and a coagulation including smoke rendering (*right*)

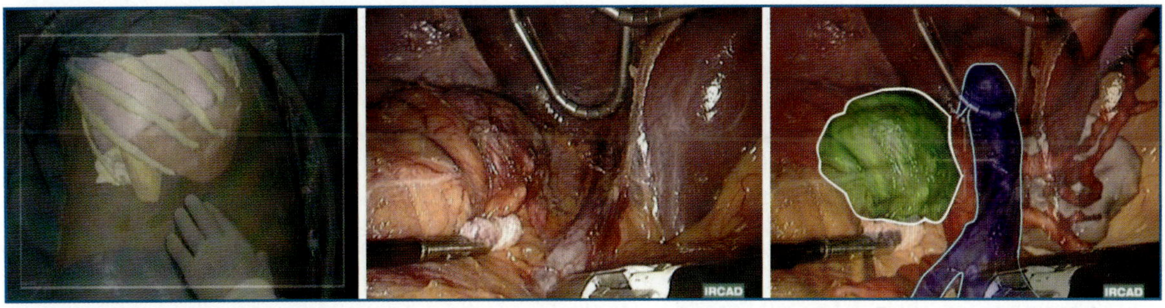

Fig. 7.8 AR makes MIS safer thanks to virtual transparency of vessels (the vena cava *in blue*), and pathologies (a tumor *in green*)

view of patients and can also guide surgeons thanks to the virtual improvement of their real surgical tools, which are tracked in real-time during the procedure. We have developed two kinds of AR software: interactive AR [41] and fully automatic AR [42, 43].

Interactive Augmented Reality is necessarily user-dependant due to manual positioning. Therefore, it is impossible to ensure accuracy for this first interesting image-guided surgical tool, which can only be used to gain a better understanding of patient anatomy using preoperative data. However, its drawback is also an advantage, due to the fact that any possible mistake from the automatic process can be manually corrected by the expert. Currently, for soft tissue or organs with large displacements, such techniques remain the easiest to apply. In the future, predictive simulation of organ motion will modify this state of the art technology by providing an efficient and accurate automatic registration of soft tissues and organs in movement. This next step of computer-assisted surgery will thus represent a revolutionary tool in any laparoscopic surgery.

Conclusion

3D Medical imaging has led to major progress in biliary lithiasis diagnosis, with MRCP and CCT being the two best modalities. From these imaging techniques, virtual reality concepts allow a new vision of the patient to be obtained thanks to the possibility of performing a virtual cholangioscopy. This virtual technology provides good sensitivity and specificity for diagnosis, and also permits the surgical procedure to be preoperatively planned, using the virtual copy of the patient. In the near future, the virtual model of the patient will also be included in preoperative surgical simulators, allowing the evaluation of surgery efficiency before the procedure. Moreover, AR will guide surgeons intra-operatively thanks to virtual transparency of the patient. This certainly represents the next revolution in biliary lithiasis therapy.

References

1. Millat B, Borie F (2000) Common bile duct stones and their complications. Rev Prat 50:2123-2129
2. Hugier M (2001) Prospective analysis of a scoring system to predict choledocholithiasis (Br J Surg 2000; 87:1176–1181). Br J Surg 88:314-315
3. Lincender L, Sadagic E, Vrcic D et al (2000) Magnetic resonance cholangiography in patients with bile duct obstruction. Radiol Oncol 34:319-324
4. Ferrari FS, Fantozzi F, Tasciotti L et al (2005) US, MRCP, CCT and ERCP: a comparative study in 131 patients with suspected biliary obstruction. Med Sci Monit 11(3): MT8-178
5. Yamakawa T, Sakai S, Mu ZB et al (2000) Laparoscopic management of common bile duct stones. J Hepatobiliary Pancreat Surg 7:9-14
6. Prat F, Meduri B, Ducot B et al (1999) Prediction

of common bile duct stones by noninvasive tests. Ann Surg 229:362-368
7. Tham TC, Lichtenstein DR, Vandervoort J et al (1998) Role of endoscopic retrograde cholangiopancreatography for suspected choledocholithiasis in patients undergoing laparoscopic cholecystectomy. Gastrointest Endosc 47:50-56
8. Ohtani T, Kawai C, Shirai Y et al (1997) Intra-operative ultrasonography versus cholangiography during laparoscopic cholecystectomy: a prospective comparative study. J Am Coll Surg 185:274-282
9. Cotton PB, Baillie J, Pappas TN et al (1991) Laparoscopic cholecystectomy and the biliary endoscopist. Editorial. Gastrointest Endosc 37:94-96
10. Falcone RA Jr, Fegelman EJ, Nussbaum MS et al (1999) A prospective comparison of laparoscopic ultrasound vs intra-operative cholangiogram during laparoscopic cholecystectomy. Surg Endosc 13:784-788
11. Sodickson DK, McKenzie CA, Ohliger MA et al (2002) Recent advances in image reconstruction, coil sensitivity calibration, and coil array design for SMASH and generalized parallel MRI. MAGMA 13:158-163
12. Wang Y (2000) Description of parallel imaging in MRI using multiple coils. Magn Reson Med 44:495-499
13. Dwyer SJ III, Stewart BK, Sayre JW et al (1992) Performance characteristics and image fidelity of gray scale monitors. Radiographics 12:765-772
14. Hangiandreou NJ, Fetterly KA, Felmlee JP (1999) Optimisation of contrast detail based method for electronic image display quality evaluation. J Digit Imaging 12:60-67
15. Hess RF, Liu CH, Wang YZ (2002) Luminance spatial scale and local stereosensitivity. Vision Res 42:331-342
16. Krissian K, Malandain G, Ayache N (1996) Directional anisotropic diffusion applied to segmentation of vessels in 3D images. INRIA France: RR-3064
17. Simone M, Mutter D, Rubino F et al (2004) three-Dimensional virtual cholengioscopy, a reliable tool for the diagnosis of common bile duct stones. Ann Surg 240:82-88
18. Vasilescu C, Filippi della Palavesa M, Coumaros D et al (2001) Cholangite sclérosante primitive: rôle de la cholangio-pancréatographie par IRM. Feuillets de Radiol 41:340-347
19. Cannard L, Leclerc JC, DeBelle L et al (2001) Exploration de la pathologie de l'ampoule de Vater en cholangio IRM. Feuillets de Radiol 41:215-222
20. Burtin P (1998) Cost-effectiveness of various diagnostic and therapeutic approaches to lithiasis of the common bile duct. Gastroenterol Clin Biol 22(Suppl 5): B30–B38
21. Scheiman JM, Carlos RC, Barnett JL et al (2001) Can endoscopic ultrasound or magnetic resonance cholangiopancreatography replace ERCP in patients with suspected biliary disease? A prospective trial and cost analysis. Am J Gastroenterol 96:2900-2904
22. Savader SJ, Lillemoe KD, Prescott CA et al (1997) Laparoscopic cholecystectomy- related bile duct injuries: a health and financial disaster. Ann Surg 225:268-273
23. Kern KA (1997) Malpractice litigation involving laparoscopic cholecystectomy. Cost, cause, and consequences. Arch Surg 132:392–397; discussion 397–398
24. Hugh TB (2002) New strategies to prevent laparoscopic bile duct injury–surgeons can learn from pilots. Surgery 132:826-835
25. Marmitt G, Friedrich H, Slusallek P (2006) Interactive volume rendering with ray tracing. Eurographics state-of-the art report 2006. STARs. Wyvill B, Wilkïe A (eds), Vienna, September 6-8, pp 115-136
26. Seong W, Kim EJ, Park JW (2004) Automatic segmentation technique without user modification for 3D visualization in medical image. CIS 2004, LNCS 3314:595-600
27. Schenk A, Prause G, Peitgen HO (2000) Efficient semiautomatic segmentation of 3D objects in medical images. MICCAI 2000. LNCS 1935:186-195
28. Young YN, Levy D (2006) Registration-based morphing of active contours for segmentation of CT scans. Math Biosci Eng 2: 79-96
29. Camara O, Colliot O, Bloch I (2004) Computational modeling of thoracic and abdominal anatomy using spatial relationships for image segmentation. Real Time Imaging 10: 263-273
30. Kitasaka T, Ogawa H, Yokoyama K et al (2005) Automated extraction of abdominal organs from uncontrasted 3D abdominal X-Ray CT images based on anatomical knowledge. Journal of Computer Aided Diagnosis of Medical Images 9:1-14
31. Soler L, Delingette H, Malandain G et al (2001) Fully automatic anatomical, pathological, and functional segmentation from CT scans for hepatic surgery. Comput Aided Surg 6:131-142
32. Simone M, Mutter D, Rubino F et al (2004) Three-dimensional virtual cholangioscopy: a reliable tool for the diagnosis of common bile duct stones. Ann Surg 240:82-88
33. Fasquel JB, Agnus V, Lamy J (2006) An efficient and generic extension to ITK to process arbitrary shaped regions of interest. Computer Methods Programs Biomed 81:1-7
34. Fasquel JB, Agnus V, Moreau J et al (2006) A medical image segmentation system based on the optimal management of the regions of interest us-

ing topological medical knowledge. Computer Methods Programs Biomed 82:216-230
35. Fasquel JB, Brocker G, Moreau J et al (2006) A modular and evolutive component oriented software architecture for patient modelling. Computer Methods Programs Biomed 83:222-233
36. Meinzer HP, Schemmer P, Schöbinger M et al (2004) Computer-based surgery planning for living liver donation. 20th ISPRS Congress, Istanbul 2004, International Archives of Photogrammetry and Remote Sensing, Vol. XXXV, Part B, pp 291-295
37. Numminen K, Sipilä O, Mäkisalo H (2005) Preoperative hepatic 3D models: virtual liver resection using three-dimensional imaging technique. Eur J Radiol 56:179-184
38. Radtke A, Nadalin S, Sotiropoulos GC et al (2007) Computer-assisted operative planning in adult living donor liver transplantation: a new way to resolve the dilemma of the middle hepatic vein. World J Surg 31:175-185
39. Koehl C, Soler L, Marescaux J (2002) A PACS based interface for 3D anatomical structures visualization and surgical planning. SPIE proceeding. 4681:17-24
40. Allard J, Cotin S, Faure F et al (2007) SOFA – an open source framework for medical simulation. Stud Health Technol Inform 125:13-18
41. Marescaux J, Rubino F, Arena M, Soler L (2004) Augmented Reality assisted laparoscopic adrenalectomy. JAMA 292:2214-2215
42. Nicolau S, Pennec X, Soler L et al (2003) Evaluation of a new 3D/2D registration criterion for liver radio-frequencies guided by Augmented Reality. IS4TM. LNCS 2673:270-283
43. Nicolau S, Garcia A, Pennec X et al (2005) An Augmented Reality system to guide radio-frequency tumor ablation. Journal of Computer Animation and Virtual Worlds 16:1-10

Chapter 8

Endoscopic Retrograde Cholangiopancreatography and Endoscopic Ultrasound

John Meenan

Introduction

Endoscopic retrograde cholangiopancreatography (ERCP) remains the mainstay of therapeutic biliary intervention; its role in diagnosis, however, has rapidly diminished with the advent of high resolution cross sectional magnetic resonance imaging (MRI) and endoscopic imaging (endoscopic ultrasound). This change has been driven mainly by an aversion to the risks of ERCP, particularly that of inducing pancreatitis [1].

Due the limited diagnostic role of ERCP in the setting of choledocholithiasis and the relative novelty of endoscopic ultrasound (EUS), the focus of this chapter will be on describing the latter technique.

ERCP

Introduction

ERCP is performed under fluoroscopy using a side-viewing endoscope ("duodenoscope") that allows for en face views of the ampulla of Vater with a "stable" scope position (i.e., the scope rests within the second part of the duodenum without falling backwards to the stomach).

Dedicated tools (mostly disposable) exist for cannulating the major ampulla, selective opacification of the common bile and pancreatic ducts, sphincterotomy, fragmentation and removal of calculi, insertion of stents and direct visualization of the biliary lumen. Much of the equipment usage is based on the Seldinger technique: instrumentation being deployed over a wire placed within the biliary tree. Since the mid 1990s, the older and more awkward "long wire" technique has been replaced by user-friendly "short wire" rapid exchange systems that permit the use of multi-functional cannulae [2].

ERCP and Detecting Choledocholithiasis

ERCP is the gold standard by which other imaging modalities are judged for the detection of ductal stones (Figs. 8.1, 8.2). Accuracy rates are in the region of 96%, with the main cause of missed stones, other than failed cannulation, being the use of too dilute contrast or a capacious, dilated common bile duct (CBD) [3].

Indications and Risks

The indications for ERCP, particularly in relation to the diagnosis and treatment of biliary lithiasis, have changed considerably since the heydays of the early 1990s. This change is the result of an increasing aversion to risk, coupled with the more widespread use of equally accurate technologies such as MRI and EUS [4, 5].

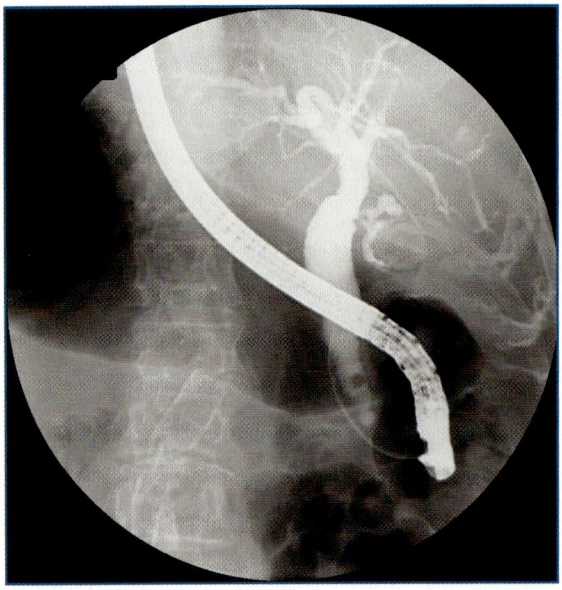

Fig. 8.1 Distal common bile duct stone at ERCP

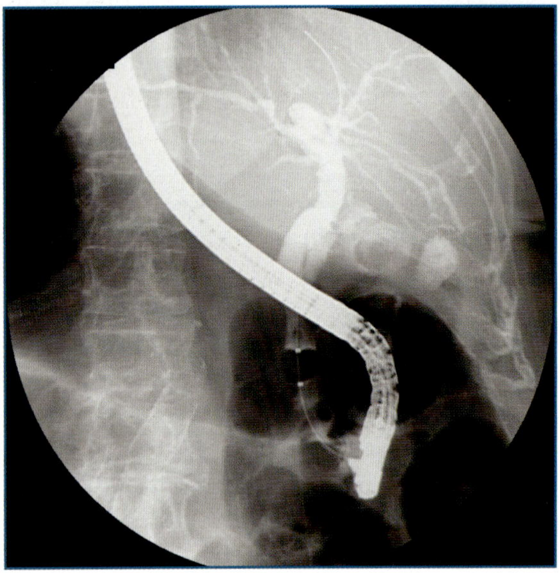

Fig. 8.2 Balloon retrieval of a distal common bile duct stone. Note large stone in gallbladder

The major risk associated with ERCP, diagnostic or therapeutic, is acute pancreatitis. This risk follows from the required cannulation of the ampulla and possible mis-opacification of the pancreatic duct. The general level of risk quoted is that about 5% of cases will develop clinically relevant pancreatitis requiring hospitalization; with one of every two hundred cases developing a life-threatening form. Those most at risk include the young, overweight females and those with a history of recent acute pancreatitis. This last group is of particular relevance, as determining the presence of choledocholithiasis in a patient presenting with acute pancreatitis is a common diagnostic dilemma [6].

The potential for inducing pancreatitis has fuelled studies seeking the Holy Grail of ERCP; namely, a method for the prevention of pancreatitis. Chemical (gabexate, somatostatin, ocreotide, glyceryl trinitrate, pentoxifilline, indomethacin) and mechanical (short-term pancreatic stenting) strategies have been tried with little or at best, mixed success [7–15]. Consequently, a detailed consent process is an absolute requirement before performing ERCP. Equally, ERCP must be seen as a therapeutic, not diagnostic, procedure. There is little or no justification for embarking on ERCP if some form of endoscopic intervention is not envisaged. Lack of local access to MRI or EUS does not alter this stance, certainly in a developed healthcare system.

Performing ERCP

Endoscopic retrograde cholangiopancreatography may be carried out in a day-case setting provided that the patient can be observed for at least 6 hours (median time to onset of acute pancreatititic symptoms) prior to discharge.

The patient fasts for at least 4 hours prior to the procedure. Baseline vital signs including peripheral oxygen saturation are measured and a prophylactic antibiotic, usually a quinolone, is given. Conscious sedation (bolus intravenous midazolam and pethidine or fentanyl) or propofol (infusion without need for intubation) is used for the procedure, which takes from 30 minutes to 2 hours. Constant monitoring of blood pressure, pulse and oxygen saturation is required throughout.

The duodenoscope is passed through to the second part of the duodenum ("D2") and "shortened" by clockwise rotation and withdrawal of the scope shaft. This brings the scope into a stable position opposite the ampulla. A smooth, blunt-tipped cannula (5 Fr), primed with non-ionic contrast is passed through the operating channel of the scope (usually 4.2 mm) and directed upwards towards 11 o'clock on the ampulla. A small bolus of contrast is injected under fluoroscopy to ensure correct cannulation of the CBD. Once deep cannulation has been achieved, a guide-wire (usually 0.035 inch) with a "slippery" hydrophilic coating can be passed deep into the biliary system. This permits the subsequent confident use of other instruments, such as sphincterotomes. Altered anatomy resulting from surgical intervention (Billroth II gastrectomy or Roux-en-y formation) or local pathology (duodenal stricture) can present a significant impediment to procedure success.

The question of what happens if biliary cannulation cannot be easily achieved is a difficult one. The options lie between persistence, persistence with adjunct usage of equipment such as guide-wire or sphincterotome, pre-cut sphincterotomy (incising the ampullary mucosa to reveal the ductal orifices), the Rendez-vous procedure (the ampulla is traversed by the trans-cutaneous placement of a trans-hepatic guide-wire, to be grabbed internally through the endoscope), or abandonment. The correct decision is often guided by the skill of the operator, as both persistence and needle knife pre-cutting carry equal risk [16].

The presence of a duodenal diverticulum can present technical difficulties to bile duct cannulation and has been associated with an increased prevalence of pigment stones [17–19]. Previous manipulation, such as the presence of an endoprosthesis, can act as a nidus for stone formation [20].

Cholangioscopy

The potential of missing small ductal calculi in capacious biliary systems can be obviated to a degree through the use of trans-papillary cholangioscopy (through the scope or wire-guided), an approach that also allows for directed lithotripsy [21]. The advent of disposable systems may widen the availability of this technique [22]. Percutaneous cholangioscopy is addressed elsewhere in this book.

EUS

Introduction

The proximity of the biliary tree to the stomach and duodenum presents ultrasound imaging with both its greatest weakness and its greatest strength. On the one hand, air in the duodenum hampers views of the distal CBD by trans-abdominal ultrasound, while on the other hand, an ability to place a (relatively) high frequency transducer within the gut lumen permits exquisitely detailed views of the biliary tree. Hence the potential value of EUS in diagnosing biliary lithiasis.

EUS Equipment

Echoendoscopes are large bore instruments with an ultrasound transducer (5–12 MHz) in addition to an optical video camera, built into a relatively long, rigid and broad tip (diameter approximately 14 mm as opposed to 8 mm for a standard gastroscope). Grooves to take a water-filled balloon are sited either side of the transducer. This balloon can be inflated/deflated using dual purpose buttons on the scope handle. The purpose of the balloon is to ensure good acoustic coupling between the transducer and the bowel wall.

The two systems that are in use yield distinct views: radial (360 degree coronal sections, analogous to a CT scan; Fig. 8.3) and linear (narrow, sectional views, similar to

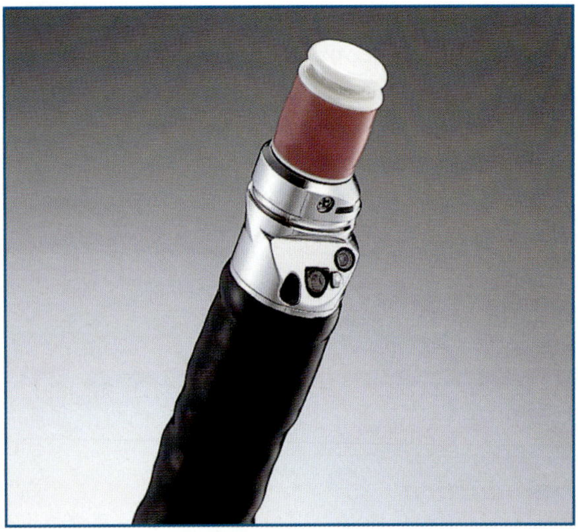

Fig. 8.3 Electronic radial endoscopic ultrasound probe. Olympus KeyMed Group Companies, Southend-on-Sea, U.K., reproduced with permission

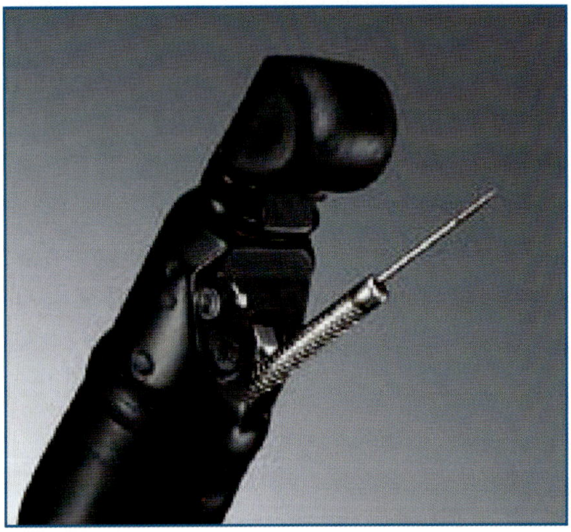

Fig. 8.4 Electronic linear endoscopic ultrasound probe with projecting fine needle aspiration needle. Olympus KeyMed Group Companies, Southend-on-Sea, U.K., reproduced with permission

those seen with traditional trans-abdominal ultrasound; Fig. 8.4). The major advantage of linear instruments is that they make it possible to perform ultrasound guided biopsy. For historical reasons, radial instruments are the most widely used.

The echoendoscope is attached to two processors, one for the endoscopic view, another for the ultrasound view. The luminal view is used only to locate pathology and to place the echoendoscope in the duodenum for views of the CBD.

Performing EUS

This is an outpatient procedure performed under conscious sedation. The procedure takes approximately 10–20 minutes to perform. The recovery time is shorter than that for ERCP, as there is no risk of acute pancreatitis.

The common bile duct is viewed from the duodenal bulb and the second part of the duodenum. The scope is passed to the duodenum, the ampulla inspected endoscopically (small adenomas might not be picked up on ultrasound unless their presence is previously known) and the transducer turned on. The CBD, cystic duct (more difficult) and right/left hepatic ducts are viewed from the duodenal bulb (angle between bulb and D2). With radial instruments, the left common hepatic duct is less easily seen. The liver hilum can be inspected from the duodenal bulb with both radial and linear instruments, whereas very detailed transgastric views (about 45–50 cm from incisors) are only yielded by linear instruments. The gallbladder is seen from the duodenal bulb and as the echoendoscope is withdrawn through the distal stomach.

EUS and Choledocholithiasis

Standard EUS is extremely accurate at detecting biliary duct stones (Fig. 8.5) and is at least equivalent to ERCP [23–27] and MR cholangiography (MRC) [28–33]. It has been suggested that EUS might be superior to MRI in detecting calculi in the face of a normal/small calibre CBD [29]. If EUS is normal, there is no indication to proceed to ERCP [35]. Although most studies have used radial instruments, linear endosonography is equally accurate [36]. The substitution of EUS for ERCP in the search for choledocholithiasis has had a significant

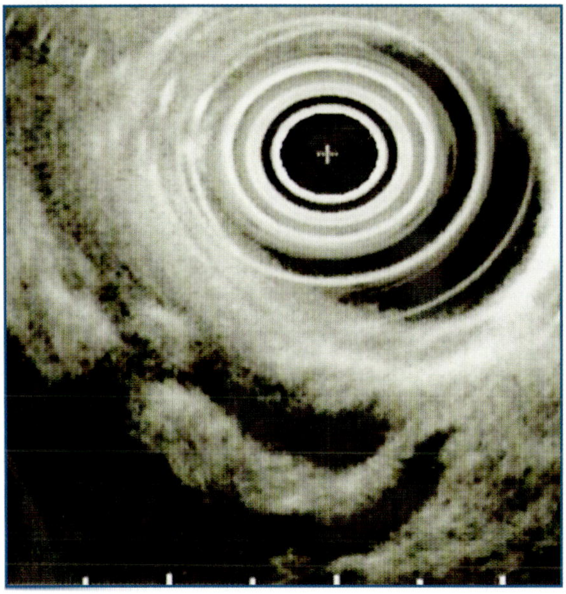

Fig. 8.5 A stone (with acoustic shadow) is seen in the mid CBD at radial EUS

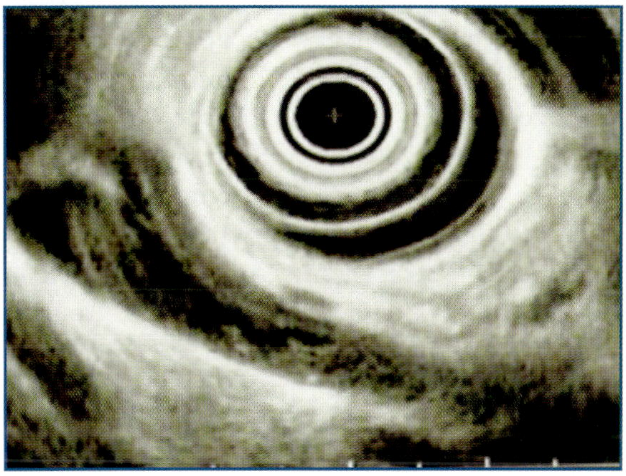

Fig. 8.6 Sludge in the distal CBD is seen as a soft, grey "cloud" with no posterior acoustic shadow

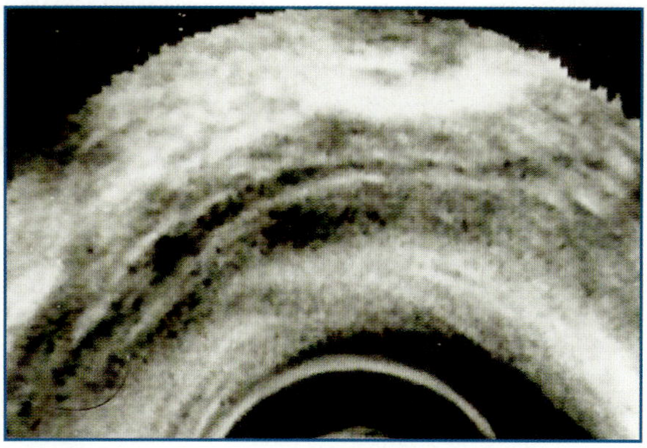

Fig. 8.7 Thickening of the CBD wall, with a slit-like lumen, is seen with primary sclerosing cholangitis

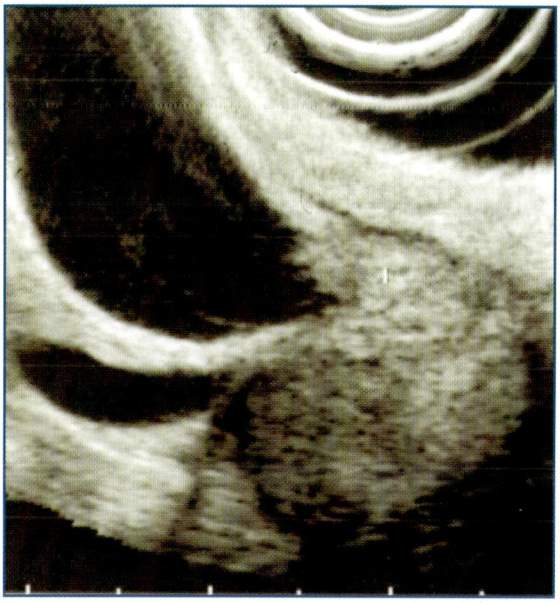

Fig. 8.8 The common bile and pancreatic ducts are seen to merge at a rounded, hypoechoic, ampullary, neuro-endocrine tumour

impact on the number of needless ERCPs as well as on overall numbers of ERCPs performed [37, 38].

The resolution of EUS allows the detection of micro-crystals and sludge (Fig. 8.6) [39]. This statement, importantly, also hold true in the specific setting of acute pancreatitis [40–45].

In addition to detecting choledocholithiasis, EUS permits the identification of co-existing pathologies where calculi might be merely a secondary phenomenon, such as primary sclerosing cholangitis (Fig. 8.7), ampullary carcinoma (Fig. 8.8), cholangiocarcinoma and pancreatic head neoplasms. Conversely, the absence of EUS findings can exclude pancreatic or ampullary cancer with a high degree of accuracy. This is important in the common situation where a dilated CBD with a short stricture may contain a stone and it is not clear whether this is only an inflammatory/fibrotic stricture or something more sinister.

Linear EUS permits the sampling by fine needle aspiration of mass lesions involving the biliary tree, e.g., a Mirizzi syndrome (a

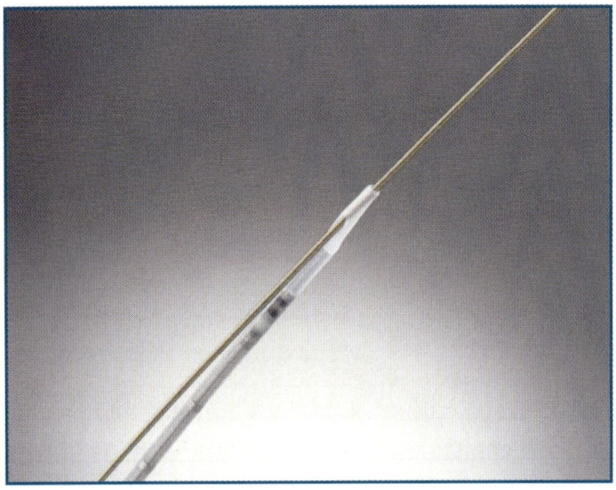

Fig. 8.9 A high frequency, wire-guided, ultrasound probe. Olympus KeyMed Group Companies, Southend-on-Sea, U.K., reproduced with permission

calculus in neck of a chronically inflamed gallbladder giving rise to obstruction of the CBD by compression, either directly from the stone or indirectly due to a phlegmon), which can be mimicked by cholangiocarcinoma.

EUS Mini-probes

The availability of small, wire-guided high frequency (12–30 MHz) mini-probes that may be deployed through a therapeutic scope, such as an ERCP duodenoscope, brings together the strengths of each technique (Fig. 8.9). These "catheter" mini-probes are approximately 2 mm in diameter and may be passed over a guide-wire through an ERCP scope to assess the problematic, dilated, "flabby" CBD in which a small stone might be obscured in a sea of contrast. Their use does improve the accuracy of stone detection [46–48]. There are no data comparing the accuracy of this technique (ERCP and EUS mini-probe) with standard EUS alone.

EUS and Access to the CBD

Cannulation of the CBD has been achieved at EUS, but this is unlikely to represent a practical, long-term approach to investigating the biliary tree [49].

The proximity to the biliary tree and a capacity for intervention afforded by linear EUS has fostered interest in the possibility of direct biliary puncture for non-transpapillary opacification of the CBD in cases where ERCP has failed [50, 51]. In terms of diagnosing choldocholithiasis, such reports are again unlikely to show the future direction of EUS, although the trans-enteric placement of stents and the like will most likely become more mainstream.

Cost Effectiveness of ERCP and EUS

Several potential strategies exist for the investigation of abnormal liver blood tests or the dilated CBD when questioning the presence or absence of choledocholithiasis. These range from ERCP (least acceptable in terms of risk but if a stone is found, it can be removed in the same procedure) to EUS or MRC (expensive and not universally available) to percutaneous cholangiography (invasive and uncomfortable for the patient).

The cost effectiveness of utilizing these various approaches has been modelled by several authors [52–54]; EUS is more accurate than MRI but is more expensive [52] and should there be a greater than 50% chance of a stone being present, then ERCP is the procedure of choice [53].

The key to accurate modelling is, however, being able to predict the likelihood of a stone being present. As discussed in another chapter, such figures are imprecise. For this reason, the choice between EUS or MRC as the investigation of choice will often be decided by factors such as equipment availability and local expertise.

Conclusion

There has been a dramatic sea-change in the utilization of ERCP. No longer can the attendant risk of acute pancreatitis be justified in the search for a ductal stone. Should the chance of a stone being present in the CBD be only low or moderate, then MRC or EUS ought to be considered. Of these two procedures, EUS is probably the better choice, as small stones in non-dilated ducts can be more accurately identified, albeit at a slightly increased level of patient discomfort.

References

1. Anonymous (2002) NIH state-of-the-science statement on endoscopic retrograde cholangiopancreatography (ERCP) for diagnosis and therapy. NIH Consens State Sci Statements 19:1-26
2. Papachristou GI, Baron TH, Gleeson F et al (2006) Endoscopic retrograde cholangiopancreatography catheter and accessory exchange using a short hydrophilic guide wire: a prospective study. Endoscopy 38:1146-1148
3. Fulcher A (2002) MRCP and ERCP in the diagnosis of common bile duct stones. Gastrointest Endosc 56:S178-S182
4. Sivak M (2002) EUS for bile duct stones: How does it compare with ERCP? Gastrointest Endosc 56:S175-S177
5. Coakley FV, Qayyum A (2002) Magnetic resonance cholangiopancreatography. Gastrointest Endosc 55:S2-S12
6. Williams EJ, Taylor S, Fairclough P et al (2007) Risk factors for complication following ERCP; results of a large, prospective, multicentre study. Endoscopy 39:793-801
7. Rudin D, Kiss A, Wetz RV, Sottile VM (2007) Somatostatin and gabexate for post-endoscopic retrograde cholangiopancreatography pancreatitis prevention: meta-analysis of randomized placebo-controlled trials. J Gastroenterol Hepatol 22:977-983
8. Manes G, Ardizzone S, Lombardi G et al (2007) Efficacy of postprocedure administration of gabexate mesylate in the prevention of post-ERCP pancreatitis: a randomized, controlled, multicenter study. Gastrointest Endosc 65:982-987
9. Hellmig S, Fölsch UR (2006) Pharmacological prevention of post-ERCP pancreatitis—an everlasting dream? Dig Liver Dis 38:596-598
10. Ito K, Fujita N, Noda Y et al (2007) Can prophylactic pancreatic duct stent placement reduce the prevalence of post-ERCP pancreatitis in patients with difficult cannulation of the bile duct? Gastrointest Endosc 65:AB239
11. Silverman WB (2007) ERCP and prophylactic pancreatic stents: raising the bar, reducing the pain. Gastrointest Endosc 65:969-970
12. Kapetanos D, Kokozidis G, Christodoulou D et al (2007) A randomized controlled trial of pentoxifylline for the prevention of post-ERCP pancreatitis. Gastrointest Endosc 66:513-518
13. Sotoudehmanesh R, Khatibian M, Kolahdoozan S (2007) Indomethacin may reduce the incidence and severity of acute pancreatitis after ERCP. Am J Gastroenterol 102:984-986
14. Li ZS, Pan X, Zhang WJ et al (2007) Effect of octreotide administration in the prophylaxis of post-ERCP pancreatitis and hyperamylasemia: a multicenter, placebo-controlled, randomized clinical trial. Am J Gastroenterol 102:46-51
15. Kaffes AJ, Bourke MJ, Ding S et al (2006) a prospective, randomized, placebo-controlled trial of transdermal glyceryl trinitrate in ERCP: effects on technical success and post-ERCP pancreatitis. Gastrointest Endosc 64:358-360
16. Tang SJ, Haber GB, Kortan P et al (2005) Precut papillotomy versus persistence in difficult biliary cannulation: a prospective randomized trial. Endoscopy 37:58-65
17. Tham TC, Kelly M (2004) Association of periampullary duodenal diverticula with bile duct stones and with technical success of endoscopic retrograde cholangiopancreatography. Endoscopy 36:1050-1053
18. Kim MH, Myung SJ, Seo DW et al (1998) Association of periampullary diverticula with primary choledocholithiasis but not with secondary choledocholithiasis. Endoscopy 30:601-604
19. Wu SD, Su Y, Fan Y et al (2007) Relationship between intraduodenal peri-ampullary diverticulum and biliary disease in 178 patients undergoing ERCP. Hepatobiliary Pancreat Dis Int 6:299-302
20. Tang SJ, Armstrong L, Lara LF, Kortan P (2007) De novo stent-stone complex after long-term biliary stent placement: pathogenesis, diagnosis, and endotherapy. Gastrointest Endosc 66:193-200
21. Piraka C, Shah RJ, Awadallah NS et al (2007) Transpapillary cholangioscopy-directed lithotripsy in patients with difficult bile duct stones. Clin Gastroenterol Hepatol 5:1333-1338
22. Chen YK, Pleskow DK (2007) SpyGlass single-operator peroral cholangiopancreatoscopy system for the diagnosis and therapy of bile-duct disorders: a clinical feasibility study. Gastrointest Endosc 65:832-841
23. Edmundowicz SA, Aliperti G, Middleton WD (1992) Preliminary experience using endoscopic

ultrasonography in the diagnosis of choledocholithiasis. Endoscopy 24:774-778
24. Norton SA, Alderson D (1997) Prospective comparison of endoscopic ultrasonography and endoscopic retrograde cholangiography in the detection of bile duct stones. Br J Surg 84:1366-1369
25. Canto MI, Chak A, Stellato T, Sivak MV (1998) Endoscopic ultrasonography versus cholangiography for the diagnosis of choledocholithiasis. Gastrointest Endosc 47:439-448
26. Amouyal P, Amouyal G, Levy P et al (1994) Diagnosis of choledocholithiasis by endoscopic ultrasonography. Gastroenterol 106:1062-1067
27. Palazzo L, Girollet PP, Salmeron M et al (1995) Value of endoscopic ultrasonography in the diagnosis of common bile duct stones: comparison with surgical exploration and ERCP. Gastrointest Endosc 42:225-231
28. Schmidt S, Chevallier P, Novellas S et al (2007) Choledocholithiasis: repetitive thick-slab single-shot projection magnetic resonance cholangiopancreaticography versus endoscopic ultrasonography. Eur Radiol 17:241-250
29. Kondo S, Isayama H, Akahane M et al (2005) Detection of common bile duct stones: comparison between endoscopic ultrasonography, magnetic resonance cholangiography, and helical-computed-tomographic cholangiography. Eur J Radiol 54:271-275
30. de Lédinghen V, Lecesne R, Raymond JM et al (1999) Diagnosis of choledocholithiasis: EUS or magnetic resonance cholangiography? A prospective controlled study. Gastrointest Endosc 49:26-31
31. Aubé C, Delorme B, Yzet T et al (2005) MR cholangiopancreatography versus endoscopic sonography in suspected common bile duct lithiasis: a prospective, comparative study. AJR Am J Roentgenol 184:55-62
32. Fernandez-Esparrach G, Ginas A, Sanchez M et al (2007) Comparison of endoscopic ultrasonography and magnetic resonance cholangiopancreatography in the diagnosis of pancreatobiliary diseases: a prospective study. Am J Gastroenterol 102:1632-1639
33. Verma D, Kapadia A, Eisen GM et al (2006) EUS vs MRCP for detection of choledocholithiasis. Gastrointest Endosc 64:248-254
34. Garrow D, Miller S, Sinha D et al (2007) Endoscopic ultrasound: a meta-analysis of test performance in suspected biliary obstruction. Clin Gastroenterol Hepatol 5:616-623
35. Napoléon B, Dumortier J, Keriven-Souquet O et al (2003) Do normal findings at biliary endoscopic ultrasonography obviate the need for endoscopic retrograde cholangiography in patients with suspicion of common bile duct stone? A prospective follow-up study of 238 patients. Endoscopy 35: 411-415
36. Kohut M, Nowakowska-Duława E, Marek T et al (2002) Accuracy of linear endoscopic ultrasonography in the evaluation of patients with suspected common bile duct stones. Endoscopy 34:299-303
37. Meenan J, Tibble J, Prasad P, Wilkinson M (2004) The substitution of endoscopic ultrasound for endoscopic retrograde cholangio-pancreatography: implications for service development and training. Eur J Gastroenterol Hepatol 16:299-303
38. Sotoudehmanesh R, Kolahdoozan S, Asgari AA et al (2007) Role of endoscopic ultrasonography in prevention of unnecessary endoscopic retrograde cholangiopancreatography: a prospective study of 150 patients. J Ultrasound Med 26:455-460
39. Mirbagheri SA, Mohamadnejad M, Nasiri J et al (2005) Prospective evaluation of endoscopic ultrasonography in the diagnosis of biliary microlithiasis in patients with normal transabdominal ultrasonography. J Gastrointest Surg 9:961-964
40. Liu CL, Fan ST, Lo CM et al (2005) Comparison of early endoscopic ultrasonography and endoscopic retrograde cholangiopancreatography in the management of acute biliary pancreatitis: a prospective randomized study. Clin Gastroenterol Hepatol 3:1238-1244
41. Liu CL, Lo CM, Chan JK et al (2000) EUS for detection of occult cholelithiasis in patients with idiopathic pancreatitis. Gastrointest Endosc 51:28-32
42. Chak A, Hawes RH, Cooper GS et al (1999) Prospective assessment of the utility of EUS in the evaluation of gallstone pancreatitis. Gastrointest Endosc 49:599-604
43. Liu CL, Lo CM, Chan JK et al (2001) Detection of choledocholithiasis by EUS in acute pancreatitis: a prospective evaluation in 100 consecutive patients. Gastrointest Endosc 54:325-330
44. Prat F, Edery J, Meduri B et al (2001) Early EUS of the bile duct before endoscopic sphincterotomy for acute biliary pancreatitis. Gastrointest Endosc 54:724-729
45. Romagnuolo J, Currie G, Calgary Advanced Therapeutic Endoscopy Center study group (2005) Noninvasive vs. selective invasive biliary imaging for acute biliary pancreatitis: an economic evaluation by using decision tree analysis. Gastrointest Endosc 61:86-97
46. Moon JH, Cho YD, Cha SW et al (2005) The detection of bile duct stones in suspected biliary pancreatitis: comparison of MRCP, ERCP, and intraductal US. Am J Gastroenterol 100:1051-1057
47. Tseng LJ, Jao YT, Mo LR, Lin RC (2001) Over-the-wire US catheter probe as an adjunct to ERCP in the detection of choledocholithiasis. Gastrointest Endosc 54:720-723

48. Das A, Isenberg G, Wong RC et al (2001) Wire-guided intraductal US: an adjunct to ERCP in the management of bile duct stones. Gastrointest Endosc 54:720-723
49. Rocca R, De Angelis C, Castellino F et al (2006) EUS diagnosis and simultaneous endoscopic retrograde cholangiography treatment of common bile duct stones by using an oblique-viewing echoendoscope. Gastrointest Endosc 63:479-484
50. Mallery S, Matlock J, Freeman ML (2004) EUS-guided Rendez-vous drainage of obstructed biliary and pancreatic ducts: Report of 6 cases. Gastrointest Endosc 59:100-107
51. Bories E, Pesenti C, Caillol F et al (2007) Transgastric endoscopic ultrasonography-guided biliary drainage: results of a pilot study. Endoscopy 39:287-291
52. Scheiman JM, Carlos RC, Barnett JL et al (2001) Can endoscopic ultrasound or magnetic resonance cholangiopancreatography replace ERCP in patients with suspected biliary disease? A prospective trial and cost analysis. Am J Gastroenterol 96:2900-2904
53. Ainsworth AP, Rafaelsen SR, Wamberg PA et al (2004) Cost-effectiveness of endoscopic ultrasonography, magnetic resonance cholangiopancreatography and endoscopic retrograde cholangiopancreatography in patients suspected of pancreaticobiliary disease. Scand J Gastroenterol 39:579-583
54. Arguedas MR, Dupont AW, Wilcox CM (2001) Where do ERCP, endoscopic ultrasound, magnetic resonance cholangiopancreatography, and intraoperative cholangiography fit in the management of acute biliary pancreatitis? A decision analysis model. Am J Gastroenterol 96:2892-2899

Chapter 9

Pre- and Intra-operative Diagnostic Fibrocholangioscopy

Gian M. Gazzaniga, Marco Filauro

Introduction

Exploration of the intra- and extra-hepatic biliary tree using small-size flexible endoscopic instruments took place in the 1980s, when technological improvement in the field of endoscopy made technically more advanced instruments available [1].

Surgeons, as well as radiologists and gastroenterologists, have all used fibrocholangioscopy with different techniques for both diagnostic and therapeutic procedures, such as the so-called 'babyscope' introduced into a 'mother' duodenoscope during endoscopic retrograde cholangiograpy, or the percutaneous approach for a trans-hepatic biliary drainage after sinus tract dilation.

Whatever the indication or the technique, the aim of the method is to explore the bile duct lumen using a direct approach that enables a magnified view even of the smaller branches of the biliary tree in the setting of both malignant and benign obstruction.

At the end of the 1980s and beginning of the 1990s the method was given a considerable boost by Japanese practitioners, who adopted the percutaneous fibrocholangioscopic approach for diagnostic purposes in cases of malignant obstruction of the biliary tract [2, 3]. The most common indication was hepatic hilar cholangiocarcinoma (Klatskin tumour) and the aim was a more precise staging of the endo-luminal extension of the tumour in order to schedule a more appropriate treatment (biliary resection with associated hepatic resection for a radical treatment). Undoubtedly, such an invasive procedure for tumoral pre-operative assessment has not been widely adopted due to the increasing accuracy of non-invasive imaging techniques, such as CT scan and magnetic resonance imaging (MRI), for the T, N and M staging of the tumour.

Differently benign biliary obstructions may still be an indication for a fibrocholangioscopic approach, although developments in noninvasive imaging and related software allow a virtual cholangiography (Cholangio CT and Cholangio MRI) to be performed.

Essentially, fibrocholangioscopy is indicated in those biliary obstructions where the precise nature of the disease is unknown and diagnosis is of importance in deciding the treatment strategy. In the cases of biliary lithiasis, such an approach has proven to be effective in the diagnostic assessment of both common bile duct and intra-hepatic lithiasis [4–6].

Fibrocholangioscopy may be performed either pre- or post-operatively by a percutaneous approach, as well as intra-operatively. In recent years the latter method has also been performed during laparoscopic surgery, leading to improved diagnostic accuracy in the biliary system.

Instruments

Both percutaneous and intra-operative techniques require the use of flexible instruments of different calibre depending on the purpose of the investigation. Exclusive biliary endoscopic investigation is performed with the thinnest instruments (with an outer diameter of 2.8 mm) that have no operative channel. For both diagnostic and therapeutic manoeuvres, larger instruments (with a diameter of 3.5 mm) are necessary since one or more operative channels are provided for the introduction of accessory instruments of different shapes and aims (Fig. 9.1).

Fibrocholangioscopic optical and light transmission systems are those of the larger calibre common endoscopic instruments used for digestive, respiratory, and urological endoscopy; fibrocholangioscopic instruments are therefore connected to light source and video-processors. The connection to cameras similar to those used in videolaparoscopy enables view onto a screen (video-fibrocholangioscopy) with undeniable advantages in terms of quality of imaging and viewing management. Images can also be captured and stored in a digital or other suitable system.

For each instrument a dedicated channel is provided to irrigate the biliary duct. Continuous irrigation is necessary throughout the examination in order to keep the lumen dilated and to prevent that biliary material from disturbing the exploration by obstructing the view. A bag containing saline solution is connected to the irrigation channel to allow irrigation to be achieved continuously under the pressure that is applied to the bag.

Given the delicacy of the optic fibres system, the instrument must be handled with extreme care, especially when it is introduced into the biliary tract percutaneously or through a trocar during laparoscopy. Even when it is introduced into the biliary tract directly during an open procedure, the quality of the fiberscope image is inevitably compromised after a number of examinations. Microscopic damage to the optic fibres may occur, causing a series of black dots to be seen on the screen. For these reasons, regular and careful maintenance of the instruments is required. The instruments should not be bent excessively in order not to damage the delicate optical fibres and the operative channels need to be cleaned properly with saline solution to prevent obstruction that otherwise may become permanent. The use

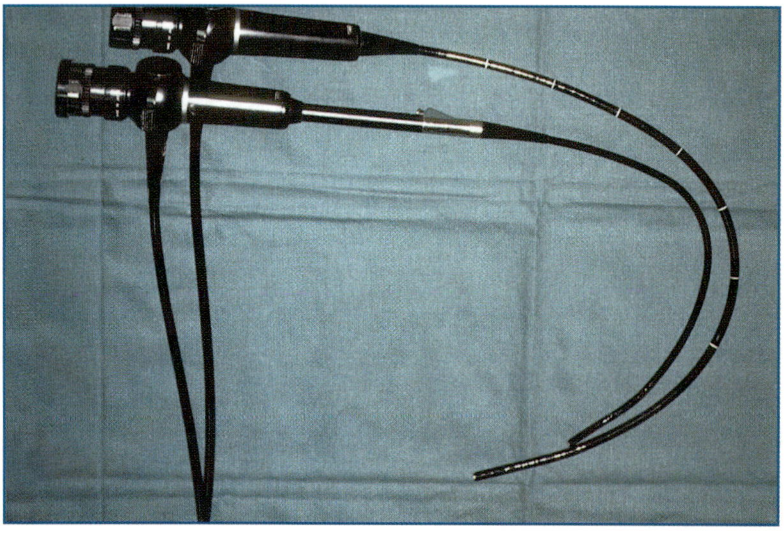

Fig. 9.1 Different caliber fibrocholangioscopic instruments (2.8 mm, E 3.5 mm)

of instruments for which operative channels are provided is supported by major digestive and extra-digestive endoscopic practice. Diagnostic accessory instruments such as brushes and bioptic forceps are provided in addition to therapeutic accessory instruments such as Dormia baskets, laser microfibers, electro-hydraulic or shock wave lithotripsy electrodes for biliary lithiasis management, all of which have a calibre which is suitable for the operative channel. Sometimes introduction of accessory instruments may be troublesome due to the curvature of the endoscope or diameter of the item being examined (intra-hepatic biliary tracts, distal tract of the common bile duct) (Fig. 9.2).

Indications and Technique

Percutaneous cholangioscopy

Indications

In the case of biliary lithiasis, the indications for carrying out percutaneous fibrocholangioscopy for diagnostic purposes are now limited to a few cases of diagnostic doubt relating to a concomitant obstructive disease, the nature of which cannot be ascertained without direct view and/or with targeted biopsy of the lesion. Percutaneous treatment of biliary lithiasis, particularly for intra-hepatic stones, has been reported previously with good therapeutic results in selected cases [7].

The most common indication for a percutaneous approach remains, in selected cases, residual lithiasis of the biliary tract after surgical treatment either by laparoscopy or open surgery after which biliary drainage has been positioned, and biliary stones in patients unfit for surgery for whom an endoscopic approach is not suitable.

Technique

Percutaneous fibrocholangioscopy is usually carried out in a radiologic unit or in an operative room adequately equipped for radiological explorations. Patient positioning allows the endoscopic instrument to be easily controlled during its insertion and simplifies all the manoeuvres that follow using endoscope and accessory instruments, along with the re-positioning of percutaneous drainage through the sinus tract, maintained by a guide wire. Patient position

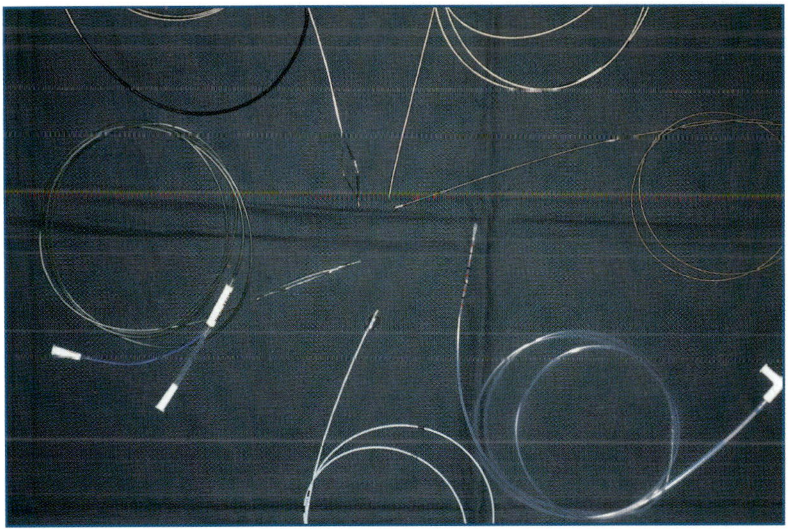

Fig. 9.2 Diagnostic and therapeutic fibrocholangioscopic instrument

may also be varied during examination in order to obtain the best radiological imaging. Radiological exploration is carried out by obtaining radioscopic and radiographic imaging with and without contrast solution.

Percutaneous access for fibrocholangioscopy is given by previous percutaneous drainage of the biliary tree or by a T-tube positioned during previous laparoscopic or open surgery on the biliary tract (Fig. 9.3).

Drainage must enable the creation of strengthened percutaneous access by way of the fibrotic reaction along the sinus tract in order to directly reach intra- or extra-hepatic biliary ducts without any transit trough the peritoneal cavity.

For this purpose the sinus tract must be (1) properly dilated by suitable dilators of increasingly large diameter and over a long enough time to prevent laceration of the hepatic parenchyma and/or biliary extrahepatic duct; and (2) properly strengthened (as stated above).

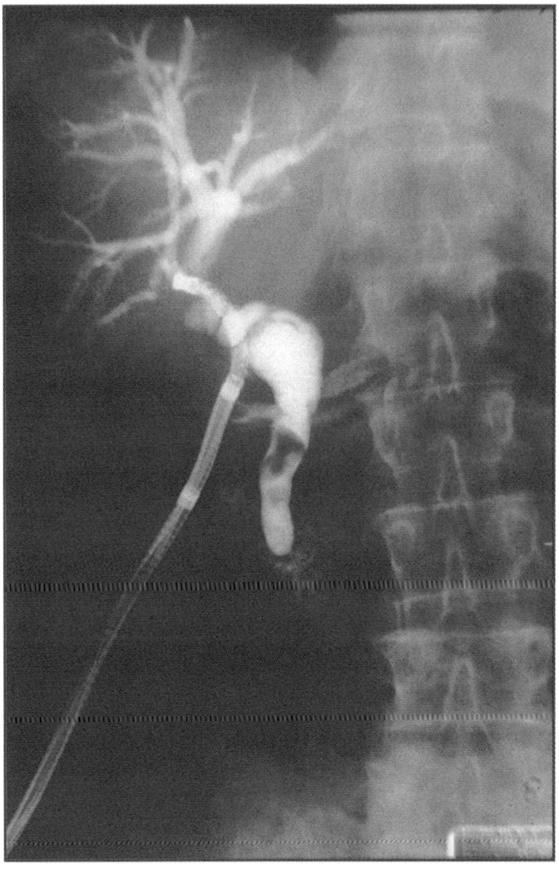

Fig. 9.3 Percutaneous fibrocholangioscopy through a T-tube

Percutaneous fibrocholangioscopy therefore requires between 15 days to 1 month of preparation time in order to achieve the above-mentioned conditions.

The dilation procedure for the chosen route is normally carried out under mild sedation and with anaesthetic cutaneous infiltration after cleaning with iodine solution. Biliary drainage is removed after a guide wire has been introduced into its lumen. The guide wire is then fitted into the irrigation or operative channel of the endoscope that is then introduced very delicately through the cutaneous orifice of the sinus tract.

Under radioscopic control, progression of the instrument is monitored throughout the sinus tract and the biliary ducts (Fig. 9.4). When the biliary lumen is reached the guide wire can be removed and the irrigation system connected so that physiological solution flows into the lumen. After connecting the optical system to the endoscope, exploration can begin.

Moving the instrument backwards and forwards with short radioscopic glimpses should enable correct endo-biliary positioning, the flexibility of the instrument allows endo-luminal withdrawal to reach either the common bile duct or the intra-hepatic biliary ducts.

It may be sometimes necessary to refit the guide wire into the operative channel in order to guide the endoscope when a right angle has to be overcome, such as may occur when the proximal tract of the common bile duct is reached with a horizontally placed endoscope. Special attention needs to be paid in cases of angles into the biliary tract in patients recovering from inflammatory processes, since even mild forcing with the endoscope may provoke wall lesions. Therefore, the endoscopic instrument must be advanced under continual direct visual control through endoscopic

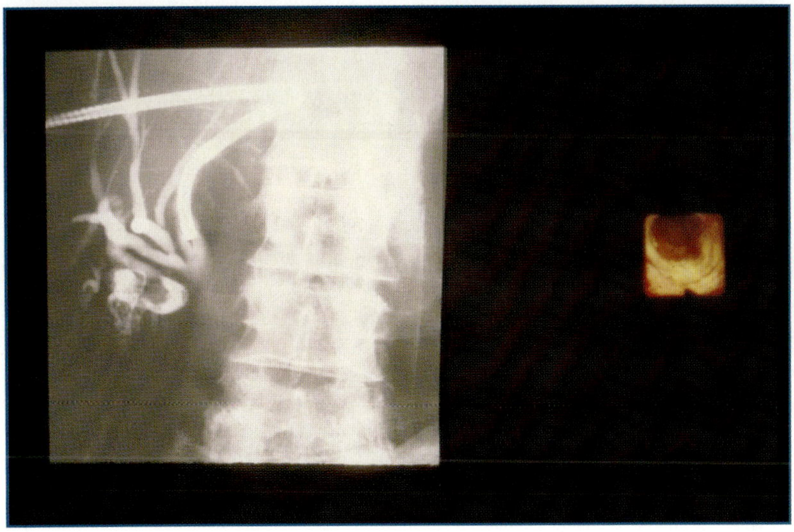

Fig. 9.4 Percutaneous fibrocholangioscopy for recurrent intra-hepatic biliary lithiasis

viewing, and the lumen of the biliary duct must be kept under constant control, as well as under radioscopic control.

Intra-operative cholangioscopy

Indications

In the course of open surgery for biliary lithiasis, there may be dual indications for intra-operative fibrocholangioscopy: (1) study of the associated obstructive diseases that have given rise to the lithiasis (inflammatory stenosis, tumours, parasite infection) with uncertain pre-operative diagnosis and for which intra-operative staging is required; (2) resolution assessment of complex biliary lithiasis such as primitive or secondary intra-hepatic lithiasis or lithiasis of the distal biliary tract with stone(s) in the pre-papillary tract. In these cases, the diagnostic phase is often strictly correlated with a therapeutic act, such as the extraction of bile stones with suitable instruments.

In the case of the laparoscopic approach, the indications for diagnostic fibrocholangioscopy are limited to an assessment of intra- or biliary stenosis extra-hepatic biliary lithiasis or biliary stenosis associated lithiasis, for the purposes of removal and diagnostic assessment with a mini-invasive method (Fig. 9.5) [8, 9].

Technique

Open surgery

The introduction of the instrument into the biliary lumen usually takes place via a longitudinal incision of the main bile duct

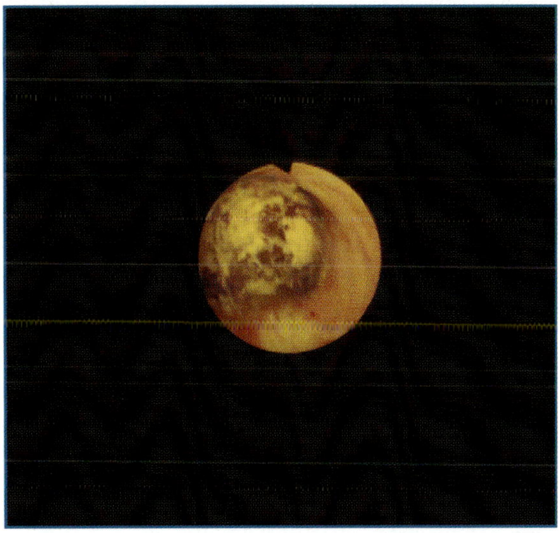

Fig. 9.5 Common bile duct stone removal by intra-operative fibrocholangioscopy with Dormia basket during laparoscopy

below the outlet of the cystic duct or, in the case of a distal implant of the duct, about 2 cm from the upper edge of the duodenum. In the case of a large lumen cystic duct, the instrument can be inserted through the latter. A progressive and careful divulsion of the cystic duct may also be carried out in order to facilitate trans-cystic access of the endoscope.

The exploration of the biliary lumen generally begins at the distal tract after the lumen has been filled by irrigation with saline solution.

The instrument is advanced slowly, without any forcing manoeuvres in areas of stenosis or sub-stenosis. For such a purpose, the primary operator modifies the angle and direction of the tip of the instrument, while an assistant is responsible for pushing or withdrawing the instrument. As stated above, it is important for the biliary lumen to be visible at all times, especially in areas of small diameter.

The study of the biliary walls involves the assessment of solid or encroaching areas in the lumen, of hyperaemic areas and/or areas that cannot be distended, as well as microlithiasis or cholesterinic deposits on the wall.

A biopsy or brushing with suitable instruments should be assessed and carried out whenever there is a diagnostic uncertainty and diagnosis is required to proceed into the subsequent therapeutic phase.

The study of the distal biliary tract must include, wherever possible, trans-papillary passage of the instrument in order to assess its patency: the duct may be obstructed/sub-obstructed by inflammation of the papilla or by tumoral lesions. Exploration has to be completed by viewing the papilla area from the duodenal side by inversion of the instrument in the duodenal lumen.

Special care should be taken to assess the presence of biliary stones in pre-papillary recesses, since they can be removed more easily and effectively by fibrocholangioscopy (Fig. 9.6). Finally, the assessment

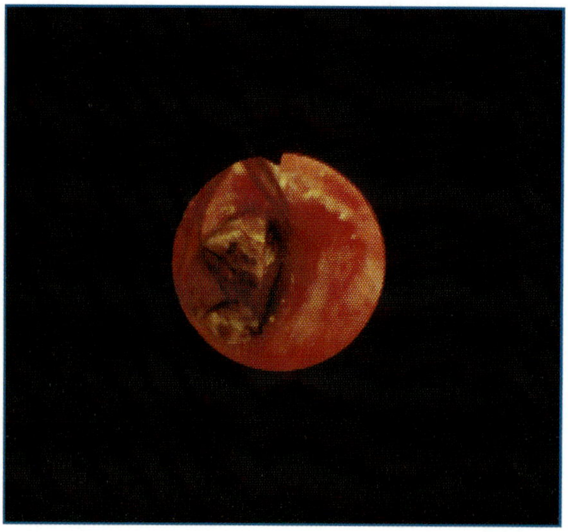

Fig. 9.6 Intra-operative fibrocholangioscopy showing a common bile duct stone

of a more or less conspicuous lithiasis of the distal biliary tract enables the benign nature of the obstruction to be confirmed and assessment of the removal methods to be determined.

For the study of the proximal biliary tract as well as for the intra-hepatic biliary branches above the confluence, the instrument must, of course, be inversely directed compared to the distal biliary tract. This manoeuvre may be difficult when the trans-cystic route is used since it is not always possible to invert in the intra-luminal direction at the level of the junction of the cystic duct with the common bile duct (e.g., in the case of a low cystic implant).

The study of the proximal part of the hepatic duct and that above the biliary convergence also involves the assessment of areas of stenosis or sub-stenosis of the lumen with biopsy or brushing, the assessment of the biliary duct wall for any kind of lesions, as well as assessment for biliary stones. It must be emphasised that the most valid indication for intra-operative fibrocholangioscopy is actually intra-hepatic lithiasis, primitive or secondary to extra-hepatic lithiasis, in relation to the current diagnostic possibilities of pre-operative imaging [10].

Management of intra-hepatic lithiasis must therefore involve the use of intra-operative fibrocholangioscopy in order to achieve definitive diagnosis and staging, as well as complete removal of stones and assessment of the complete clearance of the biliary tree. The endoscopic study must therefore be very carefully carried out in the segmentary branches, as well as in those sub-segmentary branches that are accessible to the instrument, both left and right, ensuring irrigation and removal of biliary stones by pressure flushing, retrojet, lithotripsy and tweezers. Fibrocholangioscopy allows determination of whether the presence of a biliary stenosis is the cause of biliary lithiasis formation, and if the stenosis is a secondary inflammatory process caused by the migration of stones.

The cholangioscopic study may also be associated with cholangiographic control via selective injection of contrast solution into the biliary branches through the instrument. The operative channel may be used to introduce a cholangiographic catheter and carry out an intra-operative cholangiography.

Laparoscopic surgery

Laparoscopic intra-operative fibrocholangioscopy uses the same endoscopic instruments as open surgery, although obviously a second video is needed. The technique differs in the way in which the instrument is introduced into the biliary tract.

Instruments fitted with a proper operative channel may be introduced into a 5 mm trocar, although a 10–12 mm trocar with its adaptor is more suitable. A larger trocar may reduce the risk of damaging the instrument. Dedicated atraumatic forceps for seizure and management of the endoscope into the peritoneal cavity are also available to reduce the risk of damage to the instrument.

The introduction of the endoscope into the biliary lumen may also be performed through the cystic duct (dilated if needed) or an incision in the common bile duct. Assessment and manoeuvres on the intra-hepatic and extra-hepatic biliary tract are similar to those reported for open surgery.

The videolaparoscopic approach may involve difficulty in endoscope insertion into the biliary tract due to the effect of the fixed trocar on the abdominal wall and the required bending of the instrument. Therefore it is important to place the trocar in the optimum position when intra-operative fibrocholangioscopy is scheduled.

Conclusion

Although indications to fibrocholangioscopy are actually limited due to progress in noninvasive imaging, the percutaneous and intra-operative intra-luminal endoscopic approach may be useful whenever treatment strategy is conditioned by a diagnostic uncertainty. In the case of biliary lithiasis, this mainly involves biliary stenosis associated stones, since the procedure allows direct exploration and biopsy. A percutaneous approach is also the more suitable option in patients unfit for surgery and for whom a ERCP is not feasible.

References

1. Gazzaniga GM, Faggioni A, Bondanza G et al (1983) Fibrocolangioscopia transparietoepatica Estratto da Notiziario Chirurgico 4:41-46
2. Simon T, Fink AS, Zuckermann AM (1999) Experience with percutaneous transhepatic cholangioscopy (PTCS) in the management of biliary tract disease. Surg Endosc 13:1199-1202
3. Seo DW, Kim MH, Lee SK et al (1999) Usefulness of cholangioscopy in patients with focal stricture of the intrahepatic duct unrelated to intrahepatic stones. Gastrointest Endosc 49:204-209
4. Kim HJ, Kim MH, Lee SK et al (2001) Characterization of primary pure cholesterol hepatolithia-

sis: cholangioscopic and selective cholangiographic findings. Gastrointest Endosc 53:324-328
5. Kim JH, Lee SK, Kim MH et al (2003) Percutaneous transhepatic cholangioscopic treatment of patients with benign bilio-enteric anastomotic strictures. Gastrointest Endosc 58:733-738
6. Jeng KS, Sheen IS, Yang FS (2000) Percutaneous transhepatic cholangioscopy in the treatment of complicated intrahepatic biliary strictures and hepatolithiasis with internal metallic stent. Surg Laparosc Endosc Percutan Tech 10:278-283
7. Faggioni A, Bondanza G, Filauro M et al (1985) Trattamento transcutaneo della calcolosi residua/recidiva delle vie biliari. Estratto da Minerva Chirurgica 40:489-494
8. Petelin JB (2003) Laparoscopic common bile duct exploration. Surg Endosc 17:1705-1715
9. Lyass S, Phillips EH (2006) Laparoscopic trans-cystic duct common bile duct exploration. Surg Endosc suppl 2:441-445
10. Hwang S, Lee SG, Kim MH et al (2007) Intraoperative biliary exploration through the left hepatic duct orifice during left hepatectomy in patients with left-sided hepatolithiasis. Langenbecks Arch Surg Jun 2 [Epub ahead of print]

Chapter 10

Intraoperative Cholangiography

Markus Schäfer

Introduction

Since the 1940s, intraoperative information on the individual anatomy of the biliary tree and the localization of biliary stones has been obtained through the use of radiologic contrast-based cholangiography or cholecystocholangiography [1]. At first glance, intraoperative cholangiography seems purely advantageous, but a closer look reveals many controversial issues that have been extensively discussed for several decades. While some surgeons strongly advocate the routine performance of intraoperative cholangiography, others are in favour of a selective use or have stopped using it altogether [2].

The advent of endoscopic retrograde cholangio pancreatography (ERCP) has altered the policy of routine intraoperative cholangiography. ERCP is a less invasive technique than open bile duct revision, providing excellent detection and removal of bile duct stones. The high success rate of ERCP has resulted in a more selective use of intraoperative cholangiography [2, 3]. Laparoscopic surgery has heavily impacted on biliary surgery during recent years. Laparoscopic cholecystectomy has almost completely replaced open cholecystectomy, but laparoscopic bile duct clearance has not been adopted by the majority of the surgical community. Hence, the discussion has re-emerged as to whether routine or selective intraoperative cholangiography should be used.

Some of the longstanding debates are related to the different goals of intraoperative cholangiography, which cause confusion on the value of routine versus selective use of intraoperative cholangiography. The issues that need to be analyzed separately when it comes to intraoperative cholangiography include avoidance of iatrogenic bile duct injuries, detection of bile duct stones and training of residents, as well as legal aspects [4].

History

The first clinical attempts to visualize the anatomy of the biliary tract were described by Reich in 1918 and by Tenney and Patterson in 1922 [5, 6]. They assessed biliary fistulas and bile duct stenosis using bismuth paste in patients with previous cholecystectomy. In 1930, Ginzburg and Benjamin used a lipiodol solution as a new contrast dye to detect external biliary fistula and bile duct stones [7].

Pablo Mirizzi (1893-1964, a surgeon from Argentina), who reported the first series of routine intraoperative cholangiograms using lipiodol during cholecystectomy in 1932, is recognized as the main contributor to the modern era of bile duct depiction [8]. He described the function of the sphincter of Oddi, and recommended T-tube cholangiography after bile duct exploration for bile duct stones in order to minimize bile duct leakage and injuries. A few years later, Hicken reported an incidence of 12% of retained bile duct stones that were detected using routine intraoperative cholangiography [9]. Until the end of the 1960s, only static films could be obtained, and almost 30 minutes were needed to get three to four images that were often of low quality [1]. With the advent of television fluoroscopy in recent decades, dynamic imaging, high resolution cameras, and mobile image intensifiers markedly improved the quality of intraoperative cholangiogram images, leading to more accurate detection of bile duct injuries and retained bile duct stones [10].

Modern C-arm, with its image intensifier and digital image processing capacities, currently offers real-time subtraction and mapping of the bile ducts, and decreases the duration of intraoperative cholangiography from three to five minutes [1].

Technical Aspects

Laparoscopic cholecystectomy is usually initiated with the dissection of the triangle of Calot to identify the cystic duct and the cystic artery. To this end, a grasper inserted in the right upper quadrant pulls the infundibulum of the gallbladder laterally to the right side. A second grasper lifts the fundus anteriorly. While this maneuver opens the triangle of Calot and facilitates the recognition of the insertion of the cystic duct into the gallbladder and common bile duct, the common hepatic duct will be distorted to a curved shape, thus increasing risk of injury [11].

After having cleared the gallbladder neck and the proximal part of the cystic duct, a clip is placed close to the infundibulum of the gallbladder to occlude gallbladder outflow. A small (1–3 mm) transverse incision is made on the anterior surface of the cystic duct. Prior to opening the cystic duct, the cholangiocatheter should already have been introduced into the abdominal cavity. The cholangiocatheter is inserted as far as necessary into the cystic duct, and then secured using either a clip or a special grasper, e.g., an Olsen cholangiograsper [1]. Of note, the cholangiocatheter should not be fixed too tightly in order to prevent its occlusion (Fig. 10.1).

The C-arm fluoroscope is placed over the right upper quadrant, and the first 3–5 ml of contrast media are injected under fluoroscopy. The cystic duct and its conjunction with the common bile duct must be visual-

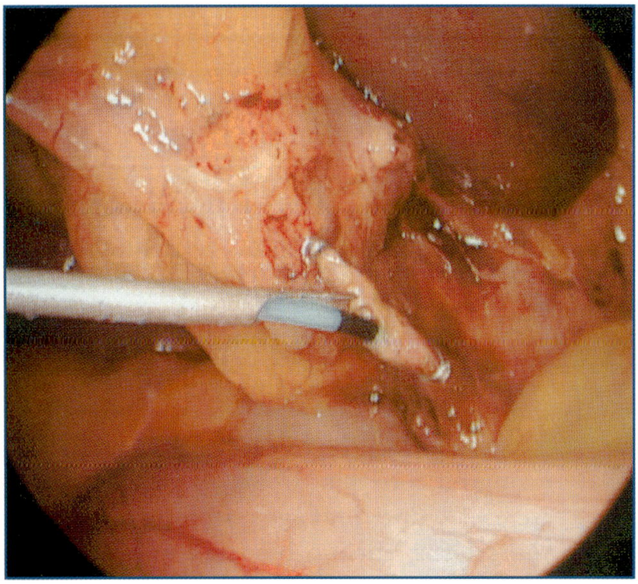

Fig. 10.1 Transcystic placement of the cholangiocatheter

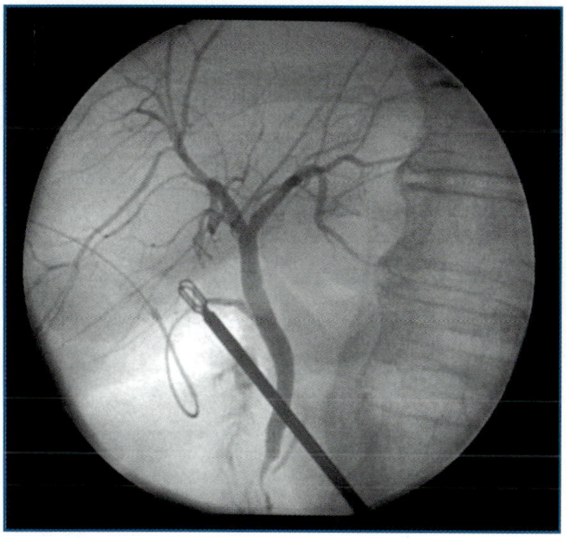

Fig. 10.2 Standard cholangiography by insertion of the cholangiocatheter into the cystic duct

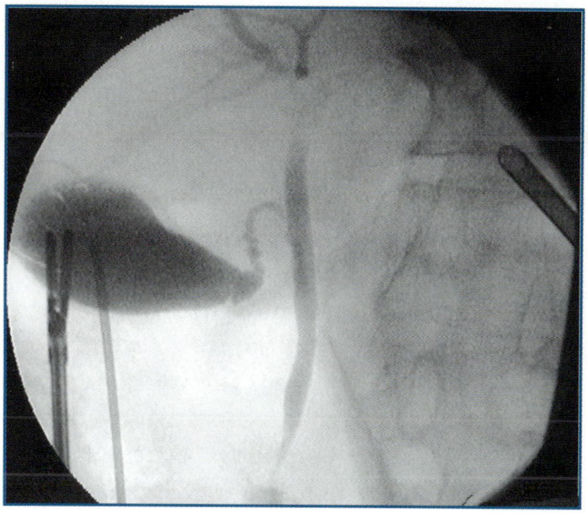

Fig. 10.3 Cholangiography through the gallbladder (cholecystocholangiography)

ized (Fig. 10.2). Since a short cystic duct and a long cystic duct lying parallel to the common bile duct are the two most important anatomical variations leading to increased risk of bile duct injuries, the length of the cystic duct and its position relative to the common bile duct need to be accurately assessed. The contrast media must clearly delineate the distal common bile duct, and then rapidly flow through the sphincter of Oddi into the duodenum. Whereas the patient is initially placed in a slight Trendelenburg position, the proximal bile duct and its main branches to the left and right hepatic lobe and segments are often better filled with contrast in a reverse Trendelenburg position. In addition to the visualization of the biliary anatomy, intraoperative cholangiography enables the detection of bile duct stones. If the contrast media does not easily pass into the duodenum, a possible spasm of the sphincter of Oddi may be relaxed by the use of 1 ml of intravenously-administered glucagon. Air bubbles may be detected by placing the patient in the reverse Trendelenburg position, so that the bubbles rise to the top. Finally, the cholangiocatheter is removed under visual control, and the cystic duct can safely be clipped and transected.

If the cholangiocatheter cannot be placed into the cystic duct, a cholecystocholangiography may be obtained by inserting the catheter into the gallbladder (Fig. 10.3) [1]. However, more contrast media is needed to distend the gallbladder and to visualize the biliary tree. This alternative technique is not successful if the cystic duct is occluded and if there is a contracted fibrotic gallbladder.

Indications

Prevention and Early Recognition of Iatrogenic Bile Duct Injuries

Until a novel surgical technique is clinically established and safely performed by the vast majority of the surgical community, there is always a danger to the target organ derived from iatrogenic lesions attributed to the handling of new devices, uncommon anatomical access and view, and limited experience with specific complications. The very rapid spreading of laparoscopic cholecystectomy during the late 1980s created an urgent need for improved safety concepts in order to minimize bile duct injuries, since early reports on laparoscopic cholecystectomy described an alarmingly high rate of such lesions [12]. This has led to the re-emergence of the discussion of routine versus selective intraoperative cholangiography [1, 2].

If the surgeon gets clear information on the anatomy of the biliary tree using intraoperative cholangiography prior to dividing any biliary duct, misidentification of the cystic duct can be markedly decreased or even completely avoided. The proponents of the routine use of intraoperative cholangiography further emphasize that only consistently repeated practice will allow surgeons to become familiar with the technical aspects as well the correct interpretation of the cholangiograms [13]. While the latter statement is obviously true and needs no further discussion, the problem of misidentification is only partially solved by the use of intraoperative cholangiography.

Why and in what circumstances does misidentification occur? First, only 75% of all patients reveal a "normal" biliary anatomy, while the remaining 25% have some minor or major anatomical variation [14, 15, 16]. Second, disease-specific anatomical changes may severely impair the safe dissection of the triangle of Calot. Mirizzi syndrome and acute cholecystitis, for example, induce major inflammatory changes and may even create cholecystobiliary fistulae, which impede any safe identification of the biliary anatomy by a laparoscopic approach. Third, iatrogenic distortion of the common bile duct may occur if the surgeon exerts too much tension by pulling the gallbladder laterally to the patient's right side. Fourth, once the surgeon has "identified" the local anatomical structures, this intraoperative information is fixed in the surgeon's mind, and will not be further scrutinized [17]. The basic issue is the fact that the local anatomy remains unclear, and there is an increased risk for bile duct injuries.

There are two main anatomical variations that place the bile duct at particular risk of injury during laparoscopic cholecystectomy. A short cystic duct leaves little space between the gallbladder and the common bile duct. Extensive dissection may lead to injury to the common bile duct. On the other hand, a long cystic duct lying parallel to the common bile duct for several centimeters and inserting inferiorly may result in a higher incidence of thermal injuries and accidental clipping of the common bile duct [12, 18, 19].

Intraoperative cholangiography most commonly starts with the dissection of the cystic duct. The cystic duct is encircled, a clip is placed near the gallbladder, and then the cystic duct is incised and a catheter is inserted for the cholangiography. In case of unclear anatomy, there is an inherent risk of bile duct injuries using this standard technique. If the common bile duct has been misidentified, it will probably be devascularized and dissected, then clipped and incised. Even if the cystic duct is successfully dissected, bile duct injuries can occur through the use of rigid catheters that may puncture the dorsal wall of the common bile duct. Thus, these types of bile duct injuries happen because an intraoperative cholangiography has been imperatively and prematurely attempted instead of or before a complete and careful surgical dissection of Calot's triangle! If the cholangiography cannot be performed, in such situations the bile duct injury may not be detected intraoperatively [2, 12].

A "fundus first" or conversion to an open approach is strongly recommended in cases where the biliary anatomy cannot be easily dissected or if there are any doubts. Intraoperative cholangiography should never replace meticulous surgical dissection using an adequate approach. The only advantage of intraoperative cholangiography is that it may allow the early recognition of a bile duct injury. The treatment options for the different types of bile duct injuries are not discussed in this chapter.

Several studies have attempted to assess the role of intraoperative cholangiography in preventing bile duct injuries. Methodological issues, e.g., only small patient groups, retrospective study design, and in particular, low incidence of bile duct injuries, make it difficult to draw reliable conclusions from the literature. In fact, to achieve a 50% reduction in bile duct injuries using intraoperative cholangiography, Massarweh and Flum [20] calculated that a sample size of 30,000 patients would be needed in order to get a sufficient statistical power. Such a study will probably never be performed, and therefore all published studies have the major drawback of lack of statistical power. Most studies based on relatively small patient groups concluded selective intraoperative cholangiography could be safely applied since routine use failed to reveal clear advantages. However, a recently published meta-analysis of 40 case series, including 327,523 laparoscopic cholecystectomies, found a statistically significant reduction in bile duct injuries using intraoperative cholangiography (incidence 0.21%) compared to a selective use (incidence 0.43%) [21]. These findings have been confirmed by an Italian survey of 56,591 laparoscopic cholecystectomies that found a 50% reduction in bile duct injuries using routine intraoperative cholangiography [22].

Detection of Bile Duct Stones

The indication for intraoperative cholangiography to detect bile duct stones is highly dependent on treatment strategy. For many decades, open bile duct revision was the only available treatment modality for bile duct calculi; thus, intraoperative cholangiography was mandatory. ERCP subsequently revealed itself as a very effective tool with which to remove bile duct stones, and open bile duct revision became less commonly used and restricted to complicated biliary stones [2, 3].

In the era of laparoscopic cholecystectomy, many surgeons still prefer ERCP to laparoscopic bile duct clearance. Laparoscopic bile duct clearance ranges from simple transcystic insertion of a balloon catheter and pushing stones through the papilla of Vater, to choledochotomy with instrumental stone removal and closure of the defect over a T-tube. While the first procedure can often be performed easily, the latter one is restricted to experienced hepatobiliary and laparoscopic surgeons. Thus, if common bile duct calculi are already suspected preoperatively, ERCP will be performed in most cases to avoid surgical bile duct revision. Moreover, small stones should simply pass, and no intervention is necessary.

In conclusion, routine use of intraoperative cholangiography is not necessary for the detection of bile duct stones in most patients. Careful preoperative assessment detects bile duct stones with a high sensitivity, and ERCP will clear the biliary system in almost every case. If intraoperatively-detected bile duct calculi cannot be removed using a simple transcystic approach, postoperative ERCP should be preferred in most cases. Bile duct clearance by a laparoscopic approach has not yet been adopted by the majority of the surgical community. However, this issue will be further discussed in next chapters.

Training

Only regular use will allow a surgeon to become familiar with the procedure of intraoperative cholangiography and ensure its correct interpretation. In particular, surgical residents need thorough training. If the procedure becomes intraoperatively necessary, it can be performed safely. This argument is often used to promote routine performance of intraoperative cholangiography [13].

It is undoubtedly true that surgeons and surgical residents must be trained in order to become familiar with intraoperative cholangiography. On the other hand, in most cases diagnostic intraoperative cholangiography is easily performed. In addition, conversion to an open approach and calling a more experienced surgeon are probably better strategies for the prevention of bile duct injuries than forcing an intraoperative cholangiography to be performed.

From a more basic point of view, there is no good justification for exposing patients to risk and increased costs merely in order to train residents [2, 4]. An intraoperative cholangiography should not be carried out without good medical reasons.

Legal Aspects

During the early years of laparoscopic cholecystectomy, there was a dramatic increase in bile duct injuries compared to the previous open era [12]. Repair of such injuries is often complex and several surgical and interventional procedures are mandatory. In addition, quality of life and survival in the long-term are often impaired. Despite the absolute number of bile duct injuries being low, they still represented a major cause for medical malpractice claims [20].

If it could have been clearly proved that routine intraoperative cholangiography reduces the number of bile duct injuries and facilitates early recognition and repair, the lack of intraoperative cholangiography could have been used as possible evidence for malpractice. Thus, the careful assessment of the role of intraoperative cholangiography heavily impacts on legal issues [4]. While the possibility of malpractice claims represents an important concern of surgeons in the United States, in many European countries surgeons can still act without major impairment. Nevertheless, lack of documentation severely hampers any surgeon in defending a malpractice accusation.

References

1. MacFayden BV (2006) Intraoperative cholangiography: past, present, and future. Surg Endosc 20:S436-S440
2. Talamini MA (2003) Routine vs selective intraoperative cholangiography during cholecystectomy. JAMA 289:1691-1692
3. Heinerman PA, Boeckl O, Pimpl W (1989) Selective ERCP and preoperative stone removal in bile duct surgery. Ann Surg 209:267-272
4. Talamini MA (1995) Selective cholangiography. In: Arregui ME, Fitzgibbons RJ, Katkhouda N, McKernan JB, Reich H (eds) Principles of laparoscopic surgery. Springer Berlin, Heidelberg, New York, pp 139-142
5. Reich A (1918) Accidental injection of bile ducts with petrolatum and bismuth paste JAMA 71:1555
6. Tenney CF, Patterson SH (1922) Injection of bile ducts with bismuth paste. JAMA 78:171
7. Ginzburg L, Benjamin EW (1930) Lipiodol studies of postoperative biliary fistulae. Ann Surg 91:233-241
8. Mirizzi PL (1932) La cholangiografia durante la operaciones de las vias biliares. Bol Soc Cir Buenos Aires 16:1133
9. Hicken NF, Best RR, Hunt HB (1936) Cholangiography. Ann Surg 103:210-229
10. Berci G, Shore JM, Hamlin JA, Morgenstern L (1978) Operative fluoroscopy and cholangiography. Am Surg 135:32-35
11. Keus F, Broeders IA, van Laarhoven CJ (2006) Surgical aspects of symptomatic cholecystolithiasis and acute cholecystitis. Best Pract Res Clin Gastroenterol 20:1031-1051
12. Connor S, Garden OJ (2006) Bile duct injury in the era of laparoscopic cholecystectomy. Br J Surg 93:158-168
13. Traverso LW (2006) Intraoperative cholangiography lowers the risk of bile duct injury during laparoscopic cholecystectomy. Surg Endosc 1659-1661
14. Kune GA (1970) The influence of structure and function in the surgery of the biliary tract. Ann Roy Coll Surg 47:78-91
15. Sackier JM, Berci G, Phillips E et al (1991) The role of cholangiography in laparoscopic cholecystectomy. Arch Surg 126:1021-1025
16. Gertsch P (2000) The technique of cholecystectomy. In: Blumgart LH, Fong Y (eds) Surgery of the Liver & Biliary Tract. Edinburgh, WB Saunders, pp 697-708
17. Way LW, Stewart L, Gantert W et al (2003) Causes and prevention of laparoscopic bile duct injuries: analysis of 252 cases from a human factors

and cognitive psychology perspective. Ann Surg 237:460-469
18. Olsen D (1997) Bile duct injuries during laparoscopic cholecystectomy. Surg Endosc 11:133-138
19. Hugh TB (2002) New strategies to prevent laparoscopic bile duct injury – surgeons can learn from pilots. Surgery 132:826-835
20. Massarweh NN, Flum DR (2007) Role of intraoperative cholangiography in avoiding bile duct injury. J Am Coll Surg 204:656-664
21. Ludwig K, Bernhardt J, Steffen H, Lorenz D (2002) Contribution of intraoperative cholangiography to incidence and outcome of common bile duct injuries during laparoscopic cholecystectomy. Surg Endosc 16:1098-1104
22. Nuzzo G, Guliante F, Giovannini I (2005) Bile duct injuries during laparoscopic cholecystectomy: results of an Italian national survey of 56,591 cholecystectomies. Arch Surg 140:986-992

Chapter 11

Laparoscopic Ultrasound during Laparoscopic Cholecystectomy

Jean-Marc Catheline, Joël Roussel

Introduction

The incidence of choledocholithiasis (CDL) has been shown to be around 10% when intra-operative cholangiography (IOC) is practised routinely during cholecystectomy [1–3]. The advent of laparoscopic cholecystectomy has enlivened the debate between those who defend systematic intra-operative opacification of the common bile duct (CBD) [4–6] and those who advocate a selective approach [7, 8] based on certain predictive factors [9, 10]. IOC remains an invaluable tool for the detection of asymptomatic stones, as well as the prevention and/or detection of possible CBD injuries [11–13]. Regarding the latter, authors such as Wright [14] have suggested that IOC is not a prerequisite for the safe performance of laparoscopic cholecystectomy and cannot be relied upon to prevent all biliary injuries. Nevertheless, IOC is routinely performed by many surgeons, despite the fact that false positive and false negative results are not uncommon both for the conventional and the laparoscopic operations [1, 3, 5]. Laparoscopic ultrasound (LU) is a relatively recent development [15, 16]. The availability of B-mode real-time ultrasound machines, combined with purpose-designed transducers, has led to renewed interest in intra-operative ultrasound for the detection of CDL, as evidenced by numerous studies [17–24].

Technique

Hardware

Ultrasound Device

The equipment used (Ultra Sonograph 3535, B&K Medical, Denmark) produces images of high resolution (< 1 mm) and is operable at multiple frequencies (5, 6.5, 7.5 MHz). A surgically ergonomic remote control, placed in a sterile plastic bag, allows the operator to zoom, measure, record, alter gain, and select the pre-programmed depth of image for the organ being examined.

Laparoscopic Sonography Probe

A multiple frequency laparoscopic ultrasound transducer (Ultrasound Laparoscopic Transducer 8555, B&K Medical, Denmark) (Fig 11.1), with a 180° flexible tip and a convex scanning angle of 60° which can be introduced via the umbilical port with the camera in the 10 mm left upper quadrant port.

Biliary Exploration

Laparoscopic Ports' Placement

Pneumoperitoneum was achieved in most cases using the "open" method with a 10

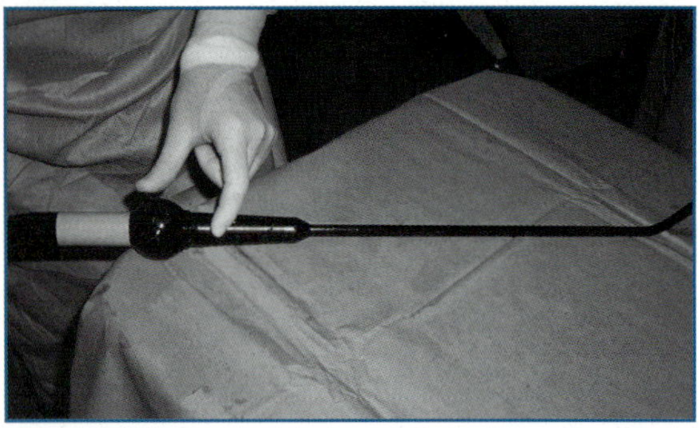

Fig. 11.1 The laparoscopic ultrasound probe allows most distal explorations. Its tip features an acoustic contact surface, with up to 180° flexibility

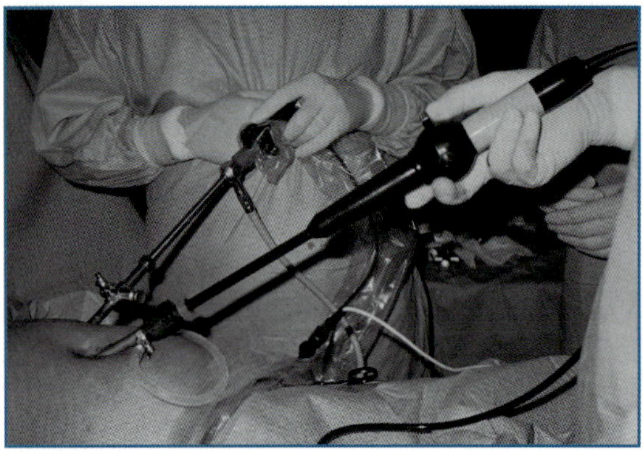

Fig. 11.2 The probe is introduced through the umbilical access port

mm umbilical port. After CO_2 insufflation to a maximum pressure of 12 mmHg, another 10 mm port was placed in the left upper quadrant. Two additional 5 mm ports were inserted to the right of the xiphisternum and at the right subcostal margin in the mid-clavicular line. The 10 mm ports had magnetic hinge valves so as not to damage the ultrasound transducer (Fig 11.2).

Biliary Ultrasonography

Laparoscopic ultrasonography is performed prior to dissection of the lower biliary confluence. Different sequences of the exploration are well codified. The gallbladder and upper biliary confluence are first explored transhepatically. Then the proximal two-thirds of the CBD is visualized by

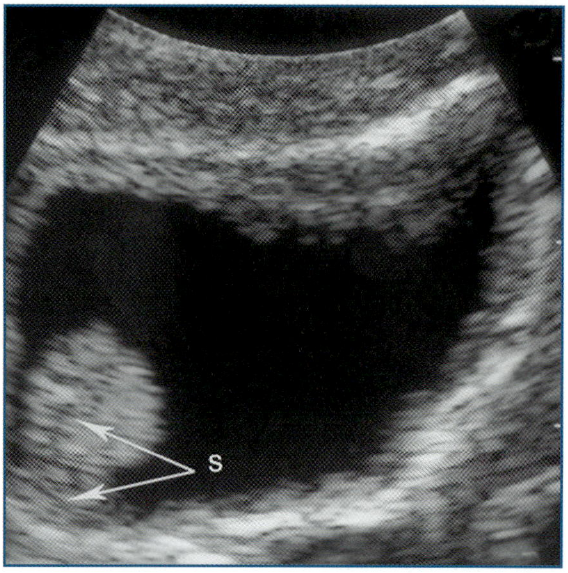

Fig. 11.3 Stones in the gallbladder seen through liver segment V (*s*, stones)

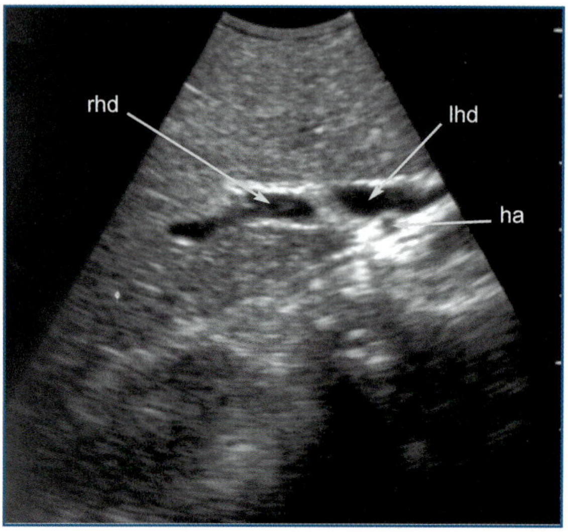

Fig. 11.4 The upper biliary confluent is best seen through segment IV (*rhd*, right hepatic duct; *lhd*, left hepatic duct; *ha*, hepatic artery)

direct contact between the probe and the hepatic pedicle. Finally, the retro-pancreatic duct segment is seen across the second duodenal portion.

Gallbladder and Upper Biliary Confluencc

The gall bladder was then viewed through the liver parenchyma (segment V) in order

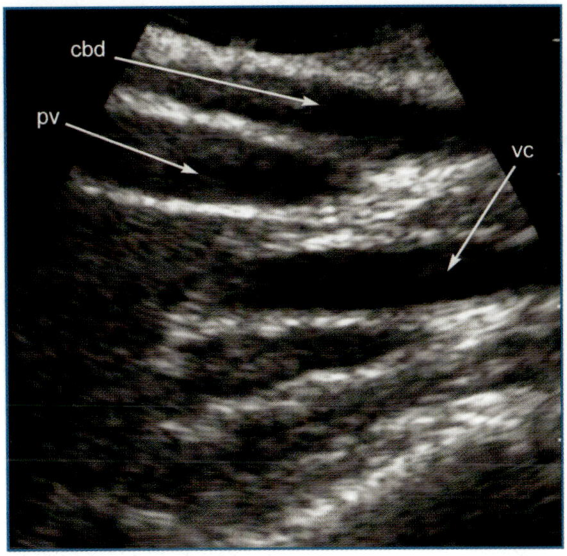

Fig. 11.5 Visualization of the hepatic pedicle shown by direct contact of the transducer with the hepatic pedicle (*cbd*, common bile duct; *pv*, portal vein; *vc*, vena cava)

to quantify the size of calculi, the number of acoustic shadow cones, and the wall thickness (Fig 11.3). The confluence of the right and left hepatic ducts was seen through segment IV (Fig 11.4).

Proximal Two-thirds of the CBD

The transducer was then placed over the anterolateral aspect of the hepatic pedicle. Axial rotation enabled identification of the CBD, portal vein, inferior vena cava and hepatic artery (Fig. 11.5). Once the bile duct was identified, the transducer was passed along its length from top to bottom. Color Doppler can be used to facilitate identification of structures through liver segment IV and within the hepatic pedicle according to the flow within them. If the surgeon feels it necessary, normal saline can be instilled into the abdomen to improve the acoustic contact with biliary structures. The calibre of the CBD was measured at the level of its confluence with the cystic duct using acoustic calipers. Any intra-ductal calculi were sought (Fig 11.6) and a note made of their number, size and location.

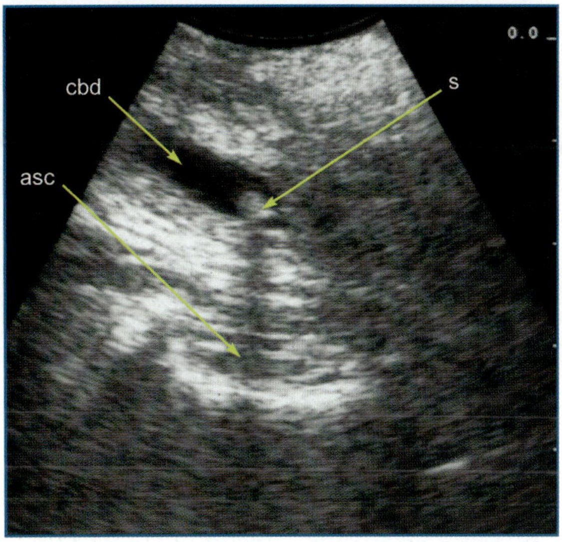

Fig. 11.6 Stone in the common bile duct shown by direct contact of the transducer on the hepatic pedicle (*cbd*, common bile duct; *s*, stone; *asc*, acoustic shadow cone)

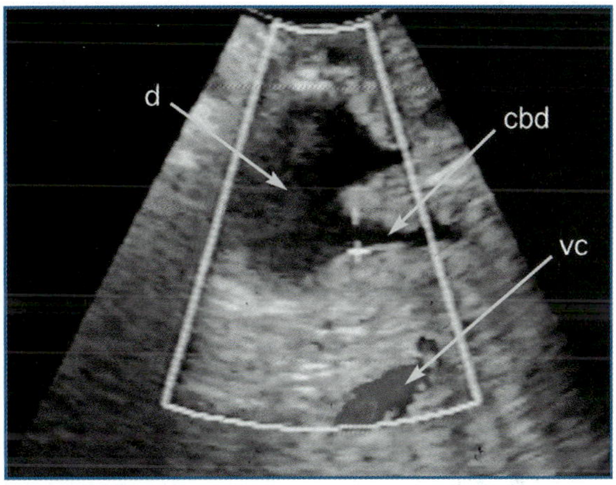

Fig. 11.7 The retropancreatic portion of the common bile duct and the ampulla of Vater seen through the duodenum (*d*, duodenum; *cbd*, common bile duct; *vc*, vena cava)

Retro-pancreatic Bile Duct

The LU probe is left in place within the umbilical port. Distal acoustic surface scans the stomach and the duodenum. The distal third of the CBD and Vater's Ampulla can only be seen through the second duodenal portion. When the duodenum is reached, the ampulla of vater and distal CBD are explored (Fig 11.7). At this point, the initially oblique view of the CBD becomes horizontal as it enters the duodenum. The duration of this exploration may be uncomfortable, depending on patient status, especially if they are overweight.

Methodology

Design

We have undertaken a prospective study of 600 consecutive laparoscopic cholecystectomies, with the aim of comparing the feasibility and diagnostic efficacy of LU and IOC. The biliary tree was routinely and successively evaluated by these two methods. Between November 1994 and August 2000, the biliary trees of 600 patients undergoing laparoscopic cholecystectomy were routinely visualized by both LU and IOC. The population consisted of 432 women and 168 men with a mean age of 54 (21–94) years and a mean weight of 73 (48–140) kg. Indications for operation were: biliary colic (376 cases), acute cholecystitis (172 cases), cholangitis (28 cases) and gallstone pancreatitis (24 cases). General fitness was assessed using the scoring system of the American Society of Anesthesiologists (ASA): 210 patients were classified as ASA I, 294 as ASA II, and 96 as ASA III. ASA IV patients were excluded from the study, as a level of ASA IV was considered a relative contraindication to laparoscopy. All patients had undergone an abdominal ultrasound examination with measurement of CBD calibre. This was performed by a sonographer experienced in hepatobiliary ultrasound on average 9 days prior to operation. Preoperative serum levels of bilirubin, alkaline phosphatase, transaminases (AST, ALT) and amylase were obtained the day before surgery. The clinical, biochemical and sonographic predictive factors for CDL are given in Table 11.1. Endoscopic retrograde cholangiography was performed in 20 patients, before they were referred to us. They had initially presented with jaundice or cholangitis. Where CDL was confirmed, endoscopic sphincterotomy and duct clearance were performed.

Training in Laparoscopic Ultrasound and Cholangiography

Laparoscopic ultrasound and cholangiography were routinely performed by seven different surgeons: two consultant surgeons

Table 11.1 Predictive factors for choledocholithiasis

Predictive factors for CDL	No. of patients (*n*=600)	%
Clinical		
Age > 70 years	72	12
Jaundice	70	12
Biochemical		
Bilirubin > 26 umol/l	58	10
Alkaline-phosphatase >200IU/l	96	16
Serum amylase > 200 IU/l	40	7
Preoperative ultrasound		
CBD diameter > 8 mm	70	12
Intraductal stones seen	40	7

CDL, Choledocholithiasis; *CBD*, Common bile duct

formally trained in these techniques and five trainee surgeons. This latter group had a pre-requisite apprenticeship of five combined sonographic and cholangiographic examinations (not included in the study). For the next 20 cases of each trainee (included in the study), the LU and cholangiograms were supervised by one of the consultants. Thereafter all examinations were performed independently by each of the operators. For each case, the interpretation of the LU was performed by the individual operator (supervised by a consultant for the first 20 cases). The cholangiogram films were developed in the radiology department and interpreted in a blind fashion, by a radiologist who was unaware of the findings of the ultrasound examination, before being returned to the surgeon in operating room.

Performance Evaluation

For the evaluation of detection of choledocholithiasis by LU and cholangiography, the ultimate reference criterion was the confirmation on CBD exploration of stones previously diagnosed by LU and/or IOC. Where CBD stones were not detected by either investigation, the reference criterion was the absence of retained stones after one year of clinical follow-up. The data (including feasibility, image quality, detection of CBD stones, and biliary tree anomalies) were coded by the authors and entered into a computerized database. Inferential analysis was performed with a statistical program utilizing Student's t-test and the chi-squared test.

Results

In this study, CBD stones were found in 54 cases (9%). Twenty endoscopic retrograde cholangiograms were performed preoperatively, 14 with stone extraction and six revealing the CBD to be free of stones. Forty cases of CDL were diagnosed intra-operatively. Twenty-eight of these were dealt with laparoscopically, eight required conversion to an open procedure, and four were treated by postoperative endoscopic stone extraction. Of the 40 cases diagnosed intra-operatively, 12 had no pre-existing risk factors (30%). Twenty-eight (70%) had at least one of the clinical, biochemical, and/or sonographic predictive factors given in Table 11.1. CDL was revealed in 15 (9%) out of 172 cases with acute cholecystitis, and seven (25%) out of 28 cases with cholangitis, but not in any of the patients who had clinical or biochemical evidence of pancreatitis. All 600 patients in the study were reviewed at 1 month, 6 months and 1 year after surgery. None were lost to follow-up. During the 12 month follow-up period, none of the patients presented with clinical evidence of retained CBD stones.

Laparoscopic Ultrasound Versus Cholangiography

Feasibility

No morbidity or mortality resulted from either technique. All 600 patients (100%) underwent LU. IOC was not achieved in 102 patients (17%). In 86 of these, this was due to failed cystic duct cannulation: narrow lumen or cystic duct valves in 36 cases, and an excessively inflamed cystic duct in 50 cases with acute cholecystitis. For the remaining 16 cases, iodine allergy presented a contraindication to cholangiography. Mean duration was 10.2 minutes (5–20) for LU and 17.9 minutes (7–38) for IOC (p=0.0001).

Image Quality and Detection of Biliary Anomalies

The mean calibre of the CBD was given as 5.5 mm (2.8–18 mm) by ultrasound and 7 mm (3.5–22 mm) by cholangiography. This difference was not statistically significant. Including the 102 cases of failed cholangiography, the intra-hepatic biliary tree was accurately visualized by LU in 97% of cases and by IOC in 77%, and the proximal two-thirds of the CBD in 100% and 80%, respectively. The distal one-third of the CBD was adequately seen by LU in only 87% of cases (particularly difficult in obese subjects) compared to 79% for IOC. Cholangiography proved better than LU in detecting variations in biliary anatomy. It detected 15 long and 12 short cystic ducts, compared to only eight long and seven short ducts diagnosed by LU. IOC also revealed other anatomical anomalies not seen at all by ultrasound, such as three cystic ducts draining into the right hepatic duct and four cholecystohepatic ducts that were subsequently identified when dissecting the gallbladder from the liver bed and divided between two clips. On the other hand, LU fortuitously detected other co-existing pathologies: 12 hepatic cysts, four liver abscesses, three pancreatic cysts and four renal cysts.

Detection of CDL

Common bile duct exploration was undertaken in 52 cases where at least one of the two investigations suggested filling defects. Forty of these (7%) confirmed the presence of stones, whereas 12 did not (2%). Subsequent follow-up to one year revealed no patients with clinical evidence of retained CBD stones. Hyper-echoic lesions were detected by ultrasound in 36 cases, of which 32 were true positives and four false positives (calculi lodged in the cystic duct near the junction with the CBD). IOC similarly showed 38 filling defects, of which 30 were true positives and eight false positives. The latter were defects suggested in at least one of the films taken for each patient and subsequently judged to be air bubbles when radiologists and surgeons later conjointly reviewed the films. There were eight false negatives for LU (due to non-visualization of the distal CBD) and ten for IOC (because of poor quality films or stones less than 3 mm). The false negatives for one investigation were nevertheless detected as true positives by the other. The 102 cases where IOC was not successful were diagnosed as true negatives by LU. This was confirmed by subsequent clinical follow-up. The results (Table 11.2) were calculated on an intention-to-perform basis. The calculation of sensitivities, specificities, and positive and negative predictive values were done with a denominator of 600 cases for both LU and IOC, with the 102 unsuccessful IOCs being counted as true negatives. In the detection of CBD stones, sensitivity was 80% for LU and 75% for IOC. Specificity was 99% for both investigations. Differences between the two methods were not statistically significant. The two investigations were in fact complementary. When combined, they achieved 100% sensitivity and 98% specificity for detection of CBD stones.

It should also be noted that LU revealed micro-bubbles of gas in the CBDs of five of the 14 patients who had had a pre-operative endoscopic retrograde cholangiopancreatography (ERCP) with sphincterotomy and stone extraction. Although these were considered an artifact, they did not result in any false negatives or positives, as such bubbles are not hyper-echoic (i.e., without shadow cones).

Effect of Operator Experience

The numerical experience and respective failure rates of each of the operators are shown in Table 11.3. For cholangiography, consultant surgeons succeeded in opacifying the biliary tree more often than trainees. False negatives occurred between the 23rd and 64th examination, and were not encountered thereafter. False positives were seen near the start of operative experience (e.g., the 18th case for one of the surgeons), but also as late as the 98th case for another surgeon. For LU, consultant surgeons who were already experienced in the

Table 11.2 Laparoscopic ultrasound versus cholangiography: results calculated on the basis of intention-to-perform

	Laparoscopic ultrasounds (n=600)	Intraoperative cholangiographies (n=600)	"p"
Adequate visualization			
Intrahepatic ducts	582 (97%)	463 (77%)	ns
Proximal 2/3 CBD	600 (100%)	478 (80%)	ns
Distal 1/3 CBD	522 (87%)	473 (79%)	ns
Detection of CDL			
True negatives	556	552*	ns
True positives	32	30	ns
False negatives	8	10	ns
False positives	4	8	ns
Sensitivity	80%	75%	
Specificity	99%	99%	ns
Positive predictive value	89%	79%	ns
Negative predictive value	99%	98%	ns

* Includes 102 cases of failed intraoperative cholangiography; *CDL*, Choledocholithiasis; *CBD*, Common bile duct

Table 11.3 Laparoscopic ultrasound versus cholangiography: results according to operator experience

Operator experience	Cholecys-tectomies	Laparoscopic ultrasounds			Intra-operative cholangiographies		
	No.	No. (%)	False + (cases)	False - (cases)	No. (%)	False + (cases)	False - (cases)
Surgeon 1 (consultant)	57	57 (100%)	0	0	53 (93%)	0	0
Surgeon 2 (consultant)	145	145 (100%)	0	0	131 (90%)	1 (98th)	1 (45th)
Surgeon 3 (trainee)	96 (trainee)	96 (100%)	1 (34th)	1 (24th)	72 (75%)	2 (48th, 65th)	2 (23rd, 44th)
Surgeon 4 (trainee)	79	79 (100%)	1 (42nd)	1 (32nd)	62 (79%)	1 (44th)	1 (52nd)
Surgeon 5 (trainee)	82	82 (100%)	0	2 (28th, 44th)	67 (82%)	2 (45th, 60th)	2 (39th, 64th)
Surgeon 6 (trainee)	75	75 (100%)	1 (23rd)	2 (36th, 38th)	63 (83%)	1 (18th)	2 (26th, 37th)
Surgeon 7 (trainee)	66	66 (100%)	11 (36th)	2 (42nd, 44th)	50 (76%)	1 (39th)	2 (33th, 53rd)
Total	600	600	4	8	498 (83%)	8	10

technique had no false negatives or positives. For trainees, false negatives occurred between the 24th and 44th cases, and false positives between the 23th and 42nd cases. There were no errors of either type with LU for any of the operators after 45 examinations had been completed.

Discussion

Routine IOC has traditionally been used for the detection of CDL during open and laparoscopic cholecystectomies. Our study has shown that LU is of comparable efficacy in this regard. The other benefit of IOC is the definition of biliary anatomy and the potential avoidance of bile duct injuries. According to Fletcher et al. [25], IOC provides a protective effect against the complications of cholecystectomy. However, it is recognized that IOC has its limitations. It is contraindicated in pregnancy and iodine allergy. It is difficult to perform in acute cholecystitis. A narrow cystic duct lumen or the presence of cystic duct valves can also prevent its realization. Even though we sought to undertake it routinely, we were unable to perform it on 102 occasions (17% of the cases in our study), the principal reason being acute cholecystitis (50 cases). The failure rate reported in the literature for unselected cases is generally less than 10% [26, 27]. This actually corresponds to the results of the two consultant surgeons in our study. The success rate was less for surgical trainees, reflecting the learning curve that is necessary, particularly for difficult cases such as acute cholecystitis. False negatives are similarly a function of operative experience, as none were noted after the 64th case for any of the surgeons. However, false positives seem to be independent of experience, as these were still occurring quite late in an operator's individual experience (the 98th examination for one of the consultants and the 65th for one of the trainees).

Laparoscopic ultrasound is a new technique that requires evaluation. It is only relatively recently that the usefulness of LU has been reported with respect to staging of hepatic and pancreatic cancers [28–32]. Multiple frequency LU enables extremely high resolution images of the liver, pancreas and biliary tree, as well as the ampulla of Vater. The flexible transducer also permits optimal acoustic contact with most surfaces. Studies on the use of intra-operative ultrasound in conventional surgery have shown it to be as viable a method as cholangiography for the detection of CDL [33–35]. In accordance with other authors [21–24], our series suggests that LU is comparable to IOC for the detection of CDL. Moreover, we noted no false negatives in cases where both investigations concurred with a negative result. This was despite a relatively exhaustive 12 month follow-up. Positivity in one of the investigations was considered an indication for CBD exploration, thus yielding 40 true positives (7%) but also 12 in which the CBD was found to be free of stones (2%)

Special training is necessary for LU, preferably supervised by someone experienced in both conventional and laparoscopic intra-operative ultrasonography [17, 19]. In our study, none of the trainees had any false positives or negatives for their first 20 cases that were supervised by a consultant. We nevertheless underestimated the length of the necessary training period. The eight false negatives and four false positives noted soon thereafter highlight the fact that there is a definite learning curve for this technique. After an individual experience of 45 cases, no further errors were noted. Until such time, as reported in other studies on this subject, we thus suggest that this figure be the recommended minimum requirement before an operator performs the investigation independently. The time taken to adequately evaluate the biliary tree progressively declined during the course of our experience. A trained operator could perform a full biliary LU in less than 10 minutes. This is confirmed by other authors [21–24]. This relatively short time reflects the user-friendly nature of this new technique. There is no patient-related restriction on the type of cases in which LU can be used. This is a great advantage in acute cholecystitis where cannulation of the cystic duct may not be possible. The 102 cases of failed cholangiography were seen to be true negatives by IOC, a fact that was confirmed by subsequent clinical follow-up. Furthermore, the false results of one method were shown to be true by the other method. In combination, the two techniques had 100% sensitivity and 98% specificity for the detection of common duct stones. It should be noted that 12 (23%) of the 52 CBD explorations were negative. These should not necessarily be seen as complications (particularly where explorations are performed transcystically), but as the acceptable price of ensuring 100% sensitivity. This leads us to recommend the performance of both investigations in order to maximize the intra-operative detection of choledocholithiasis.

LU can be used to check CBD clearance after choledochotomy. Artifacts may nevertheless be produced by air bubbles present in the biliary tree following choledochotomy. LU also permits exploration of the rest of the abdominal cavity, as evidenced by our fortuitous discovery of a liver abscess and cysts in various organs [21].

We achieved adequate visualization of the distal CBD in only 87% of cases, which is comparable to the results of other authors [21–23]. This is particularly difficult in obese subjects, in whom introduction of normal saline into the abdominal cavity only partially improves acoustic contact. The mean calibre of the CBD as measured by IOC was greater than that given by LU. This is likely due to distension of the CBD with the contrast material, as well as an intrinsic magnification factor afforded by radiography. LU cannot, according to our study, provide sufficiently clear images of biliary anatomy to allow it to replace cholangiography for this purpose. Cholangiography also revealed anatomical anomalies not seen by ultrasound. Even with color and pulse Doppler, LU does not give the same degree of biliary topographical detail as IOC [36–45].

References

1. Mansberger JA, Davis J, Scarborough C, Bowden TA (1988) Selective intraoperative cholangiography. A case for its use on an anatomic basis. Am J Surg 55:31-33
2. Ijzermans JNM, De Waard P, Merkelbach JW (1989) Cholangiography during cholecystectomy: a plea for selective use. Neth J Surg 41:79-81
3. Shively EH, Wieman TJ, Adams AL et al (1990) Operative cholangiography. Am J Surg 159:380-384
4. Corbitt JD, Cantwell D (1991). Laparoscopic cholecystectomy with operative cholangiogram. Surg Laparosc Endosc 1:229-232
5. Flowers JL, Zucker KA, Graham SM et al (1992) Laparoscopic cholangiography: results and indications. Ann Surg 215:209-216
6. Sackier JM, Berci G, Phillips E et al (1991) The role of cholangiography in laparoscopic cholecystectomy. Arch Surg 126:1021-1026
7. McEntee G, Grace PA, Bouchier-Hayes D (1991) Laparoscopic cholecystectomy and the common bile duct. Br J Surg 78:385-386
8. Trondsen E, Edwin B, Reiertsen O et al (1998) Prediction of common bile duct stones prior to cholecystectomy: a prospective validation of a discriminant analysis fonction. Arch Surg 133:162-166
9. Bogokowsky H, Slucki S, Zaidenstein L et al (1987) Selective operative cholangiography. Surg Gynecol Obstet 164:124-126
10. Huguier M, Bornet P, Charpak Y et al (1991) Selective contraindications based of multivariate analysis for operative cholangiography in biliary lithiasis. Surg Gynecol Obstet 172:470-474
11. Bagnoto VJ, McGee GE, Hatten LE et al (1991) Justification for routine cholangiography during laparoscopic cholecystectomy. Surg Laparosc Endosc 1:89-93
12. Berci L, Sackier RJ, Paz Partlow M (1991) Routine or selected intraoperative cholangiography during laparoscopic cholecystectomy. Am J Surg 161:355-360
13. Hunter JG (1991) Avoidance of bile duct injury during laparoscopic cholecystectomy. Am J Surg 162:71-76

14. Wright KD, Wellwood JM (1998) Bile duct injury during laparoscopic cholecystectomy without operative cholangiography. Br J Surg 85:191-194
15. Rothlin M, Sclumpf R, Largiader F (1991) Die technik der intra-operativen sonographie bei der laparoskopiscer cholecystektomie. Chirurg 62:899-901
16. Ascher SM, Evans RT, Goldberg JA (1992) Intraoperative bile duct sonography during laparoscopic cholecystectomy: experience with a 12,5 MHz catheter-based U.S. probe. Radiology 185:493-496
17. Castro D, Arregui ME, Brueggeman A (1995) Laparoscopic ultrasound: principles and techniques. In: Arregui ME, Fitzgibbons RJ, Katkouda N, Mc Kernam JB, Reich H (eds) Principles of laparoscopic surgery. Basic and advances techniques. New York, Springer Verlag, pp 489-505
18. Machi J, Sigel B, Zaren HA et al (1993) Technique of ultrasound examination during laparoscopic cholecystectomy. Surg Endosc 7:544-549
19. Rothlin MA (1995) Laparoscopic ultrasound of the biliary tree. In: Arregui ME, Fitzgibbons RJ, Katkouda N, MC Kernam JB, Reich H (eds) Principles of laparoscopic surgery. Basic and advances techniques. New York, Springer Verlag, pp 506–512
20. Yamamoto M, Stiegman GV, Durham J et al (1993) Laparoscopy-guided intracorporeal ultrasound accurately delineates hepatobiliary anatomy. Surg Endosc 7:325-330
21. Greig JD, John TG, Mahadaven M, Garden OJ (1994) Laparoscopic ultrasonography in the evaluation of the biliary tree during laparoscopic cholecystectomy. Br J Surg 81:1202-1206
22. Barteau JA, Castro D, Arregui ME, Telik C (1995) A comparison of intraoperative ultrasound versus cholangiography in the evaluation of the common bile duct during laparoscopic cholecystectomy. Surg Endosc 9:490-496
23. Rothlin MA, Schob R, Schlumpf R, Lagardir F (1996) Laparoscopic ultrasonography during cholecystectomy. Br J Sur 83:1512-1516
24. Yamashita Y, Kurohiji T, Hayashi J (1993) Intraoperative ultrasonography during laparoscopic cholecystectomy. Surg Laparosc Endosc 3:167-171
25. Fletcher DR, Hobbs MS, Tan P et al (1998) Complications of cholecystectomy: risks of the laparoscopic approach and protective effects of operative cholangiography: a population-based study. Ann Surg 229:449-457
26. Bouillot JL, Fernandez FJ, Dehni N et al (1995) Intraoperative systematic cholangiography in celoscopic cholecystectomy. Gastroenterol Clin Biol 19:287-290
27. Millat B, Atger J, Deleuze A et al (1997) Laparoscopic treatment for choledocholithiasis: a prospective evaluation in 247 consecutive unselected patients. Hepatogastroenterology 44:28-34
28. Miles WFA, Paterson-Brown S, Garden OJ (1992) Laparoscopic contact hepatic ultrasonography. Br J Surg 79:419-420
29. Murighia M, Paterson-Brown S, Winsor JA et al (1993) Early experience of laparoscopic ultrasonography in the management of pancreatic carcinoma. Surg Endosc 7:177-181
30. John TG, Greg D, Carter DC, Garden OJ (1995) Carcinoma of the pancreatic head and periampullary region: tumour staging with laparoscopy and laparoscopic ultrasonography. Ann Surg 221:156-164
31. John TG, Greig D, Crosbie JL et al (1994) Superior staging of livers tumors with laparoscopy and laparoscopic ultrasound. Ann Surg 220:711-719
32. Catheline JM, Turner R, Rizk N et al (1999) The use of diagnostic laparoscopy supported by laparoscopic ultrasonography in the assessment of pancreatic cancer. Surg Endosc 13:239-245
33. Lane RJ, Coupland GAE (1992) Ultrasonic indications to explore the common bile duct. Surgery 91:268-274
34. Sigel B, Machi J, Beitler JC (1983) Comparative accurancy of operative ultrasonography and cholangiography in detecting common duct calculi. Surgery 94:715-720
35. Jakimowicz JJ, Rutten H, Jurgens PJ, Carol EJ (1987) Comparison of operative ultrasonography and radiography in screening of the common bile duct for calculi. World J Surg 11:628-634
36. Foley WD, Quiroz FA (2007) The role of sonography in imaging of the biliary tract. Ultrasound 23:123-135
37. Tai CK, Tang CN, Ha JP et al (2004) Laparoscopic exploration of common bile duct in difficult choledocholithiasis. Surg Endosc 18:910-914
38. Costi R, Iusco DR, Sarli L (2005) Evaluation of the predictors of choledocholithiasis: comparative analysis of clinical, biochemical, radiological, radionuclear, and intraoperative parameters. Surg Today 35:1095-1096
39. Sgourakis G, Delemadi G, Stamatelopoulos A et al (2005) Predictors of common bile duct lithiasis in laparoscopic era. World J Gastroenterol 11:3267-3272
40. Alecu L, Corodeanu G, Costan I et al (2001) Intraoperative ultrasonography, dissection with ultrashears and trans-cystic choledochoscopy during laparoscopic apprroach in obstructive lithiasis icterus case. Chirurgia (Bucar) 96:85-90
41. Catheline JM, Turner R, Paries J (2002) Laparoscopic ultrasonography is a complement to cholangiography for the detection of choledocholithiasis at laparoscopic cholecystectomy. Br J Surg 89:1235-1239

42. Luo D, Chen X, Li S, Mao J (2002) Laparoscopic ultrasonography-assisted complicated laparoscopic cholecystectomy. Zhonghua Wai Ke Za Zhi 40:417-419
43. Halpin VJ, Dunnegan D, Soper NJ (2002) Laparoscopic intracorporeal ultrasound versus fluoroscopic intraoperative cholangiography: after the learning curve. Surg Endosc 16:336-341
44. Santambrogio R, Bianchi P, Opocher E et al (1999) Prevalence and laparoscopic ultrasound patterns of cholecocholithiasis and biliary sludge during cholecystectomy. Surg Laparosc Endosc Percutan Tech 9:129-134
45. Biffl WL, Moore EE, Offner PJ (2001) Routine intraoperative laparoscopic ultrasonography with selective cholangiography reduces bile duct complications during laparoscopic cholecystectomy. J Am Coll Surg 193:272-280

Chapter 12

Diagnostic Flow Charts for Biliary Lithiasis

Emilie Lermite, Patrick Pessaux

Gallbladder Stones

Clinical

Gallstones remain asymptomatic in nearly 80% of cases [1]. The clinical features of gallbladder stone disease include biliary colic and acute cholecystitis. Biliary colic is caused by impaction of the stone in the cystic duct with distension of the gallbladder and activation of visceral sensory neurons [2]. The pain typically arises in the right upper quadrant of the abdomen or epigastrium, rapidly increases in intensity and then plateaus, lasts for 30 min to 6 h, and occasionally radiates to the right subscapular area. Associated symptoms including nausea and vomiting are common.

Acute cholecystitis arises when a stone remains impacted in the neck of the gallbladder [3]. The symptoms begin as a biliary colic, but the pain persists for more than 12 h. The typical signs are right upper abdominal pain and tenderness, fever, leukocytosis and Murphy's sign. An inflammatory mass (the gallbladder) may be palpable in the right upper quadrant.

Diagnostic Tools

Biological

Liver function tests may be normal. Leukocytosis is seen in acute cholecystitis.

Radiological

Transabdominal ultrasonography is the gold standard for the diagnosis of gallbladder stones [4]. Its sensitivity and specificity are high: over 95% for detection of gallbladder stones more than 1.5 mm diameter in size. Ultrasonography provides information about the stone size, burden and mobility within the gallbladder, the size of the gallbladder and its wall thickness, the size of the CBD and hepatic duct, and the status of both liver and pancreas parenchyma. Wall thickness greater than 3 mm is regarded as abnormal, it is one of the signs of cholecystitis. Transabdominal ultrasonography can exhibit positive sonographic Murphy's sign.

Diagnostic Flow Chart

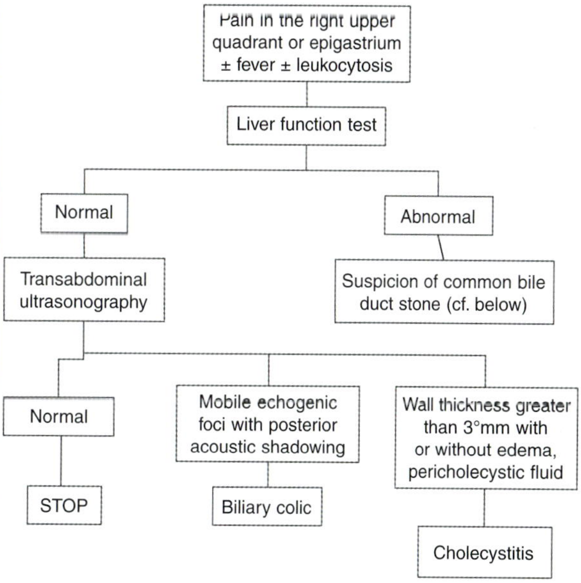

Common Bile Duct Stones

Clinical

The symptoms of CBD stones (CBDS) are variable; they range from being completely asymptomatic to involving such clinical pictures as those of biliary colic, jaundice, cholangitis, or pancreatitis. Up to 15% of patients have CBDS in combination with gallbladder stones, but the majority (73%) of CBDS will pass spontaneously into the duodenum without significant sequelae [5]. When a stone is impacted in the bile duct, obstructed jaundice ensues. When the obstructed bile becomes infected it results in cholangitis. Charcot's triad describes cholangitis as the association of jaundice, fever, and pain that is observed in up to 75% of these patients. Prolonged biliary obstruction results in secondary biliary cirrhosis after approximately 5 years [6].

Between 4% and 8% of patients with gallstones will develop gallstone pancreatitis secondary to migratory gallstones.

Diagnostic Tools

Laboratory Tests

Patients with symptomatic CBDS often have abnormal cholestatic liver function test. In a study by Anciaux, elevated serum gamma glutamyl transpeptidase (GGT) and alkaline phosphatase (ALP) were the most frequent biochemical abnormalities in patients with symptomatic choledocolithiasis (elevated in 94% and 91% of cases, respectively) [7]. In another study, by Peng et al. [8], GGT appears to be the most sensitive marker of CBDS. However, laboratory data can be normal in as many as one third of patients with choledocolithiasis.

Radiological

Transabdominal Ultrasonography

Transabdominal ultrasonography (TUS) is the most commonly used screening modality. It can provide information suggestive of the presence or absence of CBDS, specifically the diameter of the CBD. A CBD diameter greater than 7 mm on TUS is associated with a higher prevalence of choledocolithiasis than normal. Although TUS has a high sensitivity in detecting CBD dilatation (96% according to Stott and al. [9]), it has a low sensitivity in the diagnosis of CBD stones (only about 63% [10]). A negative TUS in a patient with suspected choledocholithiasis does not rule out CBDS [11], however, with a specificity of 95% TUS remains an extremely useful test if CBDS are detected.

Computed Tomography

Studies on conventional computed tomography (CT) have found sensitivities between 70% and 90% in detection of choledocolithiasis. The sensitivity, specificity, and accuracy of spiral CT vary between 85% and 88%, 88% and 97%, and 86% and 94%, respectively [12, 13]. CT can exclude the differential diagnosis of pancreatic tumor. The need for contrast medium and radiation exposure is a further drawback of CT.

Endoscopic Ultrasonography

Endoscopic ultrasonography (EUS) is an invasive procedure, but the morbidity and mortality associated with it are minimal [14]. The diagnostic accuracy of EUS for CBDS is higher than 95% and compares favorably with that of endoscopic retrograde cholangiopancreatography (ERCP). Moreover, EUS avoids the risks of pancreatitis, cholangitis, and radiation exposure [15]. EUS may play a role in detecting gallstones too small to be picked up by other investigations.

Endoscopic Retrograde Cholangiopancreatography

Endoscopic retrograde cholangiopancreatography used to be the gold standard for preoperative diagnosis of CBDS, with sensitivity between 90% and 95% in detecting choledocolithiasis [16]. ERCP has both diagnostic and therapeutic value for visualization and extraction of the impacted stones. However, complication rates associated with ERCP can be as high as 15%, and possible complications include pancreatitis, cholangitis, and perforation or bleeding of the duodenum. The mortality rate of ERCP is 0.2–0.5% [17, 18]. Therefore ERCP is recommended only for patients in whom there is a high probability of CBDS. In patients with an intermediate probability of CBDS other imaging modalities should be considered.

Magnetic Resonance Cholangiopancreatography

Magnetic resonance cholangiopancreatography (MRCP) has emerged as an accurate, noninvasive diagnostic modality for investigating the biliary and pancreatic ducts [19]. It has a sensitivity of 81–100% and a specificity of 92–100% in detecting choledocolithiasis, i.e. similar to ERCP. However, if gallstones are small (less than 4 mm) and sited close to Vater's papilla, MRCP accuracy is rather unsatisfactory [20]. Moreover, MRCP is clearly an expensive option and is not available everywhere and does not allow endoscopic extraction of stones.

Intraoperative Cholangiography

Intraoperative cholangiography (IOC) can be a useful tool to identify choledocolithiasis, but it remains controversial. Dynamic fluoroscopy imaging is the technique of choice and has a specificity of 94% and sensitivity of 98% in experienced hands [21]. When there is any suspicion of choledocolithiasis, IOC seems to be a better choice than preoperative ERCP assessment, because of its low morbidity.

Diagnostic Flow Chart

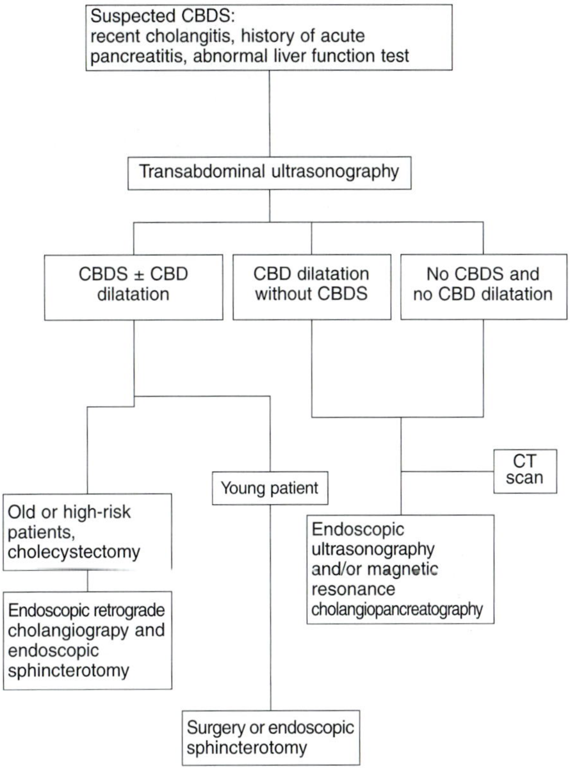

Intrahepatic Stones

Clinical

Patients suffering from hepatolithiasis can nonetheless remain free of symptoms. Symptoms of hepatolithiasis include abdominal pain, jaundice, cholangitis, or liver abscesses. Chronic cholangitis and resulting sepsis are characteristic symptoms of the disease.

Diagnostic Tools

Biological

Laboratory evaluation is usually nonspecific, confirming the obstructive nature of the jaundice. Blood cultures are positive in up to 50% of cases.

Radiological

In the diagnosis of hepatolithiasis, imaging studies should aim not only to diagnose intrahepatic stones but also to evaluate, in detail, the precise location of stones, any stricture(s) of bile ducts, and even concurrent cholangiocarcinoma [22].

Transabdominal Ultrasonography

Ultrasonograpy is free from ionizing radiation and contrast is not required. It is available everywhere and remains the first study when hepatolithiasis is suspected. Intrahepatic stones appear as echogenic spots with an acoustic shadow behind. Abdominal ultrasonography in expert hands can detect more than 90% of intrahepatic stones but cannot identify or localize biliary stricture. TUS can, however, detect gallbladder and extrahepatic bile duct stones.

Computed Tomography

Intrahepatic stones can be depicted on unenhanced CT, but the detection rate is not satisfactory (63–81%). Contrast-enhanced studies do not help in detection of the stones. CT can be less sensitive than US in detection of stones, but is useful for detecting parenchymal atrophy [23, 24] and bile duct dilatation. Dilated bile ducts appear as a low-density tubular, tortuously branching structure best appreciated on contrast-enhanced studies. CT is also helpful in the diagnosis of liver abscesses and may be useful for percutaneous drainage.

Magnetic Resonance Cholangiopancreatography

The sensitivity, specificity, and accuracy of MRCP in detecting and locating intrahepatic stones are 97%, 99%, and 98%, respectively, in some series. Stones are recognized as defective low-density areas. The sensitivity, specificity, and accuracy of MRCP in detecting and locating intrahepatic bile duct strictures are 93%, 97%, and 97%, respectively [25]. The principal advantage of MRCP is its ability to depict the entire biliary tract and to allow identification of dominant strictures without further instrumentation [26]. Moreover, it is ionizing radiation free, noninvasive, and operator-independent, and involves only negligible morbidity. However, the ability of MRCP to reveal concurrent intraductal cholangiocarcinoma associated with hepatolithiasis is limited. It is also an invaluable tool in the diagnosis and location of hepatic abscesses.

ERCP and Percutaneous Cholangiography

Until recently, cholangiography, whether percutaneous (PC) or endoscopic (ERCP), has provided the most accurate diagnosis, the information it yields including locations and shapes of stones and the site of any stricture [27]. Cholangiography has a sensitivity of almost 100% in the detection of any obstruction. However, ERCP cannot opacify peripheral intrahepatic bile ducts, because it commonly happens that several ductal strictures are present. Moreover, both PC and ERCP are invasive, with relatively high morbidity rates of 1–7% for ERCP and 3–5% for PC. As the role of MRCP evolves, the roles of both ERCP and PC become primarily therapeutic owing to their ability to provide drainage of an infected bile duct.

Diagnostic Flow Chart

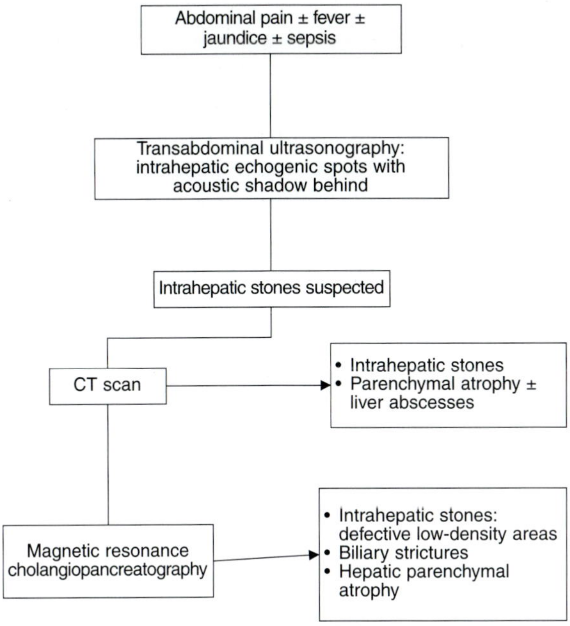

References

1. Gibney EJ (1990) Asymptomatic gallstones. Br J Surg 77:368-372
2. Diehl AK, Sugarek NJ, Todd KH (1990) Clinical evaluation for gallstone disease: usefulness of symptoms and signs in diagnosis. Am J Med 89:29-33
3. Friedman GD (1993) Natural history of asymptomatic and symptomatic gallstones. Am J Surg 165.399-404
4. Leopold GR, Amberg J, Gosink BB, Mittelstaedt C (1976) Gray scale ultrasonic cholecystography: a comparison with conventional radiographic techniques. Radiology 121:445 448
5. Tranter SE, Thompson MH (2003) Spontaneous passage of bile duct stones: frequency of occurrence and relation to clinical presentation. Ann R Coll Surg Engl 85:174-177
6. Scobie BA, Summerskill WH (1965) Hepatic cirrhosis secondary to obstruction of the biliary system. Am J Dig Dis 10:135-146
7. Anciaux ML, Pelletier G, Attali P et al (1986) Prospective study of clinical and biochemical features of symptomatic choledocolithiasis. Dig Dis Sci 31:449-453
8. Peng WK, Sheikh Z, Paterson-Brown S, Nixon SJ (2005) Role of liver function tests in predicting common bile duct stones in acute calculous cholecystitis. Br J Surg 92:1241-1247
9. Stott MA, Farrands PA, Guyer PB et al (1991) Ultrasound of the common bile duct in patients undergoing cholecystectomy. J Clin Ultrasound 19:73-76
10. Sugiyama M, Atomi Y (1997) Endoscopic ultrasonography for diagnosing choledocolithiasis: a prospective comparative study with ultrasonography and computed tomography. Gastrointest Endosc 45:143-146
11. Gross BH, Harter LP, Gore RM et al (1983) Ultrasonic evaluation of common bile duct stones: a prospective comparison with endoscopic retrograde cholangiopancreatography. Radiology 146:471-474
12. Neitlich JD, Topozian M, Smith RC et al (1997) Detection of choledocolithiasis: comparison of unenhanced helicoidal CT and endoscopic retrograde cholangiopancreatography. Radiology 203:753-757
13. Polkowski M, Palucki J, Regula J et al (1999) Helicoidal computed tomographic cholangiography versus endosonography for suspected bile duct stones: a prospective blinded study in non-jaundiced patients. Gut 45:744-749
14. Lightdale CJ (1996) Indications, contraindications, and complications of endoscopic ultrasonography. Gastrointest Endosc 43:S15-19
15. Norton SA, Alderson D (1997) Prospective comparison of endoscopic ultrasonography and endoscopic retrograde cholangiopancreatography in the detection of bile duct stones. Br J Surg 84:1366-1369
16. Frey CF, Burbige EJ, Meinke WB et al (1982) Endoscopic retrograde cholangiopancreatography. A J Surg 144:109-114
17. Ong TZ, Khor JL, Selamat DS et al (2005) Complications of endoscopic retrograde cholangiography in the post-MRCP era: a tertiary center experience. World J Gastroenterol 11:5209-5212
18. Rhodes M, Sussman L, Cohen L, Lewis MP (1998) Randomised trial of laparoscopic exploration of common bile duct versus postoperative endoscopic retrograde cholangiography for common bile duct stones. Lancet 351:159-161
19. Hallal AH, Amortequi JD, Jeroukhimov IM (2005) Magnetic resonance cholangiopancreatography accurately detects common bile duct stones in resolving gallstone pancreatitis. J Am Coll Surg 200:869-875
20. NIH state-of-the-science statement on endoscopic retrograde cholangiopancreatography (ERCP) for diagnosis and therapy. NIH Consens State Sci Statements 2002; 19: 1-26
21. Griniatsos J, Karvounis E, Isla AM (2005) Limitations of fluoroscopic intraoperative cholangiography in cases suggestive of choledocholithiasis. J Laparoendosc Adv Surg Tech A 15:312-317

22. Valls C, Guma A, Puig I et al (2000) Intrahepatic peripheral cholangiocarcinoma: CT evaluation. Abdom Imaging 25:490-496
23. Nakayama F, Koga A (1984) Hepatolithiasis: present status. World J Surg 8:9-14
24. Ohto M, Kimura K, Tsuchiva Y et al (1984) Diagnosis of hepatolithiasis. Prog Clin Biol Res 152:129-148
25. Park DH, Kim MH, Lee SS et al (2004) Accuracy of magnetic resonance cholangiopancreatography for locating hepatolithiasis and detecting accompanying biliary stricture. Endoscopy 36:987-992
26. Fulcher AS, Turner MA, Capps GW et al (1998) Half-Fourier RARE MR cholangiopancreatography: experience in 300 subjects. Radiology 207:21-32
27. Su HC, Wei HC, Liu QX, Li YB (1991) Treatment of bilateral intrahepatic stones with high duct strictures through selective central hepatic resection. Surgery 110:8-12

Chapter 13

Medical Treatment of Gallstone Disease

Piero Portincasa, Antonio Moschetta, Francesco Puglisi, Luigi Borracino, David Q.-H. Wang

Introduction

Gallstones are one of the most prevalent and costly digestive diseases [1]. About 75% of the gallstones in the United States and other westernized countries are cholesterol gallstones, which are subclassified as either pure cholesterol or mixed stones that contain at least half cholesterol by weight. The remaining gallstones are pigment stones that contain mostly calcium bilirubinate and are subclassied into two groups: black pigment stones (20%) and brown pigment stones (5%).

Gallstones may be present in the gallbladder, the extrahepatic bile duct, or the intrahepatic bile duct, and their location determines the chosen treatment strategy. In this chapter, we will mainly discuss the medical treatment of gallbladder gallstones.

Treatment of gallstones should be reserved only for a subgroup of patients because of the elevated costs of therapeutic interventions and should be based on the natural history of the disease [1, 2]. Therefore, the selection of patients for either medical or surgical therapy is of key importance. The onset of biliary pain is the only suggestive symptom of "symptomatic" gallstone disease [3, 4], although it can be problematic to distinguish between symptomatic and asymptomatic subjects in a random population of gallstone patients [5]. The diagnosis can be misleading if patients inadequately describe "typical" symptoms or suffer from highly atypical symptoms [6]. A list of practice points to be taken into account when assessing symptoms during the clinical workup of gallstone patients is depicted in Table 13.1. Of note, prior symptomatic patients who are symptom free for 5 consecutive years should be included in the group of asymptomatic subjects. After this time the risk of pain attacks gradually decreases towards values similar to those in patients with asymptomatic gallstones [7]. An overview of therapeutic options available for gallstone patients is depicted in the flow chart in Figure 13.1 [1], and shows that medical treatment is indeed limited to a small subgroup of patients with tiny cholesterol gallstones.

Asymptomatic Gallstone Patients

Expectant Management

Most gallstones are incidentally found during routine abdominal ultrasonography, and in the majority of the cases (60–80%) stones do not generate symptoms (i.e., biliary pain) [5, 8, 9]. Indeed, the average risk of developing symptomatic gallstones is as low as 2.0–2.6% per year [7, 10]. Micro stones and sludge, by contrast, put gallstone patients at risk of biliary pain and complications, and play a major role in the etiology of acute otherwise idiopathic pancreatitis [11, 12].

Table 13.1 Practice points to consider in the presence of a "symptomatic" gallstone patient. Adapted from Portincasa et al [2]

- Biliary colic is described as an intense right hypocondrium pain, irradiated to the back. This symptom is highly suggestive of symptomatic gallstone disease, and its appearance is important for prognosis and treatment
- Non-specific dyspeptic symptoms and intolerance to fried or fatty food might also be associated with colicky pain
- Given the high incidence of biliary pain recurrence and the high rate of complications (about 1–2%), the "symptomatic" gallstone patient requires treatment
- The association of pain with nausea, vomiting, fever, jaundice, leukocytosis, suggests complicated biliary pain

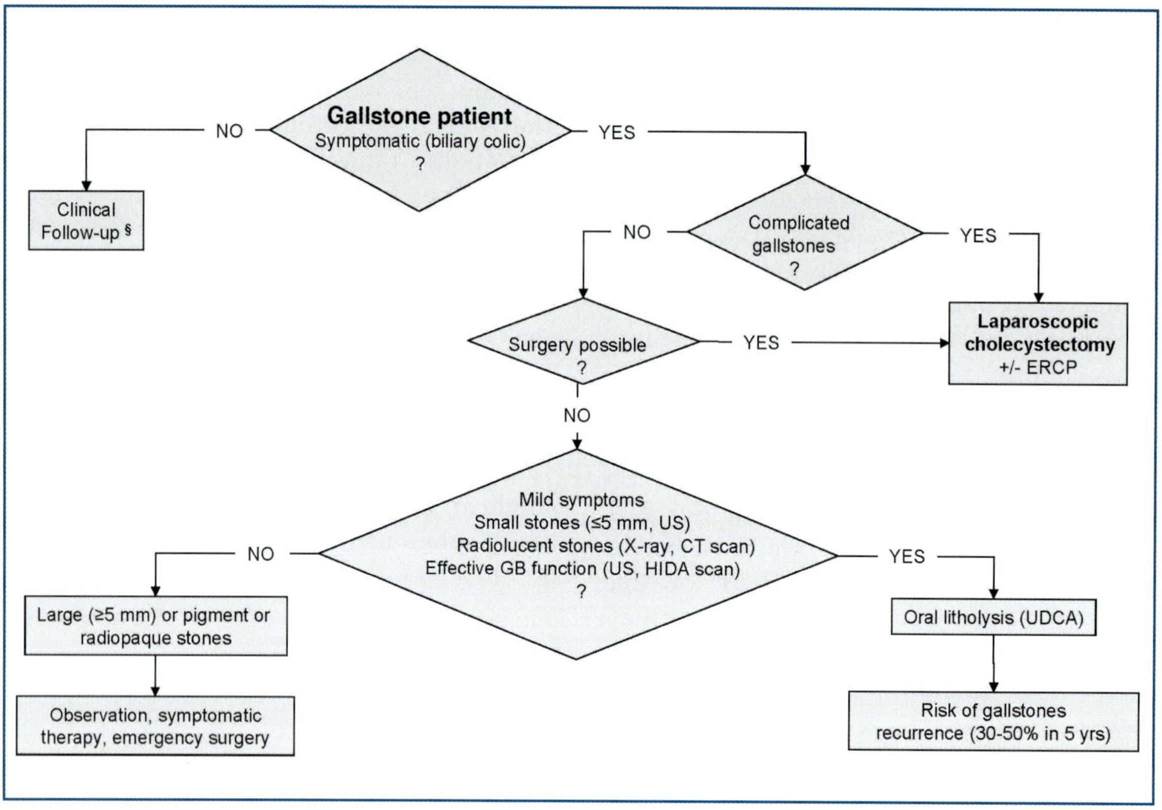

Fig. 13.1 Algorithm for the management of gallstone disease. The symbol "§" in the "Follow-up" box indicates that a subgroup of symptomatic patients may be referred for medical or surgical therapy, depending on more tailored clinical decisions (see text for explanation). Identification of the true symptomatic patient is a key point in the selection process of cholesterol gallstone treatment strategies, since following therapies rely on the presence of biliary symptoms [2]. Gallstone-induced pain is usually localized in right upper quadrant of the abdomen and/or in the epigastrium. It is often intense, with a mean visual analogue scale 90 mm on a 0–100 mm scale, as well as being typically intermittent. The duration of the pain is generally longer than 15–30 minutes and it often radiates to the angle of the right scapula and/or shoulder, or infrequently (7%) to the retrosternal area. The patient often feels the urge to walk [6], vomits, or is nauseated [3, 6, 9]. The pain can last several hours with associated non-specific symptoms of indigestion. *CT*, computerized tomography; *ERCP*, endoscopic retrograde cholangiopancreatography; *HIDA*, ^{99m}Tc-N-(2,6-dimethylacetanilide)-iminodiacetic acid; *GS*, gallstones; *GB*, gallbladder; *UDCA*, ursodeoxycholic acid; *US*, abdominal ultrasonography). Adapted from Portincasa et al. [1]

However, one should consider that the yearly incidence of complications is very low (0.3%), and the rate risk for gallbladder cancer is as low as 0.02% [13, 14]. Therefore, treatment of "asymptomatic" gallstone patients is not routinely recommended, as the overall risk of biliary colic, complications and gallbladder cancer are very low [15–17]. Moreover, routine "prophylactic" treatment, either medical or surgical, is expensive and has not improved survival even in a high-risk subgroup of patients for which such prophylactic treatment has been attempted [13, 14].

Prophylactic Treatment

Whereas expectant management is the appropriate choice in the vast majority of patients with asymptomatic gallstones, prophylactic therapy should be offered to a subgroup of asymptomatic patients at high risk of becoming symptomatic. Prophylactic theraphy will be mainly surgical (cholecystectomy) because this subgroup of patients includes (a) children [18] (exposed to the long term physical presence of stones), (b) morbidly obese gallstone patients undergoing bariatric surgery [19], as these are likely to become symptomatic during rapid weight loss, (c) patients at increased risk of gallbladder cancer [20], including those with large stones [21, 22] (a solitary stone or a stone burden greater than 3 cm in size), a "porcelain" gallbladder [23] or gallbladder polyps that are rapidly growing or that are larger than 1 cm, and (d) native Americans with gallstones (increased risk of cancer between 3 to 5%) [24]. Prophylactic cholecystectomy should also be considered in asymptomatic gallstone patients with sickle cell anemia. In these subjects, calcium bilirubinate gallstones form due to chronic hemolysis and they may become symptomatic with recurrent episodes of abdominal pain mimicking either sickle cell crisis or colicky pain [25]. Prophylactic cholecystectomy is still not widely accepted in asymptomatic gallstone patients undergoing solid organ transplantation; pre-transplant cholecystectomy may suffer a higher surgical risk in these patients but, on the other side, they are also at increased risk of post-transplant biliary infection, drug side effects and malignancies [26–28]. Morbidly obese patients undergoing bariatric surgery have a high incidence of gallbladder disease and gallstone-related complications [29, 30] and might benefit from prophylactic cholecystectomy [31]. Prophylactic cholecystectomy has also been proposed in patients with small gallstones and associated gallbladder dysmotility, conditions that increase the risk of pancreatitis [11]. Small gallstones, sludge and microlithiasis are definitively the major etiological factors for acute pancreatitis [32, 33], but prospective studies are needed to evaluate costs and risk-related benefits of prophylactic cholecystectomy. In fact, no data on incidence and occurrence of pancreatitis in patients with small gallstones are currently available.

Symptomatic Gallstone Patients

The selection of patients for non-surgical treatment of gallstone disease depends on factors such as patient characteristics and gallbladder function, as well as size, number, and composition of the stones. Dissolution therapy for gallstones should be considered as a surgical alternative in carefully selected patients. The same approach may also be useful as prophylaxis in patients at high risk of developing symptomatic gallstone disease.

Cholecystectomy

Cholecystectomy is the most important treatment strategy for symptomatic patients with gallstones or those with complicated gallstone disease, as shown in Fig. 13.1. The

National Institutes of Health consensus conference concluded that laparoscopic cholecystectomy is safe and cost-effective compared to open cholecystectomy [34]. Therefore, the correct identification of "symptomatic" gallstone patients is essential, because the cardinal indication for cholecystectomy is pain attack [13, 35, 36].

Medical Therapy of Biliary Colic

As the intensity of biliary pain is usually high patients require immediate medical attention and analgesia. This visceral pain is caused by the impaction of the stone in the cystic duct or ampulla of Vater, with distension of the gallbladder and/or biliary tract and activation of visceral sensory neurons [3]. Pain relief is obtained if the stone returns to the gallbladder lumen, and back into the common bile duct or passes through the papilla into the duodenum according to its location. Pain can be alleviated by narcotic analgesics or non-steroidal anti-inflammatory drugs (NSAIDs). Of note, besides their fast and intense effect, NSAIDs may reduce the risk of evolution towards acute cholecystitis in patients with biliary colic [37–40]. As outlined in Table 13.1, the association of nausea, vomiting, fever, jaundice and leukocytosis points to complicated biliary pain. This clinical picture requires immediate hospital admission and appropriate treatment. Acute cholecystitis, acute pancreatitis, biliary obstruction and cholangitis, abscess formation, gallbladder perforation, or mucocele of the gallbladder are the most frequent gallstone complications and require, from time to time, additional medical therapy with antibiotics or invasive procedures with or without surgical interventions. Studies on the risk of biliary pain in asymptomatic carriers are lacking, but the risk is estimated to be approximately 1% [41, 42]. In early non-randomized or placebo-controlled studies, it was reported that ursodeoxycholic acid (UDCA), the hydrophilic bile acid, reduced the risk of biliary colic [43, 44]. In a non-randomized study, Tomida et al. [45] treated patients referred for symptomatic or asymptomatic gallstones with 600 mg UDCA per day; patients who refused the treatment constituted the control group. The incidence of biliary pain was apparently reduced by UDCA in asymptomatic patients, although a bias might include a misclassification of symptoms. However, in a large randomized, double-blind, placebo-controlled trial on the effects of UDCA in highly symptomatic gallstone patients scheduled for cholecystectomy, UDCA did not exert a beneficial effect on biliary colic. The likelihood of remaining colic-free was comparable in patients with strong or weak baseline gallbladder contraction as determined by ultrasonography after a standard mixed meal [46].

Dissolution Therapy

Dissolution of cholesterol gallstones by oral bile acids following fragmentation by extracorporeal shock wave lithotripsy (ESWL) was first introduced in Munich in 1986 [47]. Contact dissolution of cholesterol gallstones by the organic solvent methyl tert-butyl ether (MTBE) via percutaneous puncture of the gallbladder was first reported in 1985 [48]. However, these techniques are no longer used due to their invasiveness, costs and high recurrence rate of gallstones following gallstone clearance [47–50]; a recent review has been published on this topic [51].

The only dissolution therapy currently available is the use of oral litholysis by bile acids. This approach, however, has a limited role in a small subgroup of patients (less than 10% of the total), i.e., those who are unfit for surgery, or have small (equal to or less than 5 mm in size), uncalcified (radiolucent), and cholesterol-enriched (i.e., > 80%) stones in a functioning gallbladder (Fig. 13.1) [52]. In other words, large, either pigment or calcified stones are poor candidates for dissolution therapy. Ultrasonography of the right upper quadrant is the best diagnostic tool for detecting gallstones [17, 53], as well as for assessing gallstone size and burden [54]. Although not routinely employed, functional ultrasonography provides additional information about time-dependent changes of both fasting and postprandial gallbladder volume as markers of gallbladder emptying and bile duct patency [55–61]. The imaging examination with ^{99m}Tc-N-(2,6-dimethylacetanilide)-iminodiacetic acid (HIDA) is an alternative tool to assess gallbladder function [1, 2]. Additional diagnostic tools include the use of abdominal plain radiography and – not routinely – computerized tomographic (CT) scan [62, 63] for detecting calcified stones as radiopaque bodies in the right upper quadrant (these stones are unfit for dissolution because they are either calcified cholesterol stones or stones made of pigment calcium bilirubinate [64]). Also, oral cholecystography might disclose the presence of floating (cholesterol) stones in the gallbladder and a preserved cystic duct patency. Well selected patients are those who have a higher chance of successful oral litholysis alone or after ESWL for stone fragmentation [57–60, 65].

Medical treatment with bile acids was first described in the late nineteenth century [66, 67] and complete dissolution of gallstones by bile acids was reported in 1937 by Rewbridge [68]. Furthermore, oral bile acid litholysis for cholesterol stones emerged in the 1970s with chenodeoxycholic acid (CDCA), [69] and in the 1980s with the hydrophilic bile acid UDCA [70]. Medical treatment lost interest after the first laparoscopic cholecystectomy performed by Mouret in 1987 [71], since then, this has been the treatment of choice for symptomatic gallstones. The UDCA dose used for cholesterol stone dissolution is usually 10–14 mg/kg body weight per day. The therapeutic effects of bile acids include the inhibition of hepatic secretion and phase separation of biliary cholesterol, the reduction of intestinal cholesterol absorption, and possibly improvement in gallbladder emptying [72, 73]. Indeed, oral administration of UDCA is associated with increased amounts of biliary UDCA, which results in a decreased hepatic secretion of biliary cholesterol and the formation of unsaturated gallbladder bile (meaning a cholesterol saturation index of less than 1) [74–76]. During UDCA treatment, more cholesterol can be transported in vesicles so that crystallization can be prevented [77]. From a pathophysiological point of view, when plotting the solubility limits for the three main bile lipids (percent mole of cholesterol vs. percent mole of phospholipids vs. percent mole of bile salts) in UDCA-enriched bile, one can observe a marked reduction in the micellar zone as well as a strong shift of all phase boundaries and crystallization pathways to the left, i.e., to a lower lecithin content (Fig. 13.2). As a result, the right two-phase E-zone is greatly enlarged and overlaps pathophysiological lipid compositions, where cholesterol is solubilized mainly in vesicles. Thus, in region E, solid cholesterol crystals are a forbidden phase transition and would be difficult to achieve. This indicates that during UDCA treatment, the chance of cholesterol crystallization is strongly reduced, because vesicles are relatively stable and have a greater ability to dissolve cholesterol in bile compared with mixed micelles [78, 79].

UDCA might also prevent gallstone formation in obese patients during rapid weight loss [80]. After one year of dissolution treatment, the success rate is not more than 50–75% complete dissilution for small stones. This is considerably lower in patients with larger stones or multiple stones, where success rates are lower than 40–50% after one year [13, 81]. Several studies found that in 30–50% of cases gallstones recur 5 years after bile acid therapy or lithotripsy [58, 82–84]. Both the high rate of gallstone recurrence after medical therapy and the unfavorable cost-benefit analysis are the main reasons why medical therapy of cholesterol gallstones has been largely abandoned.

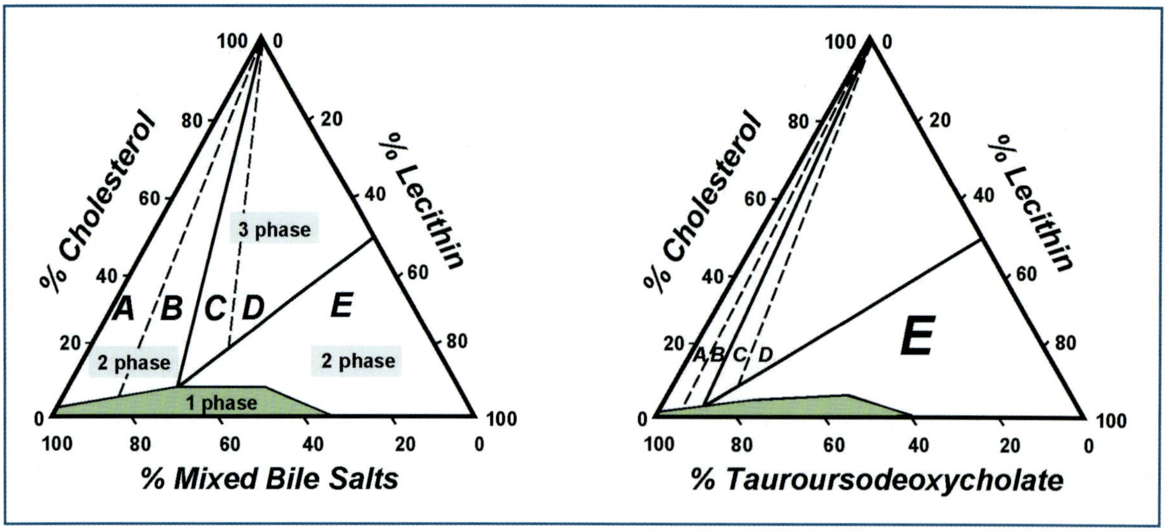

Fig. 13.2 Effects of UDCA on bile composition and cholesterol solubility are explained using the ternary phase diagram [85]. As an example, the equilibrium phase diagram of cholesterol-lecithin-mixed bile salt system (37°C, 0.15 M NaCl, pH 7.0, total lipid concentration 7.5 g/dL) displaying positions and configuration of crystallization regions is shown in the *left panel*. The lipid components are expressed in moles percent. The one-phase micellar zone at the bottom is enclosed by a shadow. Above it, two solid lines divide the two-phase zones from a central three-phase zone. Based upon the solid and liquid crystallization sequences present in the bile, the left two-phase and the central three-phase regions are divided by dashed lines into regions A to D. The number of phases given represents the equilibrium state. They are cholesterol monohydrate crystals and saturated micelles for crystallization regions A and B; cholesterol monohydrate crystals, saturated micelles and liquid crystals for regions C and D; and liquid crystals of variable compositions and saturated micelles for region E [85]. Positions of crystallization regions A-E for UDCA-enriched bile (*right panel*) induces an evident leftward shift of the E-zone. This event is followed by greatly reduced chance of crystal formation in such biles

Conclusion

The use of medical therapy for the treatment of symptomatic gallstones has dramatically declined following the introduction of laparoscopic cholecystectomy in 1987. Medical therapies for gallstones can be considered in a subgroup of patients with mild symptoms who prefer a non-surgical approach and in those with symptomatic disease who have medical conditions precluding surgery. Of course, the selection of patients in whom either medical or surgical therapy is indicated is of key importance. Based on the natural history of the disease and because of the elevated costs of therapeutic interventions, medical treatment of gallstone disease is currently indicated for the treatment of biliary colic and some complications unfit for surgery. To date, dissolution therapy has a limited role in a small subgroup of patients, i.e., they are unfit for surgery, or have small, uncalcified, and cholesterol-enriched stones in a functioning gallbladder. Both the high rate of gallstone recurrence after medical therapy and unfavorable cost-benefit analysis explains why medical therapy of cholesterol gallstones has been largely abandoned. Thus, it can be concluded that choosing medical treatment for dissolution of cholesterol gallstone represents a Grade 2B recommendation (i.e., a weak recommendation: “alternative approaches may be better for some patients under some circumstances”) [51].

Acknowledgments
The authors’ experimental work related to the topic of gallstones is supported in part by research grants “Progetti Ateneo 2005-2007” (P.P. and A.M.) from the University of Bari, “COFIN

2005-6" (P.P.), "COFIN 2006-8" (P.P.) by the Ministero Italiano dell'Università e della Ricerca and DK54012 and DK73917 (D.Q.-H.W.) from the National Institutes of Health (US Public Health Service). P.P. was a recipient of the short-term mobility grant 2005 between the University of Bari Medical School and the Harvard Medical School from the Italian National Research Council (CNR). We thank Francesca Bello and Ersilia Romanelli for skillful technical assistance.

References

1. Portincasa P, Moschetta A, Palasciano G (2006) Cholesterol gallstone disease. Lancet 368:230-239
2. Portincasa P, Moschetta A, Petruzzelli M et al (2006) Gallstone disease: symptoms and diagnosis of gallbladder stones. Best Pract Res Clin Gastroenterol 20:1017-1029
3. Diehl AK, Sugarek NJ, Todd KH (1990) Clinical evaluation for gallstone disease: usefulness of symptoms and signs in diagnosis. Am J Med 89:29-33
4. Paumgartner G, Carr-Locke DL, Roda E et al (1988) Biliary stones: non-surgical therapeutic approach. Gastroenterology International 1: 17-24
5. Jorgensen T (1989) Abdominal symptoms and gallstone disease: an epidemiological investigation. Hepatology 9:856-860
6. Berhane T, Vetrhus M, Hausken T et al (2006) Pain attacks in non-complicated and complicated gallstone disease have a characteristic pattern and are accompanied by dyspepsia in most patients: the results of a prospective study. Scand J Gastroenterol 41:93-101
7. Friedman GD, Raviola CA, Fireman B (1989) Prognosis of gallstones with mild or no symptoms: 25 years of follow-up in a health maintenance organization. J Clin Epidemiol 42:127-136
8. Gibney EJ (1990) Asymptomatic gallstones. Br J Surg 77:368-372
9. Festi D, Sottili S, Colecchia A et al (1999) Clinical manifestations of gallstone disease: evidence from the multicenter Italian study on cholelithiasis (MICOL). Hepatology 30:839-846
10. Thistle JL, Cleary PA, Lachin JM et al (1984) The natural history of cholelithiasis: the National Cooperative Gallstone Study. Ann Intern Med 101:171-175
11. Venneman NG, Renooij W, Rehfeld JF et al (2005) Small gallstones, preserved gallbladder motility, and fast crystallization are associated with pancreatitis. Hepatology 41:738-746
12. Venneman NG, Buskens E, Besselink MG et al (2005) Small gallstones are associated with increased risk of acute pancreatitis: potential benefits of prophylactic cholecystectomy? Am J Gastroenterol 100:2540-2550
13. Paumgartner G, Carr-Locke DL, Dubois F et al (1993) Strategies in the treatment of gallstone disease. Working team report. Gastroenterology International 6:65-75
14. Brugge WR (2000) The silent gallstone. In: gallbladder and biliary tract diseases. Afdhal NH (ed) New York, Basel, Marcel Dekker, Inc., pp 447-453
15. Tait N, Little JM (1995) The treatment of gall stones. BMJ 311:99-105
16. Hofmann AF, Amelsberg A, Vansonnenberg E (1993) Pathogenesis and treatment of gallstones. N Engl J Med 328:1854-1855
17. Johnston DE, Kaplan MM (1993) Pathogenesis and treatment of gallstones. N Engl J Med 328:412-421
18. Pokorny WJ, Saleem M, O'Gorman RB et al (1984) Cholelithiasis and cholecystitis in childhood. Am J Surg 148:742-744
19. Amaral JF, Thompson WR (1985) Gallbladder disease in the morbidly obese. Am J Surg 149:551-557
20. Sleisenger MH, Fordtran JS (2006) Gastrointestinal disease: pathophysiology, diagnosis, management, 8th edn. Philadelphia, W.B. Saunders
21. Lowenfels AB, Walker AM, Althaus DP et al (1989) Gallstone growth, size, and risk of gallbladder cancer: an interracial study. Int J Epidemiol 18:50-54
22. Randi G, Franceschi S, La VC (2006) Gallbladder cancer worldwide: geographical distribution and risk factors. Int J Cancer 118:1591-1602
23. Ashur H, Siegal B, Oland Y et al (1978) Calcified ballbladder (porcelain gallbladder). Arch Surg 113:594-596
24. Lowenfels AB, Lindstrom CG, Conway MJ et al (1985) Gallstones and risk of gallbladder cancer. J Natl Cancer Inst 75:77-80
25. Bonatsos G, Birbas K, Toutouzas K et al (2001) Laparoscopic cholecystectomy in adults with sickle cell disease. Surg Endosc 15:816-819
26. Graham SM, Flowers JL, Schweitzer E et al (1995) Opportunistic upper gastrointestinal infection in transplant recipients. Surg Endosc 9:146-150
27. Graham SM, Flowers JL, Schweitzer E et al (1995) The utility of prophylactic laparoscopic cholecystectomy in transplant candidates. Am J Surg 169:44-48
28. Kao LS, Kuhr CS, Flum DR (2003) Should cholecystectomy be performed for asymptomatic cholelithiasis in transplant patients? J Am Coll Surg 197:302-312
29. Shiffman ML, Sugerman HJ, Kellum JH et al

(1993) Gallstones in patients with morbid obesity. Relationship to body weight, weight loss and gallbladder bile cholesterol solubility. Int J Obes 17:153-158
30. Shiffman ML, Sugerman HJ, Kellum JM et al (1991) Gallstone formation after rapid weight loss: a prospective study in patients undergoing gastric bypass surgery for treatment of morbid obesity. Am J Gastroenterol 86:1000-1005
31. Liem RK, Niloff PH (2004) Prophylactic cholecystectomy with open gastric bypass operation. Obes Surg 14:763-765
32. Lee SP, Nicholls JF, Park HZ (1992) Biliary sludge as a cause of acute pancreatitis. N Engl J Med 326:589-593
33. Ros E, Navarro S, Bru C et al (1991) Occult microlithiasis in 'idiopathic' acute pancreatitis: prevention of relapses by cholecystectomy or ursodeoxycholic acid therapy [see comments]. Gastroenterology 101:1701-1709
34. (1993) National Institutes of Health Consensus Development Conference Statement on Gallstones and Laparoscopic Cholecystectomy. Am J Surg 165:390-398
35. Schoenfield LJ, Carulli N, Dowling RH et al (1989) Asymptomatic gallstones: definition and treatment. Gastroenterology International 2:25-29
36. Sauerbruch T, Paumgartner G (1991) Gallbladder stones: management. Lancet 338:1121-1124
37. Kumar A, Deed JS, Bhasin B et al (2004) Comparison of the effect of diclofenac with hyoscine-N-butylbromide in the symptomatic treatment of acute biliary colic. ANZ J Surg 74:573-576
38. Al-Waili N, Saloom KY (1998) The analgesic effect of intravenous tenoxicam in symptomatic treatment of biliary colic: a comparison with hyoscine N-butylbromide. Eur J Med Res 3:475-479
39. Akriviadis EA, Hatzigavriel M, Kapnias D et al (1997) Treatment of biliary colic with diclofenac: a randomized, double-blind, placebo-controlled study. Gastroenterology 113:225-231
40. Goldman G, Kahn PJ, Alon R et al (1989) Biliary colic treatment and acute cholecystitis prevention by prostaglandin inhibitor. Dig Dis Sci 34:809-811
41. Gracie WA, Ransohoff DF (1982) The natural history of silent gallstones: the "innocent" gallstone" is not a myth. N Engl J Med 307:798-800
42. Friedman GD (1993) Natural history of asymptomatic and symptomatic gallstones. Am J Surg 165:399-404
43. Tint GS, Salen G, Colalillo A et al (1982) Ursodeoxycholic acid: a safe and effective agent for dissolving cholesterol gallstones. Ann Intern Med 97:351-356
44. Meredith TJ, Williams GV, Maton PN et al (1982) Retrospective comparison of 'Cheno' and 'Urso' in the medical treatment of gallstones. Gut 23:382-389
45. Tomida S, Abei M, Yamaguchi T et al (1999) Long-term ursodeoxycholic acid therapy is associated with reduced risk of biliary pain and acute cholecystitis in patients with gallbladder stones: a cohort analysis. Hepatology 30:6-13
46. Venneman NG, Besselink MG, Keulemans YC et al (2006) Ursodeoxycholic acid exerts no beneficial effect in patients with symptomatic gallstones awaiting cholecystectomy. Hepatology 43:1276-1283
47. Sauerbruch T, Delius M, Paumgartner G et al (1986) Fragmentation of gallstones by extracorporeal shock waves. N Engl J Med 314:818-822
48. Allen MJ, Borody TJ, Bugliosi TF et al (1985) Rapid dissolution of gallstones by methyl tert-butyl ether. Preliminary observations. N Engl J Med 312:217-220
49. Hellstern A, Leuschner U, Benjaminov A et al (1998) Dissolution of gallbladder stones with methyl tert-butyl ether and stone recurrence: a European survey. Dig Dis Sci 43:911-920
50. Paumgartner G, Sauter GH (2005) Extracorporeal shock wave lithotripsy of gallstones: 20th anniversary of the first treatment. Eur J Gastroenterol Hepatol 17:525-527
51. Nunes DP (2007) Nonsurgical treatment of gallstone disease. UpToDate 1-5
52. Paumgartner G, Pauletzki J, Sackmann M (1994) Ursodeoxycholic acid treatment of cholesterol gallstone disease. Scand J Gastroenterol Suppl 204:27-31
53. Leopold GR, Amberg J, Gosink BB et al (1976) Gray scale ultrasonic cholecystography: a comparison with conventional radiographic techniques. Radiology 121:445-448
54. Portincasa P, Di Ciaula A, Palmieri VO et al (1994) Sonographic evaluation of gallstone burden in humans. Ital J Gastroenterol Hepatol 26:141-144
55. Everson GT, Braverman DZ, Johnson ML et al (1980) A critical evaluation of real-time ultrasonography for the study of gallbladder volume and contraction. Gastroenterology 79:40-46
56. Portincasa P, Moschetta A, Colecchia A et al (2003) Measurement of gallbladder motor function by ultrasonography: towards for standardization. Dig Liver Dis (già Ital J Gastroenterol Hepatol) 35 (Suppl 3):S56-S61
57. Pauletzki JG, Althaus R, Holl J et al (1996) Gallbladder emptying and gallstone formation: a prospective study on gallstone recurrence. Gastroenterology 111:765-771
58. Portincasa P, van Erpecum KJ, van de Meeberg PC et al (1996) Apolipoprotein (Apo) E4 genotype and gallbladder motility influence speed of gallstone clearance and risk of recurrence after ex-

tracorporeal shock-wave lithotripsy. Hepatology 24:580-587
59. Venneman NG, van Berge-Henegouwen GP, Portincasa P et al (2001) Absence of apolipoprotein E4 genotype, good gallbladder motility and presence of solitary stones delay rather than prevent gallstone recurrence after extracorporeal shock wave lithotripsy. J Hepatol 35:10-16
60. Festi D, Frabboni R, Bazzoli F et al (1990) Gallbladder motility in cholesterol gallstone disease. Effect of ursodeoxycholic acid administration and gallstone dissolution. Gastroenterology 99:1779-1785
61. Portincasa P, Di Ciaula A, Baldassarre G et al (1994) Gallbladder motor function in gallstone patients: sonographic and in vitro studies on the role of gallstones, smooth muscle function and gallbladder wall inflammation. J Hepatol 21:430-440
62. Pereira SP, Veysey MJ, Kennedy C et al (1997) Gallstone dissolution with oral bile acid therapy - Importance of pretreatment CT scanning and reasons for nonresponse. Dig Dis Sci 42:1775-1782
63. Pereira SP, Hussaini SH, Kennedy C et al (1995) Gallbladder stone recurrence after medical treatment. Do gallstones recur true to type? Dig Dis Sci 40:2568-2575
64. Sherlock S, Dooley J (2002) Diseases of the liver and biliary system. Oxford, Blackwell Science
65. Sackmann M, Eder H, Spengler U et al (1993) Gallbladder emptying is an important factor in fragment disappearance after shock wave lithotripsy. J Hepatol 17:62-66
66. Schiff M (1873) Il coleinato di soda nella cura dei calcoli biliari. L'Imparziale 13:97-98
67. Dabney WC (1876) The use of choleate of soda to prevent the formation of gallstones. Am J Med Sci 71:410
68. Rewbridge AG (1937) The disappearance of gallstone shadows following the prolonged admnistration of bile acids. Surgery 1:395-400
69. Danzinger RG, Hofmann AF, Schoenfield LJ (1972) Dissolution of cholesterol gallstones by chenodeoxycholic acid. N Engl J Med 286:1-8
70. Makino I, Shinozaki K, Yoshino K et al (1975) [Dissolution of cholesterol gallstones by long-term administration of ursodeoxycholic acid]. Nippon Shokakibyo Gakkai Zasshi 72:690-702
71. Mouret P (1990) [Celioscopic surgery. Evolution or revolution?] Chirurgie 116:829-832
72. van de Heijning BJM, van de Meeberg P, Portincasa P et al (1999) Effects of ursodeoxycholic acid therapy on in vitro gallbladder contractility in patients with cholesterol gallstones. Dig Dis Sci 44:190-196
73. Guarino MP, Cong P, Cicala M et al (2007) Ursodeoxycholic acid improves muscle contractility and inflammation in symptomatic gallbladders with cholesterol gallstones. Gut 56:815-820
74. van Erpecum KJ, Portincasa P, Stolk MFJ et al (1994) Effects of bile salt and phospholipid hydrophobicity on lithogenicity of human gallbladder bile. Eur J Clin Invest 24:744-750
75. van Erpecum KJ, Portincasa P, Gadellaa M et al (1996) Effects of bile salt hydrophobicity on nucleation behaviour of cholesterol crystals in model bile. Eur J Clin Invest 26:602-608
76. Portincasa P, van Erpecum KJ, Jansen A et al (1996) Behavior of various cholesterol crystals in bile from gallstone patients. Hepatology 23:738-748
77. Moschetta A, van Berge-Henegouwen GP, Portincasa P et al (2001) Cholesterol crystallization in model biles. Effects of bile salt and phospholipid species composition. J Lipid Res 42:1273-1281
78. Venneman NG, Huisman SJ, Moschetta A et al (2002) Effects of hydrophobic and hydrophilic bile salt mixtures on cholesterol crystallization in model biles. Biochim Biophys Acta 1583:221-228
79. Venneman NG, van Kammen M, Renooij W et al (2005) Effects of hydrophobic and hydrophilic bile salts on gallstone growth and dissolution in model biles. Biochim Biophys Acta 3:209-219
80. Sugerman HJ, Brewer WH, Shiffman ML et al (1995) A multicenter, placebo-controlled, randomized, double-blind, prospective trial of prophylactic ursodiol for the prevention of gallstone formation following gastric-bypass-induced rapid weight loss. Am J Surg 169:91-96
81. Paumgartner G (1996) Therapeutic options and choice of appropriate treatment. In: Bile acids - Cholestasis - Gallstones. Advances in basic and clinical bile acid research. Dordrecht, Kluwer Academic Publishers, pp 205-210
82. Sackmann M, Ippisch E, Sauerbruch T et al (1990) Early gallstone recurrence rate after successful shock-wave therapy. Gastroenterology 98:392-396
83. Villanova N, Bazzoli F, Taroni F et al (1989) Gallstone recurrence after successful oral bile acid treatment. a 12 year follow-up study and evaluation of long term postdissolution treatment. Gastroenterology 97:726-731
84. Petroni ML, Jazrawi RP, Pazzi P et al (2000) Risk factors for the development of gallstone recurrence following medical dissolution. The British-Italian Gallstone Study Group. Eur J Gastroenterol Hepatol 12:695-700
85. Wang DQH, Carey MC (1996) Complete mapping of crystallization pathways during cholesterol precipitation from model bile: influence of physical-chemical variables of pathophysiologic relevance and identification of a stable liquid crystalline state in cold, dilute and hydrophilic bile salt-containing system. J Lipid Res 37:606-630

Chapter 14

Surgical Treatment of Cholelithiasis: Exclusion Criteria

G. Paolo Spina, Giacomo Gaverini

Introduction

Surgical removal of the gallbladder and gallstones is the recommended treatment option for patients with cholelithiasis [1], but is surgical intervention always the best option? Or, as the title of this chapter suggests, are there patients presenting with gallstones for whom surgery is not the optimal therapy, which would mean there were exclusion criteria, and if so, what are these criteria?

Overall, general contraindications to surgical treatment are well-known: usually they concern symptomatic patients who are at high-risk for surgery, particularly if elderly and in emergency cases. In these patients, the use of noninvasive procedures is recommended. However, it is the management, mainly by exclusion, of patients with asymptomatic cholelithiasis that presents physicians with a real clinical dilemma and one which is likely to grow in frequency with the increasing use of ultrasonography (US) both for the study of abdominal disorders and as part of a routine check-up examinations.

Asymptomatic Cholelithiasis

A Consensus Conference held in Strasbourg (France) in 1991 [2] gave the following definition for symptomatic cholelithiasis: lithiasis is considered to be symptomatic in the presence of biliary pain or complications. Biliary pain can be distinguished on the basis of its location (usually in the epigastrium, less often in the right hypochondrium), duration (from 10 min to 5 h) and intensity (constant and severe during crisis). Symptoms may include nausea and vomiting. In the absence of these clinical symptoms, cholelithiasis is considered asymptomatic. The Strasbourg definition continues to be relevant [3, 4] and pain remains the hinge symptom, meaning that surgery is indicated, even if some observations induce a rethinking of the limits between "silent" and "non-silent" lithiasis. Some patients with non-specific symptoms improve after a cholecystectomy [5], while others with biliary pain related to gallstones do not benefit from this treatment [6]. Stones considered to be silent because of their lack of symptoms continue to undergo morphological changes in the gallbladder [7]. About 30% of people with one pain episode have no further episodes [8]. In formerly symptomatic patients who remain symptom-free for 5 consecutive years, the risk of future pain attacks gradually decreases towards values similar to those of patients with asymptomatic gallstones [9].

Although in the majority of epidemiological studies of asymptomatic patients no standard definition of biliary pain has been used, results relating to the incidence of pain can nevertheless be considered to be valid, and they confirm that 60–90% of gallstones are asymptomatic and are diagnosed "accidentally". Following diagnosis, the percentage of cases in which disease progresses from asymptomatic to symptomatic ranges from 7 to 38% [10, 11], depending on the follow-up duration and also on the population studied, with an annual risk of developing symptoms or a complication ranging between 1 and 4% [1]. Biliary pain usually occurs within the first 5 years after the initial diagnosis [8] and incidence of symptom appearance progressively decreases over time with an overall reduction in the number [12] but not severity [9] of events. The cumulative probability of developing a long-term complication is 2–6% [11], with an annual rate ranging between 0.3% and 1.2% [12]. The most common symptom is acute cholecystitis [12] and the majority of patients do not develop complications without first experiencing at least one episode of biliary pain [1].

Cholecystectomy

Over time the procedure for gallbladder surgery has evolved from laparotomic and mini-laparotomic surgery to laparoscopic surgery, which has now become the treatment of choice in the management of patients with cholelithiasis [1, 13].

Apart from differences in the period of hospital stay and convalescence, which are shorter following the use of mini-laparotomic or laparoscopic surgery, mortality rates approach zero in all these procedures (0–0.09%) [13]. Morbidity ranges from 5% to 26% [13] and the frequency of bile duct injury between 0.2% and 1.9% [13, 14]. These data derive from surgery carried out in symptomatic patients, some of whom have acute clinical pictures. One study has shown that morbidity rates and conversion rates are significantly lower, and operating time is shorter in asymptomatic subjects [15].

Patients usually fully recover without sequelae; if symptoms do occur they are typically related to the underlying pathology of the bile duct (retained gallstones, stenosis or papillary neoplasia) or of others organs (Wirsung stenosis, pancreatitis, oesophagitis, functional diseases of the intestine, psychosomatic disorders), that was pre-existing but had not previously been diagnosed [16].

Prophylactic Cholecystectomy or "Watchful Waiting"?

Taking into account the results presented above, what is the preferred management approach? Advocates of the surgical approach believe that cholecystectomy is the definitive treatment for a pathology that could develop serious and, at times, fatal complications, including pancreatitis and gallbladder carcinoma. These complications can be prevented with a surgical technique that is safe when performed in an elective manner [17], whereas it is associated with significant risk when carried out in the case of complicated cholelithiasis, particularly as the age of the patient increases [15, 18, 19].

On the other hand, advocates of the "watchful waiting" approach underline the fact that cholelithiasis has a benign history and that the surgical approach means overtreatment in the majority of patients (85–90%) who are destined to remain asymptomatic. There is also a minimal risk that the patient will develop severe complications; however, in most cases it is possible to identify these patients in advance as they normally have had at least one painful episode; in these cases it is possible to arrange surgery at a safe time. Waiting avoids the limited (but not negligible) morbidities associated with surgery and/or or the anaesthesia, particularly in elderly patients or in those with severe comorbidities [17]. While this allows savings in terms of cost and healthcare resources [20], it is not counterbalanced by the fact that delaying surgery can increase the number of emergency/urgent cholecystectomies that cost twice as much as an elective cholecystectomy and require more experienced surgeons.

Unfortunately, there is no conclusive evidence allowing a full evaluation of the relationship between the appropriateness of the use of cholecystectomy and outcomes. Quintana et al. [21] conducted a prospective observational study using a method that combines expert opinion with available scientific evidence. A procedure was considered appropriate if the "expected health benefit exceeds the expected negative consequences by a sufficiently wide margin". Outcomes were measured using two Health Related Quality of Life (HRQoL) assessments: the SF-36 Health Survey (SF-36) and the Gastrointestinal Quality of Life Index (GIQLI). Quintana proposed that patients considered appropriate for cholecystectomy would have greater improvement in HRQoL in some domains of these assessments. He concluded: "These results support a conservative approach regarding the indication of cholecystectomy for patients with silent calculi, based on the panel criteria and on the low HRQoL improvement shown".

In a recently published review [17] it emerged that to date no randomised clinical trials have been carried out in asymptomatic patients to compare the results of cholecystectomy versus clinical observation. Furthermore, the authors were unable to identify non-randomised studies that provided sufficient information to answer the question posed and they therefore concluded that there was "...no evidence in literature to either recommend or refuse surgery to patients with asymptomatic gallstones".

In light of this uncertainty, surgeons have directed their efforts towards identifying those subgroups of patients with asymptomatic gallstones who are at risk of developing symptoms or complications. Many factors have been considered.

Gallbladder Motility

It has been postulated that two distinct subgroups of patients with gallstones can be identified with regard to gallbladder emptying: strong and weak contractors [22].

Postprandial gallbladder volume changes and relative ejection fraction, determined sonographically, appear to differentiate gallstone dyspepsia from functional dyspepsia. De-Chuan et al. [23] found that dyspeptic patients, in whom symptoms improved after cholecystectomy, had stronger gallbladder contractions in response to gastric distension and fatty meals. This type of diagnostic study may help to determine the appropriate treatment for patients with gallstones and dyspepsia.

A recent study [24] correlated the gallbladder walls' motility and the onset of biliary symptoms in patients with cholelithiasis. Gallbladder emptying was higher in patients who had biliary pain than in asymptomatic subjects or in those who had not suffered from biliary pain in the previous 2 years. Similar results were observed during a 4-year follow-up in patients who became symptomatic as compared to other patients whose symptoms did not change. It seems reasonable to state that gallbladder wall motility is a predicting factor for symptom appearance. This suggests that periodic evaluation of gallbladder wall motility could represent a safe and reliable tool for the management of patients with gallstones, in order to identify those destined to remain asymptomatic. This attitude is not shared by Larsen et al. [25], whose study including patients with uncomplicated gallbladder stones concluded that gallbladder function, evaluated by hepatobiliary scintigraphy, is not related to the profile of symptoms and to the outcome 1 year after watchful waiting.

The relationship between gallbladder function and the clinical course of gallstones patients needs further study.

Age

The surgical removal of gallstones is warranted in both young and elderly patients because complications could develop during the lifetime of the former and are frequently serious and sometimes fatal in the latter [26].

The problem was approached using decision analytic models with life expectancy as the only outcome measure [20]. The choice of prophylactic cholecystectomy could reduce survival in elderly patients (70 years), albeit non-significantly. However, in younger patients, around 30 years of age, surgery was associated with an improvement in life expectancy. Survival in younger patients was even more impressive when higher incidences were assumed for biliary complications, pain, and cancer. Nevertheless, the magnitude of the survival advantage associated with cholecystectomy in younger patients is not so large as to provide unequivocal guidance in deciding whether to perform surgery [27].

Recently, Quintana et al. [21] set out to determine if there were subgroups of patients among asymptomatic subjects for whom a surgical option was more appropriate. Patients aged from 16–45 years and at low-medium surgical risk were identified as a group which could benefit from cholecystectomy. However, these results remain to be confirmed.

Microlithiasis

The relationship between microlithiasis and gallbladder disease has remained controversial in spite of several studies addressing this topic.

Prophylactic intervention seems to be justified in patients with microlithiasis because of the danger of gallstone migration and the onset of acute pancreatitis [28]. The annual incidence of acute pancreatitis in asymptomatic patients with gallstones varies in prospective studies between 0.07% and 0.2% [29]. The risk increases with age, with the course of pancreatitis often worse, especially in elderly patients [30]. Diehl et al. [31] demonstrated that patients with at least one gallstone less than 5 mm in diameter have more than a four-fold increased risk of presenting with acute biliary pancreatitis. In a recent study [32], it was found that patients with pancreatitis had greater gallbladder motility, more sludge and a greater number of small gallstones (smallest stone diameters: 2 ± 1 vs. 8 ± 2 mm; $p=0.001$) than patients with uncomplicated symptomatic gallstones. When the gallstones are small ($\leq$ 5 mm) and gallbladder motility is preserved, the stones can more easily migrate from the gallbladder to the common bile duct. In these patients the "wait and see" option appears to be inappropriate.

The potential benefit of prophylactic cholecystectomy should be considered, since complicated gallstone disease is largely prevented by cholecystectomy [33, 34]. In clinical practice, however, in a decisional analysis study, the authors concluded that prophylactic cholecystectomy was associated with some benefits only if the patient had the highest risk of developing and dying of pancreatitis (incidence of pancreatitis greater than 0.15% and a pancreatitis-related mortality rate of 7.5% or greater) [30]. Therefore, only a limited number of patients could be included, which may include younger patients because of longer life expectancy. The results of this analysis are questionable for some methodological bias implied in the study and are of limited value in assisting surgeons in deciding whether prophylactic cholecystectomy should be performed [35]. Furthermore, the same authors consider that it is too early to recommend prophylactic cholecystectomy for asymptomatic small gallstones in the general population [29] and thus the problem remains unsolved.

Chronic Haemolytic Syndromes

Chronic haemolysis, with its accelerated bilirubin turnover, leads to a high incidence of pigmented gallstones. In addition, modern management of patients with homozygous beta-thalassaemia has increased survival. As a result, more patients suffer from pigmented gallstone disease [36]. Ultrasound examination of patient populations indicate that the onset of cholelithiasis can occur from as early as 2–4 years of age and its prevalence progressively increases with age [37]: 14% in subjects under the age of 10 years, 22% at 10–14 years, 36% at 15–18 years, and a reported prevalence of 50% at 22 years [38] and over 80% after 30 years [39].

Laparoscopic cholecystectomy has been performed safely in patients with sickle cell disease (SCD) and at present is the treatment of choice in children with clinically symptomatic disease. An aggressive approach provides the benefits of reducing the risk of the morbid complications of cholelithiasis, as well as eliminating gallbladder disease as a confounding item in the differential diagnosis of right upper quadrant pain [40].

The place of surgery for asymptomatic gallstones in children with SCD must be determined by the risk of developing complications. In Walker's series [37], these risks were not high enough to justify routine surgery. Most authors, in contrast, believe that children awaiting surgery have a high risk of developing complications and that their occurrence significantly affects the preoperative and postoperative course [41–43]. The mean number of hospitalisations and outpatient visits is twice as high as those in children without cholelithiasis [43]. With a maximum delay of 2.5 years, 28% of patients experienced complications [44] increasing to 50% within 3–5 years [37]. With adequate preoperative preparation it is possible to perform laparoscopic cholecystectomy safely in a patient who has acute cholecystitis [41]; however, clearly the risks of operating on surgically well-prepared individuals are less than those in patients who are already acutely unwell [38].

At present it is generally agreed that laparoscopic cholecystectomy, when performed after appropriate preparation and with meticulous operative and postoperative care, is a safe and effective procedure in the management of patients with SCD, beta-thalassaemia and asymptomatic cholelithiasis. It prevents the potential complications of cholecystitis and choledocholithiasis that lead to major risks, discomfort, and longer hospital stay [43, 45].

Gallbladder Cancer

The precise aetiology of gallbladder cancer (GBC) is unknown, but gallstones and chronic inflammation are a key pathogenic events [46, 47] involved in the relatively well-defined sequence of flat-epithelial premalignant changes (dysplasia and carcinoma in situ) that ultimately lead to the development of an invasive carcinoma [48].

While it is possible that gallstones and GBC have common risk factors, there is actually significant evidence of a direct link between the two: in about 85% cases of GBC it is possible to identify gallstones [49]. A history of gallstones was the strongest risk factor for GBC [50, 51], with a pooled relative risk of 4.9 [51]. In fact, the increase in the number and size of gallstones among patients with GBC could simply be a result of aging, or it could be a result of the long-term presence of stones in the gallbladder rather than of any particular chemical or physical effects [52]. In certain populations there is a correlation between gallstones and GBC frequency [50]. A significant decline in mortality from GBC has followed increases in the rates of cholecystectomies performed in the United States, England,

Wales, and Canada [53]. Conversely, decreasing cholecystectomy rates in Chile have been followed by an increased mortality from GBC in subsequent years [54].

These data seem to favour the practice of prophylactic cholestectomy, but only a small proportion of patients with cholelithiasis (~1–3%) develop GBC [50]. In particular, in patients with asymptomatic cholelithiasis, the risk per year of developing GBC is negligible (0.01%) [55], while approximately 15% of patients with GBC do not have any evidence of cholelithiasis [50]. The incidence rates of GBC in specimens obtained during cholecystectomy vary from 0.9% to 6% according to geographic location and among individual institutions [49, 54]. Moreover, the percentage of gallstones associated with GBC varies from 85–90% in Chile, from 60–70% in India, and up to 50% in Japan [48].

It is therefore likely that other factors including ethnic origin, genetics, sex, geography and infective factors (biliary and systemic) may contribute to the development of GCB [48, 56] and the present level of evidence does not therefore allow definitive recommendations on the use of systematic cholecystectomy for "silent" gallstones.

Nevertheless, based on the data reported above, prophylactic cholecystectomy to prevent GBC should be strongly considered in selected subgroups of patients living in areas where GBC is highly prevalent (American Indians and Mexican Americans, patients in Colombia, Chile, Bolivia, India, Pakistan, Korea etc.), especially if the subject has a long life expectancy at the time of diagnosis of cholelithiasis [57, 58], or has a fairly low socio-economic status [58]. Patients should be more liberally selected for cholecystectomy in these high risk populations [18], even in absence of results from randomised trials [7, 18, 51, 52, 57, 59].

Moreover, prophylactic cholecystectomy is indicated in patients with large gallstones, since the risk of GBC increases according to gallstone dimension [relative risk (RR) = 2.4 if < 3 cm; RR = 10.1 if > 3 cm] [60]; in patients with thick-walled gallbladders (wall thickness > 3 mm on US), as up to 50% of these are likely to have xanthogranulomatous cholecystitis, which increases the risk of GBC in these patients [61]; and in patients with porcelain gallbladder. Porcelain gallbladder is present in less than 1% of samples of cholecystectomy but it is associated with a high incidence of GBC (7%) [62], although this is lower than previously estimated.

Diabetes

The prevalence of gallstones is high in patients with diabetes, about twice that of the general population in an Italian study [63], although the relationship is confounded by a number of co-factors including age, body mass index (BMI) and a family history of gallstones [63].

Some authors think that diabetic patients are at a higher risk of developing complications that are more serious than those in the general population [64, 65] because diabetes is frequently associated with older age, cardiovascular and renal disease [66]. In addition, diabetic neuropathy is thought to play a significant role that could mask symptoms and as a result delay correct diagnosis [67]. It was more likely that patients would undergo surgery during the acute phase of the disease (22% versus 12%) with a higher percentage of septic bile, gangrenous changes, and perforation of the gallbladder wall [68]. This might cause a higher morbidity (21% versus 9%) [68] and a moderate (although non-significant) increase in mortality [18, 68, 69]. These considerations resulted in prophylactic cholecystectomy being recommended [18, 66, 69].

However, other authors have demonstrated that the natural history of cholelithiasis has a more benign course in diabetic patients and a lower risk of complications than previously thought. Among 47 asymptomatic patients followed for 5 years, only 14.9% developed biliary pain and only 4.2% experienced complications [70]. Conversely, surgical mortality and morbidity were not different from those observed in the non-diabetic population [64, 71, 72], even allowing for the fact that cardiovascular or renal comorbidities frequently occur in this patient group [73]. At the same time, it has been reported that surgical intervention does not improve the quality of life or extend survival, and in fact may have the opposite effect [74, 75].

As a result, current opinion is that treatment of diabetic patients should follow the same criteria as the general population [64, 70, 72, 75], but surgery should be performed as soon as symptoms develop [68, 76].

Cholecystectomy during Abdominal Surgery

Bariatric surgery

There is an ongoing debate on whether prophylactic cholecystectomy should be performed in patients with "silent gallstones" undergoing bariatric surgery (11–27%) [77–84].

Morbidly obese subjects have a higher prevalence of cholelithiasis [26]. Rapid weight loss occurring after bariatric surgery is lithogenous [85, 86], and previously silent gallstones may become symptomatic and cause complications following laparotomy for unrelated conditions [87, 88]. As these patients are already undergoing surgery in the upper abdomen for obesity, the addition of cholecystectomy might incur lower costs and/or morbidity than would be expected with two separate procedures: it is both feasible and safe and it avoids both the need for subsequent cholecystectomies, and the challenges of managing choledocholithiasis because of the difficult access for endoscopic retrograde cholangiopancreatography (ERCP) after a Roux-en-Y gastric bypass (RYGB). These are some of the valid reasons advocating routine concomitant prophylactic cholecystectomy in all patients [78, 89, 90] or, for the more cautious, only in patients with gallstones regardless of the presence or absence of symptoms (selective cholecystectomy) [91–93].

Prophylactic (though selective) treatment presupposes that the natural history of asymptomatic gallbladder stones in patients who have undergone bariatric surgery is different from that of the general population.

In recent studies, the incidence of complications due to asymptomatic gallstones left in situ ranges from 8.3% to 17.6% with RYGB [80, 83, 84, 94]. In addition, obstructive jaundice and gallstone pancreatitis are rare after RYGB [79, 95, 96]. Abdominal ultrasound (AUS) in morbidly obese patients is a less sensitive method of diagnosing cholelithiasis [89, 97]. The use of intraoperative ultrasound (IOUS) is more sensitive, but it has a steep learning curve that increases the cost and time of the procedure [98]. A number of authors found no significant differences in cholecystectomy rates after bariatric surgery between asymptomatic patients with preoperative gallbladder screening and patients with no screening [80, 84] and in the first case between patients with negative and positive AUS findings [83].

The percentage of patients with symptomatic gallstones requiring cholecystectomy after bariatric surgery is not much different whether or not silent gallstone have been treated at the time of surgery. It ranges between 1.3% and 10% and from 5.5 % to 14.7% respectively after RYGB [77, 79, 81, 83, 84, 92, 93]. In patient undergoing laparoscopic adjustable gastric banding (LAGB), where weight loss is more gradual than after RYGB [85, 101], percentage ranges between 1.2% and 6.8% [82, 102] in the former and reported to be 6.8% [101] in the latter cases.

In laparoscopic techniques, concomitant cholecystectomy can be technically demanding during a concurrent operation [91, 92, 101]. In contrast, laparoscopic cholecystectomy after RYGB is easier and is associated with little morbidity or mortality [91, 94, 101] even though laparoscopic conversion rates can vary. In addition, during LAGB, removing the gallbladder while placing a prosthetic device raises the issue of possible infectious complications [103]. Finally, it has been demonstrated that the incidence of biliary diseases after RYGB increases during the first 2 years after surgery and returns to baseline thereafter, and previously documented gallstones (on AUS) may disappear [77, 104, 105]. Prophylaxis with ursodiol for 6 months after RYGB reduces the gallstone formation rate [86], although compliance with treatment is variable [80, 98, 102].

According to these data most authors suggest that there is little clinical value in "routine" preoperative ultrasonography [80, 84, 93, 100, 102] and certainly no evidence to support prophylactic cholecystectomy [79, 80, 83, 84, 93, 94, 99, 100, 102], especially in performing LAGB [101].

The methodological insufficiencies of the studies, almost all of which were retrospective and had selection bias and incomplete follow-up, make it difficult to propose recommendations based on high-quality evidence. Furthermore, information on the high-risk patient subgroups is not yet available [101]. The use of an open or laparoscopic approach, expertise in the performance of concurrent cholecystectomy and the confidence placed in the expected efficacy of ursodiol also play a role. One thing is certain: a more selective approach is needed for the management of silent gallbladder stones in patients who have undergone bariatric surgery.

Transplantation

There is a lack of consensus regarding the optimal treatment strategy (prophylactic cholecystectomy versus expectant management) for incidental gallstone management in solid organ transplant recipients. There is a wide variability in the reported mortality and morbidity rates associated with cholecystectomy at various stages of a transplant patient's life.

According to some authors, the onset of symptoms and complications related to gallstones has a very low incidence in the transplant population [106, 107] and the subsequent laparoscopic cholecystectomy is a safe procedure, with low morbidity and no negative effects on the transplanted organ [108–112]. For these reasons, the authors believe that "watchful waiting" should be exercised in transplant patients with silent gallstones.

Authors who support surgical intervention, conversely, believe that these patients are more likely to become symptomatic, especially in the first 2 years after transplantation, and especially during maximum immunosuppression (cyclosporin A is prolithogenic) or during rejection episodes [113–117]. Moreover, due to immunosuppression, diagnosis of complications of cholelithiasis may be more difficult, and these complications are associated with increased morbidity and mortality [113, 116]. Prophylactic cholecystectomy can be performed either during the pre-transplant period or—when appropriate—at the time of transplantation.

In the absence of prospective data, Kao et al. [118] developed two decisional models (one for heart transplantation, and the other for kidney and/or pancreas transplantation) to compare pre-transplantation prophylactic cholecystectomy, post-transplantation cholecystectomy, and expectant management. The primary outcome used was the probability of death. Despite all the limitations related to data heterogeneity and the quality of included studies, it seems that in transplant patients experiencing asymptomatic cholelithiasis, a prophylactic post-transplant cholecystectomy is better indicated in hearth transplant patients and a conservative approach when kidney/pancreas transplantation is involved.

Incidental Cholecystectomy

It is common to discover asymptomatic cholelithiasis during pre- or intra-operative investigations for unrelated abdominal surgery. Many clinical trials document that in this type of patient, the lithiasis becomes symptomatic after the surgery (in up to 70% of patients) and that in 23–65% it is necessary to remove the gallbladder within 6 months to 1 year of surgery, mainly due to complications, and thus in less favourable conditions [119–122].

These results should be judged considering that the morbidity rate related to incidental cholecystectomy may vary between 0.3% and 3% [88, 123]. This is why many authors believe that in these circumstances, in absence of any contraindications, the cholecystectomy should be associated with the primary surgical intervention. The best case scenario would be to have a pre-operative diagnosis of the cholelithiasis so that it could be possible to discuss and evaluate the risk/benefit profile of the surgery with the patient [88, 122, 123]. This would allow the already limited complications to be reduced further, with a screening of patients on the basis of their general conditions and possible comorbidities and with the choice of a surgical incision that allows the best exposure in the operating theatre. This is very useful, for example, in gynaecologic surgery unless laparoscopy is carried out [124]. The local conditions found at the operating table are pivotal: for example, the presence of a shrunken or scarred gallbladder, cirrhosis, extensive firm adhesions or tissue scarring [125].

Overall, there is no general agreement on interventions that involve the use of prosthetic materials such as vascular prostheses or meshes for incisional hernia repair because of the ever present risk of possible infectious complications [100].

Miscellaneous

There are a large number of other groups of patients in which surgery may be warranted.

In the case of young women of childbearing age who plan to have several pregnancies, it appears that there is a high probability that lithiasis becomes manifest during pregnancy, thus compounding the problems of diagnosis and therapy [126].

A similar situation occurs in gallstones patients with dyspeptic symptoms (common in the general population), who "wish" to have surgery, even taking into account that sometimes it may be difficult for physicians to distinguish between symptomatic and asymptomatic subjects in a random population of patients with gallstones [127]. The same applies to patients debilitated by cancerophobia.

Up to 15% of patients with gallbladder stones exhibit concomitant stones in the common bile duct [128]. The annual incidence of symptomatic choledocholithiasis in asymptomatic gallstone carriers has been estimated to be 0.2% [87, 129]. Asymptomatic cholelithiasis in association with common bile duct stones (CBDS) could be considered as another indication for selective prophylactic surgery even if the natural history of asymptomatic CBDS appears to be more benign than that of symptomatic CBDS [130].

Selective cholecystectomy should also be considered in those patients with silent gallstones who live or work in an area where it could be difficult to get medical assistance. These patients may be at risk for an adverse outcome if complications develop [131].

In all these circumstances, it is essential to have close interaction with the patients and to carefully explain the benefits and costs of surgery and those of "watchful waiting".

Conclusion

At the "*Berlin Klinische Wochenschrift*" in 1882, when the first cholecystectomy was carried out at the S. Lazzaro Hospital in Berlin on the 43-year-old male secretary of a magistrate, Carl Langenbuck explained that in his opinion this operation was indicated "only in cases in which the patient and the doctor have run out of patience" [132]. In the next century, the improvements in surgical and anesthesiologic techniques were such that most people considered it was necessary "to operate on every lithiasis for whom a medical contraindication was not present" (Fauvert), "even if it was latent, asymptomatic or fortuitously discovered" (Debray) [133].

Successive epidemiologic studies have documented that asymptomatic lithiasis is generally benign, and that complications are limited and if adequately treated, easily resolvable. The patient does not need a frequent and expensive follow-up and he can live with his disease without fear. If complications develop they are usually preceded by a biliary pain event that allows the physician to operate in favourable conditions with a morbidity and mortality rate almost equivalent to elective cholecystectomy. This information has modified a therapeutic attitude that has not changed with the introduction of laparoscopy.

Surgical intervention clearly has many advantages: it is benign, it is effective, its results are long lasting and usually without unfavourable sequelae. In clinical practice, however, it does not improve survival; it has a debatable impact on the quality of life, and it has high costs, especially if conducted laparoscopically. There is a general consensus among experts that asymptomatic lithiasis should not be operated. The decision to expose 85–90 patients to the risks of unnecessary surgery to prevent gallstone-associated complications in 10–15 patients has to be considered carefully.

In the same way, however, epidemiological, observational and cohort studies seem to document the existence, in patients affected by asymptomatic cholelithiasis, of a group at a high risk of developing symptoms and complications. For them, surgical

Table 14.1 Selective cholecystectomy for asymptomatic cholelithiasis

Accepted indications	Calcified (porcelain) gallbladder Residence in areas with high prevalence of gallbladder cancer associated with gallstones Presence of large (≥ 3 cm) gallstones Asymptomatic cholelithiasis associated with choledocholithiasis Chronic hemolytic conditions Heart transplantation
Questionable indications	Efficient gallbladder emptying Small gallstones (≤ 5 mm) and gallbladder motility preserved Life expectancy > 30 years Gallbladder wall thickness > 3 mm on US Incidental (concomitant) cholecystectomy Renal-pancreatic transplantation Bariatric surgery Residence in an area remote from medical facilities Child-bearing age Dyspeptic symptoms and "wish" for surgery

intervention may be justified even in the absence of symptoms. Who are these patients and how can they be selected? At present, there is no scientific evidence to identify them (Table 14.1).

If surgery is chosen, a careful analysis of hepatobiliary and systemic risk factors (such as advanced age and significant comorbidity) should precede any decision regarding cholecystectomy. The patient has to be well informed regarding the morbidity and mortality risks associated with surgical intervention and general anaesthesia. The patient's preferences should be taken into consideration by the surgeon, because the decision to go ahead with surgery remains an individual decision.

With this in mind, refraining from surgery is ultimately not only the more favourable approach for the patient, but also the most suitable one for the health system, which has to bear the costs of the patient's treatment.

"Observational studies, which measure outcomes such as obstructive jaundice, gallstone-associated pancreatitis, and/or gallbladder cancer for sufficient duration of follow-up, are vital. Such studies could help to determine the dimension and duration of follow-up and randomised clinical trials designed to evaluate whether cholecystectomy or no cholecystectomy is better for asymptomatic gallstones" [15].

References

1. NIH Consensus conference. Gallstones and laparoscopic cholecystectomy (1993) JAMA 269: 1018-1024
2. Conférence européenne de consensus, Strasbourg (1991) La lithiase vésiculaire: stratégie thérapeutique. Ann Chir 46:11-23
3. Berhane T, Vetrhus M, Hausken T et al (2006) Pain attacks in non-complicated and complicated gallstone disease have a characteristic pattern and are accompanied by dyspepsia in most patients: the results of a prospective study. Scand J Gastroenterol 41:93-101
4. Portincasa P, Moschetta A, Petruzzelli M et al (2006) Symptoms and diagnosis of gallbladder stones. Best Pract Res Clin Gastroenterol 20:1017-1029
5. Karam J, Roslyn J (1997) Cholelithiasis and cholecystectomy. In: Zinner MJ, Schwartz SI, Ellis H (eds) Maingot's abdominal operations. Stanford, Appleton & Lange, pp 1723–1725
6. Berger MY, Olde Hartman TC, Van Der Velden JJ et al (2004) Is biliary pain exclusively related to gallbladder stones? A controlled prospective study. Br J Gen Pract 54:574-579
7. Tewari M (2006) Contribution of silent gallstones in gallbladder cancer. J Surg Oncol 93:629-632
8. Ransohoff DF, Gracie WA (1993) Treatment of gallstones. Ann Intern Med 119:606-619
9. Friedman GD, Raviola CA, Fireman B (1989) Prognosis of gallstones with mild or no symptoms: 25 years of follow-up in health maintenance organization. J Clin Epidemiol 42:127-136
10. Halldestam I, Enell EL, Kullman E et al (2004) Development of symptoms and complications in individual with asymptomatic gallstones. Br J Surg 91:734-738
11. Sakorafas GH, Milingos D, Peros G (2007) Asymptomatic cholelithiasis: is cholecystectomy really needed? A critical reappraisal 15 years after the introduction of laparoscopic cholecystectomy. Dig Dis Sci 52:1313-1325
12. Attili AF, De Santis A, Capri R et al (1995) The natural history of gallstones: the GREPCO experience. The GREPCO group. Hepatology 21:656-660
13. Keus F, de Jong JAF, Gooszen HG et al (2006) Laparoscopic versus open cholecystectomy, laparoscopic versus small-incision cholecystectomy, small-incision versus open cholecystectomy for patients with symptomatic cholecystolithiasis. Cochrane Database of Systematic Reviews. Issue 4. Art. No.: CD006231. DOI: 10.1002/14651858. CD006231.; CD006229. DOI:10.1002/14651858. CD006229 ; CD004788. DOI: 10.1002/14651858. CD004788
14. Nuzzo G, Giuliante F, Giovannini I et al (2005) Bile duct injury during laparoscopic cholecystectomy: results of an Italian national survey on 56 591 cholecystectomies. Arch Surg 140:986-992
15. Yano H, Kinuta M, Iwazawa T et al (2003) Laparoscopic cholecystectomy for asymptomatic cholelithiasis. Digestive Endoscopy 15:190-195
16. Spina GP (1989) La colecistectomia. In: Il Fegato. Bologna, Editrice Compositori Bologna, vol 35, pp 81-94
17. Gurusamy KS, Samraj K (2007) Cholecystectomy versus no cholecystectomy in patients with silent gallstones. Cochrane Database of Systematic Reviews 2007; Issue 1: Art. No. CD006230. DOI: 10.1002/14651858.CD006230. pub216.

18. Patino JF, Quintero GA (1998) Asymptomatic cholelithiasis revisited. World J Surg 22:1119-1124
19. Bittner R, Ulrich M (2004) Gallbladder calculi - always an indication for surgery? Gallenblasensteinleiden - immer eine Operationsindikation? Der Internist 45:8-15
20. Ransohoff DF, Gracie WA, Wolfenson LB et al (1983) Prophylactic cholecystectomy or expectant management for silent gallstones. A decision analysis to assess survival. Ann Intern Med 99:199-204
21. Quintana JM, Cabriada J, Aostegui I et al (2005) Health-related quality of life and appropriateness of cholecystectomy. Ann Surg 241:110-11824
22. Maudgal DP, Kupfer RM, Zentler-Munro PL (1980) Postprandial gallbladder emptying in patients with gallstones. BMJ 280:141-143
23. De-Chuan C, Tzu-Ming C, Cheng-Jueng C et al (2004) Gallbladder contractility and volume characteristics in gallstone dyspepsia. World J Gastroenterol 10:721-724
24. Colecchia A, Sandri L, Bacchi-Reggiani ML et al (2006) Is it possibile to predict the clinical corse of gallstone disease? Usefulness of gallbladder motility evaluation in a clinical setting. Am J Gastroenterol 101:2576-2581
25. Larsen TK, Qvist N (2007) The influence of gallbladder function on the symptomatology in gallstones patients, and the outcome after cholecystectomy or expectancy Dig Dis Sci 52:760-763
26. The Rome Group for Epidemiology and Prevention of Cholelithiasis (GREPCO) (1980) The epidemiology of gallstone disease in Rome, Italy. Part I. Prevalence data in men. Part II. Factors associated with the disease. Hepatology 8:904-913
27. Kottke T, Feldman R, Albert D (1984) The risk ratio is insufficient for clinical decisions. The case of prophylactic cholecystectomy. Med Decis Making 4:177-94
28. Farinon AM, Ricci GL, Sianesi M et al (1987) Physiopathologic role of microlithiasis in gallstone pancreatitis. Surg Gynecol Obstet 164:252-256
29. Venneman NG, van Erpecum KJ (2006) Gallstone disease: primary and secondary prevention. Best Pract Res Clin Gastroenterol 20:1063-1076
30. Venneman NG, Buskens E, Besselink MGH et al (2005) Small gallstones are associated with increased risk of acute pancreatitis: potential benefits of profilactic cholecystectomy? Am J Gastroenterol 100:2540-2550
31. Diehl AK, Holleman DR Jr, Chapman JB et al (1997) Gallstone size and risk of pancreatitis. Arch Intern Med 157:1674-1678
32. Venneman NG, Renooij W, Rehfeld JF et al (2005) Small gallstones, preserved gallbladder motility, and fast crystallization are associated with pancreatitis. Hepatology 41:738-746
33. Kaw M, Al Antably Y, Kaw P (2002) Management of gallstone pancreatitis: Cholecystectomy or ERCP and endoscopic sphincterotomy. Gastrointest Endosc 56:61-65
34. Levy MJ (2002) The hunt for microlithiasis in idiopathic acute recurrent pancreatitis: should we abandon the search or intensify our efforts? Gastrointest Endosc 55:286-293
35. Barkun J, Woo D, Marcaccio M et al (2007) Small gallstones may increase the risk of pancreatitis; is there a benefit for a prophylactic cholecystecomy? J Can Chir 50:62-65
36. Kok KY, Yapp SK (2003) Techniques and clinical outcomes of laparoscopic cholecystectomy in adult patients with beta-thalassemias. Surg Laparosc Endosc Percutan Tech 13:168-172
37. Walker TM, Hambleton IR, Serjeant GR (2000) Gallstones in sickle cell disease: observations from the Jamaican cohort study. J Pediatr 136:80-85
38. Suell MN, Horton TI, Dishop MK et al (2004) Outcomes for children with gallbladder abnormalities and sickle cell disease. J Pediatr 145:617-621
39. Hendricks-Ferguson V, Nelson MA (2003) Treatment of cholelithiasis in children with sickle cell disease. AORN 77:1170-1178
40. National Institutes of Health. National Heart, Lung, and Blood Institute. Division of Blood Diseases and Resources (2002) The management of sickle cell disease. NIH publication n° 02-2117 4th edn
41. Al-Mulhim AS, Al-Mulhim FM, Al-Suwaiygh AA (2002) The role of laparoscopic cholecystectomy in the management of acute cholecystitis in patients with sickle cell disease. Am J Surg 183:668-672
42. Seleem IM, Al-Hashemy AM, Meshref SS (2005) Mini-laparoscopic cholecystectomy in children under 10 years of age with sickle cell disease. Aust NZ J Surg 75:562-565
43. Currò G, Meo A, Ippolito D et al (2007) Asymptomatic cholelithiasis in children with sickle cell disease early or delayed cholecystectomy? Ann Surg 245:126-129
44. Parez N, Quinet B, Batut S et al (2001) Lithiase biliaire chez l'enfant drepanocytaire: experience d'un hopital pediatrique parisien. Arch Pediatr 8:1045-1049
45. Marakis G, Pavlidis TE, Ballas K et al (2005) Laparoscopic cholecystectomy in adult patients with beta-thalassemia or sickle cell disease. Surg Endosc 19:1668-1669
46. Nervi F, Duarte I, Gomez G et al (1988) Frequency of gallbladder cancer in Chile, a high-risk area. Int J Cancer 41:657-660
47. de Aretxabala X, Riedeman P, Burgos L et al (1995) Gallbladder cancer. Case-control study. Rev Med Chil 123:581-586
48. Wistuba II, Gazdar AF (2004) Gallbladder cancer:

lessons from a rare tumour. Nature reviews. Cancer 4:695-706
49. Roa I, Araya JC, Villaseca M et al (1999) Gallbladder cancer in a high risk area: morphological features and spread patterns. Hepatogastroenterology 46:1540-1546
50. Lazcano-Ponce EC, Miguel JF, Munoz N et al (2001) Epidemiology and molecular pathology of gallbladder cancer. CA Cancer J Clin 51:349-364
51. Randi G, Franceschi S, La Vecchia C (2006) Gallbladder cancer worldwide: geographical distribution and risk factors. Int J Cancer 118:1591-1602
52. Csendes A, Becerra M, Rojas J et al (2000) Number and size of stones in patients with asymptomatic and symptomatic gallstones and gallbladder carcinoma: a prospective study of 592 cases. J Gastrointest Surg 4:481-485
53. Diehl AK, Beral V (1981) Cholecystectomy and changing mortality from gallbladder cancer. Lancet 2:187-189
54. Serra I, Calvo A, Maturana M et al (1990) Changing trends of gallbladder cancer in Chile, a high-risk area. Int J Cancer 45:376-377
55. Maringhini A, Moreau JA, Melton LJ et al (1987) Gallstones, gallbladder cancer and other gastrointestinal malignanncies. An epidemiologic study in Rochester, Minnesota. Ann Intern Med 107:30-35
56. Kapoor VK (2006) Gallbladder cancer: a global perspective. J Surg Oncol 93:607-609
57. Kapoor VK (2006) Cholecystectomy in patients with asymptomatic gallstones to prevent gall bladder cancer – the case against. Indian J Gastroenterol 25:152-154
58. Dutta U, Nagi B, Garg PK et al (2005) Patients with gallstones develop gallbladder cancer at an earlier age. Eur J Cancer Prev 14:381-385
59. Mohandas KM, Patil PS (2006) Cholecystectomy for asymptomatic gallstones can reduce gall bladder cancer mortality in northern Indian women. Indian J Gastroenterol 25:147-151
60. Diehl AK (1983) Gallstone size and the risk of gallbladder cancer. JAMA 250:2323-2326
61. Srikanth G, Kumar A, Khare R et al (2004) Should laparoscopic cholecystectomy be performed in patients with thick walled gall bladder? JHPB Surg 11:40-44
62. Stephen AE, Berger DL (2001) Carcinoma in the porcelain gallbladder: a relationship revisited. Surgery 129:699-703
63. Pagliarulo M, Fornari F, Fraquelli M et al (2004) Gallstone disease and related risk factors in a large cohort of diabetic patients. Dig Liver Dis 36:130-134
64. Aucott JN, Cooper GS, Bloom AD et al (1993) Management of gallstones in diabetic patients. Arch Intern Med 153:1053-1058
65. Schwesinger WH, Diehl AK (1996) Changing indications for laparoscopic cholecystectomy. Stones without symptoms and symptoms without stones. Surg Clin North Am 76:493-504
66. Gibney EJ (1990) Asymptomatic gallstones. Br J Surg 77:368-372
67. Ponte E, Pinebianco A, Morena S (1990) Diabetic neuropathy. Minerva Med 81:335-340
68. Landau O, Deutsch AA, Kott I et al (1992) The risk of cholecystectomy for acute cholecystitis in diabetic patients. Hepatogastroenterology 39:437-438
69. Ikard RW (1990) Gallstones, cholecystitis, and diabetes. Surg Gynecol Obstet 171:528-5325
70. Del Favero G, Caroli A, Meggiato T et al (1994) Natural history of gallstones in non-insulin-dependent diabetes mellitus. A prospective 5-year follow-up. Dig Dis Sci 39:1704-1707
71. Ransohoff DF, Miller GL, Forsythe SB et al (1987) Outcome of acute cholecystitis in patients with diabetes mellitus. Ann Intern Med 106:829-832
72. Babineau TJ, Bothe A (1995) General surgery considerations in the diabetic patient. Infect Dis Clin North Am Mar 9:183-193
73. Sandler RS, Maule WF, Baltus ME (1986) Factors associated with postoperative complications in diabetics after biliary surgery. Gastroenterology 91:157-162
74. Vauthey JN, Saldinger PF (2000) The natural history of gallstones and asymptomatic gallstones. In: Blumgart LH, Fong Y (eds) Surgery of the liver and biliary tract, 3rd edn. New York, Elsevier, pp 643-649
75. Friedman LS, Roberts MS, Brett AS et al (1988) Management of asymptomatic gallstones in the diabetic patient. A decision analysis. Ann Intern Med 109:913-919
76. Persson GE, Thulin AJ (1991) Prevalence of gallstone disease in patients with diabetes mellitus. A case-control study. Eur J Surg 157:579-582
77. Shiffman ML, Sugerman HJ, Kellum JH et al (1993) Gallstones in patients with morbid obesity: relationship to body weight, weight loss and gallbladder bile cholesterol solubility. Int J Obes Relat Metab Disord 17:153-158
78. Fobi M, Lee H, Igwe D et al (2002) Prophylactic cholecystectomy with gastric bypass operation: incidence of gallbladder disease. Obes Surg 12:350-353
79. Caruana JA, McCabe MN, Smith AD et al (2005) Incidence of symptomatic gallstones after gastric bypass: is prophylactic treatment really necessary? Surg Obes Relat Dis 1:564-568
80. Papasavas PK, Gagné DJ, Ceppa FA et al (2006) Routine gallbladder screening not necessary in patients undergoing laparoscopic Roux-en-Y gastric bypass. Surg Obes Relat Dis 2:41-46
81. Vanek Vincent W, Catania M, Triveri T et al (2006)

Retrospective review of the preoperative biliary and gastrointestinal evaluation for gastric bypass surgery. Surg Obes Relat Dis 2:17-23
82. Kiewiet RM, Durian MF, van Leersum M et al (2006) Gallstone formation after weight loss following gastric banding in morbidly obese dutch patients. Obes Surg 16:592-596
83. Ellner SJ, Myers TT, Piorkowski JR et al (2007) Routine cholecystectomy is not mandatory during morbid obesity surgery. Surg Obes Relat Dis 3:456-460
84. Portenier DD, M Grant JP, Blackwood HS et al (2007) Expectant management of the asymptomatic gallbladder at Roux-en-Y gastric bypass. Surg Obes Relat Dis 3:476-479
85. Everhart JE (1993) Contributions of obesity and weight loss to gallstone disease. Ann Intern Med 119:1029-1035
86. Sugerman HJ, Brewer WH, Shiffman ML et al (1995) A multicenter, placebo-controlled, randomized, double-blind, prospective trial of prophylactic ursodiol for the prevention of gallstone formation following gastric-bypass-induced rapid weight loss. Am J Surg 169:91-96
87. Friedman GD (1993) Natural history of asymptomatic and symptomatic gallstones. Am J Surg 165:399-404
88. Saade C, Bernard D, Morgan S et al (1987) Should cholecystectomy be done en passant for asymptomatic cholelithiasis? Can J Surg 30:350-353
89. Liem RK, Niloff PH (2004) Prophylactic cholecystectomy with open gastric bypass operation. Obes Surg 14:763-765
90. Schmidt JH, Hocking MP, Rout WR et al (1988) The case for prophylactic cholecystectomy concomitant with gastric restriction for morbidly obese. Am Surg 54:269-272
91. Hamad GG, Ikramuddin S, Gourash WF (2003) Elective cholecystectomy during laparoscopic Roux-en-Y gastric bypass: is it worth the wait? Obes Surg 13:76-81
92. Villegas L, Schnieder B, Provost D et al (2004) Is routine cholecystectomy required during laparoscopic gastric bypass? Obes Surg 14:60-66
93. Taylor J, Leitman M, Horowitz M (2006) Is routine cholecystectomy necessary at the time of Roux-en-Y gastric bypass? Obes Surg 16:759-761
94. Sandor A, Czerniach DR, McEananey P et al (2005) Avoidance of selective coincident cholecystectomy in patients undergoing laparoscopic bariatric surgery. Presented at SAGES, Fort Lauderdale, FL, April 13-16
95. Thiet MD, Mittelstaedt CA, Herbst CA Jr et al (1984) Cholelithiasis in morbid obesity. South Med J 77:415-17
96. Papavramidis S, Deligianidis N, Papavramidis T et al (2003) Laparoscopic cholecystectomy after bariatric surgery. Surg Endosc 17:1061-1064
97. Amaral JF, Thompson WR (1985) Gallbladder disease in the morbidly obese. Am J Surg 149:551-557.
98. Scott DJ, Villegas L, Sims TL et al (2003) Intraoperative ultrasound and prophylactic ursodiol for gallstone prevention following laparoscopic gastric bypass. Surg Endosc 17:1796-1802
99. Swartz DE, Felix EL (2005) Elective cholecystectomy after Roux-en-Y. Gastric bypass: why should asymptomatic gallstones be treated differently in morbidly obese patients? Surg Obes Relat Dis 1:555-560
100. Patel KR, White SC, Tejiran T et al (2006) Gallbladder management during laparoscopic Roux-en-Y gastric bypass surgery: routine preoperative screening for gallstones and postoperative prophlylactic medical treatment are not necessary. Am Surg 72:857-861
101. O'Brien P, Dixon J (2003) A rational approach to cholelithiasis in bariatric surgery. Arch Surg 138:908-912
102. Myers JA, Gwenyth A, Fischer, BA et al (2005) Gallbladder disease in patients undergoing laparoscopic adjustable gastric banding. Surgery for Obesity and Related Diseases 1:561-563
103. Ljungh A, Wadstrom T (2002) The role of microorganisms in biliary tract disease. Curr Gastroenterol Rep 4:167-171
104. Erlinger S (2000) Gallstones in obesity and weight loss. Eur J Gastroenterol Hepatol 12:1347-1352
105. Deitel M, Petrov I (1987) Incidence of symptomatic gallstones after bariatric operations. Surg Gynecol Obstet 164:549-552
106. Greenstein SM, Katz S, Sun S et al (1997) Prevalence of asymptomatic cholelithiasis and risk of acute cholecystitis after kidney transplantation. Transplantation 63:1030-1032
107. Jackson T, Treleaven D, Arlen D et al (2005) Management of asymptomatic cholelithiasis for patients awaiting renal transplantation. Surg Endosc 19:510-513
108. Courcoulas AP, Kelly E, Harbrecht BG (1996) Laparoscopic cholecystectomy in the transplant population. Surg Endosc 10:516-519
109. Melvin WS, Meier DJ, Elkhammas E et al (1998) Prophylactic cholecystectomy is not indicated following renal transplantation. Am J Surg 175:317-319
110. Banli O, Guvence N, Altun H (2005) Laparoscopic cholecystectomy for renal transplants. Transplant Proc 37:2127-2128
111. Sianesi M, Capocasale E, Ferreri G et al (2005) The role of cholecystectomy in renal transplantation. Transplant Proc 37:2129-2130
112. Takeyama H, Sinanan MN, Fishbein DP et al (2006) Expectant management is safe for

cholelithiasis after heart transplant. J Heart Lung Transplant 25:539-543
113. Begos DG, Franco KL, Baldwin JC et al (1995) Optimal timing and indications for cholecystectomy in cardiac transplant patients. World J Surg 19:661-665
114. Graham SM, Flowers JL, Schweitzer E et al (1995) The utility of prophylactic laparoscopic cholecystectomy in transplant candidates. Am J Surg 169:44-48
115. Cao S, Cox K, So SS et al (1997) Potential effect of cyclosporin A in formation of cholesterol gallstones in pediatric liver transplant recipients. Dig Dis Sci 42:1409-1415
116. Gupta D, Sakorafas GH, McGregor CG et al (2000) Management of biliary tract disease in heart and lung transplant patients. Surgery 128:641-649
117. Kao LS, Kuhr CS, Flum DR (2003) Should cholecystectomy be performed for asymptomatic cholelithiasis in transplant patients? J Am Coll Surg 197:302-312
118. Kao LS, Flowers C, Flum DR (2005) Prophylactic cholecystectomy in transplants patients: a decision analysis. J Gastrointest Surg 9:965-972
119. Ouriel K, Ricotta JJ, Adams JT et al (1983) Management of cholelithiasis in patients with abdominal aortic aneurysm. Ann Surg 198:717-719
120. String ST (1984) Cholelithiasis and aortic reconstruction J Vasc Surg 1:664-669
121. Bragg LE, Thompson JS (1989) Concomitant cholecystectomy for asymptomatic cholelithiasis. Arch Surg 124:460-462
122. Juhasz ES, Wolff BG, Meagher AP et al (1994) Incidental cholecystectomy during colorectal surgery. Ann Surg 219:467-472
123. Thompson JS, Philben VJ, Hodgson PE (1984) Operative management of incidental cholelithiasis. Am J Surg 148:821-824
124. Meshikhes AW (2002) Asymptomatic gallstones in the laparoscopic era. J R Coll Surg Edinb 47:742-748
125. Wolff BG (1995) Current status of incidental surgery. Dis Colon Rect 38:435-44
126. Blum A, Tatour I, Monir M et al (2005) Gallstones in pregnancy and their complications: postpartum acute pancreatitis and acute peritonitis. Eur J Intern Med 16:473-476
127. Jorgensen T (1989) Abdominal symptoms and gallstone disease: an epidemiological investigation. Hepatology 9:856-860
128. Sarli L, Iusco DR, Roncoroni L (2003) Preoperative endoscopic sphincterotomy and laparoscopic cholecystectomy for the management of cholecystocholedocholithiasis: 10-year experience. World J Surg 27:180-186
129. McSherry CK, Ferstenberg H, Calhoun WF et al (1985) The natural history of diagnosed gallstone disease in symptomatic and asymptomatic patients. Ann Surg 202:59-63
130. Caddy GR, Kirby J, Kirk SJ et al (2005) Natural history of asymptomatic bile duct stones at time of cholecystectomy. Ulster Med J 74:108-112
131. WGO (2006-2008) WGO Practice Guideline: Asymptomatic Gallstone Disease. http://www.worldgastroenterology.org/global-guidelines.html
132. Langenbuch C (1882) Ein Fall von Exstirpation der Gallenblase wegen chronischer Cholelithiasis: Heilung. Berlin Klin Wochenschr 19:725–726
133. Paris J, Salembier Y (1978) Traitment chirurgicale de la lithiase biliaire. Encycl Med Chir Paris, Foie-Pancreas 7047 G-10

Chapter 15

Anesthesia in Biliary Lithiasis

Anna M. Koivusalo

Introduction

Laparoscopy is the 'gold standard' in the treatment of symptomatic gallstones because its postoperative benefits are superior to those of open cholecystectomy. The advantages of laparoscopy over open procedures in recovery are well known and acknowledged. Postoperative pain is reduced, mobilization is easier, pulmonary function is better restored, the hospital stay is shorter, and return to daily activities is possible earlier after laparoscopy than after open surgery.

Laparoscopy is now also used in patients with underlying diseases. To be able to treat this challenging patient population we should be aware of physiological alterations caused by carbon dioxide (CO_2) insufflation and elevated intraabdominal pressure (IAP). In order to obtain an adequate surgical view, CO_2, a volatile acid, is insufflated into the abdominal cavity and the IAP is kept elevated (10–12 mmHg).

Carbon dioxide is the preferred gas for the creation of pneumoperitoneum because it is inexpensive, highly soluble, chemically stable, rapidly eliminated, and physically inert, in addition to which it suppresses combustion and also provides fairly good illumination. CO_2 is a normal product of human metabolism and is nontoxic at physiological levels.

It is now commonly accepted that pneumoperitoneum may cause adverse intraoperative cardiovascular, respiratory, and renal effects. Some of these effects are related to CO_2 and some, to elevated IAP.

Hypercarbia and Acid–Base Disturbances

During pneumoperitoneum insufflated CO_2 is very rapidly absorbed from the peritoneal cavity into the circulation. The maximal absorption rate of CO_2 is reached even at a relative low IAP, i.e., 10 mmHg. Insufflated and absorbed CO_2 is excreted only through the lungs. Not all the CO_2 absorbed is excreted during the anesthesia, so that the excess CO_2 accumulates into the body to be eliminated during the recovery phase. Up to 120 l of CO_2 can be stored in the human body. The bones serve as the largest reservoir. CO_2 is highly soluble in blood. When CO_2 dissolves the solution becomes acidic. To avoid hypercarbia and respiratory acidosis the minute volume of ventilation in anesthetized patients should be increased by about 30% during CO_2 insufflation. It seems to be more efficient to handle increased requirements for ventilation by increasing the tidal volume of ventilation and keeping the respiratory frequency low [1]. Underlying pulmonary pathology retards elimination of CO_2 during anesthesia, and this leads to the need for prolonged mechanical ventilation postoperatively [2]. Intraoperative hypercarbia is sometimes so severe that conversion to open laparotomy is needed, especially in patients with chronic obstructive pulmonary disease.

During pneumoperitoneum end-tidal (et) CO_2 concentrations increase progressively with time, reaching their maximum value after 40 min of CO_2 insufflation if ventilation is kept constant. The plateau suggests that equilibrium has been reached between the excess CO_2 absorbed and that removed by ventilation. Thereafter, CO_2 begins to accumulate in the body reservoir. Respiratory acidosis and increased CO_2 output are reported to last for up to at least 1 h postoperatively despite intraoperative normoventilation [3]. Therefore, patients with limited pulmonary reserves, i.e., with emphysema or chronic obstructive pulmonary disease, are at risk of postoperative hypercarbia and acidosis if actuation is too early and left on spontaneous breathing. During laparoscopic surgery close monitoring of et CO_2 concentrations is mandatory. Measured et CO_2 values, especially in patients with pulmonary disease, do not correlate well with arterial $PaCO_2$ values because of the intrapulmonary shunting. Slightly elevated et CO_2 values do not indicate the true, highly elevated level of arterial hypercarbia and concomitant respiratory acidosis. Therefore, arterial monitoring is strongly recommended in patients with pulmonary disease [2].

Also during the recovery phase, additional ventilatory work is needed to abolish the absorbed CO_2. Patients with chronic lung diseases may benefit from prolonged postoperative mechanical ventilation. In patients with severe pulmonary disease gasless laparoscopy is recommended if this is possible.

Pulmonary Function

Elevated IAP and abdominal expansion shift the diaphragm upward. Thus, intrathoracic pressure increases, the abdominal part of the chest wall stiffens, and expansion of the lungs is restricted. This is followed by a significant decrease up to 50% in pulmonary dynamic compliance and an increase in peak and plateau airway pressures [4, 5]. After deflation of pneumoperitoneum both the pulmonary compliance and the airway pressures return to the baseline levels [6, 7]. High airway pressures and decreased compliance can be associated with pulmonary barotrauma, which can manifest as a pneumothorax. The basal lung regions are compressed during elevated IAP, causing atelectasis and uneven ventilation–perfusion ratios that impair gas exchange. Upward shifting of the diaphragm may also require endobronchial intubation. Thus, monitoring of airway pressures and, if possible, also of pulmonary dynamic compliance is recommended during laparoscopic procedures. However, oxygenation is usually not affected during pneumoperitoneum in adults [1]. Maintenance of a constant positive end-airway pressure of 5 cmH_2O has proved effective in preserving arterial oxygenation and preventing atelectasis during prolonged pneumoperitoneum [8].

Elevated pulmonary pressures mean that the risk of aspiration is possible and therefore the use of a laryngeal mask is not advisable during CO_2 insufflation, especially in obese patients. There are other opinions on this.

Aberrant Effects of CO_2

Gas embolism during pneumoperitoneum is a well-known, potentially fatal, but fortunately very rare, complication. CO_2 bubbles can enter the circulatory system through venous rupture resulting from the raised IAP. Emboli have also been reported without vessel injury [9]. Most embolisms occur during the initial insufflation of CO_2 or during the dissection phase of the gallbladder. There is evidence that CO_2 bubbles are capable of reaching the right side of the heart [10]. When studied with transesophageal echocardiography 68% of patients are found to have CO_2 bubbles in the right chamber of the heart [11]. Transcranial Doppler has shown that CO_2 bubbles may even reach the cerebral circulation [10]. Gas emboli can escape from the venous side to the arterial circulation through the pulmonary arteriovenous shunting or through the foramen ovale. One known risk factor for embolism is hypovolemia. The patients are relatively hypovolemic during pneumoperitoneum, and the head-up tilted position is required, because venous return is decreased. Fortunately most bubbles remain without clinical manifestations.

Insufflated CO_2 can escape from the abdominal cavity to the mediastinum through the soft tissues around the vena cava and aorta. In this way, pneumothorax and pneumomediastinum can develop. Pneumothorax is more common during laparoscopic fundoplication than during cholecystectomy. Continuous side-stream spirometry has proved very useful in the diagnosis of pneumothorax. It shows a very rapid decrease in pulmonary dynamic compliance and an increase in airway pressures [12].

Subcutaneous emphysema results when trocars are incorrectly placed. The large absorption area in the subcutaneous tissue and the high partial pressure allow rapid absorption of CO_2, resulting in profound hypercarbia. Continuous capnometry is useful in detecting CO_2 emphysema. In the presence of CO_2 emphysema insufflation of CO_2 should always be discontinued and the procedure should be converted to open laparotomy.

Nitrous oxide accumulates in the cavities, e.g., the bowel, causing dilatation and thus restricting the surgical view. It has also been shown to accumulate in the abdominal cavity, and together with the intestinal gases it may form a flammable mixture. Therefore, the use of nitrous oxide is not recommended during prolonged laparoscopic procedures.

CO_2 pneumoperitoneum elevates the pressure in the inner ear and eye and raises the intracranial pressure. Clinical situations in which these pressures are known to be elevated are contraindications for CO_2 pneumoperitoneum.

An anesthetist should also be aware that CO_2 pneumoperitoneum can be associated with sudden unexpected septic complications. These septic complications may be associated with the adverse effect of CO_2 pneumoperitoneum on the function of macrophages.

Hemodynamic Effects

CO_2 pneumoperitoneum induces significant hemodynamic changes: increases in heart rate, arterial blood pressures, and systemic vascular resistance (SVR) [13–15]. The hemodynamic stress response to CO_2 pneumoperitoneum leads to an increase in myocardial oxygen consumption, which is deleterious in patients with cardiac diseases. The reason for this abrupt increase in SVR may be connected with activation of the neurohumoral vasoactive system, potent vasopressor systems, i.e., vasopressin (antidiuretic hormone, ADH), and sympathetic and renin–angiotensin–aldosterone systems (RAAS). This activation occurs in an early phase of CO_2 insufflation and may be due to CO_2 per se [14–16].

The effects of CO_2 pneumoperitoneum on the sympathetic nervous system have been studied, but no clear agreement has been reached. Elevated catecholamine levels have been measured during both induction and deflation of pneumoperitoneum [17]. However, the increases in catecholamine concentrations are quite modest, and they may only be indicators of an overall stress response.

Induction of CO_2 pneumoperitoneum leads to a rapid increase in plasma renin activity (PRA) [15, 16] and ADH [14, 18]. There is a positive correlation between mean arterial pressure (MAP) and PRA levels. The rises in PRA and ADH levels may have a role in regulating hemodynamics during laparoscopic procedures.

Recorded effects of CO_2 insufflation and pneumoperitoneum have been a progressive deterioration [19] as well as an increase [20] and no change cardiac output. A reduction in stroke volume may be due to a combination of myocardial depression and impaired contractility caused by CO_2 as well as to an increase in afterload or/and a decrease in venous return. One possible etiology of decreased cardiac output might be increased intrathoracic pressure causing cardiac compression. When patients have sufficient intravascular volume loading, i.e. 10 ml/kg before the induction of pneumoperitoneum, cardiac output increases in response to CO_2 insufflation. Therefore, generous volume loading can be recommended for all patients undergoing laparoscopic cholecystectomy, especially those with coronary artery disease [20, 21].

Treatment of Hemodynamic Response During LC

The most common method of treating the hemodynamic stress response is to enhance the depth of anesthesia during laparoscopic cholecystectomy. Owing to the prolonged recovery caused by CO_2 insufflation it might not be the best possible alternative. Other methods would, therefore, be recommended.

Vasoactive drugs, e.g., vasodilators, β_1-selective adrenoceptor antagonists [22], and α_2-agonists [17], can be successfully used during laparoscopic cholecystectomy to prevent the pressor response to induction and maintenance of CO_2 pneumoperitoneum. Patients with cardiopulmonary diseases may derive particular benefit from them when they are used in association with generous volume loading.

Rapid recovery from anesthesia and low hypnotic potency are among the characteristics of a new short-acting opioid, remifentanil. Remifentanil given as a continuous infusion might facilitate a smooth hemodynamic course and also a rapid emergence from laparoscopic cholecystectomy.

No anesthetic agent has been unequivocally shown to be superior to another in respect to hemodynamic effects, so that an optimal anesthesia does not exist. The anesthetist should use the method one is most convenient with.

Vagal nerve endings are densely distributed in the abdominal cavity. Pneumoperitoneum causes excessive stretching of the vagal nerve endings leading to bradycardia. Also, if the ventricle is dilated the risk of vasovagal reflexes is greater, so that suction of the ventricle should always be performed before CO_2 insufflation. Therefore, routine use of glycopyrronium is advisable during laparoscopic cholecystectomy.

An increase in central venous pressure (CVP) during pneumoperitoneum has been shown in many studies [7, 19]. The higher the IAP the higher is the CVP. Pneumoperitoneum with moderate IAP causes an increase in intrathoracic pressure, which results in elevated CVP values. The raised IAP forces blood out of the abdominal organs and into the venous reservoir. Under conditions of raised IAP, the CVP does not reflect venous return precisely, and falsely increased CVP values do not, therefore, describe the effective circulating blood volume [23]. Thus, normal values in CVP mean that patients may still be volume depleted during pneumoperitoneum. Intraoperative monitoring with a pulmonary artery catheter or transesophageal echocardiography may be helpful in patients with a limited cardiovascular reserve. Elevated IAP is itself also known to increase pulmonary vascular resistance, up to 65%. Thus, accurate estimation of intravascular volume is even more difficult [19, 23].

Pneumoperitoneum with the patient in the reverse Trendelenburg position decreases venous return from the lower extremities and increases femoral venous pressure. Thus, there is a potential risk of deep venous thrombosis or pulmonary embolism. Antithrombotic prophylaxis should always be used during pneumoperitoneum, in the form of low-molecular heparin and anti-thrombosis stockings.

Renal Effects

Oliguria is a common finding during laparoscopy. Renal dysfunction is caused by the elevated IAP exerting direct mechanical compression on the renal parenchyma and the renal arteries and veins [24]. When IAP increases from 0 mmHg to 20 mmHg, renal vascular resistance increases by 555% and the renal glomerular filtration rate decreases by 25% despite the expansion of blood volume [25]. The decrease in renal vein flow is reported to last for at least 2 h postoperatively.

Compression of the caval vein is one possible reason for diminished urine output. Elevated ADH [17, 18] and PRA [15, 16] levels during pneumoperitoneum may also cause diminished urine output. The only way to restore the kidney function and maintain renal perfusion is to implement generous intravascular volume loading before and during elevated IAP.

Pneumoperitoneum with cool, room temperature, CO_2 has been shown to decrease core temperature and urine output [20]. To avoid the harmful effects of pneumoperitoneum on kidney function warm insufflation gas is advisable for patients with borderline renal function.

Anti-inflammatory Analgesics and Renal Function Associated with Laparoscopy

The pain after laparoscopic cholecystectomy is moderate or severe [26]. Nonsteroidal anti-inflammatory analgesics (NSAIDs), though widely used in connection with laparoscopic cholecystectomy, cause renal medullary vasoconstriction. Together with the vasoconstriction caused by pneumoperitoneum they may be harmful to kidney function. It is not advisable to give NSAIDs to patients during pneumoperitoneum or during the early recovery phase (the first 2 h). Especially patients with borderline renal function are in danger of further deterioration in renal function. Patients with underlying renal pathology are not therefore suitable for day-case surgery, which commonly requires the use of NSAIDs.

Splanchnic Circulation

Elevated IAP is thought to cause direct mechanical compression of intraabdominal organs: the liver and gut. Previous data suggest that the effects on the perfusion of internal organs and on cardiopulmonary functions become more pronounced with increasing IAP [25, 27].

During pneumoperitoneum, a reduction in the splanchnic and hepatic perfusion has been shown with an IAP above 12 mmHg. High-pressure pneumoperitoneum has been shown to induce a more pronounced worsening of the postoperative liver function than low-pressure pneumoperitoneum, and postoperative aminotransferase levels have been shown to increase after CO_2 pneumoperitoneum [28–32]. However, conflicting data are also available: advanced transesophageal echocardiography has shown CO_2 insufflation to increase hepatic blood flow [33].

Decreased gastric intramucosal pH (pHi) is thought to reflect impaired splanchnic perfusion, both decreased [34, 35] and unchanged [36, 37] pHi values having been reported during CO_2 pneumoperitoneum. To ensure well-preserved perfusion of the gastric mucosa and splanchnic region in patients with pneumoperitoneum generous fluid loading is advisable.

Data on cytokine levels are also contradictory, and no clear conclusion is possible on the effects of elevated IAP and CO_2 pneumoperitoneum on splanchnic perfusion.

There is evidence that blood flow to intraabdominal organs may deteriorate. It would therefore be safe to perform laparoscopic procedures with a CO_2 pneumoperitoneum at a pressure of 12 mmHg or lower to avoid splanchnic microcirculatory and hepatic flow disturbances.

Postoperative Recovery

Postoperative nausea and vomiting (PONV) is a common sequela after laparoscopic cholecystectomy. Up to 62% of patients suffer from PONV, and this is the most frequent reason for patients not being discharged from hospital on the day of operation [38].

The reason for the high incidence of PONV after laparoscopic cholecystectomy is not clear. The possible causes include mechanical pressure on the gut and stomach, irritation, and stretching of the vagal nerve endings. CO_2 also has vasodilatory effects on cerebral vessels and may raise the intracranial pressure, which is known to cause nausea and vomiting.

Prophylactic antiemetics are included as a part of 'routine anesthetic management' in many centers. Ondansetron has been shown to be effective against POVN. The optimal timing of its administration is important. When ondansetron is given immediately before the end of surgery it is most efficacious in preventing PONV, facilitating early and late recovery and readiness for discharge home, and improving patient satisfaction after outpatient laparoscopic cholecystectomy. Dexamethasone has also been used to prevent PONV after laparoscopic procedures. When it is combined with ondansetron the duration of action is longer and earlier discharge from hospital is possible than with ondansetron alone.

Pain after laparoscopic cholecystectomy is multifactorial and intense. Up to 80% of patients have been reported to require opioid analgesia [39]. The following factors have been implicated: distension of the phrenic nerves, an acidic intraperitoneal milieu during the operation, residual intraabdominal gas after laparoscopy, humidity of insufflated gas, volume of insufflated gas, wound size, and sociocultural and individual factors. Staff should consider trying the following in attempts to prevent and reduce pain: infiltrating local anesthetic at port sites, keeping IAP <12 mmHg, avoiding IAP pressure peaks and prolonged insufflation, using humidified and warmed insufflation gas, evacuating residual gas at the end of laparoscopy, and using pre-emptive analgesia.

Shoulder pain is seen in 40% of patients after laparoscopic cholecystectomy. This pain is referred pain caused by distension of the phrenic nerve. The shoulder pain might be intense in the early postoperative phase. It may last for up to 2 weeks postoperatively. Intraperitoneal bupivacaine injected into the diaphragm at the end of surgery has been effective in reducing both the intensity and the frequency of shoulder pain [40].

A multimodal approach to the postoperative analgesic and PONV management is feasible and advantageous: intravenous anesthesia (propofol and ultra-short-acting opioids), targeted fluid therapy, antiemetics (ondansetron and dexamethasone), incisional bupivacaine intraoperatively, and pre-emptive analgesics (NSAIA in patients with healthy renal function and paracetamol) and treatment of transient oxygen desaturation in the early postoperative period [26].

There is increasing interest in performing laparoscopic cholecystectomy in an outpatient setting. Questions have been raised about the wisdom of this. The patients most suitable for outpatient procedures are those who are healthy and live nearby, who can be discharged on the day of the operation providing the procedure has been uncomplicated and uneventful. In selected patients outpatient laparoscopic cholecystectomy is safe and cost effective. Patients classified as ASA ≥2 or with a diagnosis of biliary pancreatitis or acute cholecystitis are most likely to require admission to hospital.

Abdominal Wall Lift Techniques

Recently a number of abdominal wall lift (AWL) methods have been developed and used for surgical laparoscopy because the adverse effects of CO_2 and elevated IAP are also well recognized by surgeons. Some of these devices are used in combination with low-pressure pneumoperitoneum and some with absolutely no gas insufflation. The advantages of these systems are the lack of hemodynamic stress response and of disturbances in the acid–base balance, better restoration of renal function, and adequate splanchnic circulation. Unfortunately, the surgical view is not always optimal, the exposure of lateral spaces being especially limited. AWL methods are inconvenient in obese patients [7, 35, 41–45]. However, the idea of using ideal lifting methods is justified and further methods are in development.

The patients for whom a gasless laparoscopy is recommended are those with restrictive and severe obstructive pulmonary pathology or underlying renal disease, pregnant patients, and patients with vascular trauma.

In conclusion, laparoscopic cholecystectomy by CO_2 insufflation and elevated intraabdominal pressure has many disadvantages that an anesthesiologist should be aware of. In the hands of an experienced surgeon and a conscientious anesthetist laparoscopic cholecystectomy is nonetheless the treatment of choice for symptomatic gallstones.

References

1. Hirvonen EA, Nuutinen LS, Kauko M (1995) Ventilatory effects, blood gas changes and oxygen consumption during laparoscopic hysterectomy. Anesth Analg 80:961-966
2. Wittgen C, Andreus C, Fitzgerald S et al (1991) Analysis of the hemodynamic and ventilatory effects of laparoscopic cholecystectomy. Arch Surg 126:997-1001
3. Kazama T, Ikeda K, Kato T, Kikura M (1996) Carbon dioxide output in laparoscopic cholecystectomy. Br J Anaesth 76:530-535
4. Bardoczky GI, Engelman E, Levarlet M, Simon P (1993) Ventilatory effects of pneumoperitoneum monitored with continuous spirometry. Anaesthesia 48:309-311
5. Kendall A, Bhatt S, Oh T (1995) Pulmonary consequences of carbon dioxide insufflation for laparoscopic cholecystectomies. Anaesthesia 50:286-289
6. Mäkinen M-T, Yli-Hankala A (1996) The effect of laparoscopic cholecystectomy on respiratory compliance as determined by continuous spirometry. J Clin Anesth 8:119-122
7. Koivusalo AM, Kellokumpu I, Scheinin M et al (1998) A comparison of gasless mechanical and conventional carbon dioxide pneumoperitoneum methods for laparoscopic cholecystectomy. Anesth Analg 86:153-158
8. Meininger D, Byhahn C, Mierdl S et al (2005) Positive end-expiratory pressure improves arterial oxygenation during prolonged pneumoperitoneum. Acta Anaesthesiol Scand 49:778-783
9. Yacoub O, Cardonaa I, Coveler L, Dodson M (1982) Carbon dioxide embolism during laparoscopy. Anesthesiology 57:533-535
10. Schindler E, Muller M, Kelm C (1995) Cerebral carbon dioxide embolism during laparoscopic cholecystectomy. Anesth Analg 81:643-645
11. Derouin M, Couture P, Boudreault D et al (1996) Detection of gas embolism by transesophageal echocardiography during laparoscopic cholecystectomy. Anesth Analg 82:119-124
12. Mäkinen MT, Yli-Hankala A, Kansanaho M (1995) Early detection of CO2 pneumothorax with continuous spirometry during laparoscopic fundoplication. Acta Anaesthesiol Scand 9:411-413
13. Struthers AD, Cuschieri A (1998) Cardiovascular consequences of laparoscopic surgery. Lancet 352:568-570
14. Joris JL, Noirot DP, Legrand MJ et al (1996) Hemodynamic changes during laparoscopic cholecystectomy. Anesth Analg 76:1067-1071

15. O'Leary E, Hubbard K, Tormey W, Cunningham A (1997) Laparoscopic cholecystectomy: haemodynamic and neuroendocrine response after pneumoperitoneum and changes in position. Br J Anaesth 76:640-644
16. Koivusalo AM, Kellokumpu I, Scheinin M et al (1996) Randomized comparison of the neuroendocrine response to laparoscopic cholecystectomy using either conventional or abdominal wall lift techniques. Br J Surg 83:1532-1536
17. Joris JL, Chiche JD, Canivet JL et al (1998) Hemodynamic changes induced by laparoscopy and their endocrine correlates: effects of clonidine. J Am Coll Cardiol 32:1389-1396
18. Ortega A, Peters J, Incarbone R et al (1996) A prospective randomized comparison of the metabolic and stress hormonal responses of laparoscopic and open cholecystectomy. J Am Coll Surg 183:249-256
19. McLaughlin J, Scheeres D, Dean R, Bonnell B (1995) The adverse hemodynamic effects of laparoscopic cholecystectomy. Surg Endosc 9:121-124
20. Backlund M, Kellokumpu I, Scheinin T et al (1998) Effect of temperature of insufflated CO2 during and after prolonged laparoscopic surgery. Surg Endosc 12:1126-1130
21. Neudecker J, Sauerland S, Neugebauer E et al (2002) The European Association for Endoscopic Surgery clinical practice guideline on the pneumoperitoneum for laparoscopic surgery. Surg Endosc 16:1121-1143
22. Koivusalo AM, Scheinin M, Tikkanen I, Ristkari S, Lindgren L (1998) Effects of esmolol on haemodynamic response to CO2 pneumoperitoneum for laparoscopic surgery. Acta Anaesth Scand 42:510-517
23. Andersson L, Wallin CJ, Sollevi A, Odeberg-Wennerman S (1999) Pneumoperitoneum in healthy humans is not associated with increased central blood volume. Acta Anaesth Scand 43:809-814
24. Miki Y, Iwase K, Kamiike W et al (1997) Laparoscopic cholecystectomy and time course changes in renal function. Surg Endosc 11:838-841
25. Harman PK, Kron IL, McLachlan HD et al (1982) Elevated intra-abdominal pressure and renal function. Ann Surg 196:594-597
26. Jensen K, Kehlet H, Lund CM (2007) Post-operative recovery profile after laparoscopic cholecystectomy: a prospective, observational study of a multimodal anaesthetic regime. Acta Anaesthesiol Scand 51:464-471
27. Schilling MK, Redaelli C, Krahenbuhl L et al (1997) Splanchnic microcirculatory changes during CO2 laparoscopy. J Am Coll Surg 184:378-382
28. Ishizaki Y, Bandai Y, Shimomura K et al (1993) Safe intraabdominal pressure of carbon dioxide pneumoperitoneum during laparoscopic surgery. Surgery 114:549-554
29. Hasukic S (2005) Postoperative changes in liver function tests: randomized comparison of low- and high-pressure laparoscopic cholecystectomy. Surg Endosc 19:1451-1455
30. Morino M, Giraudo G, Festa V (1998) Alterations in hepatic function during laparoscopic surgery. An experimental clinical study. Surg Endosc 12:968-972
31. Sato K, Kawamura T, Wakusawa R (2000) Hepatic blood flow and function in elderly patients undergoing laparoscopic cholecystectomy. Anesth Analg 90:1198-1202
32. Windberger UB, Auer R, Keplinger F et al (1999) The role of intra-abdominal pressure on splanchnic and pulmonary hemodynamic and metabolic changes during carbon dioxide pneumoperitoneum. Gastrointest Endosc 49:84-91
33. Meierhenrich R, Gauss A, Vandenesch P et al (2005) The effects of intraabdominally insufflated carbon dioxide on hepatic blood flow during laparoscopic surgery assessed by transesophageal echocardiography. Anesth Analg 100:340-347
34. Knolmayer TJ, Bowyer MW, Egan JC, Asbun HJ (1998) The effects of pneumoperitoneum on gastric blood flow and traditional hemodynamic measurements. Surg Endosc 12:115-118
35. Koivusalo AM, Kellokumpu I, Ristkari S, Lindgren L (1997) Splanchnic and renal deterioration during and after laparoscopic cholecystectomy: a comparison of the carbon dioxide pneumoperitoneum and the abdominal wall lift method. Anesth Analg 85:886-891
36. Thaler W, Frey L, Marzoli GP, Messmer K (1996) Assessment of splanchnic tissue oxygenation by gastric tonometry in patients undergoing laparoscopic and open cholecystectomy. Br J Surg 83:620-624
37. Odeberg S, Ljungqvist O, Sollevi A (1998) Pneumoperitoneum for laparoscopic cholecystectomy is not associated with compromised splanchnic circulation. Eur J Surg 164:843-848
38. Saunders C, Leary B, Wolfe B (1995) Is outpatient laparoscopic cholecystectomy wise? Surg Endosc 9:1263-1268
39. Mouton W, Bessell J, Otten K, Maddern G (1999) Pain after laparoscopy. Surg Endosc 13:445-448
40. Cunniffe M, McAnena O, Dar M, Flynn N (1998) A prospective randomized trial of intraoperative bupivacaine irrigation for management of shoulder-tip pain following laparoscopy. Am J Surg 176:258-261
41. Paolucci V, Gutt CN, Schaeff B, Encke A (1995) Gasless laparoscopy in abdominal surgery. Surg Endosc 9:497-500
42. Thoelke MH, Merkelbach D, Ehmann T et al

(1995) The abdominal lift: is there any advantage for the critically ill patient? Endosc Surg Allied Tech 3:180-182
43. Carry PY, Gallet D, Francois Y et al (1998) Respiratory mechanics during laparoscopic cholecystectomy: the effects of the abdominal wall lift. Anesth Analg 87:1393-1397
44. Galizia G, Prizio G, Lieto E et al (2001) Hemodynamic and pulmonary changes during open, carbon dioxide pneumoperitoneum and abdominal wall-lifting cholecystectomy. A prospective, randomized study. Surg Endosc 15:477-483
45. Junghans T, Modersohn D, Dorner F et al (2006) Systematic evaluation of different approaches for minimizing hemodynamic changes during pneumoperitoneum. Surg Endosc 20:763-769

Chapter 16

Cholecystectomy Techniques

Jean-François Gigot, Catherine Hubert, Benoit Navez

Introduction

The procedure of cholecystectomy was first reported in 1882 by Carl Langenbuch, who used an open approach that then remained unchanged for more than 100 years. In France in 1987, Philippe Mouret performed the procedure using a laparoscopic approach, a technique that is now considered world-wide as the "gold standard" [1–6]. However, the technique is associated with a greater incidence of bile duct injury especially, but not only, during a surgeon's learning curve [7]. The purpose of the present review is to report the technical aspects of the procedure in detail in order to allow the safe performance of laparoscopic cholecystectomy (LC). The procedure that we will discuss is the so-called "French technique" of LC.

Operative Indications and Contraindications

Symptomatic or complicated gallstones are standard indications for LC. Due to their indolent natural history, asymptomatic gallstones are not standard indications, except in some South American countries where the incidence of gallbladder cancer is high. Almost all patients can be approached laparoscopically. Severe cardiovascular compromise and uncorrectable coagulating disorders are relative contraindications to laparoscopy as well as to open surgery. The presence of severe dense intraperitoneal adhesions due to previous abdominal surgery is not a contraindication, but requires greater experience in the laparoscopic approach when peritoneal adhesions are supposed to be found. A trial of the laparoscopic approach is warranted and creation of a pneumoperitoneum using an open Hasson's technique is recommended. Chronic obstructive pulmonary disease is not a contraindication, on the contrary, in such cases post-operative recovery is easier after laparoscopy than laparotomy. Finally, patients suffering from liver cirrhosis with portal hypertension and from severe inflammation into the porta hepatis (from gangrenous cholecystitis or acute necrotizing pancreatitis) require great experience for a safe LC. Performance of LC during pregnancy should be considered with caution and avoided if possible during the third semester. Preoperative suspicion of gallbladder cancer favors a primary open approach. Regarding the surgeon, not enough laparoscopic expertise and lack of adequate instrumentation and material are strong contraindications; although this is a situation that is rarely encountered in well-developed countries. The need for preoperative informed consent is the rule, not only for medico-legal purposes but also to ensure that the patient knows that conversion in difficult cases is a sign of a wise surgical judgement and not of surgical failure.

Patient Positioning and Peritoneal Access

Patient Positioning

The patient is positioned in the supine position on the operating table, with care taken to avoid any neurological compression. Two specifications are requested for the operating table: that it is radiolucent, to allow the performance of intraoperative cholangiography and that it is electric, to allow repositioning of the patient during the procedure (especially in a reverse Trendelenburg position and a lateral tilting). The operation is performed under general anesthesia. A urinary catheter is not useful for a laparoscopic procedure within the upper abdominal quadrant unless a long procedure is anticipated. Stomach decompression by a nasogastric tube is routinely required to improve the visibility of the operative field and to avoid hollow injury during the creation of the pneumoperitoneum or the surgical dissection. For the laparoscopic technique, the surgeon stands between the patient's splayed legs (the so-called "French position"). Operating room setup for this procedure is illustrated in Figure 16.1. Conversion is always an option during LC in difficult cases, so the abdomen should be routinely prepared for a possible laparotomy.

Peritoneal Access

In the case of open approach, access to the peritoneal cavity is made through a right

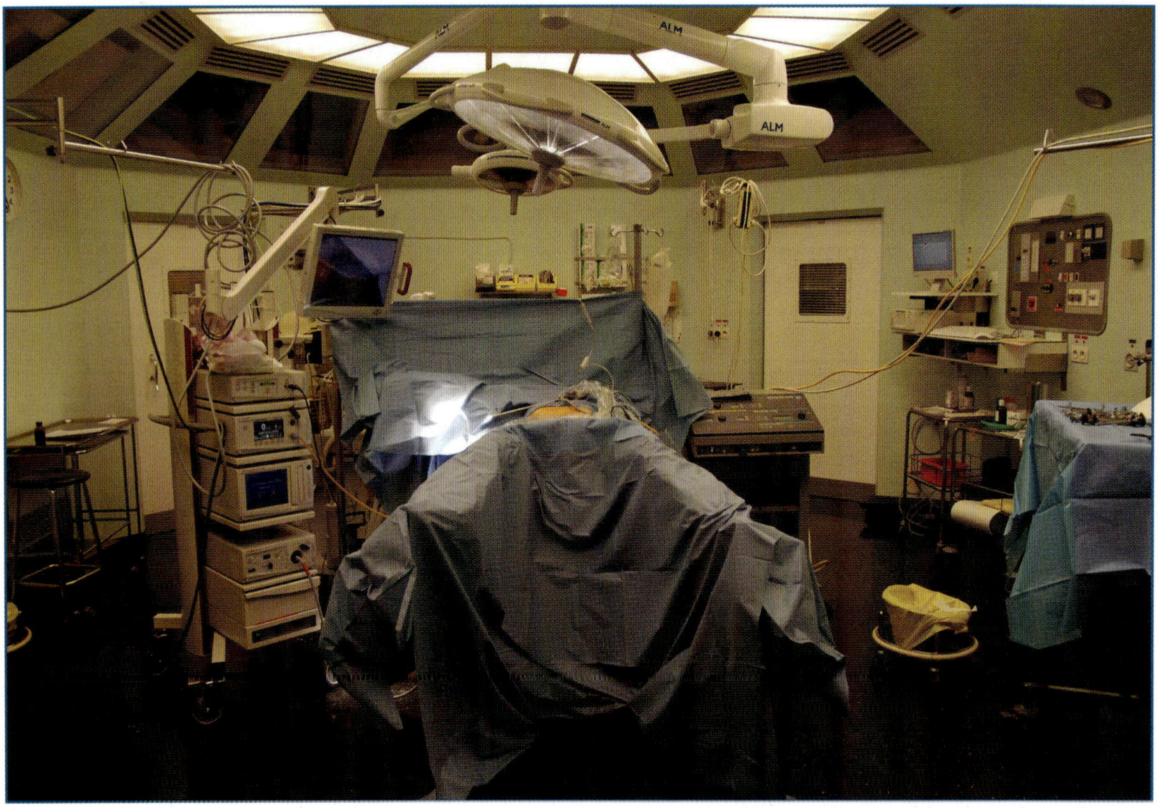

Fig. 16.1 Operative room set-up: the surgeon stands between the patient's splayed legs in the so-called "French position", with the first assistant on the left side of the patient

subcostal or transverse incision or a midline incision.

In the case of laparoscopic approach, the creation and the maintenance of an appropriate pneumoperitoneum is a prerequisite to achieve a closed peritoneal working space [8]. Carbon dioxide is usually employed because this gas is innocuous, does not support combustion during dissection with electrocautery and is highly soluble, minimizing the risk of gas embolism. The intraperitoneal pressure is increased stepwise and maintained at 12–14 mmHg by a powerful high-flow insufflator. Continuous monitoring of intra-abdominal pressure is of a paramount importance. Insufflation of the peritoneal cavity can be performed by percutaneous technique using the classical Veress needle or by introducing the first trocar under direct vision using an open Hasson's technique. We recommend the latter approach for safety reasons. Indeed, the rare but potentially lethal risk of major vascular injury (0.05%) [9] is minimized with this approach. The risk of intestinal injury (0.06%) [9] is significantly decreased but not completely abolished. Formal indications for the open Hasson's technique are patients who have undergone previous abdominal surgery and surgeons with less experience. However, the technique is not easy in morbidly obese patients who have a thick fatty abdominal wall. The principle is to choose a site for first trocar insertion far from previous abdominal scars. The best site for introduction of the first trocar is the supra-umbilical area or the left upper quadrant, usually three fingers below the left subcostal margin. This 10 mm left trocar will serve as a "dissecting port" where all dissecting, cutting and clipping instruments will be introduced. The three other trocars are introduced into the abdominal cavity under direct intraperitoneal vision. The position of trocars during LC is illustrated in Figure 16.2. The rule of a 90-degree triangulation for trocar insertion must be respected in order to achieve ergonomic manipulation of laparoscopic instruments. The 5 mm subxyphoid trocar serves as a "retracting port", especially for elevating the liver or lowering the duodeno-pancreas. A "manipulating port" for the gallbladder is provided by a fourth 5 mm trocar in the right upper quadrant (RUQ) in order to allow manipulation and retraction of the gallbladder during the surgical dissection (Fig. 16.3). Finally, in case of difficult exposition, an additional 5 mm trocar can be used, placed below the right costal margin. An alternative is the suspension of the round ligament with a transcutaneous transfixing stitch.

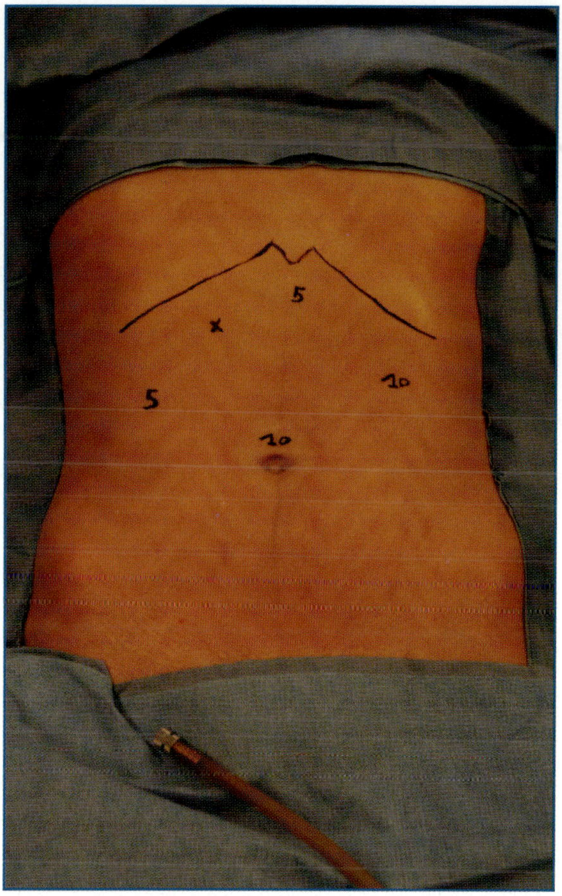

Fig. 16.2 Position of the four trocars: a 10 mm trocar at the umbilicus (optical trocar), a 10 mm trocar in the left upper quadrant (dissecting port), a 5 mm trocar in the subxyphoid area (retracting port) and a 5 mm trocar in the right upper quadrant (manipulating port) for the gallbladder (X)

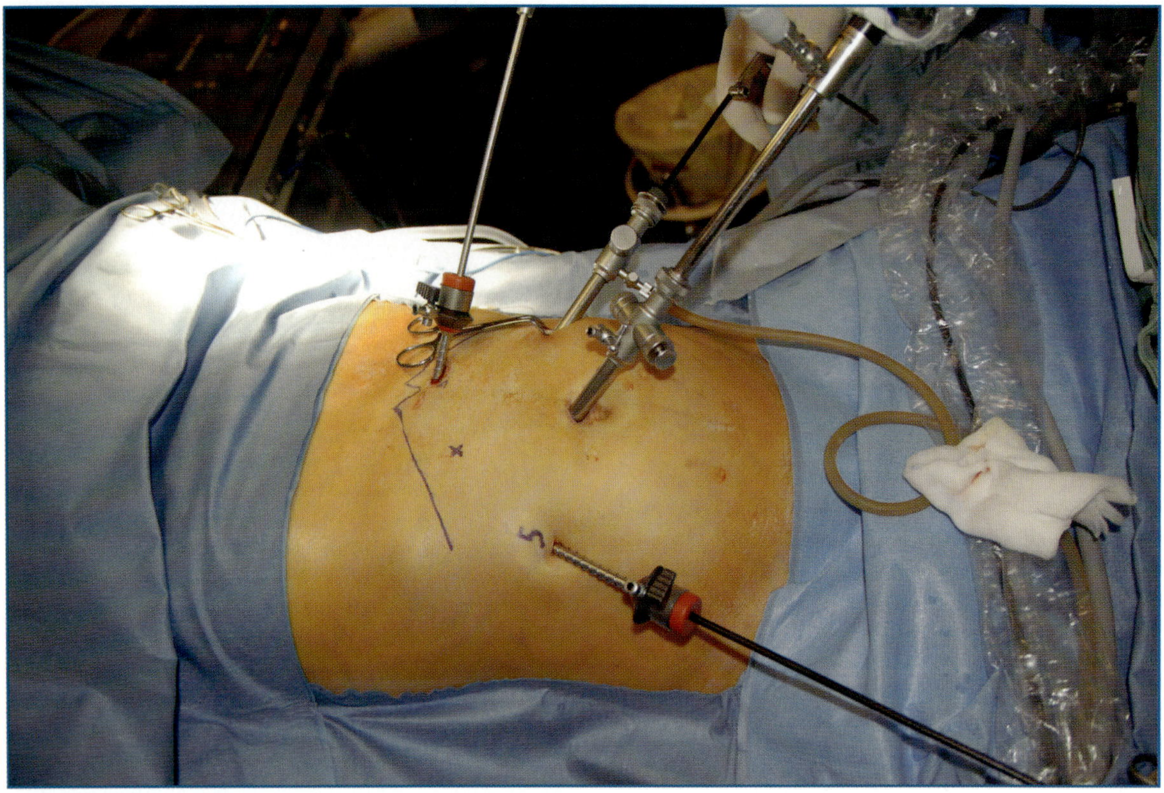

Fig. 16.3 Operative view of the trocars' positions and of the instruments

However, the trocars' positions must be tailored to the patient's intra-abdominal anatomy. In obese patients, the 10 mm optical trocar usually placed at the umbilical site must be moved upward on the middle line between the umbilicus and the sternal notch in order to get vertical access to the RUQ. The subxyphoid trocar should be placed under direct vision to the left side of the falciform ligament at a variable level on the middle line depending on the height of coexistent hepatomegaly. Similarly, the RUQ trocar is placed below the level of the inferior border of the right liver and can thus be placed low in the RUQ if a significant hepatomegaly is present. When all ports are installed, a routine visual check must be accomplished to verify the absence of complications during the trocars' insertion (e.g., bleeding, transfixing intestinal injury).

Operative Technique

Exposition of the Operative Field

The principle is to get a vertical access to the hepatoduodenal ligament and to stretch it. Both conditions are achieved either through an open or a laparoscopic approach before embarking on the surgical dissection.

During an open approach a metallic valve is installed at the right upper border of the incision to get upward retraction. The hepatoduodenal ligament is exposed by elevating the inferior edge of segment IV of the liver with a metallic retractor handled by an assistant or fixed on the metallic valve, with the assistant's hand or an atraumatic metallic valve pulling the duodenum and the pancreatic head downward.

During a laparoscopic approach, the same principles of exposure must be achieved. However, optimal exposure of the porta hepatis may be more difficult to obtain by laparoscopy than by laparotomy, especially for inexperienced surgeons. First of all, a reverse 20–30-degree Trendelenburg position of the patient allows the transverse colon, the omentum and the duodenum to fall caudally by gravity away from the gallbladder. Similar to the open approach, a flexible articulated U-retractor is placed under the inferior surface of segment IV to achieve upward liver retraction (Fig. 16.4). A 30-degree laparoscope can be employed to get a more vertical approach to the operative field, especially in obese patients. Finally, when a redundant left lateral lobe is obscuring access to the hepatoduodenal ligament by its rotation around the falciform ligament, an additional port may be required in the RUQ to elevate the left lateral segments from the right side. In this circumstance, tilting the operating table slightly to the left or suspension of the round ligament may also help to improve exposure of the gallbladder.

Exposition of Calot's Triangle

After having stretched the hepatoduodenal ligament, the basic principle is again to stretch Calot's triangle to provide a safe approach and dissection. To achieve this goal, Hartmann's pouch is grasped with atraumatic forceps introduced through the RUQ port and retracted laterally and inferiorly without excessive traction. The aim of this maneuver is also to place the cystic duct at a right angle to the common bile duct (CBD), in order to avoid misidentification and bile duct injury (Fig. 16.5). Forceful traction on the gallbladder neck exposes the cystic duct to traumatic avulsion and tenting of the CBD; both of these conditions expose also the bile duct to injury.

Dissection of Calot's Triangle

Meticulous operative technique observing strict guidelines (Table 16.1) is obviously of greatest importance in preventing bile duct injury, along with careful dissection and correct identification of the biliary anatomy.

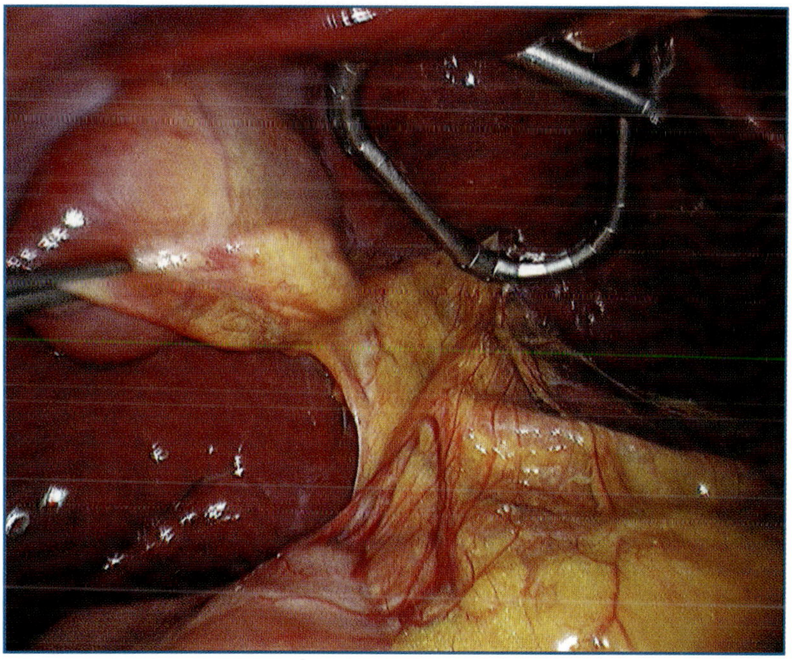

Fig. 16.4 Exposition of the operative field with a U-liver retractor under the inferior surface of segment IV, stretching the hepatoduodenal ligament

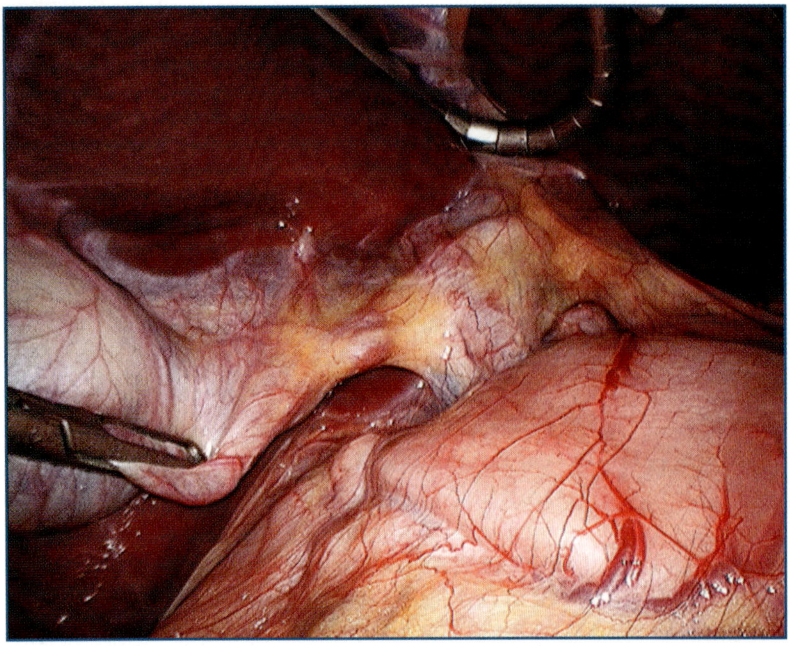

Fig. 16.5 Exposition of Calot's triangle with atraumatic forceps pulling Hartmann's pouch inferiorly and laterally, placing the cystic duct at a right angle with the common bile duct, clearly visualized in this picture

Table 16.1 Guidelines for a safe dissection during laparoscopic cholecystectomy

1. When exposing the hepatoduodenal ligament
- approach the operative field vertically
  - use a high trocar position in obese patients
  - use a 30 degree laparoscope
- make sure there is adequate visualization of the operative field
  - use high quality vision (optic) and light
  - lift up the quadrate lobe of the liver
  - use an additional trocar in case of large left liver lobe
  - use a reverse Trendelenburg position (30 degree)
  - pull down the duodenum, if necessary

2. When exposing Calot's triangle
- pull the gallbladder infundibulum laterally and inferiorly to open/stretch Calot's triangle
- avoid using excessive traction on gallbladder neck to avoid the risk of tenting the common bile duct (CBD) or traumatic rupture of the cystic duct-CBD junction.

3. When dissecting Calot's triangle
- start dissection at the gallbladder neck–cystic duct junction (and NOT at the cystic duct-CBD junction)
- visualize the entrance of cystic duct into the gallbladder
- conduct the dissection from the gallbladder neck toward the cystic duct
- avoid routine dissection of the CBD (danger with cautery)
- perform an atraumatic blunt dissection
- minimize use of electrocautery within Calot's triangle
- avoid the blind use of clips to control bleeding when hemorrhage occurs during the dissection of Calot's triangle
- completely clear Calot's triangle both ventrally and dorsally, so that the only visible structures are the cystic duct and artery
- avoid dividing any ductal structures within Calot's triangle before accurate anatomic dissection and identification by intraoperative cholangiography

cont. →

cont. **Table 16.1**

4. When dissecting Hartmann's pouch • flip Hartman's pouch up and down, to free the gallbladder neck from the liver bed • keep the dissection close to the gallbladder wall, especially at the superior part of Hartman pouch, where right biliary anomalies would be found • perform an atraumatic blunt dissection, especially in case of severe inflammation • avoid a plane of dissection that is too deep • avoid persisting in dissecting scar tissue around Hartman pouch's (in case of severe acute or chronic cholecystitis)
5. When closing the cystic duct stump • visualize both limbs of clips on the cystic duct and artery clearly • avoid tenting the CBD by clip application too close to CBD or by ligation or suture when a large cystic duct is existing

Again, the dissection of Calot's triangle starts only after adequate exposition. The dissection technique requires sharp scissors or, more commonly, a hook dissector. Great care should be taken to avoid overuse of electrocautery within Calot's triangle. Indeed, terrible thermal injury to the CBD or the hepatic hilum can occur in this setting. Similarly, blind use of clips or cautery to control bleeding in Calot's triangle should be avoided. The dissection starts far from the CBD at the presumed junction between the cystic duct and the gallbladder infundibulum, by incision of the anterior peritoneal layer, keeping the dissection close to the gallbladder (Fig. 16.6). The entrance of the cystic duct within the gallbladder must be clearly visualized. It is also important to view both the dorsal and ventral aspect of Calot's triangle by manipulating the gallbladder downwards and dissecting the gallbladder neck from above to expose the cystic duct arising from the infundibulum. The gallbladder–cystic duct junction should be completely dissected and encircled. A retrograde gentle dissection is then pursued to squelettonize the ductal structures present

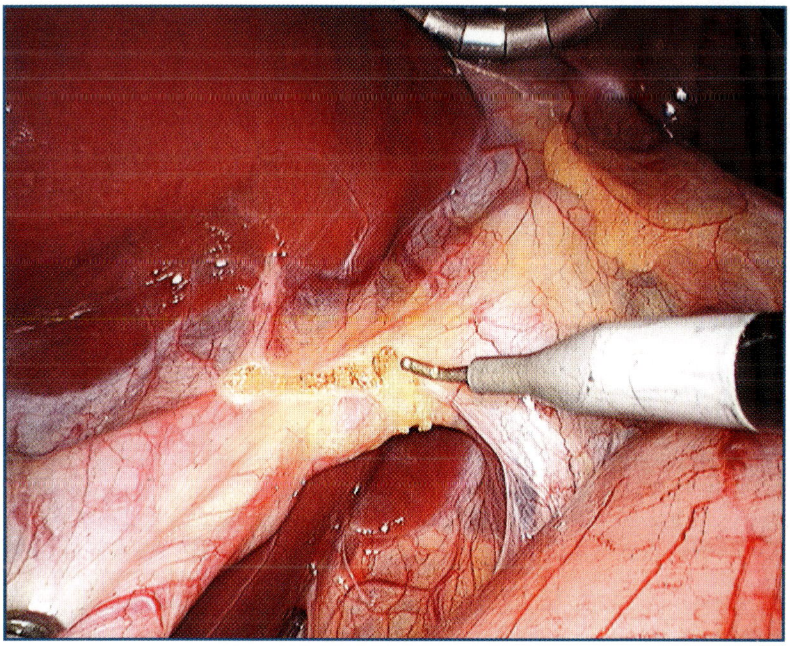

Fig. 16.6 Dissection of Calot's triangle starting at the cystic duct–Hartmann's pouch junction, with incision of the anterior peritoneal layer of Calot's triangle using a hook dissector

within Calot's triangle; namely, the cystic duct and the cystic artery (Fig. 16.7). The cystic artery is usually located cephalad to the cystic duct, running parallel to it, but there are frequently multiple variations in the arterial supply of the gallbladder. The cystic duct node is the landmark for identifying the cystic artery to which it is anatomically close. An unexpectedly large presumed cystic artery should alert the surgeon since the presumed cystic artery could be the right branch of the hepatic artery, prudence would allow to avoid hepatic artery clipping and to achieve further careful arterial dissection. Biliary dissection also needs precaution, if CBD needs to be dissected or there is a suspicion it may be involved during the dissection, electrocautery has to be avoided. A clear and complete dissection of Calot's triangle is the rule. This concept is generally accepted, being called "the flag technique" by French surgeons [10], the "critical view technique" by American surgeons [11], the "window technique" by English surgeons [12] and the "safety zone" by Asian surgeons [13, 14]. Calot's triangle is then clearly visualized anteriorly (Fig. 16.7) and posteriorly (Fig. 16.8).

Dissection of the Gallbladder Infundibulum

The dissection of Calot's triangle is then pursued along the superior border of the gallbladder infundibulum (Fig. 16.9). The gallbladder infundibulum must be dissected anteriorly and posteriorly. Close contact with the gallbladder wall should be maintained during this dissection. Indeed, an anomalous right hepatic duct draining the postero-lateral biliary sector (Fig. 16.10) may be injured if the plane of dissection is too deep and not in close contact with the gallbladder wall. At this stage, a complete dissection of Calot's triangle is achieved and the gallbladder is only attached to the gallbladder bed by the fundus. No clip should be placed on, and no incision should be made in any structure on Calot's triangle until intraoperative cholangiography (IOC) is performed. A proximal clip is then placed on the cystic duct at the gallbladder-cystic duct junction (Fig. 16.11). The cystic duct is incised with scissors (Fig. 16.12), not too close to the cystic duct–CBD junction in

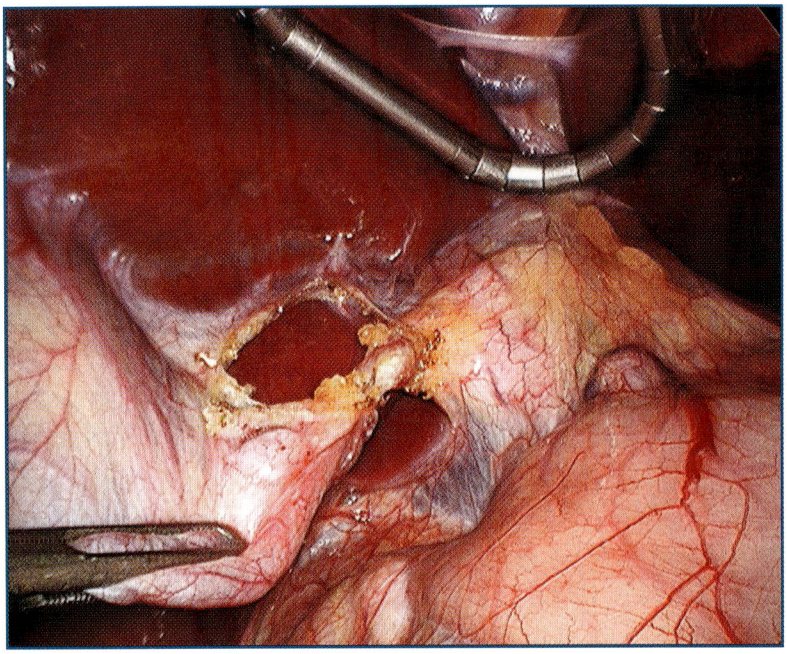

Fig. 16.7 Anterior view of the entire dissection of Calot's triangle

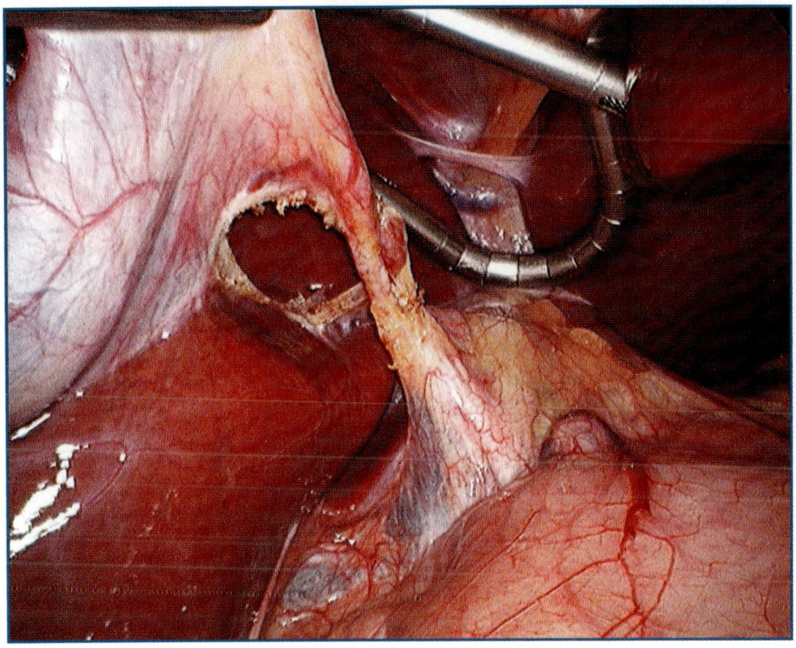

Fig. 16.8 Posterior view of the complete dissection of Calot's triangle, demonstrating the "critical view technique"

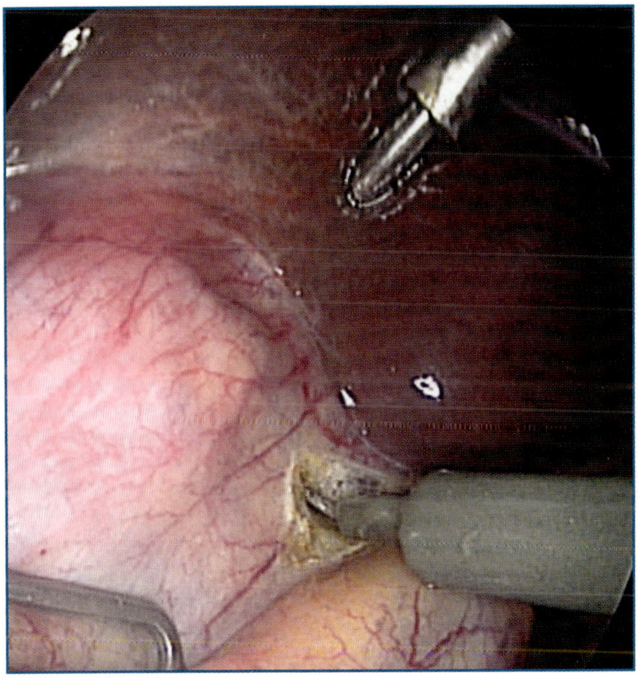

Fig. 16.9 The dissection of Calot's triangle is pursued along the superior border of the gallbladder infundibulum, keeping close contact with the gallbladder wall during the dissection

order to avoid possible bile duct injury during further manipulations, but also not too close to the gallbladder–cystic duct junction in order to avoid cystic valves precluding easy introduction of the cholangiographic catheter. The cystic duct should be routinely milked toward the gallbladder to exclude the presence of intracystic stones that will be pushed by the cholangiographic catheter into the CBD. Standard Olsen cholangiographic forceps with a soft 5 French catheter are introduced through the "manipulating port" in the RUQ. The cholangiography catheter is introduced into

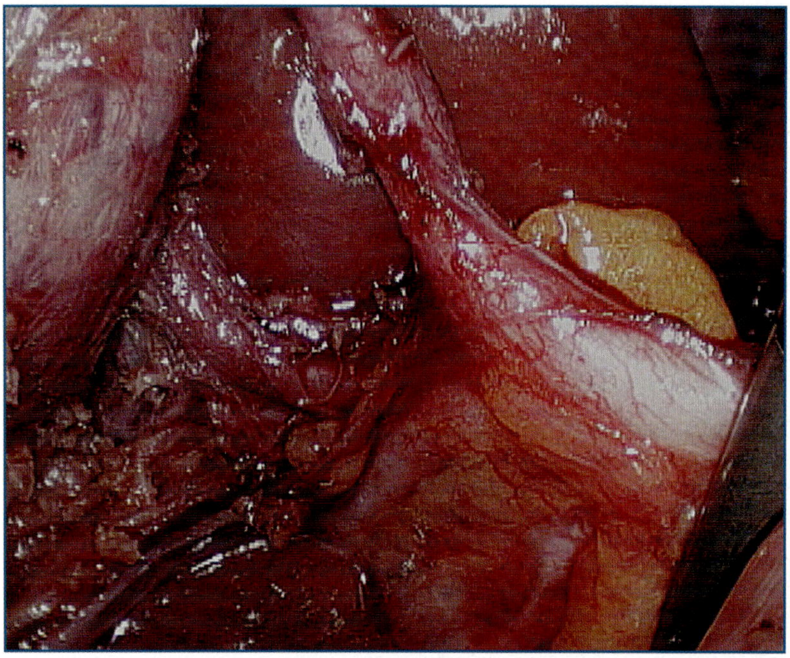

Fig. 16.10 Presence of an anomalous right hepatic duct detected during the dissection of Calot's triangle

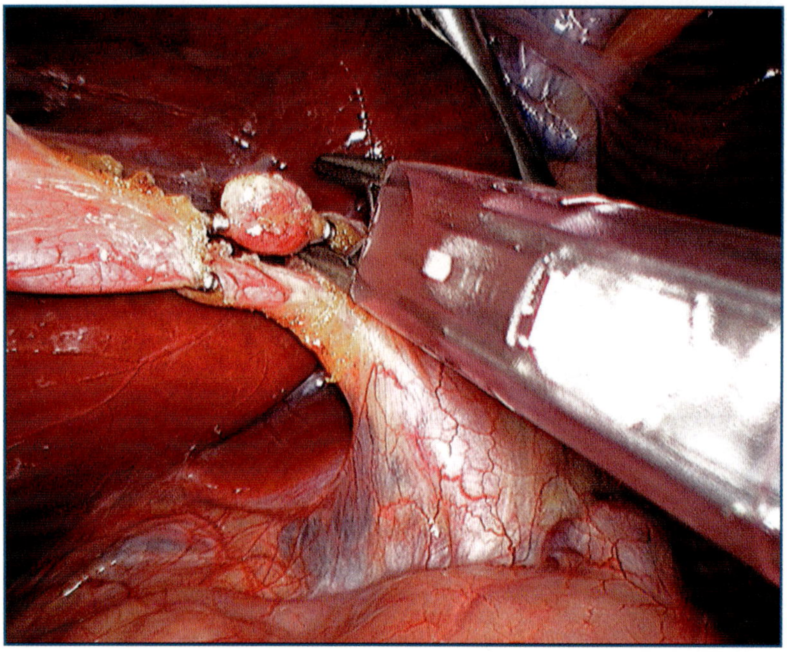

Fig. 16.11 Proximal clipping of the cystic duct close to the gallbladder–cystic duct junction and proximal and distal clipping of the cystic artery

the cystic duct aperture and gently pushed into the CBD (Fig. 16.13). The atraumatic jaws of the Olsen catheter will close the cystic duct site of catheter introduction. An alternative is to "gently" apply one clip without squeezing the cystic duct with the cholangiography catheter inside.

Intraoperative Cholangiography

A water-soluble contrast solution with a 50% dilution is slowly injected into the CBD under fluoroscopic guidance. Fluoroscopic cholangiography is preferred for dynamic

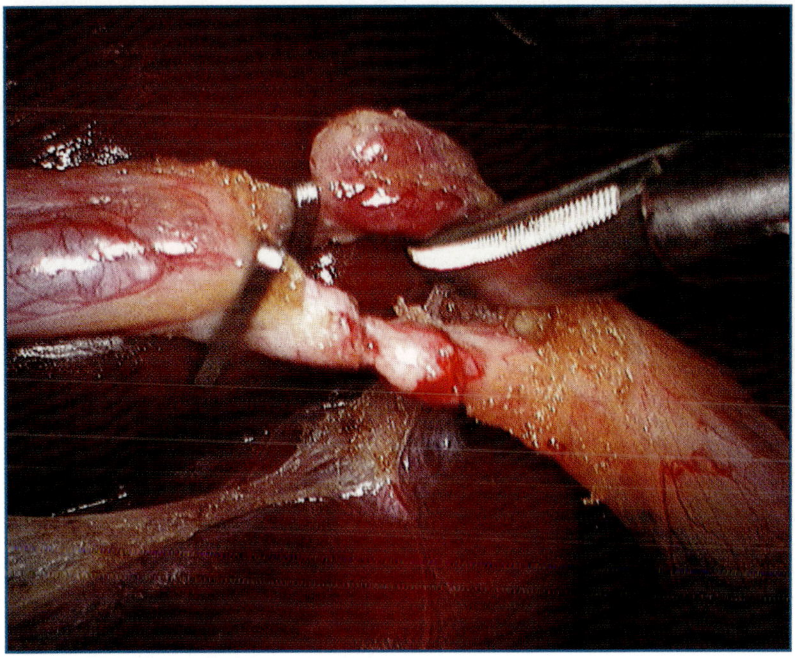

Fig. 16.12 Opening of the cystic duct with scissors in order to perform intraoperative cholangiography

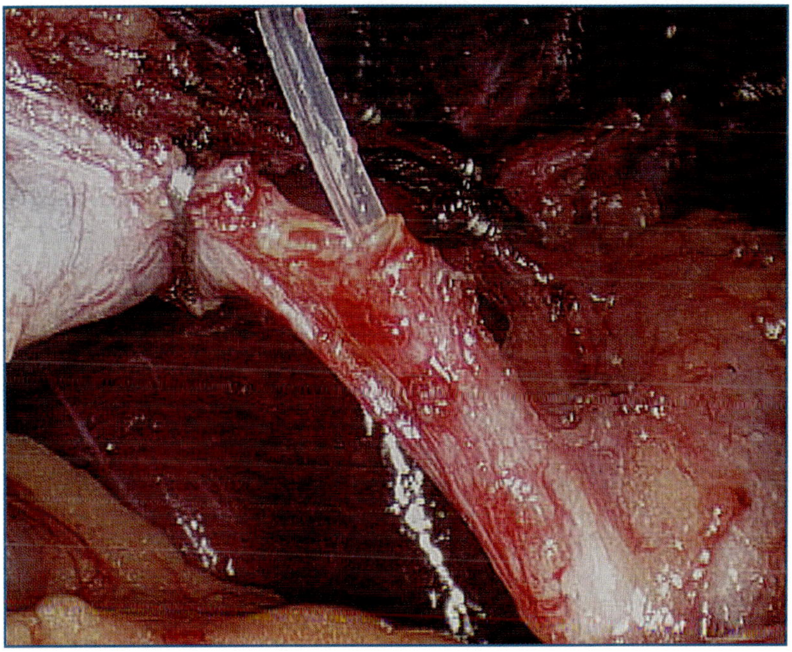

Fig. 16.13 Introduction of the cholangiographic catheter into the incised cystic duct

filling of the biliary tree. Attention should be paid to image the whole extra- and intrahepatic biliary tract as well as the trans-papillary passage of contrast. The role of IOC during LC is to detect any bile duct injury, to detect unexpected biliary anatomy (Fig. 16.14) and to diagnose occult CBD stones, strictures or other ductal pathology. When IOC is performed at the end of complete Calot's triangle dissection during LC and correctly interpreted by the surgeon, the exam is able to detect more than 90% of bile duct injuries [7], a rate significantly greater than during LC without IOC [7, 15–17]. It should be

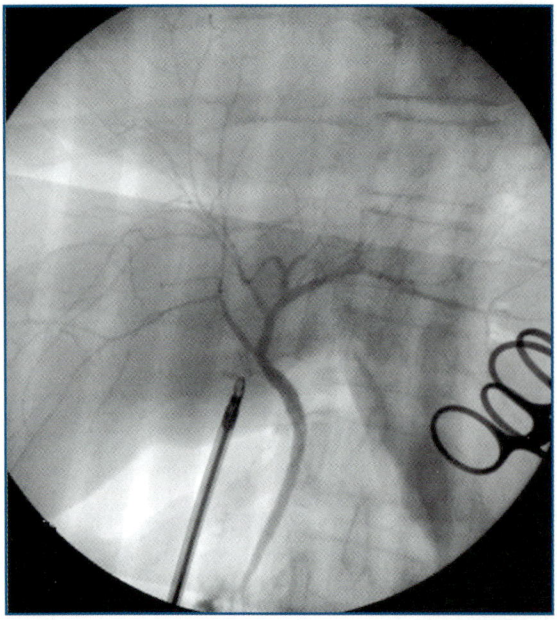

Fig. 16.14 Intraoperative cholangiography demonstrating the presence of unexpected biliary anatomy, such as an anomalous right hepatic duct

emphasized that half of bile duct injuries following LC are not diagnosed at the time of primary operation, leading to increased related morbidity and mortality [7, 15, 16]. Features at IOC that should raise suspicion of a bile duct injury are the presence of extrabiliary contrast material extravasation, the lack of opacification of the proximal bile duct system and the incomplete opacification of the right posterior intrahepatic bile ducts. IOC also plays a role in decreasing the severity of bile duct injury in case of misidentification between the cystic duct and the CBD. A completed and correctly interpreted IOC will diagnose a lateral ductal injury caused by a presumed cysticotomy during IOC, avoiding the occurrence of a complete transsection or excision [7, 16, 18]. However, a normal IOC may be encountered in spite of bile duct injury in the following cases: (1) if the injury occurs later in the cholecystectomy, after the performance of cholangiography, during the dissection of the gallbladder bed; (2) if the IOC is misinterpreted; (3) if there is thermal injury due to electrocautery leading to postoperative localized biliary necrosis or late stricture; or (4) if biliary leak originates from the cystic duct after the performance of IOC and after gallbladder removal [7, 15, 16, 18]. These data support the routine use of IOC for early detection and correction of LC-induced bile duct injury, especially during the surgeon's learning curve when the risk is known to be the greatest [7, 15, 16].

After completion of IOC, the cholangiography catheter is withdrawn from the cystic duct. The cystic duct and artery are double clipped (Fig. 16.15) with a multi-fire, spring-loaded titanium clip applier inserted through the "dissecting port". Great care should be taken to control the proper position of clips to avoid lateral clipping of the CBD. When the cystic duct is wide, thick or inflamed, closure is accomplished by intra- or extracorporeal ligation or suture or by the means of an Endoloop. The cystic artery and then the cystic duct are subsequently transected with scissors.

Dissection of the Gallbladder from the Liver Bed

The gallbladder neck is grasped with atraumatic forceps introduced through the "manipulating port". Then the gallbladder is retracted to the right and maintained under tension, exposing its medial and lateral surfaces. The hook dissector is employed to dissect the avascular plane between the gallbladder fundus and the liver bed both anteriorly (Fig. 16.16) and posteriorly (Fig. 16.17). If an accessory Luschka duct is encountered within the gallbladder bed, it must be electively clipped or ligated. A plane of dissection that is too deep within the liver bed entering the liver parenchyma is the most common cause of bleeding during this step of the operation. However, in severe acute or chronic cholecystitis, this plane is usually obscured by inflammation and the dissection is not easy, so bleeding is not uncommon. In this circumstance, electrocautery or Argon beam coagulation control the bleeding paying atten-

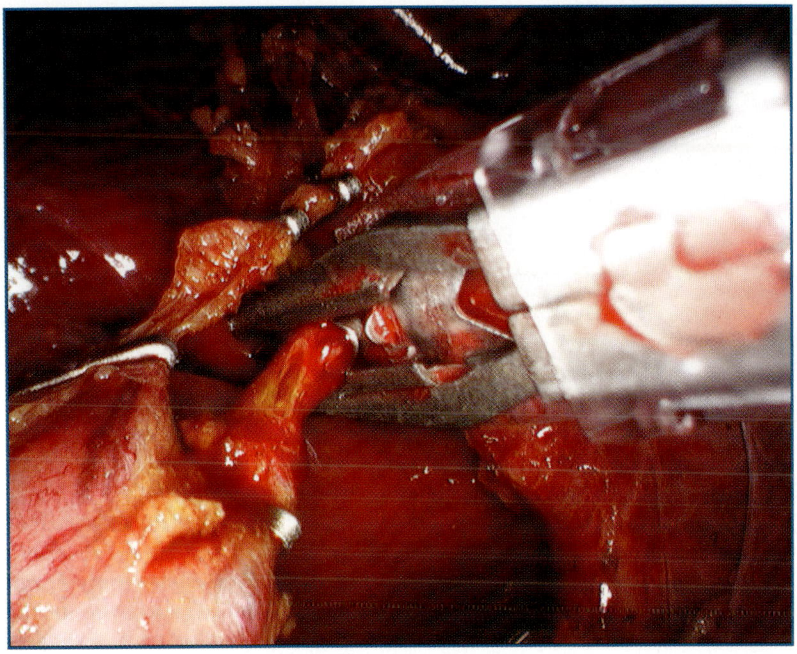

Fig. 16.15 Distal clipping of the cystic duct with a clip applier

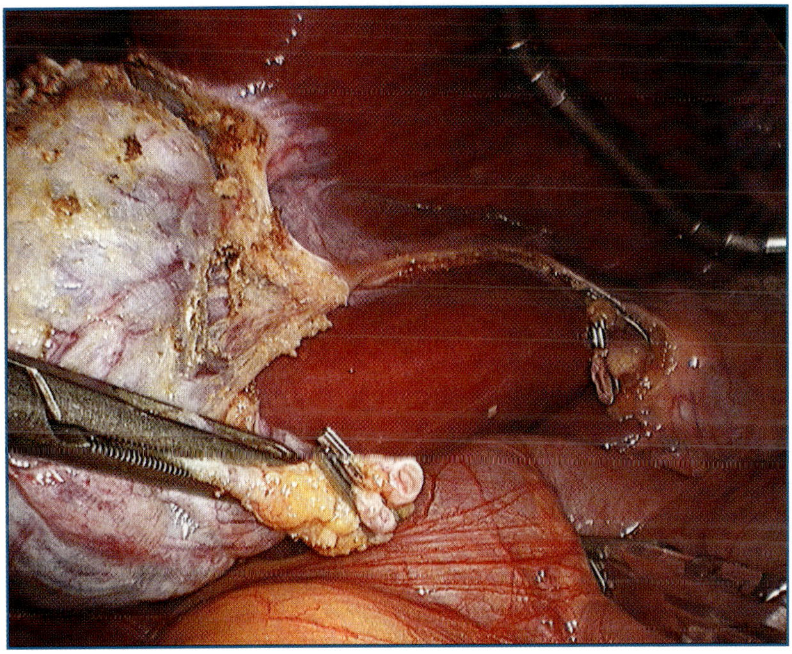

Fig. 16.16 Anterior exposition of the gallbladder fundus for completing cholecystectomy from the liver bed with the hook dissector

tion with the latter to the risk of elevated intra-abdominal pressure.

Delivery of the Surgical Specimen

When divided, the gallbladder is grasped with a heavy forceps introduced through the "dissecting port" and externalized at this trocar site (Fig. 16.18). Another alternative is to extract the specimen through the umbilical port after having exchanged the optic to the "dissecting port". While apparent at the level of the skin, the gallbladder neck is incised with scissors, the bile is aspirated and stones are extracted

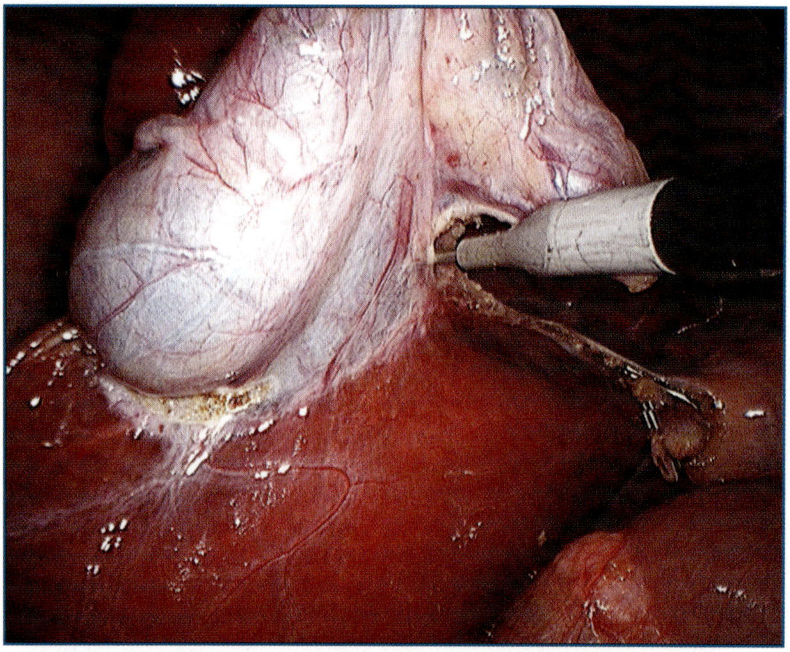

Fig. 16.17 Posterior exposition of the gallbladder for completing cholecystectomy from the liver bed with the hook dissector

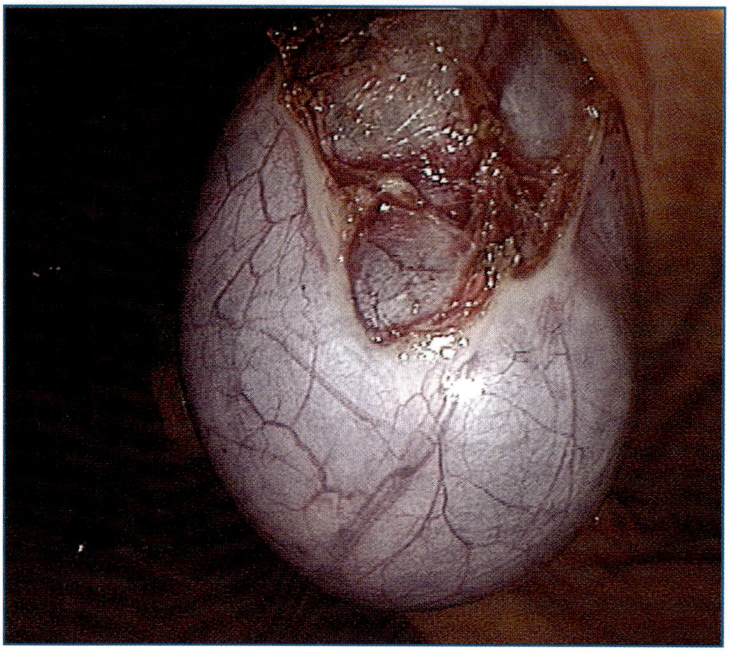

Fig. 16.18 Extraction of the gallbladder specimen through the trocar site in the left upper quadrant

after instrumental crushing, if necessary. Then the collapsed gallbladder is extracted from the abdomen. Widening the trocar incision is often necessary in case of huge gallstones or gallbladder wall thickening. If a perforation of the gallbladder has occurred during the procedure or in case of cholecystitis, the specimen is placed before extraction into a heavy plastic bag (Fig. 16.19) to avoid bile contamination and stone spillage into the peritoneum or the abdominal wall. If this complication occurs, great care must be taken to wash the site of bile contamination and to completely remove all spilled stones, in order to avoid further intraperitoneal or intra-

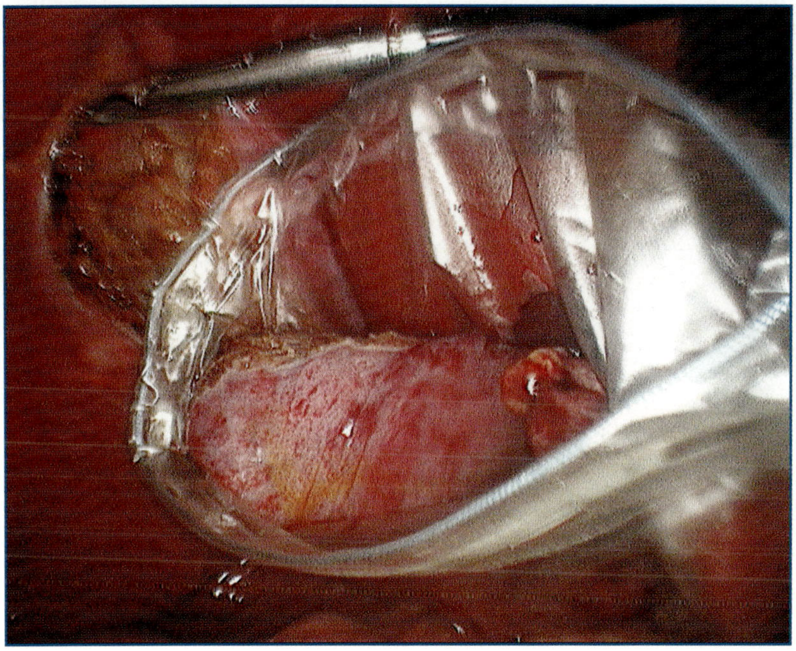

Fig. 16.19 Introduction of the gallbladder into a plastic bag for extraction in case of acute cholecystitis

parietal infectious complications. When extracted, the gallbladder must be carefully inspected to detect occult neoplastic changes that should then be confirmed by frozen section.

End of the Procedure

At the end of the procedure, the operative field is carefully inspected to check that the clips are well positioned on cystic arterial and ductal structures and that there is no bleeding or bile leakage (Fig. 16.20). A Silastic drain is placed in the sub-hepatic space, exteriorized through the "manipulating port" and secured to the skin. Peritoneal drainage is indicated in difficult operations or in cases of severe cholecystitis. In simple cases, the peritoneal drain can be omitted. Finally, the trocars are removed under vision to ensure that no bleeding from the trocar sites occurs. Attention should be paid to completely vent the peritoneum, in order to avoid postoperative shoulder pain. The fascias of the 10 mm trocars sites are closed to avoid further hernia formation.

Conversion to Laparotomy

The key principle during LC is to keep the procedure safe throughout the operation. When difficulties are encountered due to local conditions or complications that cannot be resolved laparoscopically, conversion to an open approach should be considered without any hesitation. Appropriate informed consent from the patient should help the surgeon to decide to convert without being disturbed by his surgical ego or any promises made to the patient. A low threshold for conversion should be the rule. The most common indications for conversion during LC are detailed in Table 16.2 [19].

Difficult Situations: Severe Cholecystitis

In case of severe acute or chronic cholecystitis, the operation is significantly more difficult and time-consuming due to local con-

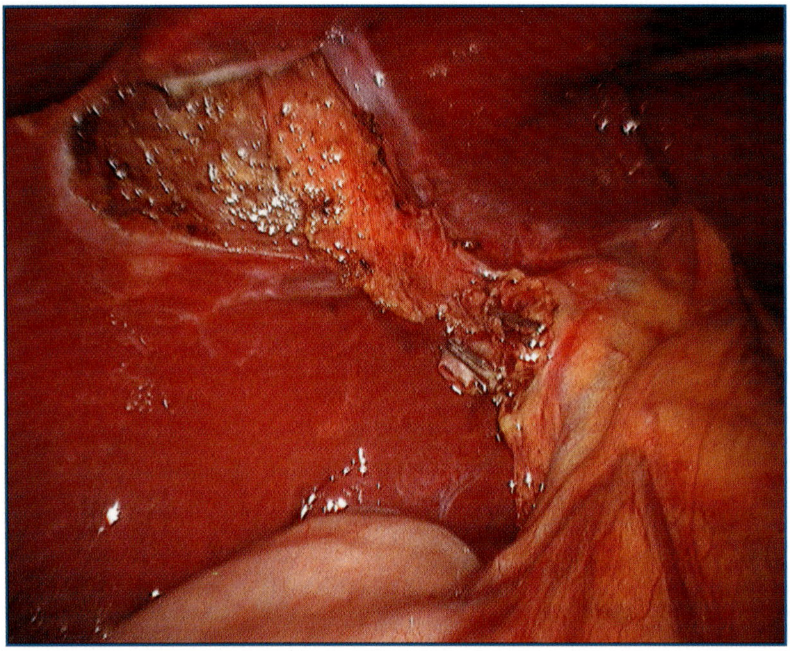

Fig. 16.20 Careful inspection of the operative field at the end of the dissection checking the correct positioning of the clips on the cystic duct and artery and the absence of bleeding or bile leakage

Table 16.2 Indications for conversion during laparoscopic cholecystectomy

1. Related to the surgeon
- when the surgeon is not confident with the dissection,
- when material or equipment are deficient.

2. Related to the patient
- when patient's anatomy or status (morbid obesity) preclude a safe technique

3. Related to the disease (difficult cases such as acute or chronic inflammation)
- when visualization or exposure is poor
- when inflammation obscures the anatomy within Calot's triangle
- when extensive use of electrocautery is employed

4. Related to the technique
- when massive bleeding is not controllable laparoscopically
- if there is questionable bile duct injury
  - during the surgical dissection
  - on intraoperative cholangiography
  - in case of continuous and unexplained leakage of bile during the operation
  - when the anatomy is confusing (e.g. multiple cystic ducts)

ditions, and has been reported to be associated with a greater incidence of conversion and bile duct injuries [20]. Poor local conditions predisposing to bile duct injury are detailed in Table 16.3. However, even in cases of acute cholecystitis, the laparoscopic approach remains the best management option [21], but early operation is strongly recommended [22, 23]. In these circumstances, the surgical technique must be adapted with the use of specific maneuvers at different steps of the dissection or by employing a completely different approach for cholecystectomy: no longer an "extrav-

Table 16.3 Details of poor local conditions predisposing to bile duct injury during laparoscopic cholecystectomy

- Due to the PATIENT: anatomical risk factors:
  - short or absent cystic duct
  - cystic duct entering the right hepatic duct
  - extrahepatic biliary anomaly such as an anomalous right hepatic duct
  - presence of arterial anomalies
- Due to the DISEASE: local risk factors:
  - acute or severe chronic inflammation
  - large impacted stone in the Hartmann's pouch
  - Mirizzi syndrome +/- bilio-biliary fistula
  - morbid obesity
- Due to the TECHNIQUE:
  - bleeding from arterial injury
  - overuse of monopolar electrocautery within Calot's triangle
  - transcystic instrumental common bile duct exploration

esicular" approach for dissecting the gallbladder, but an "endovesicular" approach with subtotal cholecystectomy [24–26].

Specific Maneuvers for Acute or Sclero-atrophic Cholecystitis

Throughout the LC, additional or specific maneuvers can be used when severe inflammation is present. These are detailed in Table 16.4. A high threshold for conversion should be adopted in such difficult cases if visualization or exposure of Calot's triangle is poor, if the anatomy is obscured by inflammation or if the dissection is not clear or not progressing in inflamed or scar tissues after a reasonable amount of time.

The "Endovesicular" Approach and Subtotal Cholecystectomy

In difficult cases due to severe inflammation within Calot's triangle an alternative approach is to dissect the gallbladder from

Table 16.4 Additional maneuvers during surgical dissection for severe acute or sclero-atrophic cholecystitis

- During exposition of the gallbladder:
  - suspend the round ligament with a suture to improve exposure
  - decompress the gallbladder with a needle to improve grasping
  - add a trocar for exposition
  - atraumatically dissect the perivesicular inflammatory mass
- During the dissection of Calot's triangle:
  - avoid use of electrocautery within Calot's triangle
  - use only atraumatic blunt dissection (peanuts swab on a fenestrated forceps, irrigation cannula, etc)
  - regularly wash an operative field obscured by diffuse oozing from inflamed tissues
  - perform intraoperative cholangiography to improve recognition of biliary anatomy and to confirm safe dissection
- During the dissection of Hartmann's pouch:
  - dissect as close as possible to the gallbladder wall
  - use a partial antegrade "fundus first approach" to mobilize the gallbladder fundus and body, but with the formal condition of stopping the antegrade dissection at the level of the gallbladder neck, avoiding access the porta hepatis
  - avoid persisting in dissecting scar tissues around Hartman pouch (in case of severe acute or chronic cholecystitis)
  - in case of huge impacted stone within Hartmann's pouch, open the gallbladder neck to extract the impacted stone
- During closure of the cystic duct:
  - close a thick, inflamed cystic duct by the means of an Endoloop or an extracorporeal ligation
- During extraction of the gallbladder:
  - routinely place the gallbladder into a heavy protective plastic bag for extraction
- At the end of the procedure:
  - wash the operative field copiously to remove blood, debris and bile contamination
  - routinely place a sub-hepatic peritoneal drain

inside (the so-called "endovesicular" approach), to skip the dissection of Calot's triangle and to complete the operation by subtotal cholecystectomy [24–26]. This original approach should not be routinely performed but is indicated when technical difficulties make the dissection unsafe and prevent the surgeon from progressing safely within Calot's triangle.

The concept of the technique is to incise the ventral surface of the gallbladder from the fundus to Hartmann's pouch (Fig. 16.21). The gallbladder content must be evacuated into a plastic bag previously introduced through the "dissecting" port and placed in a waiting position above the liver. Great care should be taken to avoid peritoneal stone spillage, a situation that is not uncommon if the gallbladder is full of small stones. A partial cholecystectomy is achieved at the level of gallbladder fundus and body, assessing the dissection from outside and from inside the gallbladder wall (Figs. 16.22, 16.23). The posterior wall of the gallbladder at the level of the infundibulum and Calot's triangle is not dissected from outside (and will be later left in place). Then, after careful inspection from inside of the Hartmann's pouch and instrumental exploration (Fig. 16.24), the cystic duct is catheterized from inside with a cholangiographic catheter without any dissection of Calot's triangle (Fig. 16.25). In the absence of obstructive cystic valves, routine IOC is attempted. The technique is useful when severe cholecystitis is associated with the existence of an anomalous right hepatic duct (a situation at high risk for bile duct injury) or Mirizzi syndrome (Fig. 16.26), features that can be detected by routine magnetic resonance (MR)-cholangiography in case of delayed cholecystectomy [27]. After completion of IOC, the cystic duct is sutured from inside the Hartmann's pouch. A subtotal cholecystectomy ends the procedure, a patch of gallbladder wall being left in place (Fig. 16.27) but destroyed by the Argon beam Coagulator (Fig. 16.28). A routine sub-hepatic drain is placed because a small bile leakage from the secured cystic duct is common. A coexistent cancer must be excluded by macroscopic examination and, when indicated, by frozen section examination of the inner gallbladder wall; in such a case laparoscopy becomes a contraindication, an open surgical treatment may be necessary according to the stage of the tumor.

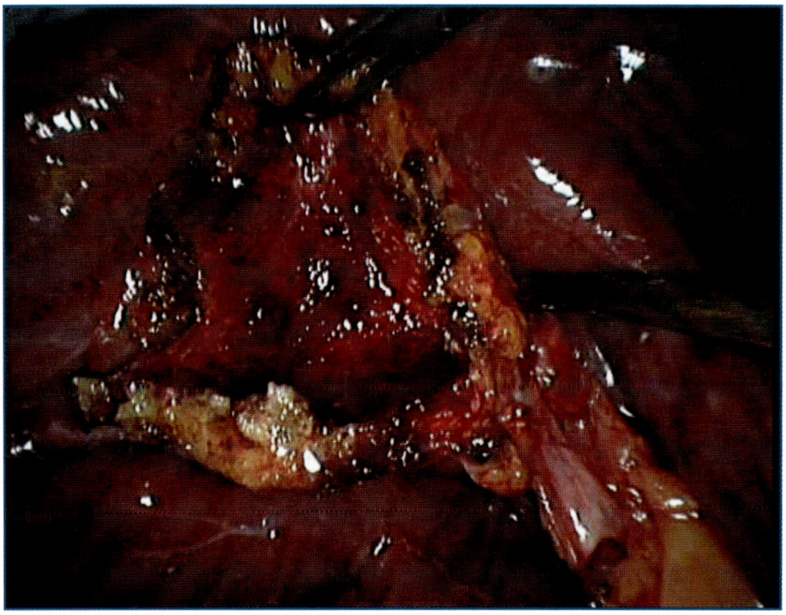

Fig. 16.21 During laparoscopic subtotal cholecystectomy: incision of the ventral surface of the inflamed gallbladder from the fundus to Hartmann's pouch

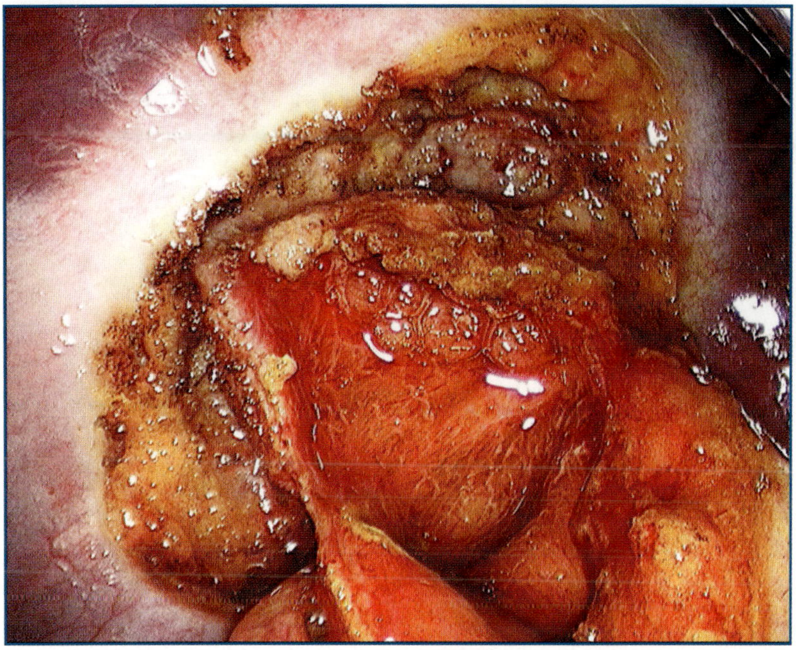

Fig. 16.22 Laparoscopic subtotal cholecystectomy at the site of the liver bed

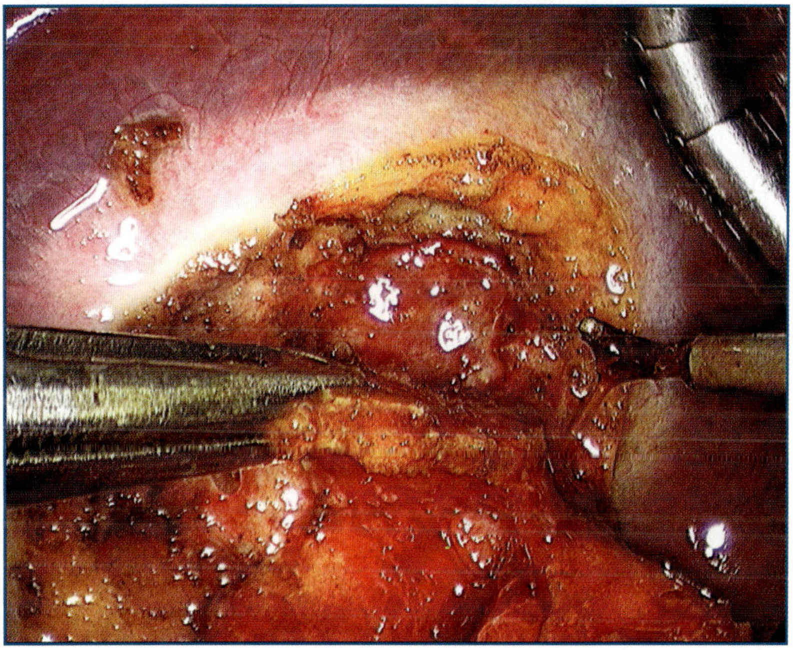

Fig. 16.23 Same operative view: the dissection of the gallbladder wall is assessed from inside and from outside, keeping the dissection with the hook dissector close to the gallbladder wall

Postoperative Care

The postoperative course after LC is usually simple. In the absence of nausea, the patient is able to eat the day following the operation and is usually discharged 1 or 2 days later. Ambulatory LC is an option. The postoperative requirement for analgesics is minimal. Irradiated scapular pain occurs when the pneumoperitoneum has not been incompletely vented at the end of the operation and disappears progressively. The patient's abdomen is clinically assessed to exclude

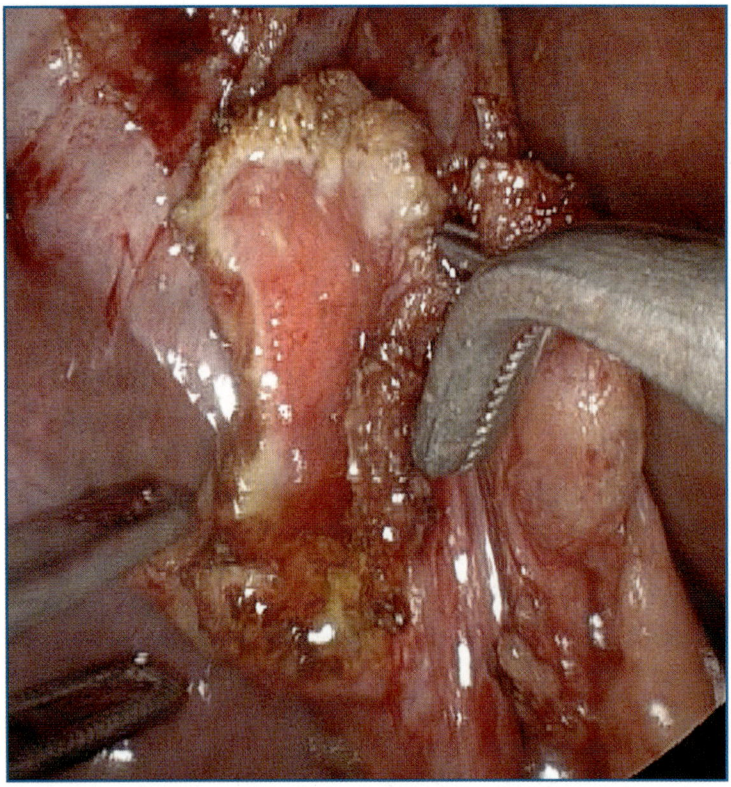

Fig. 16.24 During laparoscopic subtotal cholecystectomy, Hartmann's pouch is explored from inside by an "endovesicular approach" using instrumental identification of the cystic duct orifice

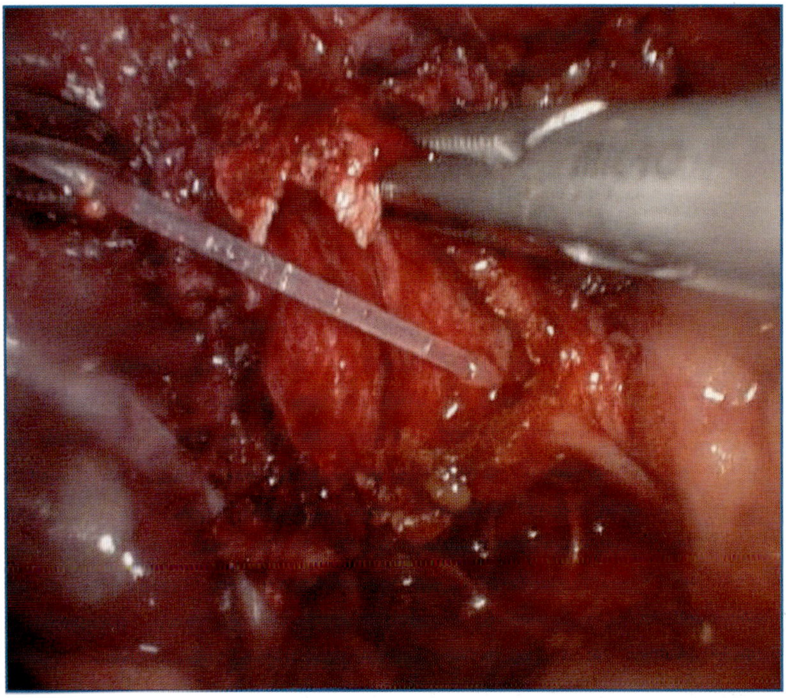

Fig. 16.25 Intraoperative cholangiography by introducing the cholangiographic catheter by an "endovesicular approach"

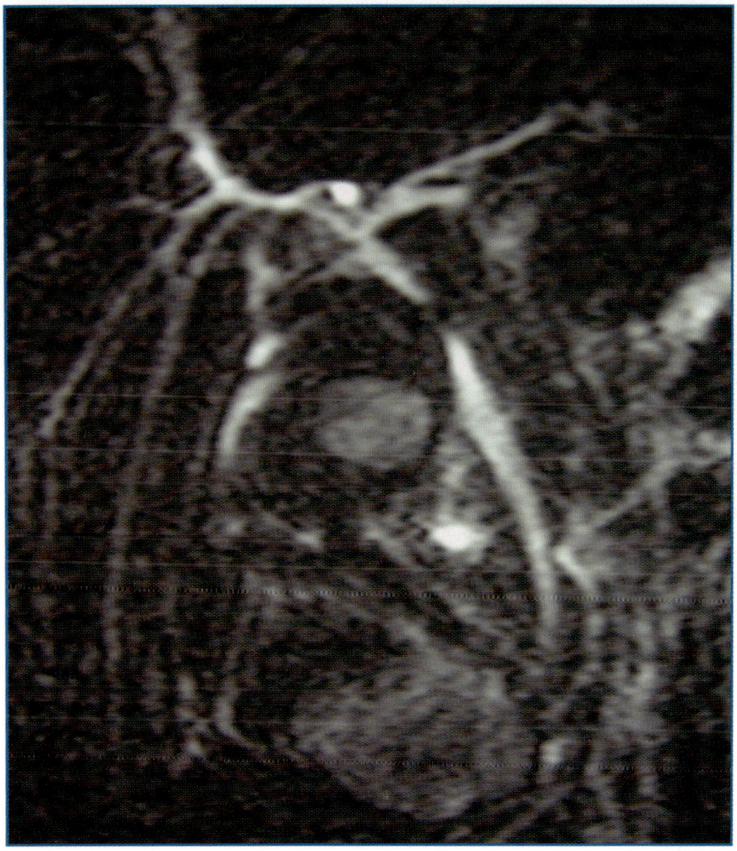

Fig. 16.26 Preoperative MR-cholangiography demonstrating Mirizzi syndrome from an enflamed gallbladder at the level of common hepatic duct

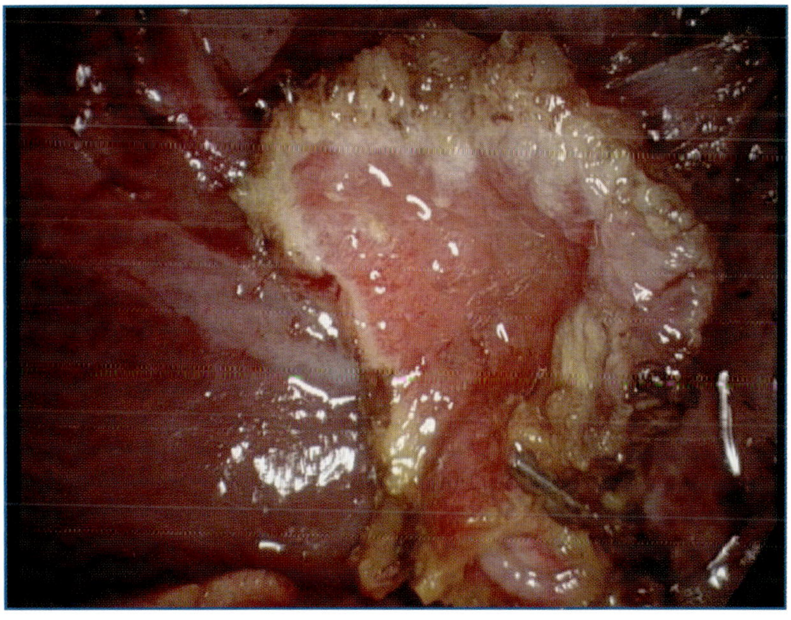

Fig. 16.27 During laparoscopic subtotal cholecystectomy, a patch of gallbladder wall is left on the right part of the hepatic hilum, protecting the common hepatic duct in case of Mirizzi syndrome or of an anomalous right hepatic duct

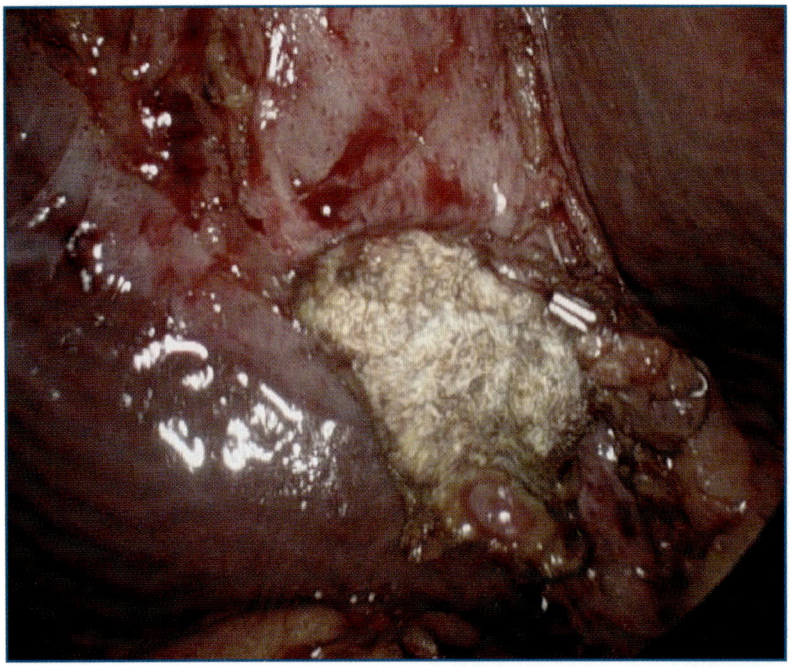

Fig. 16.28 During laparoscopic subtotal cholecystectomy the residual patch of gallbladder wall is destroyed by means of an Argon Beam coagulator at the end of the procedure

complications. The aspect and colour of the sub-hepatic drain fluid is carefully inspected to exclude postoperative bleeding or bile leak. Blood tests are useful to exclude biliary obstruction. It should be emphasized that a persisting or worsening painful postoperative course should alert the surgeon to possible complications and may mandate further investigation. At discharge, the patient should be informed about the signs of possible complications to allow early hospital consultation, if necessary.

References

1. National Institutes of Health Consensus Conference: Gallstones and laparoscopic cholecystectomy (1993) JAMA 269: 1018-1024
2. Neugebauer E, Troidl H, Kum CK et al (1995) The EAES Consensus Development Conferences on laparoscopic cholecystectomy, appendectomy, and hernia repair. Consensus statements - The Educational Committee of the European Association for Endoscopic Surgery. Surg Endosc 9:550-563
3. Neugebauer E, Sauerland S, Troidl H (2000) Recommendations for evidence-based endoscopic surgery. The updated EAES Consensus Development Conferences, Springer-Verlag
4. Barkun JS, Barkun AN, Sampalis JS et al (1993) Randomised controlled trial of laparoscopic versus mini cholecystectomy. Lancet 341:1214-1215
5. McMahon AJ, Russel IT, Baxter JN et al (1994) Laparoscopic versus minilaparotomy cholecystectomy: a randomised trial. Lancet 343:135-138
6. Majeed AW, Troy G, Nicholl JP, Smythe A et al (1996) Randomised, prospective, single-blind comparison of laparoscopic versus small-incision cholecystectomy. Lancet 347:989-994
7. Gigot JF, Etienne J, Aerts R et al (1997) The dramatic reality of biliary tract injury during laparoscopic cholecystectomy: an anonymous multicentric belgian survey of 65 patients. Surg Endosc 11:1171-1178
8. Neudecker J, Sauerland S, Neugebauer E et al (2002) The E.A.E.S. clinical guidelines on the pneumoperitoneum for laparoscopic surgery. Surg Endosc 16:1121-1143
9. Champault G, Cazacu F, Taffinder N (1996) Serious trocar accidents in laparoscopic surgery: a French survey of 103852 operations. Surg Laparosc Endosc 6:367-370
10. Mouiel J, Katkhouda N (1991) La cholécystectomie par laser en coeliochirurgie. In: Testas P, Delaitre B (eds) Chirurgie digestive par voie coelioscopique. Paris, Maloine, pp 113-119
11. McMahon AJ, Fullarton G, Baxter JN, O'Dwyer PJ (1995) Bile duct injury and bile leakage in laparoscopic cholecystectomy Br J Surg 82:307-313

12. Strasberg SM, Hertl M, Soper NJ (1995) An analysis of the problem of biliary injury during laparoscopic cholecystectomy J Am Coll Surg 180:101-125
13. Taniguchi Y, Ido K, Kimura K et al (1993) Introduction of a "Safety Zone" for the safety of laparoscopic cholecystectomy. Am J Gastroenterol 88:1258-1261
14. Ido K, Isoda N, Kawamoto C et al (1996) Confirmation of a "safety zone" by intraoperative cholangiography during laparoscopic cholecystectomy. Surg Endosc 10:798-800
15. Woods MS, Traverso LW, Korzarek RA et al (1994) Characteristics of biliary tract complications during laparoscopic cholecystectomy: a multi-institutional study. Am J Surg 167:27-34
16. Woods MS, Traverso LW, Kozarek RA et al (1995) Biliary tract complications of laparoscopic cholecystectomy are detected more frequently with routine intraoperative cholangiography. Surg Endosc 9:1076-1080
17. Flum D, Dellinger E, Cheadle A et al (2003) Intraoperative cholangiography and risk of common bile duct injury during cholecystectomy. JAMA 289:1639-1644
18. Rantis PC, Greenlee HB, Pickleman J, Prinz RA (1993) Laparoscopic cholecystectomy bile duct injuries: more than meets the eye. Am Surg 59:533-540
19. Bingener-Casey J, Richards ML, Strodel WE et al (2002) Reasons for conversion from laparoscopic to open cholecystectomy:a 10-year review. J Gastrointest Surg 6:800-805
20. Kum CK, Eypasch E, Lefering R et al (1996) Laparoscopic cholecystectomy for acute cholecystitis: is it really safe? World J Surg 20:43-49
21. Kiviluoto T, Siren J, Luukkonen P, Kivilaakso E (1998) Randomised trial of laparoscopic versus open cholecystectomy for acute and gangrenous cholecystitis. Lancet 351:321-325
22. Navez B, Mutter D, Russier Y et al (2001) Safety of laparoscopic approach for acute cholecystitis: retrospective study of 609 cases. World J Surg 25:1352-1356
23. Garber SM, Korman J, Cosgrove JM, Cohen JR (1997) Early laparoscopic cholecystectomy for acute cholecystitis Surg Endosc 11:347-350
24. Bornman PC, Terblanche J (1985) Subtotal cholecystectomy:for the difficult gallbladder in portal hypertension and cholecystitis. Surgery 98:1-6
25. Michalowski K, Bornman PC, Krige JE et al (1998) Laparoscopic subtotal cholecystectomy in patients with complicated acute cholecystitis or fibrosis. Br J Surg 85:904-6
26. Palanivelu C, Rajan PS, Jani K et al (2006) Laparoscopic cholecystectomy in cirrhotic patients: the role of subtotal cholecystectomy and its variants. J Am Coll Surg 203:145-51
27. Ausch C, Hochwarter G, Taher M et al (2005) Improving the safety of laparoscopic cholecystectomy: the routine use of preoperative magnetic resonance cholangiography. Surg Endosc 19:574-80

Chapter 17

Robot-assisted Cholecystectomy

Cinthya Solano, Monica Gualtierotti, Ronan Cahill, Jacques Marescaux

Introduction

After being first performed by Carl Langenbuch in 1882, open cholecystectomy became the accepted means of treating symptomatic cholecystolithiasis and proved itself a safe procedure with low complication rates. Then, 20 years ago, laparoscopy kick-started a revolution in abdominal surgery that has been continued with other minimally invasive techniques. The first laparoscopic cholecystectomy was performed in 1987 by Dr. Phillipe Mouret and, because of its advantages (e.g., smaller incisions, quicker recovery time, improved cosmetic results and shorter stay in costly hospital beds), became accepted within a few years as the new standard therapy for gallstone disease. However, the technology it uses can actually be viewed as a step backward from certain perspectives. In laparoscopy, instrument manoeuvrability is limited and the seven degrees of motion freedom available in open surgery (i.e., up and down, in and out, left and right and rotate) are downgraded to the four degrees possible at laparoscopy. Endoscopic movements are in addition generally neither ergonomic nor intuitive. Moreover, the surgeons' hands are relatively distant from the operative field while the instruments employed actually amplify natural tremor as well as reduce both tactile sense and force feedback appreciation [1–9].

In order to reduce these limitations, researchers have developed new tools that have led to the development of robotic telemanipulation systems. These systems represent a form of computer-assisted surgery utilising a "master-slave relationship" in which the surgeon is able to control the actions of the robot in real time. In this way, a range of advantages have been offered to the surgeon, including restoration of full dexterity and stereoscopic vision, increased surgeon comfort and ergonomics as well as tremor eradication and scaling opportunities [1–5, 7–11]. These may allow easier and more accurate tissue dissection. Even though robotic surgery has inherent disadvantages such as lack of tactile feedback, prolonged set-up and operating time (particularly early in a unit's experience) as well as added expense [12, 13] and a requirement for larger operating rooms (in order to accommodate the robotic unit and cumbersome equipment), there are now many studies that demonstrate its feasibility in standard laparoscopic procedures [3, 6, 7, 9, 13–15].

History of Robotics

The term robot was first coined in 1920 as a derivative of the Czech word "robota" (meaning compulsory labour) although the term robotic did not come into popular use until 1942 when Isaac Asimov's "Three Laws" captured the public's imagination. Since then, the success of industrial machines has stimulated interest in applying robotics to other areas, including medicine. A "surgical robot" has been defined as a self-powered computer-controlled device that can be programmed to aid in the positioning and manipulation of surgical instruments [2, 8, 16, 17]. In other words, a computer provides the digital interface between the surgeon's hands and the surgical instruments, thereby widening the skill and scope of surgical procedures. This new alliance has led to many innovations and possibly represents the beginning of a new era in medicine. The main objective in the development of robotic devices, however, is not to replace the surgeon but rather to help him perform difficult tasks more accurately and repetitive tasks more precisely. Recently, surgical robots have further evolved into telerobotic devices that may allow surgeons to operate at a distance from remote locations.

The first specialties to use such devices were neurosurgery (Neuromate®) and orthopaedic surgery (RoboDoc®). In Belgium in 1998, Himpens, Cadiere and colleagues made the first report of a successful clinical implementation of telerobotics in general surgery when they performed a robot-assisted laparoscopic cholecystectomy using the MONA® system (a prototype of the current Intuitive Surgical da Vinci ® system) [7]. Today, clinical and experimental experience suggests that the use of robotic systems does not add specific complications and can achieve outcomes similar to those of the standard laparoscopic approach.

System Description

Since 2003 (after the acquisition of Computer Motion by Intuitive Surgical), of the two advanced surgical robotic systems originally developed, only the da Vinci robot remains and will thus be described exclusively here [1, 3, 8, 16–18]. This system consists of three separate parts: the surgeon console, the robotic cart and the video endoscopic unit connected by cables (Fig. 17.1).

Surgeon Console

The surgeon sits in a comfortable and ergonomic position at the console, remote from the patient. The console is composed of "masters" as controls, a binocular display screen, foot pedals and a keyboard. The surgeon's hands fit into the free-moving "masters" or finger controls that are similar to joysticks. These convert the movements of the surgeon's wrist and finger tips into electrical signals that are then translated to the computer to direct the robotic instruments in order to perform the same movements in the operative field. The digitalisation of the surgeon's hand movements on the controls also provides the ability to eliminate physiologic tremor and produce motion scaling in

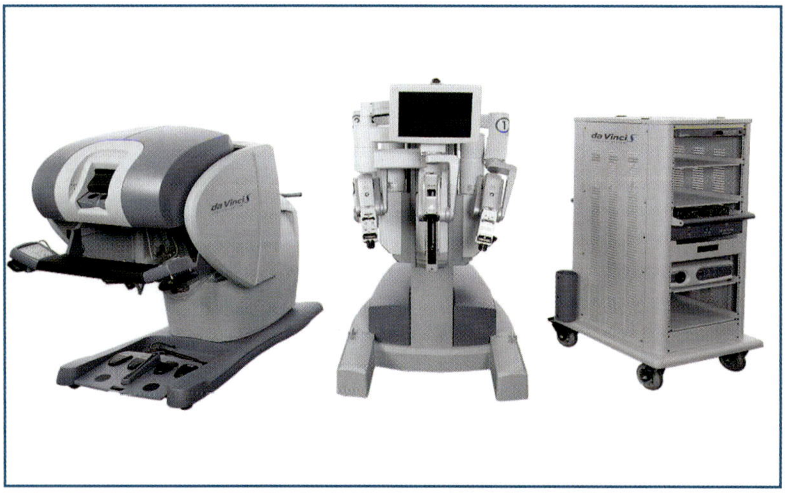

Fig. 17.1 Da Vinci robot components comprising the surgeon control, robotic cart and video-endoscopic unit

the order of 1:1, 3:1, 5:1. (i.e., the units of motion of the surgeon's hands reduced to one unit of motion for the instrument).

The da Vinci system supplies true three-dimensional (3D) imaging. The telescope for this console is 12 mm in diameter and contains two separate 5 mm telescopes. Two 3 CCD (Charged Coupled Device) cameras then send the image to two separate cathode ray tube (CRT) screens. Mirrors then reflect the images from the CRT screens up to the binocular viewer in the surgeon's console (i.e., the console displays the two camera views onto separate monitors directed to the surgeon's left and right eyes). As the left and right images are presented separately to the surgeon's eyes, visual depth is produced by the human brain's ability to integrate offset images. For safety reasons the system goes directly into stand-by modus whenever the surgeon moves away from the 3D binoculars. The camera is itself controlled by a Navigator system that enables the surgeon to pick up and move the camera by manipulating the master controllers after pressing a foot pedal. During camera movement, the slave instruments stay in position to allow repositioning of the controllers to more ergonomically favourable positions.

Video Endoscopic Unit

The video endoscopic unit consists of the tower holding the videoelectronic equipment and an insufflator for the pneumoperitoneum.

Robotic Cart

The current da Vinci robot model has four arms: one central to hold the camera, two outer arms for the surgical instruments that mimic the surgeon's left and right hands and a fourth arm that can optionally be used for exposition/traction. A screen for the assistant and the nurse is positioned on top of the robotic cart. The articulating laparoscopic instruments have a complex cable-driven joint at their distal end, which moves with the same seven degrees of freedom as does the human wrist in open surgery [8, 9]. This Endowrist® system therefore allows the surgeon to perform his manipulations intuitively. The telerobot's computer also checks the number of uses of each instrument and will not allow further loading of an instrument after its tenth use in order to ensure that their condition does not deteriorate.

Surgical Technique as Applied to Laparoscopic Cholecystectomy

The performance of laparoscopic cholecytsectomy with robot-assistance will now be discussed. Cholecystectomy is chosen as a model because the laparoscopic approach for this procedure is considered to be a gold standard and its performance is relatively standardised throughout the world. Therefore, comparison between computer-assisted and the conventional laparoscopic technique makes the advantages and disadvantages of both approaches transparent (Table 17.1) [15, 19].

Robot and Patient Position

The robot-assisted cholecystectomy is performed by the surgeon, who controls the robotic arms. It is not a job completed "automatically" by the robot. The surgeon must follow the operative principles of conventional laparoscopic cholecystectomy being also familiar with robotic systems.

Operating Room Configuration

When a surgical team plans to start robot-assisted cholecystectomy, the first issue

Table 17.1 Advantages and disadvantages of robotic surgery over conventional laparoscopic procedures

Characteristic	Robot-assisted surgery	Conventional laparoscopic operation
Vision	3-D	2-D
Instrument manipulation	360°	Limited
Set-up time	Long	Short
Ergonomics once in position	Very good	Poor
Port diameter	8 mm	> 2 mm
Telesurgery potential	Yes	No
Cost	High	Low

they must take in account is the positioning of the operating field since it is different from the standard laparoscopic cholecystectomy [20]. The robot is brought close to the table and positioned by the assistant surgeon. The bearing column of the robot works as the vertical central axis of the robot and is positioned behind the right shoulder of the patient (Fig. 17.2). In every procedure the optimal placement of the slave arm trolley also has to be determined in order to accommodate the operating table and to avoid crowding by the slave's arm volume [7]. Line-of-sight must be optimised, so it is important to locate the console for the surgeon in a place that allows him full view of the operative field. As the maximum video cable length from the Vision Cart camera control unit (CCU) is 13 feet, it is therefore recommended that both carts be positioned in a way that the cabling is loose in order to minimise any interference with traffic as well as the risk of twisting. All positional changes of the operating table after the robot has been connected require either careful guidance of the robotic arms simultaneously or else their disconnection and reconnection. The robotic arms

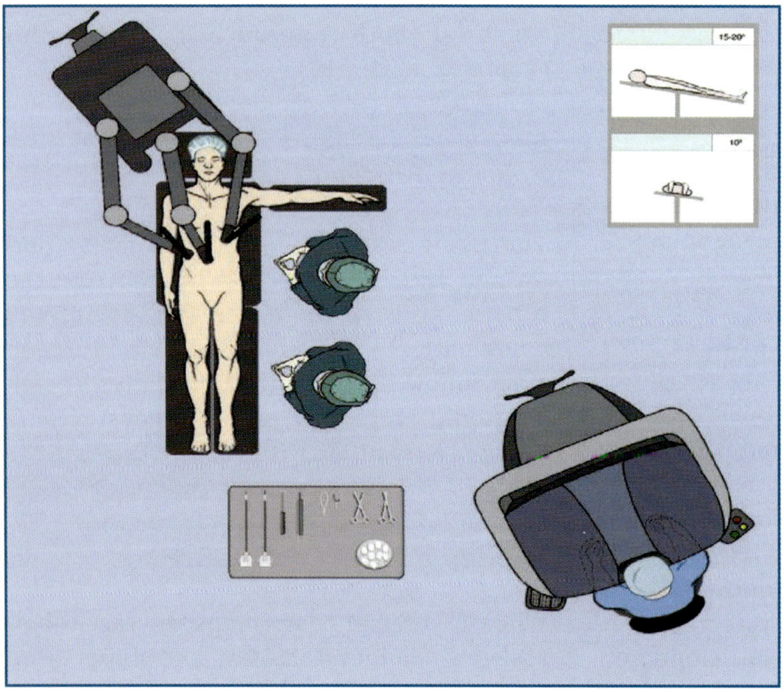

Fig. 17.2 Operating room setup for robotic-assisted cholecystectomy demonstrating both the positioning of the surgical table and of the patient

are then draped in a sterile fashion by the nurse during the preparation for surgery (there must therefore be enough space around the robot to avoid contact with the operating room staff).

Procedure

The abdomen is prepared and draped in a sterile fashion. The pneumoperitoneum can be initiated by either an open or closed technique. With the open technique, a small incision is made above the umbilicus and through the fascia. After inserting the 12 mm trocar at this supraumbilical position, the abdomen is insufflated with carbon dioxide to a pressure of 12 mmHg. A survey of the abdominal cavity must then be performed using either a 0-degree or 30-degree endoscope.

The instrument trocar positioning then mimics that of the pure laparoscopic approach and so can be adapted according to surgeon preference. Three trocars are used for the robotic instruments and scope while one additional trocar is used by the assistant surgeon for different tasks (e.g., to introduce a clip applier, suction-irrigation device and/or sutures into the abdominal cavity). We prefer to use the 12 mm disposable trocar inserted above the umbilicus as the camera port. In the left upper quadrant on the midclavicular line approximately one hand's breadth away (about 10 cm) above the level of the umbilicus, we place an 8 mm reusable trocar for the da Vinci's left arm. The 8 mm trocar for the da Vinci's right arm is positioned in the right midclavicular line at the level of the umbilicus, one hand's breath away from the camera port. The accessory port (5 mm) for use by the assistant surgeon is on the patient's right side, between the camera port and the right instrument port (Fig. 17.3 and Table 17.2).

After the pneumoperitoneum is established and the ports are inserted, the robotic cart is brought into the operating field at a 45-degree angle near the right shoulder of the patient. The da Vinci central robotic arm is attached to the 12 mm trocar to hold the camera and the two operative arms are aligned to the two 8 mm trocars. A Cadiere forceps is loaded into the left arm while an electrocautery device to accomplish dissection is placed onto the right arm. The assis-

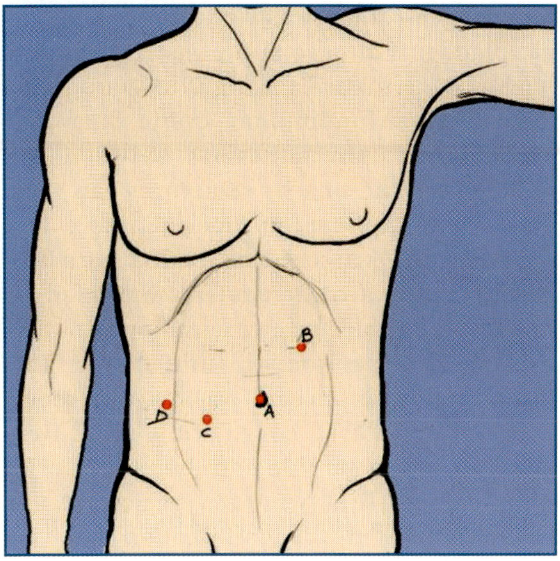

Fig. 17.3 Suggested trocar positioning in robotic-assisted cholecystectomy. *A*, camera port; *B*, left robotic arm; *C*, accessory port; *D*, right robotic arm

Table 17.2 Suggested instrumentation for a robot-assisted cholecystectomy

Instrument requirements
0° or 30 endoscope
Cadiere forceps
Long-tip forceps
Cautery hook
Round-tip scissors
Large needle driver
Suction-irrigation device
Clip applier
Endoscopic specimen bag

tant surgeon then grasps the fundus of the gallbladder with a separate instrument and pushes it up toward the right diaphragm to expose the infundibulum, cystic duct and cystic artery. Any adhesions between the gallbladder and nearby structures can then be divided. The cautery hook, Cadiere forceps and the scissors (all loaded onto the robotic arms) are then telemanipulated to dissect and ensure proper anatomic identification. The peritoneal lining over the infundibulum is incised by our preference with an articulated coagulating hook, first along its posterior side and then anteriorly. This opens the window between the infundibulum of the gallbladder and the liver and allows access to Calot's triangle. The infundibulum of the gallbladder is followed to its junction with the cystic duct in order to avoid inadvertent injury to the right hepatic duct. The cystic artery and the cystic duct are ligated both proximally and distally to the point of transection using 2-0 silk or clipped with a clip applier via the accessory port and then transected with scissors. The gallbladder is dissected off the liver using the hook cautery. It can then be placed in an endoscopic specimen bag and removed under direct vision through the umbilical port. A drain can be introduced and left in the gallbladder bed to monitor potential haemorrhage or bile leakage. The port incisions are closed in the standard fashion.

Telerobotic, Telesurgery, and Telepresence

Telerobotic surgery or telepresence surgery is the next step in the evolution of robotic surgery as these systems uniquely provide the ability to perform surgery in remote locations. To illustrate this, in September 2001, our group performed the first clinical application of remote surgery via surgeons located in New York operating on a patient in Strasbourg. This project, named Lindberg Operation, demonstrated both efficacy and safety in the use of existing high-bandwidth telecommunication lines for performing intercontinental surgery on humans [21–24]. The potential benefits of such a facility are multiple [16, 25]. Geographical limitations would not determine the type of treatment the patient receives because of lack of surgical expertise. Surgeons on call in small rural hospitals would be able to get assistance even in emergency settings from specialists located elsewhere. Furthermore, the capability to perform remote surgery may allow operation in combat zones (indeed, this is the purpose for which it was first developed) [1]. Future applications include surgery in space at the International Space Station for astronauts and perhaps space tourists. There are, however, important limitations to be considered, including the reliability of telecommunication lines as well as speed of transmission factors and the issue of latency. The latter two aspects are influenced by the distance, the intrinsic speed of the transmission system and the speed of computer interfaces in compressing and decompressing data [22–24].

These advances open new avenues for surgical education. The purpose of performing remote procedures is not to replace surgeons, but to improve training through teaching and mentoring and to reduce the learning curve of surgeons for new procedures. Assistance of an expert may range from complete performance of a procedure to simple assistance and exposure of structures that might reduce errors caused by the lack of experience or related to the early phase of the learning curve for new procedures [3]. In this way, a better standardisation of surgical outcomes between different areas of the same country as much as between different countries may be accomplished.

Although the safety of remote surgery has been assessed, some limitations remain [21, 25]. These include the availability of high-speed telecommunications lines (most hospitals are not equipped with asynchronous transfer mode technology), cost, ethical and legal issues, clinician-patient relationships and lack of surgeons with appropriate dedicated training. If remote surgery achieves its goal of increasing access to health care and enhancing outcomes, however, it may prove less costly than expected and it may even prove cost-effective. Important legal aspects also need be considered, such as whether the surgeon should be responsible for errors related to transmission or equipment failure as well as the impact of international borders on medical licensing. An ethical problem is that the traditional patient-surgeon relationship would have to be restructured due to the lack of contact between the patient and clinician.

Other Applications

Integration of virtual reality and simulation may also help the practice and rehearsal of surgical procedures based on a 3D model of the specific patient before the surgery [18, 19, 21, 25–27]. This may reduce the problems that derive from the lack of physical contact between the patient and the surgeon and as well allow both anticipation of potential problems and perfection of their solutions ahead of time [28, 29].

Conclusion

Through new technology, surgeons can operate for therapeutic intervention without using large incisions. Minimally invasive surgery has dramatically altered the route of access and has changed the surgical treatment of most disease processes. Robotic surgery now provides the technology to confront the limitations of standard minimally invasive techniques such as loss of natural 3D imaging, articulated movements and depth perception and may precipitate a new era of surgery by allowing surgeon placement remote from the site of operation.

References

1. Ballantyne G (2002) Robotic surgery, telerobotic surgery, telepresence, and telementoring. Review of early clinical results. Surg Endosc 16:1389-1402
2. Corcione F, Esposito C, Cuccurullo D et al (2005) Advantages and limits of robot-assisted laparoscopic surgery. Surg Endosc 19:117-119
3. Giulianotti P, Coratti A, Anelini M et al (2003) Robotic in general surgery. Arch Surg 138:777-784
4. Vidovzky T, Smith W, Ghosh J et al (2006) Robotic cholecystectomy: learning curve, advantages, and limitations. J Surg Res 136:172-178
5. Perez A, Zinner M, Ashley S et al (2003) What is the value of telerobotic technology in gastrointestinal surgery? Surg Endosc 17:811-813
6. Nio D, Bemelman W, Busch O et al (2004) Robot-assisted cholecystectomy vs conventional laparoscopic cholecystectomy. Surg Endosc 18:379-382
7. Cadiere G, Himpens, Germay O et al (2001) Feasibility of robotic laparoscopic surgery: 146 cases. World J Surg 25:1467-1477
8. Diodato M, Prosad S, Klingensmith M et al (2004) Robotics in surgery. Curr Probl Surg 41:752-810
9. Ruurda J, Broeders I (2001) Feasibility of robot-assisted laparoscopic cholecystectomy. International Congress Series 1230:160-165
10. Frecker M, Snyder A (2005) Surgical robotics: multifunctional end effectors for robotic surgery. Operative Techniques In General Surgery 165 169
11. Hanly E, Talamini M (2004) Robotic abdominal surgery. Am J Surg 188:19S-26
12. Hanly E, Bachman S, Marohn M (2005) Value of the SAGES Learning Center in introducing new technology. Surg Endosc 19:477-483
13. Talamini M, Chapman S, Horgan S et al (2003) A prospective analysis of 211 robotic-assisted surgical procedures. Surg Endosc 17:1521-1524
14. Kornprat P, Wekgartner G, Cerwenka H et al (2006) Prospective study comparing standard and robotically assisted laparoscopic cholecystectomy. Langenbecks Arch Surg 391:216-221
15. Bodner J, Hoeller E, Wykypiel H et al (2005) Long-term follow-up after robotic cholecystectomy. Am Surg 71:281-285
16. Dharia S, Falcone T (2005) Robotics in reproductive medicine. Fertility and Sterility 84:1-11

17. Kim H, Schulam P (2004) The PAKY, HERMES AESOP, ZEUS and da Vinci robotic systems. Urol Clin N Am 31:659-669
18. Marohn C, Hanly E (2004) Twenty-first century surgery using twenty-first century technology: surgical robotics. Curr Surg 61:466-473
19. Marescaux J, Smith M, Folscher D et al (2001) Telerobotic laparoscopic cholecystectomy: initial clinical experience with 25 patients. Ann Surg 234:1-7
20. Hourmont K, Chung W, Pereira S et al (2003) Robotic versus telerobotic laparoscopic cholecystectomy: duration of surgery and outcomes. Surg Clin N Am 83:1445-1462
21. Marescaux J, Rubino F (2004) Robot-assisted remote surgery: technological advances, potential complications, and solutions. Surgical Technology International 12:23-26
22. Marescaux J, Leroy J, Gagner M et al (2001) Transatlantic robot-assisted telesurgery. Nature 413:379-380
23. Marescaux J, Leroy J, Rubino F et al (2002) Transcontinental robot-assisted remote telesurgery: feasibility and potential applications. Ann Surg 235:487-492
24. Marescaux J (2002) Nom de code: Opération Lindbergh. Ann Chir 127:2-4
25. Marescaux J, Rubino F (2003) Remote surgery: present and future. Problems in General Surgery 20:73-78
26. Mack M (2001) Minimally invasive and robotic surgery. JAMA 285:568-572
27. Keus F, Broeders I, Laarhoven C (2006) Surgical aspects of symptomatic cholecystolithiasis and acute cholecystitis. Best Pract Res Clin Gastroenterol 20:1031-1051
28. Taylor G, Jayne D (2007) Robotic applications in abdominal surgery: their limitations and future developments. Int J Med Robotics Comput Assist Surg 3:3-9
29. Drasin T, Dutson E, Gracia C (2004) Use of robotic systme as surgical first assistant in advanced laparoscopic surgery. J Am Coll Surg 199:368-373

Chapter 18

Day Surgery Laparoscopic Cholecystectomy

Manuel Planells Roig, Rafael Garcia Espinosa, Consuelo Arnal Bertomeu, Angel Sanahuja Santafé, Miguel Carrau Giner, Maria Cervera Delgado, Jose Bueno Lledó, Eduardo Escarti Carbonell, Africa Sanchez Salas

To our patients, for choosing and believing in our team for their treatment

Introduction

With public health spending under growing social and administrative pressure and continuous efforts focusing on enhancing the efficiency of operating procedures, it is very attractive, albeit initially challenging, to consider laparoscopic cholecystectomy (LC) as an ambulatory procedure, although its development and implementation should be based on professional involvement and commitment.

Whether or not LC could safely be performed as an outpatient procedure was once a subject of controversy, but it has been performed regularly as outpatient surgery in uncomplicated gallstone disease in the United States, showing that it is a safe procedure with similar morbidity rates to standard LC.

Nevertheless, ambulatory LC (ALC) has still not been generally accepted in Europe, and few surgical groups here perform it routinely. The main reasons for this low performance rate are the potential risk of early severe complications (mainly bleeding) and events requiring readmission, and the argument that patients might feel safer when observed for one night [1].

Now, in 2007, whether LC should be performed as an outpatient procedure is no longer the subject of discussion, and increasing numbers of surgical groups are performing ALC as a routine procedure. Even though ALC is safe and cost effective, this approach still needs to become more widely accepted in Europe, as it has been demonstrated that it offers the advantages of convenience to patients and financial savings to healthcare institutes [2].

The question is: why should surgeons perform ALC?

In 1975 Zollinger wrote: "Cholecystectomy is a so frequent operation that surgeons should investigate anything that could increase its results. Each surgeon must review its [*sic*] own experience and question if he is offering their patients the most effective and efficient procedure."

LC is the most effective and efficient surgical procedure for patients. Classically demonstrated advantages of LC include less and milder pain and quicker recovery than with open cholecystectomy [3]. With LC, the postoperative period is different in quality and shorter than after classic cholecystectomy, a development that has been fostered by increased surgical experience and by advances in anesthesiology and analgesia. Since patient recovery is quicker, the feasibility of ALC has gained support among surgeons, but only when patient satisfaction is confirmed [4] and morbidity and mortality rates are similar to those observed with standard LC.

Although the main argument in favor of ALC seems to be the lower health-related costs, this should be second in importance (from the surgeon's point of view), the most important being the possibility of achieving a painless, safe, and satisfactory (from the patients' viewpoint) surgical procedure that is the most effective and efficient procedure for the patients' disease.

Moreover, as ALC means the use of less hospital resources it confers a significant benefit in terms of hospital costs and available bed capacity [5]. It also improves quality management in the LC procedure, as it is continuously analyzed in terms of improving quality assurance practices from the aspects of anesthetic and surgical performance [6–8].

Although Muhe in Germany published a first series of LC in 1986 [9], the earliest published experience of ALC is that reported by Reddick and Olsen in 1990 [10]. Since then, new reports of ALC and increasing rates of ALC among series have been published (Table 18.1) [1, 3, 10–43].

Nevertheless, its impact in Europe has been low in comparison with USA (51% of LC performed as ALC in 1997, as against 0.8% in the UK) [44].

Between 1997 and February 2007 we performed 1,000 consecutive programmed LCs as ALC. Of these patients, 820 were operated on as day patients, while 145 required one overnight (ON) stay and 35 were admitted as inpatients. The evolution of the proportions of ON stays, planned admissions, and unplanned admissions is shown in Table 18.2, where our experience is briefly summarized.

In a preliminary study performed by our group between 1999 and 2004, which involved 504 consecutive patients scheduled for ALC, we found an ambulatory index of 88.8% (448 patients); the median postoperative stay in hospital for ambulatory patients was 6.1 (1.2) hours; the unplanned admission rate was 11%, made up of ON admission in the case of 51 patients (10.1%) and hospital admission as inpatients for 5 (0.9%); the readmission rate was 1.2% (6 patients) [43]. Nevertheless, our experience has not stimulated acceptance in the University- or the non-University-affiliated part of the Spanish surgical community. Even worse: the National Health System has not shown any interest in this new treatment modality, and worst of all, private insurance companies have not considered a reimbursement plan for this new treatment, which is the most cost-effective modality cholecystectomy. Therefore, we are still applying this procedure with a view to patient benefit rather than for any economic or institutional reasons.

Table 18.1 Published reports on ambulatory laparoscopic cholecystectomy

Authors [ref.]	Year	No. of patients
Reddick et al. [9]	1990	83
Arregui et al. [11]	1991	106
Stephenson et al. [12]	1993	15
Smith et al. [13]	1994	266
Farha et al. [14]	1994	55
Saunders et al. [15]	1995	506
Prasad et al. [16]	1996	103
Fiorillo et al. [17]	1996	149
Taylor et al. [18]	1996	108
Lam et al. [19]	1997	213
Mjaland et al. [20]	1997	200
Narain et al. [3]	1997	60
Voitk et al. [21]	1997	273
Zegarra et al. [22]	1997	286
Keulemans et al. [1]	1998	37
Hollington et al. [23]	1999	60
Lillemoe et al. [24]	1999	130
Critchlow et al. [25]	1999	60
Fleming et al. [26]	2000	45
Siu et al. [27]	2001	60
Calland et al. [28]	2001	177
Bringman et al. [29]	2001	100
Richardson et al. [30]	2001	847
Serralta et al.[a] [31]	2001	271
Lau et al. [32]	2002	888
Curet et al. [33]	2002	80
Johanet et al. [34]	2002	100
Amarnath et al. [35]	2002	170
Serralta et al.[a] [36]	2002	381
Bal et al. [37]	2003	383
Ammori et al. [38]	2003	140
Leeder et al. [39]	2004	154
Vuilleumer et al. [40]	2004	136
Chok et al. [41]	2004	73
Jain et al. [42]	2005	269
Bueno et al.[a] [43]	2005	504

[a]ICAD group

Table 18.2 Istituto de Cirugía General y Aparato Digestivo (ICAD): experience of ambulatory laparoscopic cholecystectomy (ALC)

Year	No. of patients	ALC	Overnight stay (*n* / %)	Admission (*n* / %)	Unplanned admissions (%)
1997	35	8	25 / 74.3	2 / 3.7	77.1
1998	73	49	20 / 27.4	4 / 5.5	32.9
1999	84	62	14 / 16.7	8 / 9.5	26.1
2000	82	74	4 / 4.9	4 / 4.9	9.8
2001	109	98	7 / 6.4	4 / 3.7	10.1
2002	122	112	9 / 7.4	1 / 0.8	8.2
2003	99	88	10 / 10.1	1 / 1.01	11.1
2004	154	138	12 / 7.8	4 / 2.6	10.4
2005	96	76	16 / 16.7	4 / 4.2	20.9
2006	108	82	24 / 22.2	2 / 1.9	24.1
2007	38	33	4 / 10.5	1 / 2.6	13.1
Total	1,000	820 (82.0)	145 / (14.5)	35 / (3.5)	18.0

Difficulties in the implementation of ALC in surgical departments is one of the most important reasons for the low rate of ALC, worsen by a rather low acceptance of ALC among the surgical community. Nonacceptance of ALC by surgeons is due to concerns about the risk of immediate postoperative life-threatening complications related to hemorrhagic and biliary iatrogenic lesions. Therefore, most surgeons feel that clinical observation for 24 h is generally preferable to ALC.

LC morbidity rates vary between 4% and 20%. Delay in diagnosis and early management are important arguments against ALC [16, 45]. The incidence of iatrogenic biliary injuries varies from 0.30% to 1%, which is higher than in the case of open cholecystectomy [46, 47], and laparoscopic identification of intraoperative injuries seems to be achieved in a lower proportion of cases than during open surgery [1, 48], both of which are important reasons to refuse ALC.

Nevertheless, life-threatening postoperative bleeding is relatively rare (1/2,000 cases), and it is usually symptomatic during the early postoperative hours, being easily detected during the inpatient period in hospital [26, 49]. Moreover, nonemergency complications (biliary tree injuries) usually become symptomatic by 24–48 h after the procedure [50–52]. Therefore, it has been concluded that observation in hospital for 6–10 hours or less is enough to allow early detection of postoperative complications, and this is considered a safe policy [1, 49].

Clinical monitoring of the postoperative course is essential after ALC. Patients have minimal abdominal pain or none at all, tolerate oral intake with minimal nausea and/or vomiting, and are capable of independent ambulation as they do not have the feeling of having undergone surgery or of being ill, so that if they are offered discharge from hospital they usually accept even when cultural concerns about the performance of LC as day surgery have been put forward by patients or relatives earlier during initial appointments in the office.

Acceptance of ALC depends on clinical recovery after surgery, but also, and sometimes more relevantly in terms of patients' and their relatives' social and cultural expectations of LC, on medical and surgical knowledge of the feasibility and safety of ALC and clear and full postoperative instructions; therefore it is very important to gain each patient's confidence. Continuity of clinical care by the same team is mandatory, to make patients feel they are regarded as individuals [53, 54].

Ambulatory surgery patients must meet established criteria before being discharged, but not all patients meet the discharge criteria; the most usual reasons for ON admission of ALC patients for further observation and treatment are pain that has not yet been controlled, inability to walk, and uncontrolled nausea and vomiting. Therefore, a reduction in the side-effects of anesthesia and surgery, including postoperative nausea and vomiting (PONV) and abdominal pain, is essential for an ALC program to be successful and should be the target of all surgeons and anesthesiologists involved in the development of such a program.

PONV and abdominal pain are the two main causes of unplanned admissions, readmissions, emergency room visits, and telephone assistance among patients undergoing ALC [53, 55].

The incidence of PONV ranges from 12% to 52% of patients [8], or from 25% to 42% if no antiemetic prophylaxis is performed [53, 56]. PONV is mainly related to anesthetic factors, duration of surgery [57], intraperitoneal insufflation of CO_2 [58], and/or abdominal pain [59]. As a rule, narcotic use should be minimized to prevent PONV in ALC programs.

Postoperative abdominal pain varies widely between individual patients [15, 60]. In the first postoperative day almost 30% of patients report some degree of abdominal pain [61]. Unexpected admissions due to abdominal pain have been reported to occur in as many as 24–41% of patients [17, 62].

Postoperative abdominal pain includes abdominal wall pain (mainly in the umbilical wound), deep visceral pain, and pain at the tip of the shoulder, and it affects 30–50% of LC patients [63, 64]. The frequency of the latter is lower when reduced abdominal pressure is applied [65].

Factors related to surgical technique are very important in postoperative abdominal pain. Absence of residual blood in the abdominal cavity, careful dissection, and minimal trauma are key factors in minimizing abdominal pain (all this is meant when the term 'exquisite surgery' is used). Therefore, the learning curve experienced as more LC procedures are performed is a relevant factor, as the decline in the duration of surgery as a surgeon gains experience is important to the success of ALC even in difficult hilar gallbladder dissection [36, 66].

Decreasing PONV and Abdominal Pain in LC

After years of experience with ALC it has been demonstrated that short-acting anesthetics with quick patient recovery combined with exquisite surgical technique are the main key factors in decreasing PONV and abdominal pain [20, 31, 36].

Preemptive analgesia based on afferent nerve block achieved by means of anesthetic agents [67] is a very important tool in ALC [68]. Local anesthetics can be administered either into wounds or intraperitoneally (i.p.), bupivacaine being the one most frequently used. Administration i.p. induces a somatovisceral blockade [69–72], decreasing postoperative abdominal pain and also pain at the tip of the shoulder. Ropivacaine has also been introduced, with similar results [73].

Wound preincisional instillation of local anesthetic has been shown [74] to decrease parietal pain; the effect is more pronounced when it is administered before the skin incision is made rather than after [75, 76]. Levobupivacaine has been compared to ropivacaine, and has proved to offer greater advantages in terms of pain relief [77].

Multimodal administration, i.e., both wound instillation and i.p. administration, has been shown to enhance the effects in pain control and has been recommended as a routine policy in ALC [78–80].

The anesthetic technique is an independent and significant key factor in the success of ALC. Inhalatory anesthetics such as sevofluorane and desfluorane are considered the agents of choice for fast-track procedures such as ALC [81]. Combinations of propofol with fentanyl and/or remifentanyl are widely used in ALC owing to their combined intravenous action [82]. Decreasing doses of opiates or using short-acting opiates (remifentanyl) lowers the probability of PONV and enhances postoperative recovery [83, 84].

For antiemetic prophylaxis, metoclopramide administration is more cost effective than ondansetron [85] and has been recommended as the routine prophylactic agent against PONV, to be administered at the time of anesthesia induction [86], particularly in patients with gastric reflux and hiatus hernia, in whom PONV is more frequent.

Selection Criteria for ALC

The unanticipated admissions rate, like the readmission rate, is an index of the quality of ambulatory surgery [87]. Other variable outcomes that should be included in ALC analysis are: length of observation period (in hospital), unplanned admissions, emergency room consultations, nonscheduled consultations with general practitioners or in the surgical unit within 7 days after surgery, use of pain medication, quality of life, period of convalescence, time off work, and treatment preferences compared with ON LC. Finally, financial costs should be considered in association with all the above variables, to ensure that financial conclusions do not discount extra costs related to unplanned admissions and readmissions, as can happen with brief procedure studies.

Published unanticipated admission rates vary from 1% to 39% of patients, the main reasons for such admissions being uncontrolled postoperative nausea, vomiting, or abdominal pain, conversion to open surgery, and patients' subjective feeling of being unfit for discharge [88].

Identification of patients suitable for ALC is required to clarify how to select patients. Studies focused on identifying factors predicting unanticipated admissions have identified ASA class I or II, age under 65 years, absence of previous abdominal surgery, absence of previous complicated gallbladder disease (mostly acute cholecystitis), absence of gallbladder wall thickening, and duration of surgery lower than 60 min as the key factors in successful selection of patients for ALC [4, 10, 15, 88, 89]. All these are important factors in clinical care and surgery, but one of the most important factors is giving patients careful and complete information about the procedure to be performed, including extensive preoperative and postoperative counseling and instructions.

Quality Control in ALC

ALC should be safe and feasible, with morbidity rates similar to or lower than other outpatient procedures that are accepted by the community and with also a similar rates of readmission and unanticipated admission. Also, and sometimes most importantly, however, it should be perceived by patients and doctors as a better procedure than the standard LC involving an overnight stay as a matter of course.

When a new procedure is introduced as day surgery, social, medical, and surgical education is mandatory if real acceptance of the new method is to be achieved. Patients should be monitored extremely carefully to allow early detection of any adverse side-effects of the new method. Quality control of every aspect of the new process should be extremely meticulous, to avoid missing any information related to adverse effects.

Therefore, to gain patient, social and medical confidence, quality analysis should include both the patients' perception of the procedure and its outcome (subjective) and the clinical results (objective) [54]. Total quality management will include both aspects of quality, and therefore patients' expectations and needs should be carefully analyzed in terms of perceived satisfaction with the new process [90] in order to identify elements of the new method that might be modified.

ALC is accepted by 65–95% of patients [24, 30, 38, 40, 91]. In contrast, 20% of patients would prefer to have LC as inpatients [24, 38] even in the absence of any postoperative complications or side-effects of the anesthetic or surgery.

The acceptance of ALC is based on adequate anesthetic management, excellent surgical technique and continuity of clinical management by the surgical team, which creates an individualized profile of management in patients, thereby enhancing the confidence of patients and relatives. The task is to make outpatient management to be perceived as an impatient management but with domestic commodities and above all with the same levels of safety [54].

Establishing ALC as a Hospital Routine

Implementation of ALC implies the development of a list of correctable factors that may lead to an unplanned hospital admission. The most important factors considered are: preoperative patient selection, patient's position on the operating list and variations in anesthetic and surgical practice. Outpatient cholecystectomy is now a safe hospital routine for all elective procedures, even without rigorous selection methods.

Identifying and correcting modifiable factors leads to a significant increase in the institutional outpatient rate, making it comparable to reported individual rates [92].

Inclusion Criteria for ALC

Patients suitable for ALC include those with: (1) symptomatic gallbladder lithiasis, including previous cholecystitis, pancreatitis, endoscopic retrograde cholangio-pancreatography (ERCP) or obstructive jaundice, but only when preoperative choledocolithiasis has been excluded or treated; (2) symptomatic nonlithiasic gallbladder disease (chronic nonlithiasic cholecystitis) [93], (3) ASA class I, II, or even III with controlled underlying disease; and (4) absence of previous anesthetic complications. In addition, the following conditions should be met: (1) adult care facilities at home for at least the first 24 h postoperatively; (2) distance between home and hospital less than 100 km and if possible availability of a lift; (3) full preoperative examination, including recent gallbladder ultrasound (US) examination and complete liver function tests; and (4) signed informed consent to ambulatory anesthesia and ALC.

If common bile duct (CBD) stones are suspected on the grounds of liver function tests and/or ultrasound examination, magnetic resonance (MR) cholangiography is indicated, and if doubt persists preoperative ERCP with or without sphincterotomy should be performed.

A surgeon's initial experience of performing ALC should be gained exclusively in patients in whom cholecystectomy is expected preoperatively to be "easy," identified by means of US examination (absence of gallbladder wall thickening, shrunken gallbladder, nondistended gallbladder) and also by taking into account all past history related to gallbladder disease. Experience with LC is mandatory, in order to avoid the learning curve for LC incidence in addition to the learning curve for ALC, which could have adverse results on ALC development and implementation. It is recommended that during the initial development period only those criteria that identify patients who are suitable for ALC or for a short hospital stay after LC should be routinely used for adequate patient selection [94].

Ultrasound is a key preoperative examination that can predict technical difficulties in LC. A nondistended gallbladder following fasting, a thickened gallbladder wall (threefold normal value), a contracted or shrunked gallbladder, and a poorly defined gallbladder wall or a poorly defined gallbladder on US are key factors in the prediction of difficult cholecystectomies [88]. These US variables should be routinely assessed, as use of the US classification makes it possible to predict which patients will be at low risk for conversion or for technical difficulties, that is a key point when planning day case surgery [95].

Past History of Gallbladder Disease

Documented earlier cholecystitis with inpatient treatment is an important marker of a difficult cholecystectomy. Previous ERCP with or without sphincterotomy is also associated with increased technical difficulty during LC [37, 94, 96]. We do not consider these factors as contraindications for ALC, but such patients are scheduled for operation early in the morning session and allocated to more experienced surgeons as a higher than average level of technical difficulty is highly probable.

CBD Stones

Although CBD stones have become less frequent since the development of LC, preoperative screening for occult or silent CBD stones is mandatory. Preoperative ultrasound examination looking for an increase in CBD diameter or CBD stones, and also liver function tests, are mandatory in the preoperative workup of patients undergoing ALC. We apply a predictive scoring system based on clinical and laboratory tests and ultrasound findings to reach a preoperative estimate of the probability of CBD stones [97]. Nevertheless, occult or silent CBD stones are usually not diagnosed if intraoperative cholangiography (IOC) is not routinely performed, and therefore this probability should be explained to ALC patients, and the need for postoperative ERCP-ES (ERCP with endoscopic sphincterotomy) should also be discussed as part of the preoperative information.

Age

Although age is not considered an independent factor in ambulatory surgery, we have demonstrated that it is one of the most important factors influencing success of ALC. The cut-off age for ON stay or admission for ALC differs in published series, ranging from 50 to 65 years [1, 89, 98].

Although age is not per se an independent factor in selection for ALC in our series, we have found that increasing age is connected with: (1) increased frequency of undiagnosed comorbidity, (2) increased frequency of 'difficult cholecystectomies' owing to more frequent gallbladder adhesions and thickened gallbladder wall, both related to a past history of complicated biliary disease, such as cholecystitis, pancreatitis, or recurrent biliary colics. In our series, in a group of 107 patients older than 65 years almost 20% required ON admission, mostly because of longer than average operating times secondary to greater technical difficulty, and also to more frequent cultural and social arguments against early discharge.

Age should be considered an important factor in whether or not ALC could be successful. Patients over 65 years of age are significantly at risk of undiagnosed and untreated conditions, the frequency rising with advancing age. The frequency of diagnosed comorbidities also increases with age, and multiple medications are frequent. Therefore, the probability of decompensating previously diagnosed or undiagnosed illnesses is an important factor for ALC [99]. Moreover, although LC is regarded as low-trauma surgery, anesthesia, even when extremely carefully adapted for an elderly patient, also involve a higher rate of adverse effects and a slower recovery than in younger patients.

We recommend that older patients should also be scheduled early in the surgical list so that they can have a longer postoperative observation period allowing for early recognition or diagnosis of uncontrolled medical conditions and side-effects of anesthesia.

We have noticed a significant impact of social or cultural considerations against early discharge following uncomplicated ALC in aged patients. Communication with the patients, and even more important with their relatives, is absolutely mandatory to deal with social or cultural arguments against hospital discharge. The anesthetic and surgical teams should be constantly concerned to decrease the frequency of PONV and abdominal pain in this group of patients, so as to guarantee the success of their ALC operations.

Obesity

Morbid obesity should not be regarded as a contraindication for ALC. Obese patients derive even greater benefit from LC than patients with average body weight, although the surgical technique is usually more complex and the duration of surgery is usually longer [100, 101]. Although some authors do specify morbid obesity as a contraindication, it is only if severe comorbidities are associated mainly with the respiratory tract that it should be considered a formal contraindication for ALC.

Scarred abdomen

Previous abdominal surgery, even if in the upper abdomen, also should not be considered a formal contraindication for LC or ALC. In our experience patients can be safely operated on by laparoscopy, and the only factor obviously related to ON stay has been the time it takes to perform adhesiolysis of previous surgical adhesions in the gallbladder area, which leads to a 30% increase in the duration of surgery. Therefore, in contrast to other authors [4, 10, 14], we do not consider previous surgery on the upper gastrointestinal tract a formal contraindication to LC or ALC.

High-risk Patients

At first, only patients classified as ASA I or II were considered suitable for ALC [38, 40, 41]. However, ASA III patients whose disease is controlled are also suitable for ALC. Patients over the age of 70 or with an ASA classification of III are considered high-risk patients, however the study of Voikt et al. [21] shows that outpatient cholecystectomy is also safe for this subpopulation of patients. We also subscribe to this policy and regard ALC as the procedure of choice for high-risk patients.

Heartburn, Regurgitation, Hiatus Hernia, and Gastroesophageal Reflux

Heartburn and regurgitation and chronic omeprazol therapy should be routinely assessed to decrease the incidence of PONV with appropriate treatment or preoperative prophylaxis, as in this subpopulation of patients rates of PONV are higher even in the case of noncomplicated LC.

Antiaggregant Therapy and Anticoagulation

Antiaggregant therapy is discontinued for at least 14 days before the procedure; according to the main clinical indication for it, it should be substituted with low-molecular-weight heparin (LMWH) when appropriate and restarted 72–96 h after the operation, but chronic administration of antithrombotic agents should not be seen as a formal contraindication for ALC.

Patients undergoing anticoagulation are put back on LMWH treatment and on the day of surgery are scheduled for a preoperative coagulation examination before surgery.

If preoperative INR – the ratio between controlled plasma and tested plasma in relation to coagulation status – is in the normal range, these patients can also be operated on as outpatients, but account must be taken of the underlying disease for which anticoagulation was originally indicated.

Although early in our experience such patients were routinely scheduled for ON admission, they are now scheduled for surgery as outpatients, although postoperative observation is maintained for at least 8 h and they are therefore scheduled early on the surgical list.

Surgical programmation and informed consent

Rules for Inclusion Criteria

One important rule is that the most difficult cases should be scheduled for the morning or early afternoon surgery to allow patients to be discharged no later than 6:00–7:00 p.m. and to ensure a longer postoperative observation period whose standard must not be shorter than 2-3 hours when patients are obese or aged over 65, in anticoagulated patients, and when a difficult cholecystectomy has been predicted on the grounds of an ultrasound or clinical examination.

Informed consent is mandatory for the ambulatory process, as in most countries ALC is still under evaluation by the surgical and medical community and not yet fully accepted, recommended, or even considered as a plausible and safe method of performing cholecystectomy. Therefore specific informed consent to ALC is mandatory.

Although inclusion criteria should be strict at the initial experience of ALC, a rigorous preoperative selection is not necessary for ALC programs as experience grows and a more liberal policy can safely be adopted without compromising the safety of ALC [102].

Prediction of Success or Failure of ALC

Preoperative Factors

Factors related to the failure of outpatient LC are poorly defined.

The factors most frequently identified include age, ASA classification, surgery start time and duration of surgery [89]. In most studies unplanned admissions have been related to operative duration longer than 60 min and a finding of a thickened gallbladder wall on ultrasonography, although the duration of surgery has proved to be the only independent predictive factor. Therefore, duration of surgery is the best predictive factor for unplanned or unanticipated admission after ALC, and during selection of patients ultrasonographic demonstration of a thickened gallbladder wall or US risk factors suggesting a difficult cholecystectomy should be routinely evaluated [88]. In our preliminary study of 305 consecutive patients, factors related to failure in ALC identified by multivariate analysis were: age over 65 years, past history of complicated biliary disease, and previous admission to hospital because of cholecystitis or the need for ERCP, previous upper gastrointestinal surgery, and US evidence of a thickened gallbladder wall or other US risk factors for a difficult LC [43].

Intraoperative Factors

Duration of surgery is a crucial factor in success of ALC [88]. A duration of over 60 min is related to ON admission or admission to hospital as an inpatient [15, 103].

With increasing duration of surgery, the period of anesthesia also increases, as then does the probability of side-effects of anesthesia, accounting for the slower postoperative recovery and the higher rate of PONV.

Difficulties with abdominal cavity access are usually associated with obesity and previous abdominal surgery, and they account for extra surgery time [20, 24, 104].

When surgical dissection is difficult owing to inflammatory scarring of Calot's triangle or the gallbladder bed, identification of cystic duct and artery is more often difficult and increasing rates of bleeding occur more frequently [34, 39, 41], leading to longer operating times.

Therefore, scoring systems that allow easy clinical calculation of the risk of technically difficult cholecystectomies are needed for identification of patients who are suitable for ALC.

The technical difficulty of the operation should be judged according to the time required for gallbladder dissection. The quantification of technical difficulty using a scoring system would be useful for a preoperative prediction since knowing the probability of such technical difficulties may be of help in conducting a safe intervention [105]. Even more, a surgical scoring system considering all the individual patient variables in relation to intraoperative difficulties and potential postoperative development of medical complications or longer recovery should be considered a mandatory clinical tool for preoperative estimation of how successful an ALC program will be.

We have developed a simple scoring system that correlates well with operating time and surgical difficulty score. The Surgical Complexity Classification Index (SCCI) for LC allows simple and quick classification of individual patients in relation to the global complexity of the surgical process and correlates with duration of surgery, surgical complexity, and the probability of outpatient success. Moreover, with rising SCCI score more appropriate combinations of surgeons (junior or senior) can be allocated to individual patients. Our surgical program is based on the SCCI score: patients with higher SCCI scores are scheduled early on the day's list.

This system considers age, obesity, any comorbidity, and intrinsic or evolutive characteristics of gallbladder disease, with the aim of predicting preoperatively the global complexity of the procedure and thus the probability of discharging the patient the same day, the appropriate composition of the surgical team and, finally, the best time for the operation in the surgical schedule (morning versus afternoon; Table 18.3). When variables were considered in relation to same-day discharge, the SCCI was found to be the best predictive value in a previous nonpublished study conducted by our group, and since 2006 we have therefore programmed patients and the surgical team on the basis of the SCCI scores.

Surgical Procedure

Most procedures are scheduled for morning or early afternoon surgery. Cases classified as

Table 18.3 Surgical complexity classification index for laparoscopic cholecystectomy (SCCI score)

Variable	Scoring value
Comorbidity	
NIDM	1
IDDM	3
Antiaggregation	2
Anticoagulation	5
Heart disease	ASA II 1 ASA III 2
Lung disease	ASA II 1 ASA III 2
Liver disease	Child A 1 B 2 C 4
Age group (years)	
≤60	0
60–65	1
65–75	2
75–85	3
>85	4
Intrinsic conditions	
Previous cholecystitis	3
Previous biliary pancreatitis	3
Previous ERCP-ES	3
Repeated biliary colics	2
US: shrunked gallbladder	5
US: thickened gallbladder wall	2
US: contracted nondistended gallbladder	1
US: nondefined gallbladder	3
Previous upper GI surgery	4
Obesity	3
Extreme obesity	5
Male sex	2

ERCP, endoscopic retrograde cholangiopacreatography; *ERCP-ES*, endoscopic retrograde cholangiopacreatography with endoscopic sphincterotomy; *NIDM*, noninsulin-dependent diabetes mellitus; *IDDM*, insulin-dependent diabetes mellitus; *ASA*, American Society of Anesthesiologists; *GI*, gastro-intestinal

'probably difficult' and those in patients who have comorbidities and/or are over 65 years of age should be scheduled for early in the day, as postoperative recovery may take more time. Prediction of technical difficulties and/or the probability of decompensating for preexisting medical conditions is based on the SCCI system.

Patients come to the hospital on the morning of surgery having fasted for a minimum of 8 h.

The surgical procedure includes routine antibiotic prophylaxis with amoxicillin-clavulanic, or clindamicin for patients with penicillin allergy. Antithrombotic prophylaxis is selectively administered when SSAT criteria [106] are met, i.e., in the case of obesity, cardiac disease, or chronic antiaggregation medication, or if the scheduled time of the procedure is more than 60 min (beniparin DCI 3,500 IU s.c). We do not give antiemetic prophylaxis routinely: in patients with heartburn or regurgitation only, a single dose of metoclopramide and omeprazol is given during anesthetic induction.

Anesthesia is a key factor in ALC. The anesthetic team should include only committed anesthesiologists who are in close contact with the surgical team. The anesthetic protocol includes the use of atropine, propofol, and fentanyl in low doses (0.10 mg/kg). Propofol-opiate (remifentanyl/fentanyl)-rocuron-sevofluorane anesthesia and preemptive analgesia are routinely administered in all cases.

Ventilation is maintained to obtain end tidal carbonic ($ETCO_2$) values of 35–40 mmHg. Propofol and sevofluorane are used in balanced concentrations. The evolution of anesthetic protocols during our experience has included the use of ketoprofen, somatovisceral blockade with bupivacaine splashed over the subphrenic and gallbladder area, and the use of preemptive wound block with bupivacaine [107].

A nasogastric tube is routinely introduced to empty the stomach and also to allow gastric decompression if the stomach is filled with air during ventilation. The nasogastric tube is routinely retrieved before extubation.

Surgical Technique

The surgical team should include experienced laparoscopic surgeons and should be an appropriate combination of junior and senior surgeons in terms of ability in preoperative estimation of the complexity of the patient's case and of surgical experience.

The surgical technique used is the European one with four trocars and the Hasson technique for performance of the pneumoperitoneum. Our experience has shown no benefits of the three trocars technique or use of the only 5 mm trocars. Moreover, ALC should be considered an exquisite LC, and in our opinion careful and exquisite dissection of Calot's triangle requires a four-trocar technique.

Preemptive blockade of abdominal wounds is routinely performed with bupivacaine before the skin incision is made and the trocars introduced.

After pneumoperitoneum is reached with pressures no higher than 13 mmHg bupivacaine is routinely splashed into the gallbladder area to obtain a preemptive visceral blockade.

Cholecystectomy is performed with standard dissection of Calot's triangle and selective clipping of the cystic artery and duct after exquisite dissection of both structures. This means that both these structures are clipped and sectioned only after 'beyond all doubt' identification. Moreover if minimal doubt persists, a fundus-Hartman dissection is performed so as to leave the gallbladder free of any attachments other than the cystic duct and artery. We routinely apply two clips in the proximal part of the cystic duct and artery.

Intraoperative cholangiography is not performed routinely. It is only indicated if: (1) there are anatomical concerns during dissection owing to unclear anatomy and technical concerns, (2) the CBD is unexpectedly dilated, and (3) CBD stones are suspected and the result of magnetic cholangiography has been inconclusive.

At the end of the procedure, once the gallbladder has been dissected away from the liver bed, hemostasis is exhaustively checked, after which the subhepatic area including the gallbladder bed is filled with saline to detect the minimum bleeding point. If no bleeding or bile leak is detected we introduce a solution of icodextrin with bupivacaine into the abdominal cavity to enhance postoperative analgesia (somatovisceral blockade).

Prior to trocar retrieval all trocar wounds are also carefully inspected to exclude any bleeding from the trocar port sites. At the end of the procedure all CO_2 is retrieved and abdominal skin wounds are closed with staples.

The surgical report sheet records the entire surgical procedure step by step, and each step is scored for grade of difficulty (normal, easy, difficult, or very difficult), so that everyone in the surgical team has a quick view of the surgical complexity of the individual patients' cases when postoperative recovery is reviewed and at the time of discharge.

Intraoperative Cholangiography, CBD Stones, and Biliary Injuries in LC

The present trends suggest that routine use of IOC is not justified in the average patient who presents for LC with no history of jaundice or recent pancreatitis and has normal liver function tests and a normal-size CBD on ultrasonography. In these conditions, the chance of an unsuspected stone being left in the CBD is less than 1%; if it does happen the stone can be easily retrieved by endoscopic sphincterotomy, also as an outpatient procedure [108]. Therefore, in most series, the frequency of residual stone after LC without routine IOC has been estimated at 1.5–2.4% [109].

Moreover, in the context of normal preoperative imaging and laboratory work the incidence of CBD stones is not significantly higher among patients recovering from acute mild or moderate pancreatitis than among patients with no history of pancreatitis [110].

The use of IOC routinely rather than selectively during LC is controversial, the main argument for its routine use being the prevention or detection of bile duct injuries.

There was a small to moderate long-term increase in the risk of bile duct injuries after the introduction of LC compared with the prelaparoscopic era [111], but the biliary injuries rate has normalized with gathering surgical experience. It is not uncommon for intraoperative complications, particularly bile duct injuries, to be more frequent at the beginning of a surgeon's LC experience. This risk is expected to decline as the surgeon gains experience. The risk of complications increases with patient age, is higher in male patients and in teaching hospitals, but is lower when IOC is performed and, more importantly, with increasing surgical experience [112].

With reference to detection of to bile duct injuries, IOC offers the opportunity of preventing error through extensive knowledge of biliary diversity and real-time imaging [113], thereby lowering the risk of bile duct injury during cholecystectomy, even though cannulation of the cystic duct is only possible in 90% of cases [114].

We are not in agreement with the opinion that excellent results in LC have to be attributed to the routine performance of IOC. IOC might prevent bile duct transection, but this should not be an argument for its routine use. IOC should be performed if anatomical concerns arise during operation before any duct or any hilar structure is transected or if the suspicion of CBD stones arises intraoperatively [115]. Moreover, if dissection of Calot's triangle is extremely difficult and there is room for doubt in some cases, repeated attempts at cystic duct cannulation may result in bile duct injury, and then conversion to an open procedure should be considered rather than repeated maneuvers directed at cystic cannulation.

The rate of CBD injury is significantly lower when IOC is used, although this effect is magnified during surgeons' early experience. Therefore, routine IOC should be reserved for less experienced surgeons and high-risk operations [116].

Postoperative Management

Postoperative management is performed according to a fast-track protocol [117]. After extubation the patient is kept in an intermediate care area close to the operating room. As soon as the patient is fully conscious oral fluid intake is resumed with a carbonated drink [118]. If nausea or vomiting is present a single dose of metoclopramide is administered. If the patient feels pain a single dose of metamizol is given.

Once the patient is fully recovered and sitting is tolerated, he/she is returned to the ward, where he/she remains seated and oral fluid intake is resumed. Free nonassisted mobilization is encouraged by the nurses. At this point any pain and nausea are controlled with oral metoclopramide and metamizol.

Patients are routinely examined by the surgical team prior to hospital discharge, a modified Aldrete scoring system [119] being used, and discharge is preceded by an observation period ranging from 2 to 8 hours. Rigorous conditions for hospital discharge include absence or control of pain, tolerance of oral fluid intake, and free unaided ambulation.

Patients and relatives receive full written instructions for the postoperative period and a list of symptoms they should be alert to. Oral analgesia includes oral metamizol. Metoclopramide is only prescribed if nausea or vomiting have been observed during recovery and in patients with diagnosed gastroesophageal reflux.

A daily recovery sheet is given to patients, on which they are asked to report analgesic use, severity of pain, and performance of daily activities so that the postoperative recovery profile of each individual patient can be analyzed during outpatient visits.

Telephone contact at 10:00 p.m. is mandatory in all discharged patients to ensure that postoperative information has been fully understood and the patient is symptom free.

Patients are admitted in any of the following circumstances: (1) complex and difficult procedure and surgeon concern about early discharge, (2) uncontrolled abdominal pain, (3) uncontrolled PONV, and finally (4) 'social reasons', which include miscellaneous arguments against early discharge arising out of cultural considerations about LC as day surgery.

In addition, all patients are routinely contacted by telephone the day after discharge. Patients are considered outpatients if they are discharged before 6.00–7.00 p.m. and as ON stay patients if they are discharged before 9:00 a.m. the next day. Hospital admission patients are those who need a longer stay in hospital.

Learning Curve of Postoperative Management

As ALC reduces the postoperative observation time to 2–8 h, surgeons need to gain experience with the recovery profile following successful ALC. If preemptive anesthetics and postoperative anesthetics are used, pain is usually absent or responds to a single dose of an intravenous analgesic or even to oral pain medication. Shoulder tip pain may be significant, but it becomes milder during sitting and worsens when the patient is lying in bed; how it responds to analgesics is variable, and it is sometimes confused with pneumothorax or symptoms of acute respiratory failure. Therefore, if it is present patients should be given information about its nature and control, and they usually do not refuse discharge despite the pain.

A normal ALC means that patients are fully mobile, tolerate oral feeding and require minimal analgesic medication or none at all. If the patient is examined and the local blockade has been correctly performed wound pain is almost absent, except at the umbilical port, which seems to be more sensitive than other wounds. The abdomen can be explored with little or no discomfort. Orthostatic hypotension should not be present except perhaps in older patients. Hemodynamics and urine output should be normal.

In summary, at the time of discharge patients are almost symptom free, and in most cases it is they or their relatives who suggest discharge.

Uncontrolled pain or uncontrolled PONV should be regarded as alarm signals even if an operation has been classified as an easy technical procedure, as this may be the only clinical symptom in a patient with an underlying but undiagnosed complication. If this is the case a prolonged period of observation is mandatory, and therefore an ON stay should be indicated in association with other medical prescriptions consistent with the clinical status of the patient (intravenous fluids, ondansetron therapy, etc.).

It should be stressed that the high achievement of day case treatment even in patients with ASA grade III is based on the association of multimodal anesthetic regimens and excellent surgical technique, but close follow-up of patients is also essential [20].

Emergency Postdischarge Call and Readmission Management of Patients Following ALC

Nonplanned ambulatory visits and emergency call and readmissions are not rare in patients who have undergone successful ALC. Most of them are secondary to uncontrolled pain, with or without uncontrolled PONV, and most often due to inadequate information on relation to postoperative self-management.

The great importance of continuous clinical care in the management of ALC patients should be stressed; this becomes extremely important in any patient with postoperative symptoms. Adequate management of these patients should be directed by surgeons experienced in ALC. Otherwise nonspecific symptoms may be passed over and normal postoperative pain may be overestimated.

Ambulatory pain management includes oral metamizol analgesia. If pain is not controlled or acute pain develops after a brief normal postoperative period an emergency visit is strongly recommended, as intractable pain is one of the most outstanding signs of an abnormal postoperative course in ALC and therefore points to a potential complication.

Although PONV can also indicate an abnormal postoperative course there may be associated conditions, mainly hiatus hernia or reflux esophagitis, that increase its postoperative occurrence. Appropriate treatment with proton pump inhibitors associated with metoclopramide should be enough to eliminate the symptoms. Otherwise, emergency assistance should be indicated for further investigations.

When both conditions are present, that is uncontrolled pain and PONV, the probability that an underlying complication has developed should be seriously considered even in the absence of abdominal signs. Plain abdominal films (intestinal obstruction), examination and complete blood analysis including liver function tests should always be routinely performed.

If no abnormalities are found ON stay and analgesic and antiemetic treatment are appropriate as the initial treatment. A new evaluation of the patient should be performed next day, and if the patient is not fully recovered he/she should be fully re-evaluated.

If liver function tests (LFT) – (alkaline phosphatase and bilirubin) are abnormal even with normal ultrasound findings the operation record should be reviewed in order to check each of the intraoperative steps, and even if no abnormality during the operation has been recorded, MR cholangiography should be performed to exclude retained stones or biliary leakage. If either of these is suggested by MR imaging ERCP should be the next step toward diagnosis and treatment, in association with ultrasound drainage of bile collections when necessary.

In our early experience in the first 504 consecutive ALC only two patients were readmitted with postoperative subhepatic collections, which were successfully managed by US drainage. Both were related to Luschcka ducts, and results of MR cholangiography were normal. Recovery was uneventful after US drainage.

Postoperative Follow-up

Postoperative visits are routinely scheduled for 72 h after surgery, 1 and 2 weeks later, 1 month after the operation, and then 3 months, 6 months and 1 year after surgery.

At the first postoperative visit skin staples are removed and a quality interview is performed by a surgical trained nurse. Patients are reviewed again 7 days later in order to review the pathological report and then 7 days after that in order to review the postoperative recovery sheet on which patients daily graded pain, analgesic consumption, and activities of daily living in order to complete the over view of the recovery period. Visits scheduled at 3, 6 and 12 months are focused on the potential occurrence of biliary colics, retained stones or abdominal wound hernia. Heartburn and regurgitation are assessed and compared with the preoperative status.

Quality and Patient Acceptance

Although ALC has been performed as a day-case procedure for many years, few studies have been conducted with the primary focus on patient acceptance and preferences in terms of quality of life for this practice compared with an ON stay. LC can be performed as a day-case procedure, and patient acceptance is similar to that for ON stay [120]. Evaluation of patients' experience after ALC should be routine in ALC programs, and most studies that have focused on this aspect have shown a high acceptance and satisfaction rate. Quality perception by patients is mandatory in an ALC program, in order to detect any modifiable aspect of the treatment that could have a negative influence on the success of ALC.

During the period 1999–2004, 404 consecutive patients of 504 consecutive ALC were prospectively analyzed with respect to their experience of being discharged the same day after LC performed by our group. The interview was conducted 72 h after the procedure.

Some degree of abdominal pain (controlled with oral analgesics) was related by 39.9% of patients. Postoperative nausea was experienced at home by only 23.5% of cases, and only 9.7% reported vomiting at home. Almost 33% considered they were fully recovered and even for work by the first postoperative visit.

A small proportion, 2.7%, of patients had to contact the emergency general practitioner during the early convalescence period. Only 2.2% of patients attended the emergency room, and an anticipated telephone contact with the surgeon was required by 5.9% of the patients.

Despite these good clinical results, only 74.3% of patients rated same-day discharge as excellent or good, as against 25.7% who considered they would have chosen ON stay.

Moreover, in the group of patients who considered same-day discharge excellent or good, 16.0% felt somehow unsafe and 23.4% considered the time of discharge too early.

Nevertheless, patients' scores for the medical attention they received were 8–10 (excellent or very good) in 92.5% of cases. These results were similar to those recorded in a short series of 100 consecutive patients previously published by our group [121].

How can we reconcile these good clinical results and the less good patient acceptance? Patients arguing that discharge was too early or that they felt unsafe when discharged were older than 65 years (78%), with previous complicated biliary problems and hospital admission (31.2%) and with some degree of recovery problems in relation to PONV (79%). Advanced age is related to previous surgical or medical experiences of patients or relatives, who could have old-fashioned attitudes to new ambulatory procedures and therefore not feel confident about procedures classically performed as inpatient surgery when they are offered as day-case surgery (adverse cultural factors).

Our quality results compare favorably with those in previous studies of patient acceptance, which has been rated between 60% and 95% [20, 24, 28, 91].

The new gold standard for cholecystectomy should be ALC, but how viable this is depends on short-term postoperative complaints of pain and PONV. An evidence-based multimodal approach to anesthetic-analgesic management in ALC is feasible and advantageous in the early postoperative phase, and it is mandatory for any ALC program. Uncontrolled pain and PONV are significant predictors of a complicated recovery profile and deserve further attention, as they may indicate an underlying but as yet undiagnosed postoperative complication. Development and implementation of ALC programs in surgical units will give general practitioners, gastroenterologists, patients, and relatives a new view of cholecystectomy by contributing to the definitive development of ALC as the option of first choice for gallbladder diseases.

References

1. Keulemans Y, Eshuis J, de Haes H et al (1998) Laparoscopic cholecystectomy: day-care versus clinical observation. Ann Surg 228:734-740

2. Jain PK, Hayden JD, Sedman PC et al (2005) A prospective study of ambulatory laparoscopic cholecystectomy: training, economic and patient benefits. Surg Endosc 19:1082-1085
3. Narain PK, DeMaria EJ (1997) Initial results of a prospective trial of outpatient laparoscopic cholecystectomy. Surg Endosc 11:1091-1094
4. Voyles CR, Berch BR (1997) Selection criteria for laparoscopic cholecystectomy in an ambulatory care setting. Surg Endosc 11:1145-1146
5. Topal B, Peeters G, Verbert A, Penninckx F (2007) Outpatient laparoscopic cholecystectomy: clinical pathway implementation is efficient and cost effective and increases hospital bed capacity. Surg Endosc 21:1142-1146
6. Brazier JE, Johnson AG (2001) Economics of surgery. Lancet 358:1077-1081
7. Fleisher L, Yee K, Lillemoe K et al (1999) Is outpatient laparoscopic cholecystectomy safe and cost-effective? Anesthesiology 90:1746-1755
8. Lehmann HP, Fleisher LA, Lam J et al (1999) Patient preferences for early discharge after laparoscopic cholecystectomy. Anesth Analg 88:1280-1285
9. Muhe E (1986) Die erste Cholecystektomie durch das Laparoskop. Langenbecks Arch Klin Chir 359:804-802
10. Reddick E, Olsen DO (1990) Outpatient laparoscopic laser cholecystectomy. Am J Surg 160:485-487
11. Arregui ME, Davis CJ, Arkush A, Nagan RF (1991) In selected patients outpatient laparoscopic cholecystectomy is safe and significantly reduces hospitalization charges. Surg Laparosc Endosc 1:240-245
12. Stephenson B, Callender C, Sage M, Vellacott K (1993) Feasibility of "day case" laparoscopic cholecystectomy. Ann R Coll Surg Engl 75:249-251
13. Smith R, Kolyn D, Pace R (1994) Outpatient laparoscopic cholecystectomy. HPB Surg 7:261-264
14. Farha GJ, Green BP, Beamer RL (1994) Laparoscopic cholecystectomy in a freestanding outpatient surgery center. J Laparoendosc Surg 4:291-294
15. Saunders CJ, Leary BF, Wolfe BM (1995) Is outpatient laparoscopic cholecystectomy wise? Surg Endosc 9:1263-1268
16. Prasad A, Foley R (1996) Day case laparoscopic cholecystectomy: a safe and cost effective procedure. Eur J Surg 162:43-46
17. Fiorillo MA, Davidson PG, Fiorillo M et al (1996) 149 ambulatory laparoscopic cholecystectomies. Surg Endosc 10:52-56
18. Taylor E, Gaw F, Kennedy C (1996) Outpatient laparoscopic cholecystectomy feasibility. J Laparoendosc Surg 6:73-77
19. Lam D, Miranda R, Hom SJ (1997) Laparoscopic cholecystectomy as an outpatient procedure. J Am Coll Surg 185:152-155
20. Mjaland O, Raeder J, Aasboe V et al (1997) Outpatient laparoscopic cholecystectomy. Br J Surg 84:958-961
21. Voitk AJ (1997) Is outpatient cholecystectomy safe for the higher-risk elective patient? Surg Endosc 11:1147-1149
22. Zegarra RF, Saba AK, Peschiera JL (1997) Outpatient laparoscopic cholecystectomy: safe and cost effective? Surg Laparosc Endosc 7:487-490
23. Hollington P, Toogood GJ, Padbury RT (1999) A prospective randomized trial of day-stay only versus overnight-stay laparoscopic cholecystectomy. Aust N Z J Surg 69:841-843
24. Lillemoe KD, Lin JW, Talamini MA et al (1999) Laparoscopic cholecystectomy as a "true" outpatient procedure: initial experience in 130 consecutive patients. J Gastrointest Surg 3:44-49
25. Critchlow JT, Paugh LM (1999) Is 24-hour observation necessary after elective laparoscopic cholecystectomy? South Med J 92:1089-1092
26. Fleming WR, Michell I, Douglas M (2000) Audit of outpatient laparoscopic cholecystectomy. Universities of Melbourne HBP Group. Aust N Z J Surg 70:423-427
27. Siu WT, Leong HT, Law BK et al (2001) Outpatient laparoscopic cholecystectomy in Hong Kong: patient acceptance. Surg Laparosc Endosc Percutan Tech 11:92-96
28. Calland JF, Tanaka K, Foley E et al (2001) Outpatient laparoscopic cholecystectomy: patient outcomes after implementation of a clinical pathway. Ann Surg 233:704-715
29. Bringman S, Anderberg B, Heikkinen T et al (2001) Outpatient laparoscopic cholecystectomy. A prospective study with 100 consecutive patients. Ambul Surg 9:83-86
30. Richardson WS, Fuhrman GS, Burch E et al (2001) Outpatient laparoscopic cholecystectomy. Outcomes of 847 planned procedures. Surg Endosc 15:193-195
31. Serralta A, Garcia Espinosa R, Martinez P et al (2001) Cuatro años de experiencia en colecistectomía laparoscópica ambulatoria. Rev Esp Enferm Dig 93:207-210
32. Lau H, Brooks DC (2002) Transitions in laparoscopic cholecystectomy: the impact of ambulatory surgery. Surg Endosc 16:323-326
33. Curet MJ, Contreras M, Weber DM, Albrecht R (2002) Laparoscopic cholecystectomy. Surg Endosc 16:453-457
34. Johanet H, Laubreau C, Barei R et al (2002) Outpatient laparoscopic cholecystectomy. Ann Chir 127:121-125
35. Amarnath TS, Coulthard RA, Tate JJ (2002) Laparoscopic cholecystectomy as a "session" surgery. Ambul Surg 10:33-36

36. Serralta A, Planells M, Bueno J et al (2002) Learning curve in ambulatory laparoscopic cholecystectomy. Surg Laparosc Endosc Percutan Tech 12:320-324
37. Bal S, Reddy LG, Parshad R et al (2003) Feasibility and safety of day laparoscopic cholecystectomy in a developing country. Postgrad Med J 79:284-288
38. Ammori B, Davides D, Vezakis A et al (2003) Day-case laparoscopic cholecystectomy: a prospective evaluation of an 6-year experience. J Hepatobil Pancreat Surg 10:303-308
39. Leeder P, Matthews T, Krzeminska K, Dehn T (2004) Routine day-case laparoscopic cholecystectomy. Br J Surg 91:312-316
40. Vuilleumer H, Halkic N (2004) Laparoscopic cholecystectomy as a day surgery procedure: implementation and audit of 136 consecutive cases in a university hospital. World J Surg 28:737-740
41. Chok S, Yuen W, Lau H et al (2004) Outpatient laparoscopic cholecystectomy in Hong Kong Chinese—An outcome analysis. Asian J Surg 27:313-316
42. Jain PK, Hayden JD, Sedman PC et al (2005) A prospective study of ambulatory laparoscopic cholecystectomy. Training economic and patient benefits. Surg Endosc 19:1082-1085
43. Lledó JB, Planells Roig M, Arnal Bertomeu C et al (2005) Preoperative predictive factors of ambulatory laparoscopic cholecystectomy. Ambul Surg 12:45-49
44. Jarret PE (2000) Day case laparoscopic cholecystectomy. Can it be done? Should it be done? CMA 5:123-125
45. Boerci G (1990) Editorial comment. Am J Surg 160:488-489
46. Topal B, Aerts R, Penninckx F (1999) The outcome of major biliary tract injury with leakage in laparoscopic cholecystectomy. Surg Endosc 13:153-156
47. Targarona EM, Marco C, Balagué C et al (1997) Lesión quirúrgica de la vía biliar: análisis comparativo entre la colecistectomía laparoscópica y la convencional. Cir Esp 62:195-202
48. Bueno J, Serralta A, Planells M et al (2001) Colecistectomia laparoscópica y sus complicaciones. Nuestra experiencia en nueve años. Cir Esp 69:467-472
49. Deziel DJ, Millikan KW, Economou SG et al (1993) Complications of laparoscopic cholecystectomy: a national survey of 4,292 hospitals and an analysis of 77,604 cases. Am J Surg 165:9-14
50. Callery MP, Strasberg SM, Soper NJ (1996) Complications of laparoscopic general surgery. Gastrointest Endosc Clin N Am 6:423-444
51. Strasberg S, Hertl M, Soper N (1995) An analysis of the problem of biliary injury during laparoscopic cholecystectomy. J Am Coll Surg 180:101-125
52. Davidoff A, Branum G, Meyers W (1993) Clinical features and mechanism of major laparoscopic biliary injury. Semin Ultrasound CT MR 14:338-345
53. Bisgaard T, Klarskov B, Rosenberg J, Kehlet H (2001) Factors determining convalescence after uncomplicated laparoscopic cholecystectomy. Arch Surg 136:917-921
54. Planells M, Sánchez A, Sanahuja A et al (2002) Gestión de la calidad total en colecistectomía laparoscópica. Calidad asistencial y calidad percibida en colecistectomia laparoscópica ambulatoria. Rev Esp Enferm Dig 94:319-325
55. Trondsen E, Reiertsen O, Andersen O, Kjaersgaard P (1993) Laparoscopic and open cholecystectomy. A prospective, randomized study. Eur J Surg 159:217-221
56. Santon JM (1991) Anaesthesia for laparoscopic cholecystectomy. Anaesthesia 46:317
57. Tramer M, Moore A, McQuay H (1997) Propofol anesthesia and postoperative nausea and vomiting: quantitative systematic review of randomized controlled studies. Br J Anaesth 78:247-255
58. Neudecker J, Sauerland S, Neugebauer E et al (2002) The European Association for Endoscopic Surgery clinical practice guideline on the pneumoperitoneum for laparoscopic surgery. Surg Endosc 16:1121-1143
59. Klockgether A, Piorek V, Crozier T, Kettler D (1996) Nausea and vomiting after laparoscopic surgery: a comparison of propofol and thiopentone/halothane anaesthesia. Eur J Anaesthesiol 13:3-9
60. Joris J, Thiry E, Paris P et al (1995) Pain after laparoscopic cholecystectomy: characteristics and effect of intraperitoneal bupivacaine. Anesth Analg 81:379-384
61. Pasqualucci A, de Angelis V, Contardo R et al (1996) Preemptive analgesia: intraperitoneal local anesthetic in laparoscopic cholecystectomy. A randomized, double-blind, placebo-controlled study. Anesthesiology 85:11-20
62. Tuckey JP, Morris GN, Peden CJ, Tate JJ (1996) Feasibility of day case laparoscopic cholecystectomy in unselected patients. Anaesthesia 51:965-968
63. Cunnife M, McAnena O, Dar M et al (1998) A prospective randomized trial of intraoperative bupivacaine irrigation for management of shoulder-tip pain following laparoscopy. Am J Surg 176:2582-2561
64. Scheinin B, Kellokumpu I, Lindgren L et al (1995) Effect of intraperitoneal bupivacaine on pain after laparoscopic cholecystectomy. Acta Anaesthesiol Scand 39:195-198
65. Sarli L, Costi R, Sansebastiano G et al (2000) Prospective randomized trial of low-pressure

pneumoperitoneum for reduction of shoulder-tip pain following laparoscopy. Br J Surg 87:1161-1165

66. Kama N, Doganay M, Dolapci M et al (2001) Risk factors resulting in conversion of laparoscopic cholecystectomy to open surgery. Surg Endosc 15:965-968
67. Woolf CJ (1983) Evidence for a central component of post-injury pain hypersensitivity. Nature 306:686-688
68. Kehlet H (1999) Surgical stress response: does endoscopic surgery confer an advantage? World J Surg 23:801-807
69. Pasqualucci A, Contardo R, Da Broi U et al (1994) The effects of intraperitoneal local anesthetic on analgesic requirements and endocrine response after laparoscopic cholecystectomy: a randomized double-blind controlled study. J Laparoendosc Surg 4:405-412
70. Mraovic B, Jurisic T, Kogler-Majeric V, Sustic A (1997) Intraperitoneal bupivacaine for analgesia after laparoscopic cholecystectomy. Acta Anaesthesiol Scand 41:193-196
71. Weber A, Munoz J, Garteiz D, Cueto J (1997) Use of subdiaphragmatic bupivacaine instillation to control postoperative pain after laparoscopic surgery. Surg Laparosc Endosc 7:6-8
72. Chundrigar T, Hedges AR, Morris R, Stamatakis JD (1993) Intraperitoneal bupivacaine for effective pain relief after laparoscopic cholecystectomy. Ann R Coll Surg Engl 75:437-439
73. Maestroni U, Sortini D, Devito C et al (2002) A new method of preemptive analgesia in laparoscopic cholecystectomy. Surg Endosc 16:1336-1340
74. Sarac AM, Aktan AO, Baykan N et al (1996) The effect and timing of local anesthesia in laparoscopic cholecystectomy. Surg Laparosc Endosc 6:362-366
75. Hasaniya NW, Zayed FF, Faiz H, Severino R (2001) Preinsertion local anesthesia at the trocar site improves perioperative pain and decreases costs of laparoscopic cholecystectomy. Surg Endosc 15:962-965
76. Inan A, Sen M, Dener C (2004) Local aesthesia use for laparoscopic cholecystectomy. World J Surg 28:741-744
77. Papagiannopoulou P, Argiriadou H, Georgiou M et al (2003) Preincisional local infiltration of levobupivacaine vs ropivacaine for pain control after laparoscopic cholecystectomy. Surg Endosc 17:1961-1964
78. Michaloliakou C, Chung F, Sharma S (1996) Preoperative multimodal analgesia facilitates recovery after ambulatory laparoscopic cholecystectomy. Anesth Analg 82:44-51
79. Bisgaard T, Klarskov B, Kristiansen VB et al (1999) Multi-regional local anesthetic infiltration during laparoscopic cholecystectomy in patients receiving prophylactic multi-modal analgesia: a randomized, double-blinded, placebo-controlled study. Anesth Analg 89:1017-1024
80. Lee IO, Kim SH, Kong MH et al (2001) Pain after laparoscopic cholecystectomy: the effect and timing of incisional intraperitoneal bupivacaine. Can J Anaesth 48:545-550
81. Song D, Joshi GP, White PF (1998) Fast track eligibility after ambulatory anesthesia: a comparison of desflurane, sevoflurane and propofol. Anesth Analg 86:267-270
82. Lezoche E, Antognini F, Paganini A (1994) Proposal of an anesthetic technique for day-hospital laparoscopic cholecystectomy. Surg Endosc 8:422
83. Kehlet H, Rung G, Callesen T (1996) Postoperative opioid analgesia: time for a reconsideration? J Clin Anesth 8:441-445
84. Song D, Whitten CW, White PF (2002) Remifentanyl infusion facilitates early recovery for obese outpatient undergoing laparoscopic cholecystectomy. Anesth Analg 90:1111-1113
85. Wilson E, Bass C, Abrameit W et al (2001) Metoclopramide versus ondansetron in prophylaxis of nausea and vomiting for laparoscopic cholecystectomy. Am J Surg 181:138-141
86. Liberman MA, Howe S, Lane M (2000) Ondasetron versus placebo for prophylaxis of nausea and vomiting patients undergoing ambulatory laparoscopic cholecystectomy. Am J Surg 179:60-62
87. Greenburg AG, Greenburg JP, Tewel A et al (1996) Hospital admission following ambulatory surgery. Am J Surg 172:21-23
88. Lau H, Brooks DC (2001) Predictive factors for unanticipated admissions after ambulatory laparoscopic cholecystectomy. Arch Surg 136:1150-1153
89. Robinson T, Biffl W, Moore E et al (2002) Predicting failure of outpatient laparoscopic cholecystectomy. Am J Surg 184:515-519
90. Kriwanek S, Armbruster C, Beckerhinn P et al (1998) Patients' assessment and recall of surgical information after laparoscopic cholecystectomy. Dig Surg 15:669-673
91. Fassiadis N, Pepas L, Grandy-Smith S et al (2004) Outcome and patient acceptance of outpatient laparoscopic cholecystectomy. JSLS 8:251-253
92. Voitk AJ (1997) Establishing outpatient cholecystectomy as a hospital routine. Can J Surg 40:284-288
93. Planells M, Bueno J, Sanahuja A, Garcia Espinosa R (2004) Quality of life (GIQLI) and laparoscopic cholecystectomy usefulness in patients with gallbladder dysfunction or chronic non-lithiasis biliary pain (chronic acalculous cholecystitis). Rev Esp Enferm Dig 96:442-451

94. Planells M, García R, Anaya P et al (1999) Factores predictivos de colecistectomía laparoscópica dificultosa. Cir Esp 65:48-53
95. Jansen S, Jorgensen J, Caplehorn J, Hunt D (1997) Preoperative ultrasound to predict conversion in laparoscopic cholecystectomy. Surg Laparosc Endosc 7:121-123
96. Lau H, Brooks DC (2002) Contemporary outcomes of ambulatory laparoscopic cholecystectomy in a major teaching hospital. World J Surg 26:1117-1121
97. Planells M, García R, Moya A, Rodero D (1993) Score predictivo de coledocolitiasis. Una aproximación a la colangiografía selectiva intraoperatoria. Cir Esp 53:460-464
98. Voitk AJ (1996) Outpatient cholecystectomy. J Laparoendosc Surg 6:79-81
99. Thomas EJ, Brennann TA (2000) Incidence and types of preventable adverse events in elderly patients: population-based review of medical records. BMJ 320:741-744
100. Simopoulos C, Polychronidis A, Botatitis S et al (2005) Laparoscopic cholecystectomy in obese patients. Obes Surg 15:243-246
101. Pillai SB, van Rij AM, Williams S et al (1999) Complexity and risk-adjusted model for measuring surgical outcome. Br J Surg 86:1567-1572
102. Metcalfe MS, Mullin EJ, Maddern GJ (2006) Relaxation of the criteria for day surgery laparoscopic cholecystectomy. A N Z J Surg 76:142-144
103. Voitk AJ (1995) Routine outpatient laparoscopic cholecystectomy. Can J Surg 84:262-265
104. Lichten J, Reid J, Zahalsky M, Friedman R (2001) Laparoscopic cholecystectomy in the new millennium. Surg Endosc 15:867-872
105. Sakuramoto S, Sato S, Okuri T et al (2000) Preoperative evaluation to predict technical difficulties of laparoscopic cholecystectomy on the basis of histological inflammation findings on resected gallbladder. Am J Surg 179:114-121
106. National Guideline Clearinghouse. SSAT Patient Care Guidelines 2000. www.guideline.gov
107. Serralta Serra A, Bueno Lledo J, Sanahuja Santafe A et al (2002) Course of postoperative pain in laparoscopic cholecystectomy under multimodal anesthesia-analgesia in ambulatory care. Rev Esp Anestesiol Reanim 49:461-467
108. Cervantes J, Rojas G, Anton J (1997) Changes in gallbladder surgery: a comparative study 4 years before and 4 years after laparoscopic cholecystectomy. World J Surg 21:201-204
109. Lepner U, Grunthal V (2005) Intraoperative cholangiography can be safely omitted during laparoscopic cholecystectomy: a prospective study of 413 consecutive patients. Scand J Surg 94:197-200
110. Shayan H, Kopac D, Sample CB (2007) The role of intraoperative cholangiogram in the management of patients recovering from acute biliary pancreatitis. Surg Endosc 21:1549-1552
111. Waage A, Nilsson M (2006) Iatrogenic bile duct injury: a population-based study of 152776 cholecystectomies in the Swedish Inpatient Registry. Arch Surg 141:1207-1213
112. Hobbs MS, Mai Q, Knuiman MW et al (2006) Surgeon experience and trends in intraoperative complications in laparoscopic cholecystectomy. Br J Surg 93:844-853
113. Traverso LW (2006) Intraoperative cholangiography lowers the risk of bile duct injury during cholecystectomy. Surg Endosc 20:1659-1661
114. Borie F, Millat B (2003) Intraoperative cholangiography by laparoscopy. Why and how to do it. J Chir 140:90-93
115. Sarli L, Costi R, Roncoroni L (2006) Intraoperative cholangiography and bile duct injury. Surg Endosc 20:176-177
116. Flum DR, Flowers C, Veenstra DL (2003) A cost effectiveness analysis of intraoperative cholangiography in the prevention of bile duct injury during laparoscopic cholecystectomy. J Am Coll Surg 196:385-393
117. Kehlet H, Dahlj B (2003) Anaesthesia, surgery and challenges in postoperative recovery. Lancet 362:1921-1928
118. Candela M (1886) Abdominal hysterectomy (original contributions). Gynecol Process Pediatr 25 October 1886, pp 186-187
119. Aldrete JA (1995) The post-anesthesia recovery score revisited. J Clin Anesth 7:89-91
120. Johansson M, Thune A, Nelvin L, Lundell L (2006) Randomized clinical trial of day-care versus overnight-stay laparoscopic cholecystectomy. Br J Surg 93:40-45
121. Planells Roig MV, Sanchez Salas A, Bueno Lledó J et al (2002) Total quality management in laparoscopic cholecystectomy. Clinical quality and perceived quality in ambulatory laparoscopic cholecystectomy. Rev Esp Enf Digest 94:213-218

Chapter 19

Diagnosis and Treatment of Acute Cholecystitis

Giuseppe Borzellino, Edoardo Saladino, Manuela De Luca, Claudio Cordiano

Historical Aspects

Since the first cholecystectomy was performed by Langenbuch in 1882 [1], surgery has been the treatment of choice for acute gallstone cholecystitis. However, patients who underwent urgent surgery suffered from high mortality and morbidity mainly due to their general condition, to difficulties arising from the inflammatory changes in Callot triangle dissection and open common bile duct exploration when choledocolithiasis made it necessary [2–4]. Delayed surgery was advocated as a result, but reported complications of acute cholecystitis in up to 18% of patients awaiting surgery led to questions about the timing of surgery [5, 6]. The randomised controlled trials (RCTs) on early versus delayed surgery performed in the eighties show better outcomes with urgent cholecystectomy [7–10], but the issue of critically ill patients and severe acute cholecystitis was still a problem. Furthermore, other non surgical techniques appeared: Radder [11] published a first report on percutaneous cholecystostomy under ultrasound (US) guidance for treatment of gallbladder empyema, and Classen and Demling [12] described treatment of common bile duct stones by endoscopy.

The first laparoscopic cholecystectomy in 1987 opened new perspectives for the treatment of acute gallstone cholecystitis. Initially considered as a contraindication, the laparoscopic approach was rapidly reported as a feasible option. However, some initial reports are not very conclusive because of patient selection – exclusion criteria were not always clearly reported – while others highlighted the limits of a procedure for which the conversion rate was significantly higher. The introduction of laparoscopy made it therefore necessary not only to review the question of timing, but it also added new issues to the debate.

Evidence from the Literature

A search of the literature reveals a great number of publications on acute cholecystitis, but if the search is narrowed to select only those supposed to provide the best evidence, the number of relevant studies falls dramatically. We have uncovered some randomised studies and meta-analyses on timing and a few randomised studies on surgical approach and the use of cholecystostomy.

Timing

Seven randomised studies have been published on timing of laparoscopic cholecystectomy: six comparing early versus delayed cholecystectomy [13–18], one comparing delayed cholecystectomy versus observation [19], and there are four meta-analyses [20–23], one of which is from the Cochrane database [23].

Randomised controlled trials are not completely comparable because of different criteria for the timing of urgent surgery, which ranges from 24 to 72 hours, and on delayed surgery, ranging from 5 to 12 days. Meta-analyses further differ because of different studies inclusion criteria. However, while no significant difference was found on conversion, post-operative complications and post-operative complications and mortality, a longer overall hospital stay was evenly reported in the randomised trials and meta-analysis. Randomised trials also uniformly show that initial medical therapy in delayed surgery is not effective in all cases, with a failure rate ranging from 15.7 to 26%, and estimated to be 17% in a meta-analysis [23].

Surgical Approach

Three randomised studies compared open and laparoscopic cholecystectomy [24–26], and another one compared mini-laparoscopic versus conventional laparoscopic cholecystectomy [27]. One of the clinical trials [24] on open versus laparoscopic cholecystectomy suffers some bias since the experience of the surgeons who performed the laparoscopy or laparotomy differed (consultant versus resident). In addition, there was no information concerning the timing of surgery; i.e., whether it was considered from the appearance of symptoms or from admission, nor was the rate of severe acute cholecystitis reported. The other clinical trial [25] was blind and found no difference between laparoscopic and open cholecystectomy, besides in the length of post-operative stay, although this was only on a statistical basis, since it was 2 days in both groups. However, severity of cholecystitis in the two groups was not described and a 23% conversion rate was reported in the laparoscopic group. A third RCT [26] found better results after laparoscopic cholecystectomy with significantly less post-operative pain, shorter hospital stay and better pulmonary function.

Cholecystostomy

Three randomised trials have been published on the subject of cholecystostomy.

An RCT [28] compared two treatment regimens: percutaneous cholecystostomy followed by laparoscopic cholecystectomy (PCLC group) versus medical treatment followed by delayed laparoscopic cholecystectomy (DLC group) in high risk patients. Definition of risk was based either on co-morbid conditions or on the severity of cholecystitis, using the APACHE II score. Symptom relief time was significantly shorter in the PCLC group: 24 hours versus 48–72 hours in the DLC group ($P=0.001$). Two patients in the DLC group experienced mild pancreatitis during the waiting period. Results of laparoscopic cholecystectomies did not show differences in conversion rate (6.5% in PCLC versus 13.4% in DLC, $p=0.42$) or in post-operative hospital stay (1.58 SD 0.72 in PCLC versus 1.66 SD 0.72, $p=1$), while total hospital stay was shorter in the PCLC group: 5.3 days versus 15.2 days ($p=0.001$).

The trials on cholecystostomy [29] versus medical treatment included both calculus and acalculus cholecystitis, and cholecystostomy was performed if medical treatment failed on the third day. Extrapolation of data on gallstone cholecystitis showed a reduction in mortality rate in the cholecystostomy group: 6.8% versus 16% in the medical treatment group.

A trial on drainage cholecystostomy versus single aspiration showed better results in terms of clinical response in the cholecystostomy group for the treatment of severe acute cholecystitis [30].

Clinical Features and Surgical Outcomes

Background Literature

Evidence from the literature is limited to comparison of two different approaches in homogenous groups of patients, but a complete description of the samples studied is not always reported. The questions of timing and of surgical approach have been investigated, but it remains unclear whether the results are valid for all patients with acute cholecystitis. Observed wide exclusion criteria, high conversion or morbidity rates make the laparoscopic approach questionable even if comparison shows differences in its favour. Evaluation of outcomes of a definite approach for different grades of severity of cholecystitis would give further information, but such a study would have to be observational and not randomised.

A recent meta-analysis [31] on observational studies showed a higher conversion rate and a higher overall post-operative morbidity for severe acute cholecystitis. Severity can be only suspected pre-operatively when acute cholecystitis is gangrenous or there is an empyema of the gallbladder, while perforated cholecystitis with peri-cholecystic abscess or acute cholecystitis with liver abscess may be recognised pre-operatively by radiological exploration. In such cases liver abscess may be intra-parenchymal but contiguous with the gallbladder bed or distant in the right lobe of the liver. Dissemination through the right portal vein branch has been hypothesised in these cases [32].

The concept is very old, in 1888 Riedel published a paper that diligently described different clinical problems related to acute cholecystitis [33]. More recent observational studies have shown a correlation between severity of cholecystitis, general patient condition and surgical results. Severe clinical features of acute cholecystitis, due to different grades of severity or to associated diseases, have been reported to correlate statistically with conversion of laparoscopic cholecystectomy [34–37] and morbidity [34, 38–40]. This appears more evident in elderly patients [41, 42] in whom associated systemic diseases and common bile duct stones are more frequently observed.

The prevalence of common bile duct stones in acute cholecystitis has been reported in 1–18.5% of cases [14–16, 35, 39, 42–47], but such a complication is an exclusion criterion for many authors [14, 17, 36, 48–50]. Associated acute biliary pancreatitis has also been reported by some authors [41, 51, 52] and may be included in the biblio-pancreatic complications of acute gallstone cholecystis.

Based on results of observational studies it seems therefore quite obvious that different clinical features may require a differently scheduled treatment.

Personal Experience

In a previous report [47], the hypothesis that different clinical features require a different treatment strategy was tested and treatment strategy was based on the clinical pictures reported in Table 19.1. None of the expected differences due to severity of cholecystitis, systemic associated diseases or bilio-pancreatic complications were observed with a specific treatment policy for each clinical feature. A further analysis of our results (unpublished data on 300 patients) show that the only statistically significant difference between patients that

Table 19.1 Clinical features of observed acute cholecystitis in a series of 300 patients

Clinical feature	No. patients	%
Uncomplicated cholecystitis	72	24%
Predictive severe acute cholecystitis ASA I/II	51	17% 17%
Associated disease ASA III/IV	75	25%
Predictive bilio-pancreatic complications	77	25.7%
Perforated cholecystitis -Peri-cholecystic abscess -Liver abscess	17	5.7%
Acute cholecystitis and peritonitis syndrome	8	2.6%

ASA, American Society of Anesthesiologists grading

presented with uncomplicated acute cholecystitis and those with some complication of the cholecystitis, either systemic or bilio-pancreatic, is in the length of hospital stay.

A critical revision of our results with these first 300 patients led us to modify our approach. The US criteria used for severe acute cholecystitis have been published in a previous report [53] and are reported in Table 19.2. However, US alone may be source of misdiagnosis for severity of acute cholecystitis [54], so diagnosis of severe acute cholecystitis was modified to include at least two of the following clinical criteria: gender, age over 65 years, cardiovascular disease, diabetes, fever, leucocytosis, erythrosedimentation rate (ESR) or protein C. Due to the acquired experience with laparoscopy and the lack of evidence on the efficacy of cholecystostomy in patients with severe acute cholecystitis without systemic disease, patients with such a clinical feature were randomised to receive or not receive cholecystostomy prior to laparoscopic cholecystectomy.

Indications for cholecystostomy in patients with an American Society of Anesthesiologists (ASA) grading of ASA III were also revised and restricted to those with decompensated chronic diseases, with undercurrent acute illness such as pneumonia or predictive severe cholecystitis.

Finally, the acquired possibility of treating common bile duct stones intra-operatively by the way of a combined laparoscopic trans-cystic and endoscopic trans-papillary approach with the Rendez-vous technique has made accurate pre-operative diagnosis unnecessary. This new approach with a subsequent series of 250 patients allows a simplification of diagnostic patient categorisation and allows some hypotheses on surgical treatment of acute gallstone cholecystitis to be formed.

Diagnostic Uncertainty in Acute Cholecystitis

The major problems with diagnosis of acute cholecystitis are the sensitivity of acute cholecystitis diagnosis, prevision of the severity of the cholecystitis and pre-operative diagnosis of common bile duct stones.

Diagnosis of Acute Cholecystitis

If recommended diagnostic criteria for acute cholecystitis are used, 100% specificity is reached [55]. However, in our opinion sensitivity is of major concern since a missed diagnosis of acute cholecystitis may be much more dangerous than urgent intervention. Even if a patient does not have a true cholecystitis with relative pathological damage, he may still be suffering from gallstones in the gallbladder that need to be removed. A patient with an underestimated acute cholecystitis may evolve towards the dramatic picture of septic shock, with its attendant very high mortality. Testing of our

Table 19.2 US diagnostic criteria for severe acute cholecystitis

Stage I Mild	Cholelithiasis, thickening of the gallbladder wall ≥ 4 mm and < 8 mm and positive sonographic Murphy sign
Stage II Moderate	Stage I + hypoechoic band in the gallbladder wall or thickening of the gallbladder wall > 8 mm
Stage III Severe	Thickening of the gallbladder wall > 8 mm and/or peri-cholecystic fluid collection and or intra-luminal echoeic mass

diagnostic criteria may be biased, since a number of patients were treated by cholecystostomy and may have been operated on few days after the diagnosis; furthermore, the group of patients not treated by cholecystostomy had a high probability of suffering mild cholecystitis. Sensibility of US for diagnosis of acute cholecystitis has been reported to be 37.5% with a negative predictive value (NPV) of 58.3% in a recent study [56]; in our experience a total of 56 negatives US examinations were carried out in patients with pathologically proven acute cholecystitis.

In order to improve diagnostic accuracy, contrast enhanced sonography has also been proposed [57], but results are not yet conclusive.

Diagnosis of Severe Acute Cholecystitis

While diagnosis of acute cholecystitis suffers from some imprecisions, recognition of severe acute cholecystitis is much more difficult to reach pre-operatively. Accuracy of 31% with US and cholescintigraphy has been reported in a clinical series [58], a sensitivity of 83% with a NPV of 96% was obtained only by way of a predictive equation including biochemical and radiological data [54]. We initially used only US criteria to predict severity of acute cholecystitis, but in order to gain sensitivity, clinical criteria were added to US criteria. As shown in Table 19.3., accuracy has not been dramatically improved, the only result is a positive likelyhood (LH) ratio, but this does not reach statistical difference (p=0.07).

Pre-operative Diagnosis of Common Bile Duct Stones

Liver function tests alone are not sufficient to reach acceptable pre-operative accuracy. Other criteria such as clinical examination and US findings have been proposed, but results have been disappointing. When we combined clinical, biological and US data, sensitivity was 72% and specificity 81.3%, but a positive LH ratio of 3.8 (95% CI: 3.1–4.8) and a negative LH ratio of 0.3 (95% CI: 0.2–0.5) was found using endoscopic or intra-operative cholangiography as a reference test.

Therapeutic Indications for Acute Cholecystitis

Tratment should be based on clinical features of acute cholecystitis, however some uncertainties in diagnosis, physiopathology and natural history of the disease have also to be taken into account. Based on the above-mentioned clinical features, different treatment modalities may be proposed.

Table 19.3 Diagnostic accuracy for severe acute cholecystitis

	US criteria	US and clinical criteria	p-value
Sensitivity	46.3%		
	58.1%	0.24	
Specificity	69.8%		
	76.5%	0.17	
Positive LH ratio	1.5 (95% CI:1-2.3)	2.4 (95% CI:1.7-3.5)	0.07
Negative LH ratio	0.8 (95% CI:0.6-1)	0.5 (95% CI:0.4-0.8)	0.13

LH, likelihood; *US*, ultrasound

Uncomplicated Cholecystitis

Uncomplicated cholecystitis is the main indication for urgent laparoscopic cholecystectomy. However, timing of urgent intervention should be based on the natural history of acute cholecystitis rather than on results of studies in which exact timing of urgent intervention was based on surgical results of laparoscopic cholecystectomy [44, 45, 59]. Acute cholecystitis may evolve into a severe form if medical treatment fails to improve the clinical picture in the acute phase. Due to the unknown evolution and timing for each patient, laparoscopic cholecystectomy should be performed as soon possible after admission [60].

Severe Acute Cholecystitis without Associated Diseases

Predictive Severe Acute Cholecystitis

The use of cholecystostomy has been reported in the literature both in severe cholecystitis and in high surgical risk patients with every form of cholecystitis [61–64]. Small series comparing cholecystostomy with no cholecystostomy prior to laparoscopic cholecystectomy in acute cholecystitis and suppurative cholecystitis have reported a reduction in complications and conversion rates [65, 66].

We compared patients presenting with such a clinical picture to be treated or not by cholecystostomy prior to laparoscopic cholecystectomy. The results show no differences in conversion, post-operative complications, mortality and post-operative and overall hospital stay as shown in Table 19.4. However, in this series the laparoscopic cholecystectomies were performed by a surgeon experienced in the laparoscopic treatment of acute cholecystitis. Since systematic percutaneous cholecystostomy (PC) proved useful in our early experience, such a procedure should be considered when stating indications for treatment of predictive severe acute cholecystitis.

Perforated Acute Cholecystitis

Indications for perforated acute choecystitis are based on the extent of peri-cholecystic abscess; there is no evidence that preoperative drainage improves feasibility of laparoscopic cholecystectomy, but it has the advantage of resolving systemic signs prior to surgery. In our experience, preoperative drainage was performed in three of 12 cases, ten patients were approached by open surgery, and in two patients a laparoscopic approach proved feasible, with

Table 19.4 Comparative results in predictive severe acute cholecystitis without associated disease treated by pre-operative PC or untreated before laparoscopic cholecystectomy

	PC + cholecystectomy group	Cholecystectomy group	p-value
No. cases	23	34	
Cholecystectomy: Laparotomy/laparoscopy	0/23	1/33	
Conversion	1 (4.4%)	1 (3%)	1
Complications	1 (4.4%)	3 (8.8%)	0.64
Post-operative stay (days)	2.7 SD 1.3	3.3 SD 2.9	0.358
Total hospitalisation (days)	5.6 SD 1.8	4.6 SD 3.4	0.2<

PC, percutaneous cholecystotomy

drainage being performed during laparoscopic cholecystectomy.

Acute Cholecystitis and Liver Abscesses

We have observed five cases of acute cholecystitis and liver abscesses [32]. A percutaneous treatment was performed in all patients with resolution of the abscess in all cases. Cholecystectomy was performed on four patients: by open surgery in two and by laparoscopy in the other two patients with neither conversion nor post-operative morbidity.

Acute Cholecystitis with Associated Diseases

Acute cholecystitis with associated diseases is the main indication reported in the literature for pre-operative or definitive treatment by PC [29, 61, 63, 64]. Evaluation of results on a comparative basis is not allowed in our series because patients treated by PC differ significantly from those operated on without PC treatment. The use of PC is justified by the physiopathology of acute cholecystitis: the distension of the gallbladder is the underlying process of the inflammation, acting through autonomic nerves and mediators and it may lead to possible complications in distant organs whose functions are impaired due to co-morbidities. Urgent intervention is therefore advocated to avoid worsening of clinical conditions and the risk of ongoing sepsis and death, but may play an additional role in overall complications and mortality [39, 40, 51]. Urgent cholecystostomy may be indicated in such cases, allowing a delayed cholecystectomy after local and systemic signs of the inflammatory process have disappeared. Due to the proven efficacy of such an approach, a randomised study would not be ethical. In our experience we have not found the expected differences between patients with and without associated disease when ASA III/IV patients were treated by properative PC. The results reported in Table 19.5 from the more recent series allow indications to be redefined, in a group of patients classified ASA III without decompensated disease or recurrent acute illness, no differences were observed in PC treatment versus loparoscopic cholecystectomy.

Acute Cholecystitis with Bilio-pancreatic Complications

Despite increasing incidence of common bile duct stones and acute biliary pancreati-

Table 19.5 Comparative results in ASA III patients without decompensated chronic disease or severe cholecystitis either treated by pre-operative PC or not treated

	PC + cholecystectomy group	Cholecystectomy group	p-value
No. cases	31	27	
Cholecystectomy: Laparotomy/laparoscopy	4/27	0/27	
Conversion	3.7%	0	1
Complications	8 (25.8%)	5 (18.5%)	0.541
Post-operative stay (days)	4.5 SD 3.4	3.4 SD 3.3	0.234
Total hospitalisation (days)	10.1 SD 6	4 SD 3.6	<0.001

PC, percutaneous cholecystotomy

tis in association with AGC, due to a higher population mean age [41, 42] no randomized trials have been conducted on this topic. Randomised studies have been published in non acute cholecystitis cases to evaluate laparoscopic treatment versus pre-operative endoscopy or laparoscopic treatment with intra-operative endoscopy [67–69]. Laparoscopic treatment for common bile duct stones is related to the experience of the surgeon; it is not yet the gold standard treatment [70] and has not been evaluated in acute cholecystitis. We introduced intra-operative endoscopic treatment with the Rendez-vous technique in 2002. Such a trans-papillary approach is preferred since the risk related to choledocotomy may be increased by local inflammation in acute cholecystitis. The intra-operative Rendez-vous technique has been evaluated in an historical comparative analysis with pre-operative endoscopic retrograde cholangiopancreatography (ERCP) that was adopted in the early stages. The results reported in Table 19.6 do not show differences in conversion rate and morbidity, but reveal a longer post-operative stay in the Rendez-vous group and a significant longer overall hospital stay in the historical group.

Peritonitis Syndrome with Haemodynamic Instability

Urgent surgery is advocated due to very high mortality. A laparoscopic approach needs to be evaluated due to the possible consequences of pneumoperitoneum in such patients.

Conclusion

Treatment of acute cholecystitis needs to be modulated on the basis of its clinical features; treatment strategies may be stated as follows:

1. Uncomplicated cholecystitis: urgent laparoscopic cholecystectomy with intra-operative cholangiography.
2. Predictive severe acute cholecystitis without acute or chronic systemic diseases: pre-operative PC or urgent laparoscopic cholecystectomy with intra-operative cholangiography.
3. Perforated acute cholecystitis or liver abscess: pre-operative percutaneous drainage and cholecystectomy open or laparoscopic on the basis of extent of collections.

Table 19.6 Historical comparison of patients treated by pre-operative ERCP followed by cholecystectomy (historical group) and patients treated intra-operatively with the rendez-vous technique

	ERPC + cholecystectomy group	Cholecystectomy + rendez-vous group	p-value
No. cases	53	53	
Cholecystectomy: Laparotomy/laparoscopy	1/47	2/50	
ASA III with predictive severe acute cholecystitis	9	6	
Conversion	4 (8.5%)	3 (6%)	0.7
Complications	5 (10.7%)	7 (14%)	0.76
Post-operative stay (days)	3.6 SD 1.6	5.3 SD 4.1	0.01
Total hospitalisation (days)	12.7 SD 5.6	8.9 SD 5.6	0.001

ERCP, endoscopic retrograde cholangiopancreatography

4. Acute cholecystitis complicated with liver abscess: pre-operative percutaneous drainage and cholecystectomy open or laparoscopic.
5. Acute cholecystitis in ASA III/IV patients:
   - urgent PC as definitive treatment in patients unfit for surgery with trans-catheter cholangiography and endoscopic treatment of common bile duct stones when required.
   - pre-operative PC with trans-catheter cholangiography and laparoscopic cholecystectomy after treatment of associated acute conditions in decompensated patients.
   - urgent cholecystectomy for ASA III patients without decompensated diseases or predictive severe cholecystitis.
6. Acute cholecystitis with bilio-pancreatic complications without systemic disease: intra-operative endoscopic treatment with the Rendez-vous technique on the basis of intra-operative cholangiography.
7. Peritonitis syndrome: urgent surgery.

References

1. Langenbuch C (1882) Ein fall von exstirpation der gallenblase wegen chronischer cholelithiasis Heilung Berl Klin wochenschr 19:725-727
2. Duron JJ, Roux JM, Imbaud P et al (1987) Biliary lithiasis in the over seventy-five age group: a new therapeutic strategy. Br J Surg 74:848-849
3. Inglesakis JA, Migliori G, Chabannes B (1981) Facteurs de gravité de la lithiase de la voie biliaire principale après 75 ans. Chirurgie 107:34-43
4. Greenburg AG, Saik RP, Coyle JJ, Peskin GW (1981) Mortality and gastrointestinal surgery in the aged: elective vs emergency procedures. Arch Surg 116:788-791
5. Houghton PWJ, Jenkinson LR, Donaldson LA (1985) Cholecystectomy in the elderly: a prospective study. Br J Surg 72:220-222
6. Addison NV, Finan PJ (1988) Urgent and early cholecystectomy for acute gallbladder disease. Br J Surg 75:141-143
7. Lahtinen J, Alhava EM, Aukee S (1978) Acute cholecystitis treated by early and delayed surgery. A controlled clinical trial. Scand J Gastroenterol 13:673-678
8. Jarvinen HJ, Hastbacka J (1980) Early cholecystectomy for acute cholecystitis: a prospective randomized study. Ann Surg 191:501-505
9. Schaefer D, Barth H, Thon K et al (1980) Early or delayed operation in patients with acute cholecystitis. Results of a prospective randomized controlled clinical trial. Chir Forum Exp Klin Forsch pp 149-153
10. Norrby S, Herlin P, Holmin T et al (1983) Early or delayed cholecystectomy in acute cholecystitis? A clinical trial. Br J Surg 70:163-165
11. Radder RW (1980) Ultrasonically guided percutaneous catheter drainage for gallbladder empyema. Diagn Imaging 49:330-333
12. Classen M, Demling L (1974) Endoskopische sphikterotomie der papilla vateri und steinextraktion aus dem ductus choledocus. Dtsch Med Wochenschr 99:496
13. Lo CM, Liu CL, Fan ST et al (1998) Prospective randomized study of early versus delayed laparoscopic cholecystectomy for acute cholecystitis. Ann Surg 227:461-467
14. Lai PB, Kwong KH, Leung KL et al (1998) Randomized trial of early versus delayed laparoscopic cholecystectomy for acute cholecystitis. Br J Surg 85:764-767
15. Chandler CF, Lane JS, Ferguson P et al (2000) Prospective evaluation of early versus delayed laparoscopic cholecystectomy for treatment of acute cholecystitis. Am Surg 66:896-900
16. Johansson M, Thune A, Blomqvist A et al (2003) Management of acute cholecystitis in the laparoscopic era: results of a prospective, randomized clinical trial. J Gastrointest Surg 7:642-645
17. Kolla SB, Aggarwal S, Kumar A et al (2004) Early versus delayed laparoscopic cholecystectomy for acute cholecystitis: a prospective randomized trial. Surg Endosc 18:1323-1327
18. Davila D, Manzanares C, Picho ML et al (1999) Experience in the treatment (early vs delayed) of acute cholecystitis via laparoscopy. Cirugia Espanola 66(Suppl 1):233
19. Vetrhus M, Soreide O, Nesvik I, Sondenaa K (2003) Acute cholecystitis:delayed surgery or observation. A randomized clinical trial. Scand J Gastroenterol 38:985-990
20. Papi C, Catarci M, D'Ambrosio L et al (2004) Timing of cholecystectomy for acute calculous cholecystitis: a meta-analysis. Am J Gastroenterol 99:147-155
21. Lau H, Lo CY, Patil NG, Yuen WK (2006) Early versus delayed-interval laparoscopic cholecystectomy for acute cholecystitis: a metaanalysis. Surg Endosc 20:82-87

22. Shikata S, Noguchi Y, Fukui T (2005) Early versus delayed cholecystectomy for acute cholecystitis:a meta-analysis of randomized controlled trials. Surg Today 35:553-560
23. Gurusamy KS, Samraj K (2006) Early versus delayed laparoscopic cholecystectomy for acute cholecystitis. Cochrane Database Syst Rev 18(4):CD005440
24. Kiviluoto T, Siren J, Luukkonen P, Kivilaakso E (1998) Randomised trial of laparoscopic versus open cholecystectomy for acute and gangrenous cholecystitis. Lancet 351:321-325
25. Johansson M, Thune A, Nelvin L et al (2005) Randomized clinical trial of open versus laparoscopic cholecystectomy in the treatment of acute cholecystitis. Br J Surg 92:44-49
26. Hendolin HI, Paakonen ME, Alhava EM et al (2000) Laparoscopic or open cholecystectomy:a prospective randomised trial to compare postoperative pain, pulmonary function, and stress response. Eur J Surg 166:394-399
27. Hsieh CH (2003) Early minilaparoscopic cholecystectomy in patients with acute cholecystitis. Am J Surg 185:344-348
28. Akyürek N, Salman B, Yüksel O et al (2005) Management of acute calculous cholecystitis in high-risk patients: percutaneous cholecystotomy followed by early laparoscopic cholecystectomy. Surg Laparosc Endosc Percutan Tech 15:315-320
29. Hatzidakis AA, Prassopoulos P, Petinarakis I et al (2002) Acute cholecystitis in high-risk patients: percutaneous cholecystostomy vs conservative treatment. Eur Radiol 12:1778-1784
30. Ito K, Fujita N, Noda Y et al (2004) Percutaneous cholecystostomy versus gallbladder aspiration for acute cholecystitis: a prospective randomized controlled trial. AJR 183:193-196
31. Borzellino G, Sauerland S, Minicozzi AM et al (2007) Laparoscopic cholecystectomy for severe acute cholecystitis. A meta-analysis of results. Surg Endosc, in press
32. Zerman G, Bonfiglio M, Borzellino G et al (2003) Liver abscess due to acute cholecystitis. Report of five cases. Chir Ital 55:195-198
33. Scheele S, Miller DA, Hardy KJ (1999) The early operation for acute severe cholecystitis: the Riedel paper; an introduction and translation. Aust NZ J Surg 69:871-877
34. Koperna T, Kisser M, Schulz F (1999) Laparoscopic versus open treatment of patients with acute cholecystitis. Hepatogastroenterology 46:753-757
35. Schafer M, Krahenbuhl L, Buchler MW (2001) Predictive factors for the type of surgery in acute cholecystitis. Am J Surg 182:291-297
36. Brodsky A, Matter I, Sabo E et al (2000) Laparoscopic cholecystectomy for acute cholecystitis: can the need for conversion and the probability of complications be predicted? A prospective study. Surg Endosc 14:7557-60
37. Prakash K, Jacob G, Lekha V et al (2002) Laparoscopic cholecystectomy in acute cholecystitis. Surg Endosc 16:180-183
38. Araujo-Teixeira JP, Rocha-Reis J, Costa-Cabral A (1999) Laparoscopie ou laparatomie dans la cholécystite aigue (200 cas). Comparaison des résultats et facteurs prédisposants à la conversion. Chirurgie 124:529-535
39. Arvieux-Barthelemy C, Mestrallet J, Bouchard F et al (1999) Traitement chirurgical de la cholécystite aigue. Ann Chir 53:472-481
40. Navez B, Mutter D, Russier Y et al (2001) Safety of laparoscopic approach for acute cholecystitis: retrospective study of 609 cases. World J Surg 25:1352-1356
41. Kunin N, Letoquart JP, La Gamma A et al (1994) La cholécystite aigue chez le sujet agé. J Chir 131:257-260
42. Borzellino G, de Manzoni G, Ricci F et al (1999) Emergency cholecystostomy and subsequent cholecystectomy for acute gallstone cholecystitis in the elderly. Br J Surg 86:1306-1311
43. Borzellino G, Tasselli S, Zerman G et al (2002) Results of surgical treatment of acute cholecystitis. Prospective study of 280 cases. G Chir 23:79-84
44. Pessaux P, Tuech JJ, Regenet N et al (2000) Laparoscopic cholecystectomy in the treatment of acute cholecystitis. Prospective non-randomized study. Gastroenterol Clin Biol 24:400-403
45. Willsher PC, Sanabria JR, Gallinger S et al (1999) Early laparoscopic cholecystectomy for acute cholecystitis: a safe procedure. J Gastrointest Surg 3:50-53
46. Glavic Z, Begic L, Simlesa D, Rukavina A (2001) Treatment of acute cholecystitis. A comparison of open vs laparoscopic cholecystectomy. Surg Endosc 15:398-401
47. Teixeira JP, Saraiva AC, Cabral AC et al (2000) Conversion factors in laparoscopic cholecystectomy for acute cholecystitis. Hepatogastroenterology 47:626-630
48. Serralta AS, Bueno JL, Planells MR, Rodero DR (2003) Prospective evaluation of emergency versus delayed laparoscopic cholecystectomy for early cholecystitis. Surg Laparosc Endosc Percutan Tech 13:71-75
49. Madan AK, Aliabadi-Wahle S, Tesi D et al (2002) How early is early laparoscopic treatment of acute cholecystitis? Am J Surg 183:232-236
50. Lujan JA, Parrilla P, Robles R et al (1998) Laparoscopic cholecystectomy vs open cholecystectomy in the treatment of acute cholecystitis: a prospective study. Arch Surg 133:173-175
51. Suter M, Meyer A (2001) A 10-year experience with the use of laparoscopic cholecystectomy for

acute cholecystitis: is it safe? Surg Endosc 15:1187-1192
52. Puggioni A, Wong LL (2003) A metaanalysis of laparoscopic cholecystectomy in patients with cirrhosis. J Am Coll Surg 197:921-926
53. de Manzoni G, Furlan F, Guglielmi A et al (1992) Acute cholecystitis: ultrasonographic staging and percutaneous cholecystostomy. Eur J Radiol 15:175-179
54. Nguyen L, Fagan SP, Lee TC et al (2004) Use of a predictive equation for diagnosis of acute gangrenous cholecystitis. Am J Surg 188:463-466
55. Trowbridge RL, Rutkowski NK, Shojania KG (2003) Does this patient have acute cholecystitis? JAMA 289:80-86
56. De Vargas Macciucca M, Lanciotti S, De Cicco ML et al (2006) Ultrasonographic and spiral CT evaluation of simple and complicated acute cholecystitis: diagnostic protocol assessment based on personal experience and review of the literature Radiol Med 111:167-180
57. Adamietz B, Wenkel E, Uder M et al (2007) Contrast enhanced sonography of the gallbladder: a tool in the diagnosis of cholecystitis? Eur J Radiol 61:262-266
58. Wilson AK, Kozol RA, Salwen WA et al (1994) Gangrenous cholecystitis in an urban VA hospital. J Surg Res 56:402-404
59. Eldar S, Sabo E, Nash E et al (1997) Laparoscopic cholecystectomy for acute cholecystitis: prospective trial. World J Surg 21:540-545
60. Sauerland S, Agresta F, Bergamaschi R et al (2006) Laparoscopy for abdominal emergencies: evidence-based guidelines of the European Association for Endoscopic Surgery. Surg Endosc 20:14-29
61. Welschbillig-Meunier K, Pessaux P, Lebigot J et al (2005) Percutaneous cholecystostomy for high-risk patients with acute cholecystitis. Surg Endosc 19:1256-1259
62. Tseng LJ, Tsai CC, Mo LR et al (2000) Palliative percutaneous transhepatic gallbladder drainage of gallbladder empyema before laparoscopic cholecystectomy. Hepatogastroenterology 47:932-936
63. Chikamori F, Kuniyoshi N, Shibuya S, Takase Y (2002) Early scheduled laparoscopic cholecystectomy following percutaneous transhepatic gallbladder drainage for patients with acute cholecystitis. Surg Endosc 16:1704-1707
64. Tsumura H, Ichikawa T, Hiyama E et al (2004) An evaluation of laparoscopic cholecystectomy after selective percutaneous transhepatic gallbladder drainage for acute cholecystitis. Gastrointest Endosc 59:839-844
65. Kim KH, Sung CK, Park BK et al (2000) Percutaneous gallbladder drainage for delayed laparoscopic cholecystectomy in patients with acute cholecystitis. Am J Surg 179:111-113
66. Mo LR, Yau MP, Tsai CC et al (1995) Ultrasound-guided percutaneous transhepatic gallbladder drainage followed by laparoscopic cholecystectomy: a new trial in the treatment of severe acute suppurative cholecystitis. Hepatogastroenterology 42:51-54
67. Morino M, Baracchi F, Miglietta C et al (2006) Preoperative endoscopic sphincterotomy versus laparoendoscopic Rendez-vous in patients with gallbladder and bile duct stones. Ann Surg 244:889-893
68. Suc B, Escat J, Cherqui D et al (1998) Surgery vs endoscopy as primary treatment in symptomatic patients with suspected common bile duct stones: a multicenter randomized trial. French Associations for Surgical Research. Arch Surg 133:702-708
69. Hong DF, Xin Y, Chen DW (2006) Comparison of laparoscopic cholecystectomy combined with intraoperative endoscopic sphincterotomy and laparoscopic exploration of the common bile duct for cholecystocholedocholithiasis. Surg Endosc 20:424-427
70. Shamiyeh A, Wayand W (2005) Current status of laparoscopic therapy of cholecystolithiasis and common bile duct stones. Dig Dis 23:119-126

Chapter 20

Incidental Carcinoma of the Gallbladder

Lorenzo Capussotti, Andrea Muratore, Alessandro Ferrero, Luca Viganò

Introduction

Gallbladder cancer is the most common malignant neoplasm of the biliary tract [1, 2]. The reported incidence of incidental gallbladder carcinoma during or after laparoscopic cholecystectomy ranges from 0.2% to 0.6% [3–5]. Most incidental gallbladder carcinomas are T1 (tumor invading the lamina propria or muscle layer). Despite recent progress in diagnostic techniques and equipment, preoperative diagnosis of gallbladder cancer is often difficult, especially if gallstone disease is present and tumor invasion is limited to the gallbladder wall [6]. If gallbladder cancer is suspected intraoperatively, the diagnostic accuracy of the frozen section is high, but the frozen section yields less reliable information about the depth of tumor invasion (T) [7]. However, depth of tumor invasion is the only staging parameter available when diagnosis of gallbladder carcinoma is reached intra- or postoperatively. The subsequent treatment of the gallbladder cancer is determined with reference both to T and to the status of the cystic duct margin (infiltration or no infiltration).

Tis-1 Tumors

Tis (in situ cancer) and T1 gallbladder cancers are usually diagnosed at the final pathology after cholecystectomy. Tis and T1 tumors account for 4% and 10–15%, respectively, of all patients with a diagnosis of gallbladder cancer [8, 9].

If the cystic duct margin is negative for infiltration, simple cholecystectomy is an adequate treatment for Tis and T1a (lamina propria invasion) gallbladder cancers: the 5-year survival rates range from 83% to 100% [8, 10–12].

Whether simple cholecystectomy is an adequate treatment for T1b (muscle layer invasion) gallbladder cancer is still a matter of discussion. Wakai has reported a good long-term outcome regardless of whether simple or extended cholecystectomy (cholecystectomy + liver resection + lymph node dissection) was performed [13]. However, a multicenter retrospective French study revealed high recurrence rates (26%) after simple cholecystectomy for T1b disease [8]. Similarly, high recurrence rates have recently been confirmed by Wagholikar [14]. These findings are supported by the results of a multicenter Japanese study in 1,686 patients who underwent extended cholecystectomy for gallbladder cancer: the rate of lymph node metastases was 2.5% in T1a patients (n=201), but was 15.5% in T1b patients (n=165) [15]. However, a recent paper does not report lymph node metastases in any of 12 T1b patients who underwent extended cholecystectomy; moreover, the long-term outcome after simple cholecystectomy was comparable to that after extended cholecystectomy [13].

In conclusion, Tis and T1 gallbladder cancers are usually incidental discoveries during or, more often, after laparoscopic cholecystectomy performed for gallstone disease: simple cholecystectomy is an adequate treatment for patients with Tis or T1a tumors, and no further reoperation is necessary if the cystic duct margin is negative for infiltration. Literature data about the best treatment for T1b patients are contradictory. In our opinion, if the patient is otherwise healthy, liver resection (gallbladder bed resection or resection of segments 4b–5) + lymph node dissection of N1 station nodes (N1 stations: cystic duct, pericholedochal, and common hepatic artery nodes) as well as excision of the port sites should be recommended.

If the cystic duct margin is positive at final pathology, the patient should undergo reoperation regardless of the T1 status.

T2 Tumors

T2 gallbladder cancers (invasion of perimuscular connective tissue without extension into the serosa or the liver) are usually diagnosed during or, more often, after laparoscopic cholecystectomy [16]. Simple cholecystectomy is not an adequate treatment. The most appropriate treatment is resection of segments 4b–5 (Sg 4b–5) and both N1 and N2 dissection of lymph node stations (N1 stations: cystic duct, pericholedochal and proper hepatic artery nodes; N2 stations: caudal retroportal nodes, retropancreaticoduodenal nodes, common hepatic artery nodes) plus excision of the port sites [17]. If the diagnosis is made postoperatively, the patient concerned should undergo computed tomography of the chest and abdomen before reoperation. The rationale for segment 4b–5 resection and N1–2 lymph node dissection is as follows:

1. some authors have shown that angiolymphatic invasion of segments 4b–5 is possible in up to 10% of these patients, even in the absence of direct liver invasion [18, 19];
2. the lymph node metastases rate of T2 gallbladder cancers is around 40% [15, 16]. The lymph nodes most commonly affected are the cystic and pericholedochal nodes (N1 stations), followed by the retroportal, retropancreaticoduodenal, and common hepatic artery nodes (N2 stations) [20].

The 5-year survival rates of T2 patients are 22–40% after simple cholecystectomy, increasing to 60–100% after a more extensive resection [8, 21–26]. In our series of 30 patients with T2 gallbladder cancer, 25 underwent extended cholecystectomy, whereas 5 did not because of poor performance status or refusal of reoperation: the median survival rates in these two subgroups were 63 and 16 months, respectively (p=0.2). If T2 gallbladder cancer is discovered postoperatively, reoperation should be done as soon as possible, before the appearance of a macroscopic recurrence, as this is associated with a dismal prognosis even when a subsequent radical reoperation is performed; if this is done shortly after the simple cholecystectomy the presence of residual disease (i.e., regional lymph node metastases) in the specimen does affect long-term outcome [16].

In conclusion, T2 gallbladder cancers discovered incidentally during or after simple cholecystectomy should be treated by segment 4b–5 resection, dissection of N1–2 lymph nodes, and excision of the port sites. If T2 gallbladder cancer is discovered postoperatively, reresection should be performed as soon as possible. The treatment of the cystic duct is explained in the section, "*Cystic Duct and Bile Duct Resection.*"

T3-T4 Tumors

T3 (extension into gallbladder serosa and/or infiltration of the liver and/or of one adjacent organ) and T4 (infiltration of the portal vein or of the hepatic artery or of more than one extrahepatic structure) gallbladder cancers are usually diagnosed preoperatively.

However, in our series one third of T3 gallbladder cancers were diagnosed from incidental findings during or after simple cholecystectomy. The reason is the difficulty of the differential diagnosis between chronic cholecystitis with a thick-walled gallbladder and cancer (Fig. 20.1). The appropriate treatment is segment 4b–5 resection combined with N1–2 lymph node dissection and with excision of the port sites. If the gallbladder cancer invades the hepatic pedicle (hilum type), extended right hepatectomy yields a higher rate of negative margins than does segment 4b–5 resection, but the type of resection does not seem to improve survival [19]. The lymph node metastasis rate of T3–4 gallbladder cancers is around 80% [15, 20]. Moreover, involvement of N2 lymph nodes is significantly more frequent than in the case of T2 gallbladder cancers [20]. The treatment of the cystic duct is explained in the section, "*Cystic Duct and Bile Duct Resection.*

Port Site Excisions

The rate of port site recurrence after laparoscopic cholecystectomy and incidental diagnosis of gallbladder cancer ranges from 10% to 19% [25, 27–29]. Port site recurrence usually occurs in T2 or more advanced gallbladder cancers and is significantly more frequent if the gallbladder is perforated during the cholecystectomy [25, 27]. Experimental studies have shown that pneumoperitoneum significantly increases tumor implantation and growth at trocar sites and that peritoneal injuries, e.g., by trocar insertion, enhance peritoneal implantation of carcinoma cells [30–32]. Thereafter, if gallbladder cancer is diagnosed intraoperatively, the laparoscopic procedure should be converted to an open procedure. The trocar port sites should be routinely excised.

Cystic Duct and Bile Duct Resection

If the gallbladder cancer is diagnosed intraoperatively, a frozen section of the cystic duct margin should be prepared for pathology. If it is positive, further resection of the cystic duct and, probably, of the bile duct must be performed in order to obtain a negative margin. If the gallbladder cancer is diagnosed postoperatively, the status of the cystic duct margin at the final pathology of the gallbladder specimen must be checked; if the status of the margin is positive or

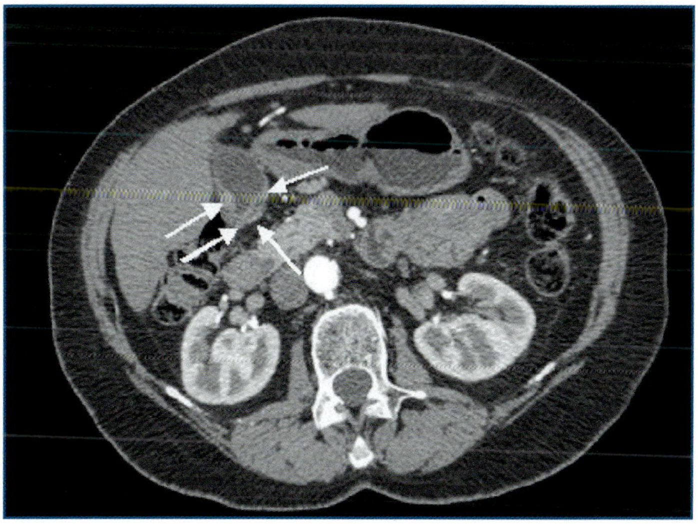

Fig. 20.1 Chronic cholecystitis with thick-walled gallbladder mimicking a gallbladder cancer on CT scan

unknown the patient should be operated on again regardless of the depth of tumor invasion. Further resection and frozen section of the cystic duct should be performed until a negative margin is obtained.

Japanese authors have advocated routine resection of the common bile duct among patients with advanced gallbladder cancer even in the absence of direct infiltration [33, 34]. However, Kosuge analyzed 55 patients with gallbladder cancer and without bile duct infiltration and shown that bile duct resection improves overall survival only in T4 patients [35]. More recently, other authors have shown that routine resection of the common bile duct does not improve long-term survival providing the surgical margins are negative [36].

We do not perform resection of the bile duct unless either direct bile duct infiltration is suspected or a negative margin cannot be achieved by further resection of an infiltrated cystic duct.

References

1. Misra S, Chaturvedi A, Misra NC, Sharma ID (2003) Carcinoma of the gallbladder. Lancet Oncol 4:167-176
2. Reid KM, De la Medina AR, Donohue JH (2007) Diagnosis and surgical management of gallbladder cancer: a review. J Gastrointest Surg 11:671-681
3. Antonakis P, Alexakis N, Mylonaki D et al (2003) Incidental finding of gallbladder carcinoma detected during or after laparoscopic cholecystectomy. Eur J Surg Oncol 29:358-360
4. Chan CP, Chang HC, Chen YL et al (2003) A 10-year experience of unsuspected gallbladder cancer after laparoscopic cholecystectomy. Int Surg 88:175-179
5. Contini S, Dalla Valle R, Zinicola R (1999) Unexpected gallbladder cancer after laparoscopic cholecystectomy. An emerging problem? Reflections on four cases. Surg Endosc 13:264-267
6. Onoyama H, Yamamoto M, Takada M et al (1999) Diagnostic imaging of early gallbladder cancer: retrospective study of 53 cases. World J Surg 23:708-712
7. Yamaguchi K, Chijiva K, Saiki S et al (1997) Reliability of frozen section diagnosis of gallbladder tumor for detecting carcinoma and depth of its invasion. J Surg Oncol 65:132-136
8. Benoist S, Panis Y, Fagniez PL and the French University Association for Surgical Research (1998) Long-term results after curative resection for carcinoma of the gallbladder. Am J Surg 175:118-122
9. Muratore A, Polastri R, Bouzari H et al (2000) Radical surgery for gallbladder cancer: a worthwhile operation? Eur J Surg Oncol 26:160-163
10. Shirai Y, Yoshida K, Tsukada K et al (1992) Early carcinoma of the gallbladder. Eur J Surg 158:545-548
11. Cubertafond P, Mathonnet M, Gainant A, Launois B (1999) Radical surgery for gallbladder cancer. Results of the French Surgical Association Survey. Hepatogastroenterology 46:1567-1571
12. Ouchi K, Sugawara T, Ono H et al (1999) Diagnostic capability and rational resectional surgery for early gallbladder cancer. Hepatogastroenterology 46:1557-1560
13. Wakai T, Shirai Y, Yokoyama N et al (2001) Early gallbladder carcinoma does not warrant radical resection Br J Surg 88:675-678
14. Wagholikar GD, Behari A, Krishnani N et al (2002) Early gallbladder cancer. J Am Coll Surg 194:137-141
15. Ogura Y, Mizumoto R, Isaji S et al (1991) Radical operations for carcinoma of the gallbladder. World J Surg 15:337-343
16. Muratore A, Amisano M, Viganò L et al (2003) Gallbladder cancer invading the perimuscular connective tissue: results of reresection after prior non-curative operation. J Surg Oncol 83:212-215
17. Muratore A, Polastri R, Capussotti L (2000) Radical surgery for gallbladder cancer: current options. Eur J Surg Oncol 26:438-443
18. Hirai Y, Tsukada K, Ohtani T et al (1995) Hepatic metastases from carcinoma of the gallbladder. Cancer 75:2063-2068
19. Yoshikawa T, Araida T, Azuma T, Takasaki K (1998) Bisubsegmental liver resection for gallbladder cancer. Hepatogastroenterology 45:14-19
20. Tsukada K, Kurosaki I, Uchida K et al (1997) Lymph node spread from carcinoma of the gallbladder. Cancer 80:661-667
21. Bartlett DL, Fong Y, Fortner JG et al (1996) Long-term results after resection for gallbladder cancer: implications for staging and management. Ann Surg 5:639-646
22. Cubertafond P, Gainant A, Cucchiaro G (1994) Surgical treatment of 724 carcinomas of the gallbladder; results of the French Surgical Association Survey. Ann Surg 219:275-280
23. Yamaguchi K, Chijiiwa K, Saiki K et al (1997) Retrospective analysis of 70 operations for gallbladder carcinoma. Br J Surg 84:200-204

24. Shirai Y, Yoshida K, Tsukada K, Muto T (1992) Inapparent carcinoma of gallbladder. An appraisal of radical second operation after simple cholecystectomy. Ann Surg 215:326-331
25. Wakai T, Shirai Y, Hatakeyama K (2002) Radical second resection provides survival benefit for patients with T2 gallbladder carcinoma first discovered after laparoscopic cholecystectomy. World J Surg 26:867-871
26. De Aretxabala X, Roa I, Burgos L et al (2006) Gallbladder cancer: an analysis of a series of 139 patients with invasion restricted to the subserosal layer. J Gastrointest Surg 10:186-192
27. Paolucci V, Schaeff B, Schneider M, Gutt C (1999) Tumor seeding following laparoscopy: international survey. World J Surg 23:989-997
28. Lundberg O, Kristofferson A (1999) Port site metastases from gallbladder cancer after laparoscopic cholecystectomy. Results of a Swedish survey and review of published reports. Eur J Surg 165:215-222
29. Yamaguchi K, Chijiiwa K, Ichimiya H et al (1996) Gallbladder carcinoma in the era of laparoscopic cholecystectomy. Arch Surg 131:981-984
30. Doudle M, King G, Thomas WM, Hewett P (1996) The movement of mucosal cells of the gallbladder within the peritoneal cavity during laparoscopic cholecystectomy. Surg Endosc 10:1092-1094
31. Bouvy ND, Marquet RL, Jeekel J, Bonier HJ (1997) Laparoscopic surgery is associated with less tumor growth stimulation than conventional surgery: an experimental study. Br J Surg 84:358-361
32. Aoki Y, Shimura H, Li H et al (1999) A model of port-site metastases of gallbladder cancer: the influence of peritoneal injury and its repair on abdominal wall metastases. Surgery 125:553-559
33. Tsukada K, Hatakeyama K, Kurosaki I et al (1996) Outcome of radical surgery for carcinoma of the gallbladder according to the TNM stage. Surgery 120:816-822
34. Shimada H, Endo I, Togo S et al (1997) The role of lymph node dissection in the treatment of gallbladder carcinoma. Cancer 79:892-899
35. Kosuge T, Sano K, Shimada K et al (1999) Should the bile duct be preserved or removed in radical surgery for gallbladder cancer. Hepatogastroenterology 46:2133-2137
36. Yokomizo H, Yamane T, Hirata T et al (2007) Surgical treatment of pT2 gallbladder carcinoma: a reevaluation of the therapeutic effect of hepatectomy and extrahepatic bile duct resection based on the long-term outcome. Ann Surg Oncol 14:1366-1373

Chapter 21

Complications of Laparoscopic Cholecystectomy

Gennaro Nuzzo, Felice Giuliante, Francesco Ardito

Epidemiology

The most serious cause of morbidity occurring during cholecystectomy is bile duct injury (BDI) [1, 2]. In fact, major BDIs (involving the common bile duct (CBD), main biliary confluence, or main bile ducts) can have a substantial impact on quality of life and survival of injured patients, who often are young people (mean age 44–55 years) [1, 3–5]. It has been reported recently that after injury there was a nearly threefold increase in the risk of death in the short term compared with patients without BDI [2].

After the introduction of laparoscopic cholecystectomy, together with the increase in the overall number of cholecystectomies [6], an increase in the overall incidence of BDI and in particular of major BDI was reported, compared to that observed during prelaparoscopic era (0.1–0.3%). The incidence of reported BDI varies from 0.25% to 0.74% (Table 21.1), but its true incidence is unknown [9, 16–22]. Since the introduction of laparoscopic cholecystectomy more than 10 years ago, the rate of BDI does not seem to have substantially changed [14, 23, 24], even if some authors report a decreasing trend [8, 9]. In a very recent report from a tertiary care center in the Netherlands analyzing 500 patients with BDIs treated over 15 years, it was reported that 35–40 patients are referred annually to the center, and there is no sign of any recent decrease [24].

Moreover, evaluation not only of the surgical literature but also of the literature on endoscopic and radiological treatment of BDI, suggests indirectly that the actual rate of BDI may be higher than commonly estimated. In fact, the reported incidence of BDI probably underestimates the true incidence for several reasons: 1) a tendency not to report all the injuries, as shown by limit-

Table 21.1 Incidence rates of major BDIs reported in multicentric surveys or population-based studies

Source	Country	Year	No. of cholecystectomies	Incidence of BDI (%)
Wherry DC et al [7]	USA	1996	9,130	0.41
Russel JC et al [8]	USA	1996	15,221	0.25
Richardson MC et al [9]	Scotland	1996	5,913	0.33
Adamsen S et al [10]	Denmark	1997	7,654	0.74
Gigot JF et al [11]	Belgium	1997	9,959	0.50
Mac Fadyen BR et al [12]	USA	1998	114,005	0.50
Z'graggen K et al [13]	Switzerland	1998	10,174	0.31
Nuzzo G et al [14]	Italy	2005	56,591	0.31
Waage A et al [15]	Sweden	2006	152,776	0.40

ed adhesions to the majority of the surveys and by the higher rates from studies based on anonymous responses; 2) an increased number of patients directly referred to endoscopy or radiology units without surgical evaluation; 3) an unknown number of patients treated in the same hospital, without referral to dedicated centers; and 4) an unknown related mortality rate before referral to dedicated centers.

In spite of the precise quantification of the incidence of BDI, it has been suggested that around half of all general surgeons may encounter BDI during their career [25].

Prevention

No cholecystectomy can be considered as a simple routine procedure immune to the risk of BDI [26], and over 70% of surgeons consider BDI unavoidable [25]. Indeed, in a recent Italian national survey [14] which collected 235 BDIs from a series of 56,591 cholecystectomies, about half of the injuries occurred during a laparoscopic cholecystectomy described by surgeons as "technically easy"; furthermore, 80% of the patients with injuries had no risk factors.

However, if it is true that each cholecystectomy can become difficult during the procedure without warning, it is also true that often there are clinical situations in which difficulties during the operation are predictable.

Risk factors for BDI can be related to the patient, to the presence of cholecystitis, to anatomy of the hepatic pedicle and biliary tree and to the experience of the surgeon.

Risk Factors Related to the Patient

Regarding the patient, the main clinical risk factors for BDI are obesity, cirrhosis with portal hypertension, acute or chronic cholecystitis and history of recurrent complications of cholelithiasis (cholecystitis, cholangitis, pancreatitis, increase of alkaline phosphatase and gamma-glutamyl transpeptidase), previous surgical procedures in upper abdominal quadrants and advanced age. At ultrasound, morphological risk criteria are the following: increase in the thickness of gallbladder wall, sclerosis of the wall, distension of the gallbladder with stone impacted at the infundibulum (Fig. 21.1), and modified morphology of the liver (hepatomegaly, lobar hypotrophy or atrophy).

Presence of more than one of these criteria increases both the possibility that the cholecystectomy will be difficult and the possibility of the presence of stones in the CBD. The prevalence of choledocholithiasis has decreased during the last 10 years and currently is less than 10% [27], probably related to the increase in the number of cholecystectomies in young and often asymptomatic patients. The main risk factors for choledocholithiasis are age greater than 60 years and onset of biliary symptoms over a long period. This is a relevant issue because unrecognized choledocholithiasis can cause postoperative

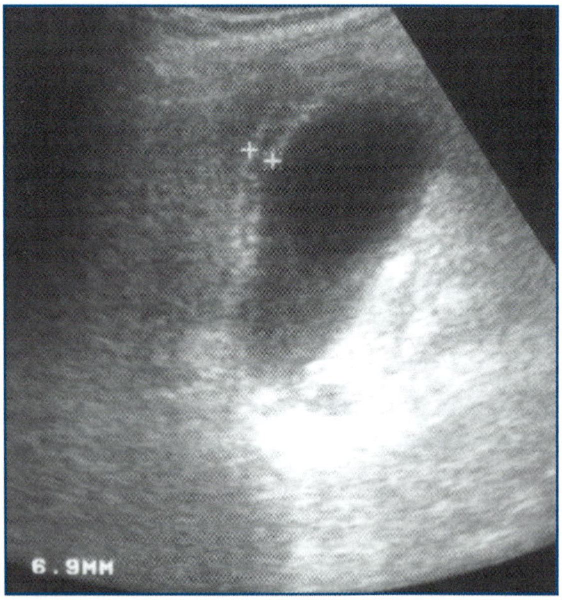

Fig. 21.1 Ultrasound: acute cholecystitis with increase in thickness of the gallbladder wall. Reproduced with permission from [42]

bile leak from the cystic duct, which is one of the most frequent cause of biliary peritonitis after laparoscopic cholecystectomy (Fig. 21.2) [28]. If the presence of stones in the CBD is suspected, preoperative study of the biliary tree is mandatory. Magnetic resonance cholangiography (MRC) is the best imaging technique, with a diagnostic accuracy rate for choledocholithiasis of around 95% [29] and for anatomic variations of cystic duct and of the main biliary confluence of 93–95% [30]. In case of stones in the CBD, the most common response is to perform an endoscopic retrograde cholangiopancreatography (ERCP) to confirm the diagnosis and to remove the stones. In some cases, when clinical and ultrasonographic criteria for a "difficult" cholecystectomy are also present, at the end of ERCP a naso-biliary drain can be left in place (Fig. 21.3). This can be useful during laparoscopic or open cholecystectomy to help recognize the CBD, particularly in cases with acute inflammation of the infundibulum of the gallbladder and of the hepatic pedicle. In this case it is probably safer to proceed from the fundus of the gallbladder toward the neck, to open the gallbladder, to remove the stones and to continue the dissection under the guidance of the finger through an open approach (Fig. 21.4). The presence of a naso-biliary drain into the CBD can be extremely useful for the completion of the cholecystectomy; it can be easily used for intraoperative cholangiography (IOC) and can be useful also as an external biliary drain during the postoperative course.

Obesity [31] and steatotic hepatomegaly increase the difficulty of the procedure because it is more difficult to expose the hepatic pedicle in obese patients and to retract the

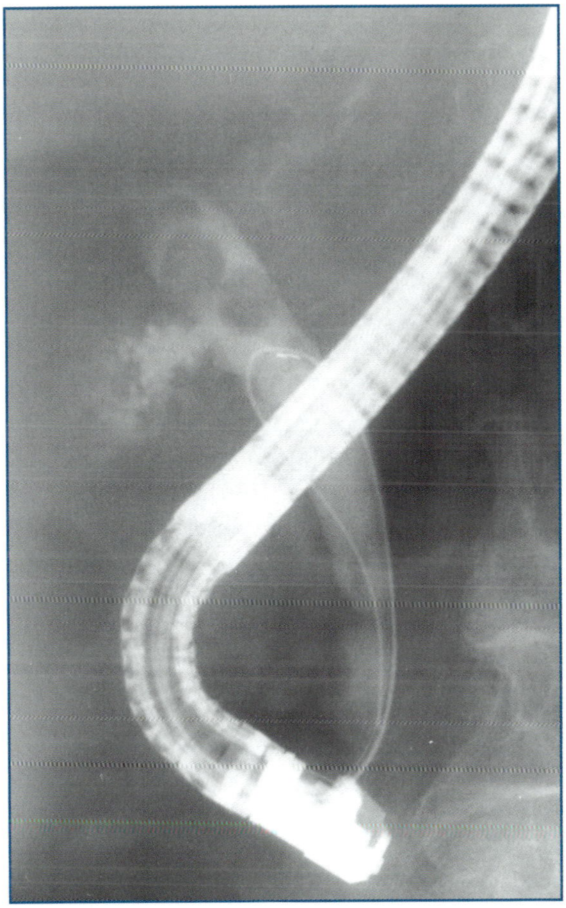

Fig. 21.2 ERCP of a 79-year-old male for biliary fistula on postoperative day 28 after cholecystectomy for gallbladder empyema: leak from the cystic duct stump with choledocholithiasis. Endoscopic sphincterotomy with stones removal; placement of naso-biliary drainage and resolution of leak 5 days after ERCP. Reproduced with permission from [42]

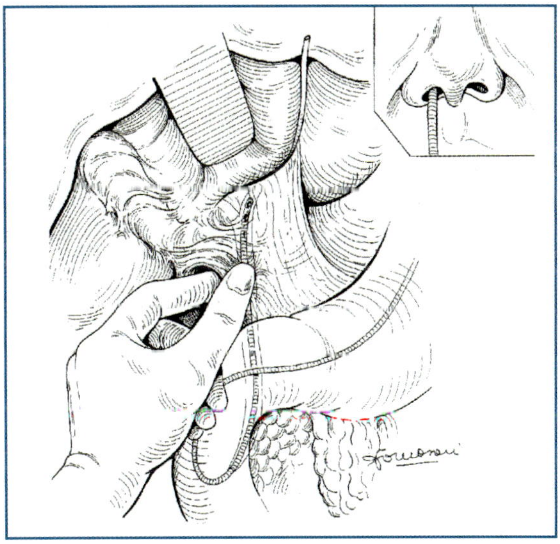

Fig. 21.3 In case of acute or chronic cholecystitis, when inflammation extends to the hepatic pedicle, naso-biliary drainage left in place during preoperative ERCP may help the surgeon to find the CBD. Reproduced with permission from [42]

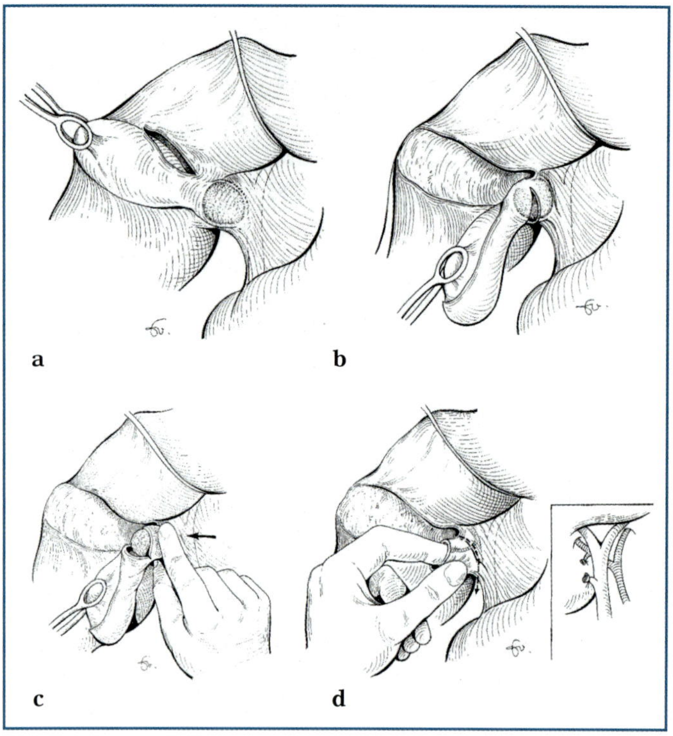

Fig. 21.4 a The presence of a large stone impacted at the infundibulum makes dissection of Calot's triangle dangerous although the attempt at finding an anterograde dissection plane also after laparotomy. **b** It is safer to open the gallbladder, (**c**) to remove the stone and (**d**) to continue cholecystectomy under finger guidance. Reproduced with permission from [42]

fragile and easily bleeding steatotic liver. Cirrhosis is not a contraindication to laparoscopic cholecystectomy, but increases the difficulty of the procedure because the liver is hard, hypomobile, and often with a hypertrophied left lobe that covers the hepatic pedicle. Controlling the bleeding can be difficult because of the presence of venous collateral branches in the hepatic pedicle, severe portal hypertension and portal cavernomatosis can however contraindicate the laparoscopic approach for cholecystectomy (Fig. 21.5). Furthermore, biliary complications in cirrhotic patients can be particularly dangerous, because a simple bile leak can easily cause infection of postoperative ascites with possible severe septic complications [32].

Risk Factors Related to Inflammatory Changes of the Gallbladder

Acute cholecystitis is not a contraindication to laparoscopic cholecystectomy, but since 1994 the European Association for Endoscopic Surgery (EAES) has recommended that patients with acute cholecystitis should be operated upon by expert surgeons [33].

This recommendation was confirmed by Navez and colleagues [34], who analyzed 609 patients with acute cholecystitis operated upon by laparoscopy. The rate of minor BDI was 1.9% and of major BDI was 0.6%, with a conversion rate of 19.8%. The conclusions of this study were that laparoscopy is indicated in acute cholecystitis if performed by a very expert surgeon and confirmed that the best time for operation is within 4 days of symptom onset.

Habib and colleagues [35] analyzed 281 patients submitted to laparoscopic cholecystectomy for acute cholecystitis (20% of whom had gangrenous cholecystitis), and reported a conversion rate of 32% and one BDI (0.35%). Also in this study, the higher degree of difficulty of the procedure than that of simple cholelithiasis was highlighted by a higher conversion rate.

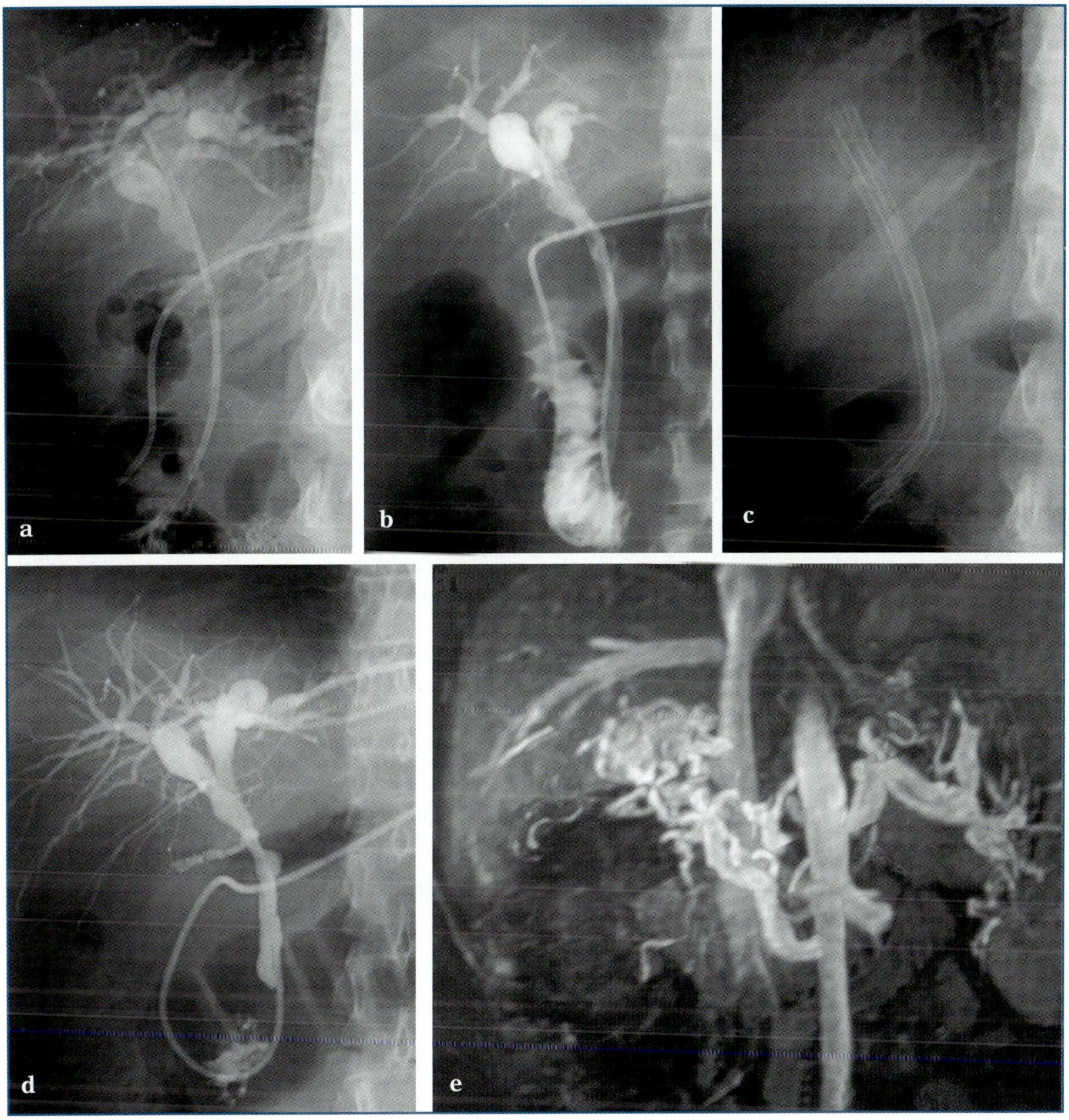

Fig. 21.5 Lithiasis of the gallbladder with increased cholestasis in a 39-year-old female. Portal hypertension and portal cavernomatosis due to neonatal pylephlebitis. Normal preoperative ERCP. Laparoscopic cholecystectomy. Severe intraoperative bleeding, conversion to laparotomy and hemostasis. On postoperative day 2 there was appearance of biliary fistula from abdominal drainage (500–800 mL/day). Reoperation on postoperative day 14, drainage of biliary fistula and its resolution on postoperative day 30. After 5 months, obstructive jaundice occurred (total bilirubin 12.4 mg/dL with increase up to 22 mg/dL). **a** ERCP shows CBD stricture below main biliary confluence, with dilation of right and left hepatic ducts. **b** Placement of one biliary stent and then (**c**) of three stents that were changed after 7, 9 and 11 months. **d** Cholangiography through naso-biliary drain fourteen months after cholecystectomy and removal of stents. **e** MR with vascular reconstruction: large portal cavernomatosis. Reproduced with permission from [42]

In the already mentioned recent Italian survey [14], the overall reported incidence of BDI was 0.42%. The incidence of injury was 0.32% after laparoscopic cholecystectomy performed for simple cholecystectomy and was 0.56% after those performed for acute cholecystitis (p<0.001). Interestingly, teams that were more experienced reported a lower overall incidence of BDI, but BDIs were more frequently observed during procedures performed for cholecystitis. On the contrary, less experienced teams reported a higher overall incidence of BDI, but during operations performed for cholecystitis the incidence of BDI was lower compared to that reported by the more experienced teams (Fig. 21.6). These results are probably related to the higher number of cholecystectomies performed for cholecystitis and to a more aggressive attitude of experienced surgeons in the presence of cholecystitis, and, on the contrary, to a lower number of procedures for cholecystitis and to a more cautious attitude of less experienced surgeons in these settings, with a higher conversion rate. In other words, it could be argued that experienced surgeons have a lower overall incidence of BDI, but cause BDIs more frequently during complex procedures, such as cholecystitis, probably because of their enlarged indications to laparoscopy and their lower conversion rate.

Technical problems during acute cholecystitis are related to: 1) the presence of adhesions, which can be easily divided if the procedure is performed as soon as symptoms occur; 2) distension of the gallbladder, which can be reduced by aspirating its content; 3) the thickening of the wall, which can hamper the traction of the gallbladder; 4) the inflammation of the tissues around Calot's triangle, which can cause bleeding during dissection; 5) the presence of a big, inflamed lymph node, which can bleed or hamper exposure of the cystic duct. In these cases it is important to distinguish the area between the neck of the gallbladder and the cystic duct clearly, to start the dissection at very high level close to the wall of the gallbladder, and then to proceed along both sides of the neck up to reach the liver bed. Detachment of the gallbladder from the liver is easier if cholecystectomy is performed early [36].

Risk Factors Related to the Anatomy of the Hepatic Pedicle

Biliary anatomic variations are frequently described in operative reports of cholecys-

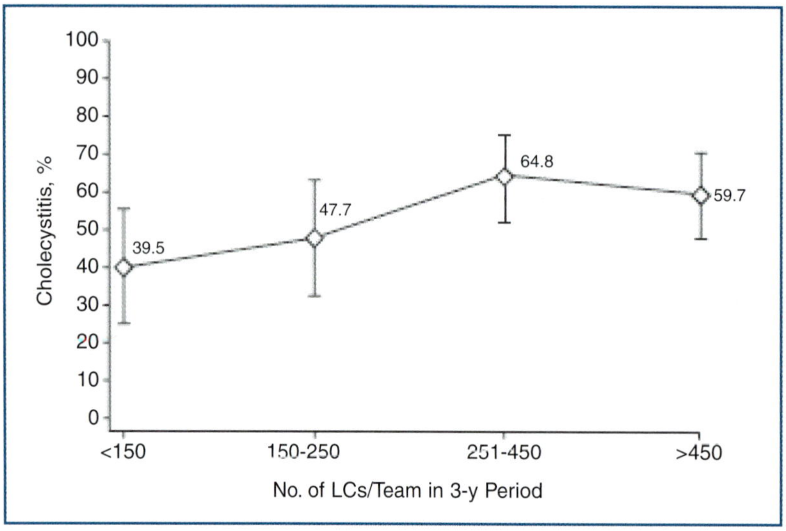

Fig. 21.6 Mean rate of cholecystitis in patients with BDI reported by surgical teams with different volumes of laparoscopic cholecystectomy (LC) in a 3-year period. The change in rate was significant (p = 0.04). Reproduced with permission from [42]

tectomy during which a BDI occurred, but the true impact of these variations is difficult to define and is probably overestimated. Recently, anatomic variations were reported as a cause of BDI in only 12.9% of 235 BDIs collected in the recent national Italian survey [14].

The occurrence of anatomic variations of the biliary tree is frequent, ranging from 30% to 50% [37–40]. This high frequency should be carefully evaluated by the surgeon who should consider any unrecognized biliary duct as an aberrant duct rather than an "accessory" duct. In fact, these ducts drain a portion of liver parenchyma, the amount of which is unknown although often limited, and do not have other communications with the biliary tree. Knowing that the likelihood of encountering such a biliary variation is high, the surgeon should proceed with extreme caution, and always perform an accurate exposure of Calot's triangle, without dividing any unidentified structure. In case of anatomical doubts, the possibility of IOC and conversion should be quickly evaluated.

The most relevant variations are those involving the cystic duct and the main biliary confluence. A truly "dangerous" variation is the junction of the cystic duct in the upper portion of the CBD, close to the main biliary confluence, which is described in 4% of cases (Fig. 21.7) [41]. If an injury to the cystic duct occurs at this level, surgical repair should be very accurate because possible failure will also involve the main biliary confluence.

A long cystic duct, parallel to the CBD, or which usually passes behind the CBD and enters its left side (Fig. 21.8), is an anatomical variation which was more dangerous in the past when avoidance to leave a long cystic stump after cholecystectomy was widely recommended. Laparoscopic technique has modified this attitude, and longer cystic stumps, provided that stones are not present, are now more frequently left behind [42].

The anatomical variations that are truly difficult to recognize are the following: 1) confluence of a right sectorial biliary duct into the gallbladder; and 2) confluence of the cystic duct into the right hepatic duct or into a right sectorial biliary duct (Figs. 21.9, 21.10), but these variations are extremely rare.

Anatomical variations of the main biliary confluence occur in 20–25% of patients and the anatomy of the right hepatic duct is more frequently involved [38, 43, 44]. More often one right sectorial bile duct, the right anterior in 16% of cases and the right posterior in 4%, directly enters the CBD. This slipped-down bile duct passes out of the hilum, where the surgeon, after division of cystic duct, does not usually expect to find other biliary structures. When a sectorial

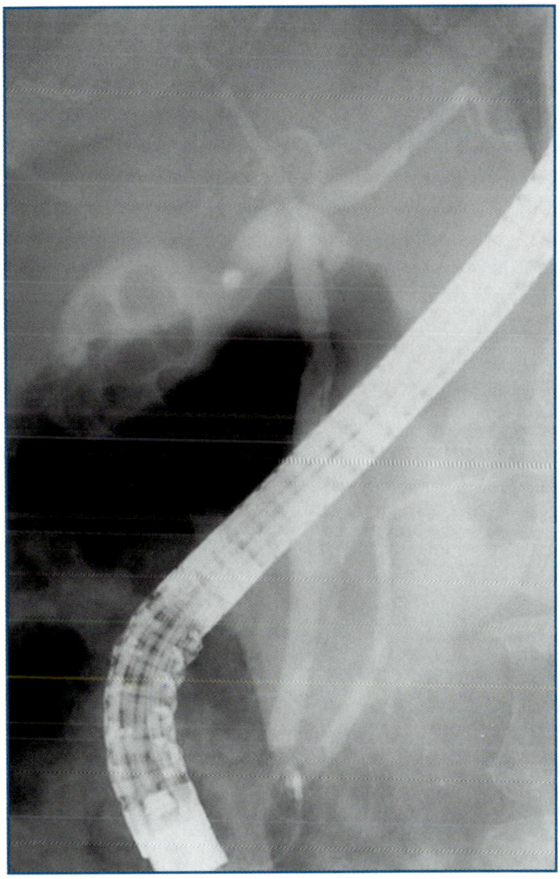

Fig. 21.7 ERCP: cystic duct enters the CBD just below the main biliary confluence. Reproduced with permission from [42]

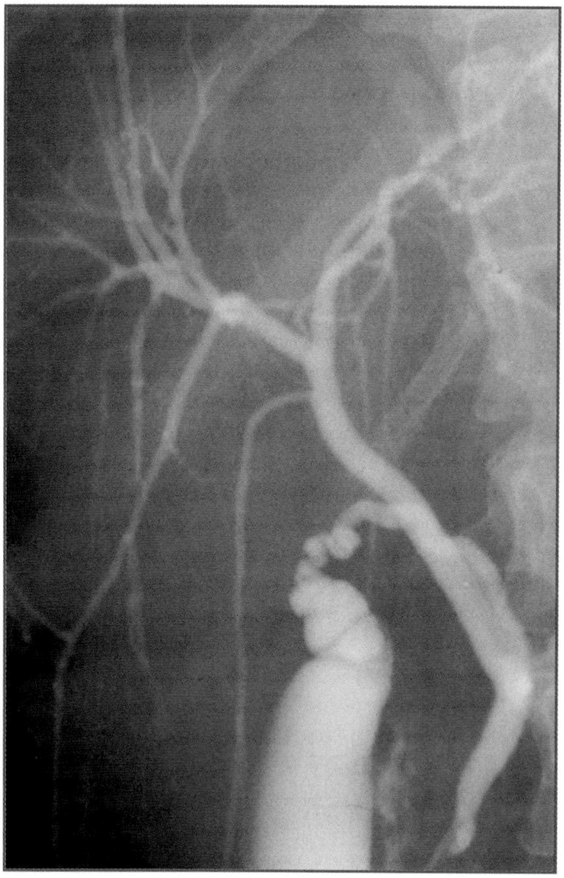

Fig. 21.8 Long cystic duct, parallel to the CBD, which enters its left side. Reproduced with permission from [42]

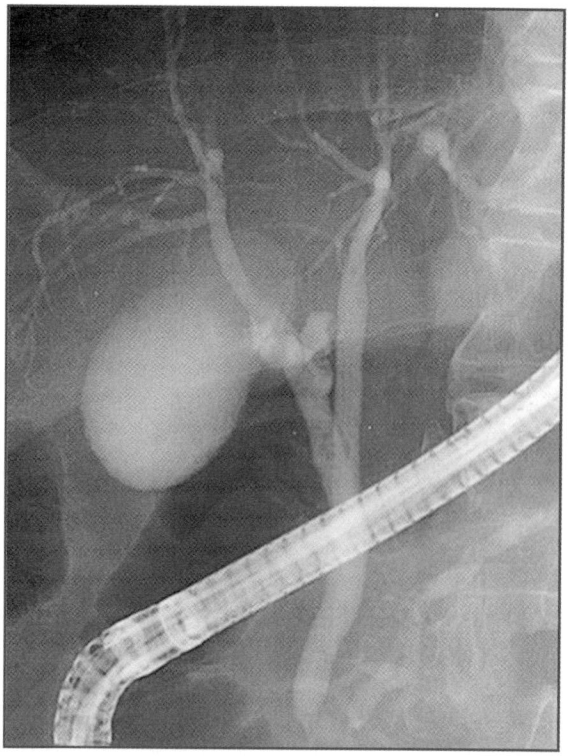

Fig. 21.9 ERCP. "Low" main biliary confluence with cystic duct entering the right hepatic duct. Reproduced with permission from [42]

bile duct is divided, around 30% of functional liver parenchyma is excluded from the biliary drainage into the CBD, and a biliary repair is necessary. Simple closure of the duct would certainly be followed by a biliary fistula, which, if well drained, could take even months to close and would cause atrophy of the involved liver sector.

A "low" main biliary confluence can deceive the surgeon, who may mistake the right hepatic duct for the cystic duct during dissection of Calot's triangle (Fig. 21.9).

Luschka's bile ducts occur in the liver bed as well as it occurs with other small aberrant bile ducts. The incidence of these small ducts is unknown [45]. The most frequently involved areas are the central zones of the liver bed and peritoneal sheaths along the borders of the liver bed [46]. Injuries of these ducts cause intraperitoneal bile leaks. In order to prevent these injuries, the dissection plane should strictly adhere to the gallbladder, away from the fibrous tissue of the liver bed (Fig. 21.10).

Vascular variations around the CBD more frequently involve arterial branches (13–20% of cases [44, 47]) and include an anomalous course of the hepatic artery along the right side of the CBD, or of the right hepatic artery and cystic artery along the anterior wall of the CBD. Arterial injury can cause liver ischemia and possible subsequent atrophy of the correspondent portion of liver parenchyma (Fig. 21.11), or pseudoaneurysms of the right hepatic artery, a possible cause of hemobilia (Fig. 21.12). Knowledge of these vascular variations is essential in order to avoid bleeding that could be difficult to control in laparoscopy and may force the surgeon towards improper blind attempts at hemostasis, with possible complex injuries of both the artery and the CBD. It has been reported that 5% of BDIs can be related to sudden intraoperative bleeding [14]. This complication is facilitated by the laparoscopic technique in itself; in fact, the operative field is quickly covered even if bleeding is limited, and magnification of images may cause a limited bleed to be mistaken for a more severe one. This can occur during dissection of the neck of the gallbladder where the surgeon may injure a posterior branch of the cystic artery if division of its anterior branch is misidentified as a cystic artery.

Tedious bleeding can occur in obese patients during dissection of Calot's triangle, but this bleeding can usually be easily controlled by simple compression with the gallbladder or small gauzes, rather than excessive use of diathermy.

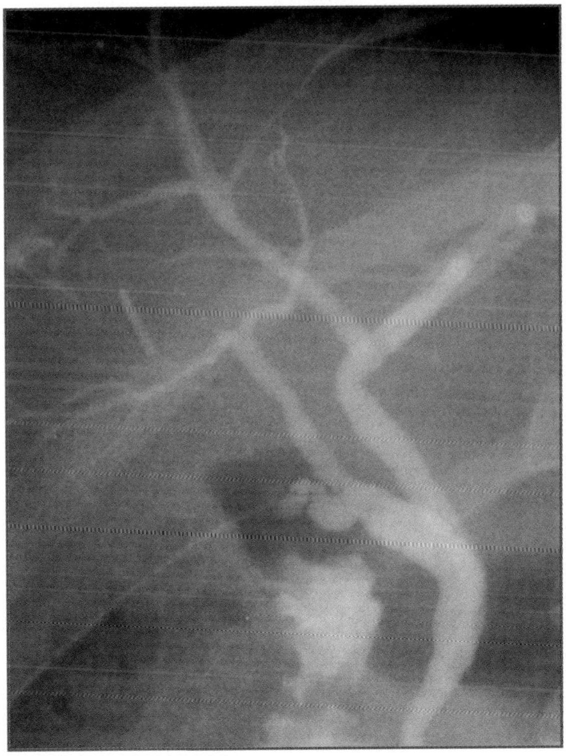

Fig. 21.10 Intraoperative cholangiography. The cystic duct enters the right sectorial bile duct, which has slipped down. Reproduced with permission from [42]

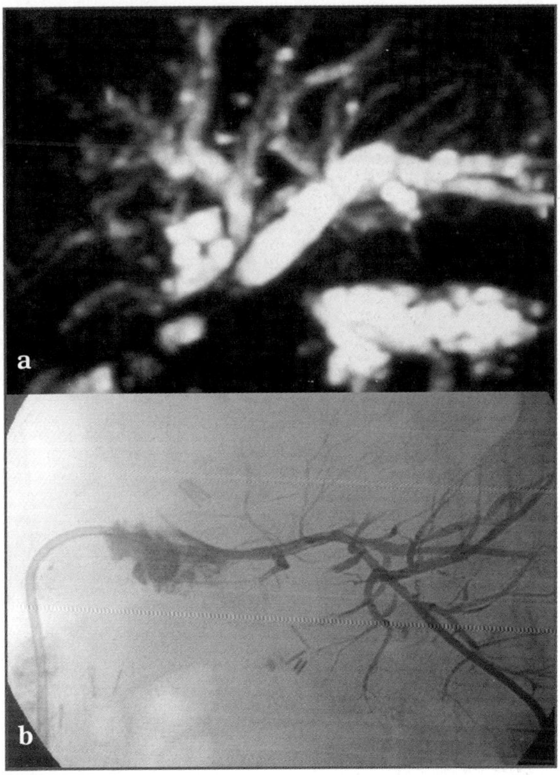

Fig. 21.11 Laparoscopic cholecystectomy converted for intraoperative bleeding in a 74-year-old old male, with difficult hemostasis (suspected injury to right hepatic artery). Occurrence of biliary fistula on postoperative day 3. Reoperation for drainage of choleperitoneum: diagnosis of proximal CBD transection. On postoperative day 15 the patient was referred to our Unit with biliary fistula and sepsis. Treatment of sepsis and progressive removal of the abdominal drainage until bile leak disappeared. After biliary fistula closure, recurrent cholangitis. **a** MR-cholangiography: type 4 stricture according to Bismuth's classification with atrophic right lobe and hypertrophied and dilated left biliary tree. At operation: presence of multiple hepatic abscesses in the right lobe; hepatectomy with left hepatic duct jejunostomy were performed. **b** Postoperative cholangiography through left percutaneous biliary drainage. Reproduced with permission from [42]

In cases of severe hemorrhage it should be evaluated whether hemostasis can be laparoscopically performed, or if it is necessary to convert to open procedure. After hemostasis, IOC should be carried out if it is not routinely performed.

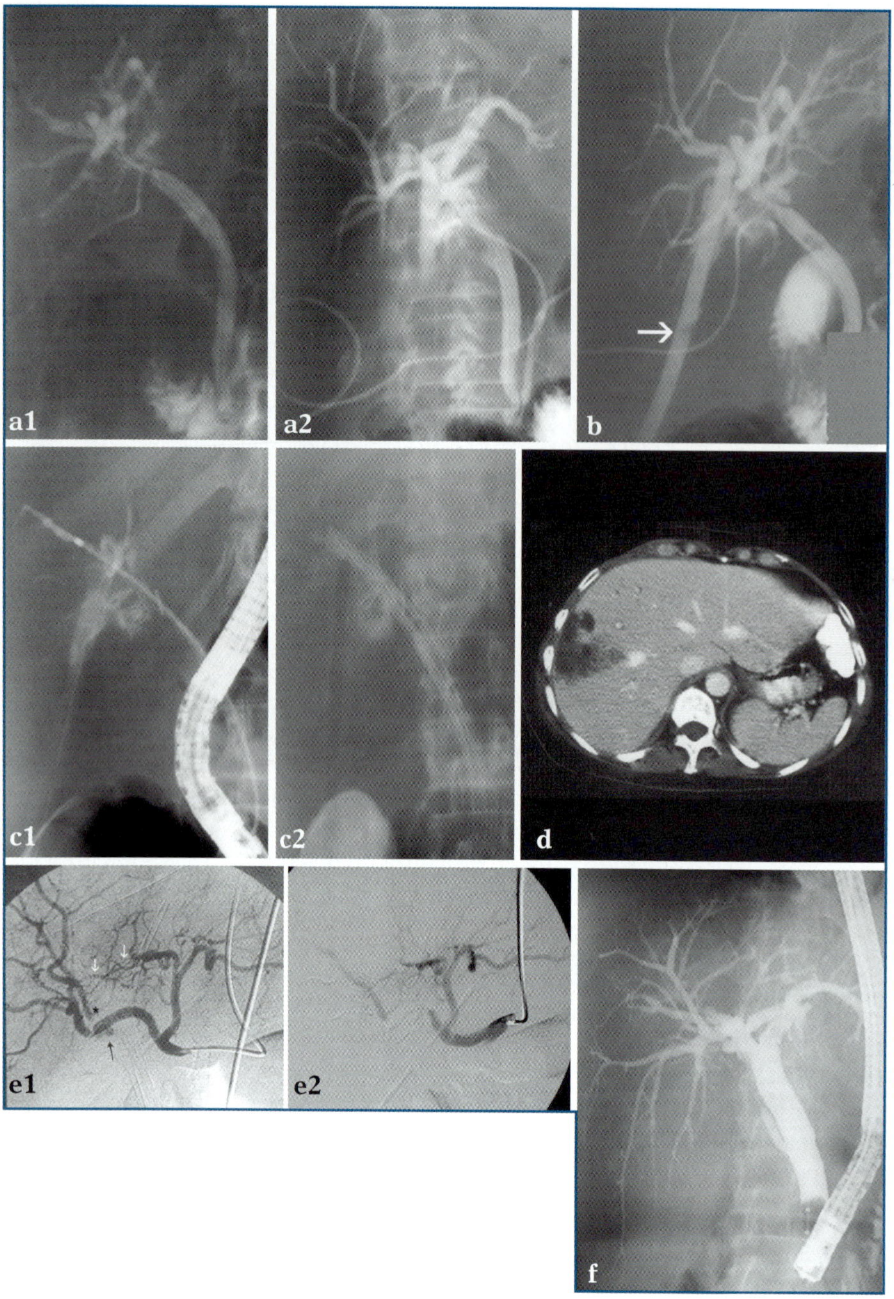

Fig. 21.12 Cholecystectomy in a 48-year-old female. Conversion to laparotomy because of occurrence of bile in the operative field. Intraoperative cholangiography referred as "non diagnostic" and suture of CBD injury". On postoperative day 4, reoperation because of biliary peritonitis; diagnosis of lateral injury to CBD (Type 3 according to Bismuth's classification) and repair over T-tube. The patient was referred to our Unit on postoperative day 14. **a1, a2** Cholangiography through the T-tube: persistence of biliary fistula sustaining the persistent choleperitoneum. Relaparotomy and drainage of biliary fistula. **b** Cholangiography through the T-tube on postoperative day 20: bile leak from the T-tube and well drained biliary fistula (*white arrow*: surgical drainage). **c1, c2** T-tube removal and endoscopic placement of 5 biliary stents (8.5 Fr). **d** Septic fever on postoperative day 24; at abdominal CT scan there was a hepatic abscess in segments 5–8. On postoperative day 31, there was severe bleeding from the subhepatic abdominal drain and emergency reoperation was performed: bleeding was stopped without cause recognition, the hepatic artery was encircled with a tourniquet that was placed outside the abdominal wound and surgical drainage of the hepatic abscess was performed. On postoperative day 39, hemobilia; hepatic artery was temporary clamped by the tourniquet and emergency angiography was performed. **e1** Pseudoaneurysm of right hepatic artery (*black arrow*), interruption of right sectorial arterial branch (*), arterial plexus from left hepatic artery to the right arterial sectorial branch (*white arrows*). **e2** Angiography showing the revascularization of right arterial sectoral branch through the arterial plexus, after embolization of right hepatic artery for bleeding from the pseudoaneurysm. **f** ERCP after stent removal (6 months after placement) showing no stricture of CBD. Reproduced with permission from [42]

Risk Factors Related to the Surgeon's Experience

Injury of the biliary tract can also occur during an "easy" cholecystectomy performed by an experienced surgeon. Therefore, it is obvious that the risk of BDI increases during "difficult" cholecystectomy and in the case of an inexperienced surgeon.

Cholecystectomy is a well known and codified surgical procedure even when performed with new technical modalities, and surgical experience should be considered not only with regard to the number of procedures carried out, but also to the capability of the surgeon to distinguish the limits of this new technique. In other words, experience is estimated also by being able to decide when to convert the procedure to an open cholecystectomy.

Since the early days of laparoscopic cholecystectomy a higher incidence of injury has been related to the learning curve of the surgeons [11]. In the already mentioned Italian survey [14] an overall incidence of 0.42% of BDI was reported. The overall incidence of BDI significantly decreased with increasing number of laparoscopic cholecystectomies performed, ranging from 0.9 for surgical teams who had performed fewer than 150 laparoscopic cholecystectomies in the 3-year period analyzed in the study, to 0.3% for those who had performed more than 450 ($p<0.01$) in the same period. A similar result was observed for major injuries (0.86% vs. 0.19%) (Fig. 21.13).

However, experience alone is not sufficient to fully understand the overall higher rate of BDI. In fact, although most BDIs occur within a surgeon's first 100 laparoscopic cholecystectomies [48], currently biliary injuries occur even with surgeons beyond the learning curve [49]. With regard to this issue, in a recent survey [48] it was reported that one third of injuries occurred after 200 laparoscopic cholecystectomies, i.e., after stabilization of the learning curve, and therefore still related to technical mistakes. A critical component is indeed the correct operative technique [48, 50, 51].

Considerations of Surgical Technique

Before any technical consideration, the surgeon must have safe, reliable, and properly maintained equipment [49]. For example, thermal injuries to bile ducts may occur because of incompletely electrically isolated hooks, so laparoscopic equipment should

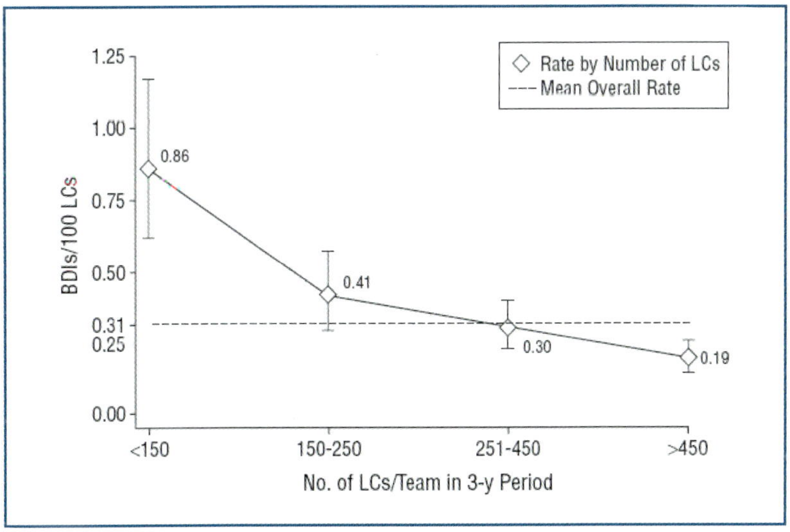

Fig. 21.13 Mean rate of major BDIs for surgical teams with different volumes of laparoscopic cholecystectomy (LC) in a 3-year period. The rate significantly decreased ($p = 0.02$) with the increasing number of laparoscopic cholecystectomy LCs. The number of teams in each group was similar. Reproduced with permission from [14]

be routinely scrutinized before use. With regard to the choice of the French or the United States technique, it seems that neither one, if correctly used, is associated with an increased risk of injury [50]. With both techniques, the use of the same principles applied to laparotomic cholecystectomy is mandatory. The critical points are good exposure of the cystic duct and hepatic pedicle, and absolutely avoiding division of any structure before the clear identification of anatomy. This was emphasized recently by Strasberg and colleagues [52] who reported that in more than 80% of cases of a series of BDIs, the cystic duct had been interrupted before completing identification and preparation of anatomical structures. Therefore, the best prevention of BDI is preliminary exposure of the hepato-cystic triangle before structure division (Figs. 21.14, 21.15).

Anatomic extensive dissection may be laborious in cases of "difficult" cholecystectomy. A "difficult" cholecystectomy is characterized by the presence of acute or chronic inflammatory changes involving the gallbladder, hepatic pedicle and hilum. In these cases it is essential to dissect away from the hepatic pedicle and along the infundibulum of the gallbladder before dissecting the cystic duct. One problem is the difficult traction of the gallbladder because of the thickness of the wall and ease with which inflamed tissues bleed, which may hamper exposure of the peritoneum around the cystic duct and incision of the anterior and posterior peritoneal sheaths. After completion of this double peritoneal incision, dissection can be performed gently in order to further mobilize the neck of the gallbladder from the hepatic pedicle. Diathermy should be used with caution, and with low intensity during this dissection because the risk of BDI is particularly high.

In conclusion, regarding risk factors for BDI in the laparoscopic era, it is confirmed that: 1) cholecystitis remains a difficult clinical situation with a higher risk of BDI compared to that of simple cholelithiasis; 2) increased surgical experience is associated with a reduced risk of BDI, but in this setting also expert surgeons are at risk of caus-

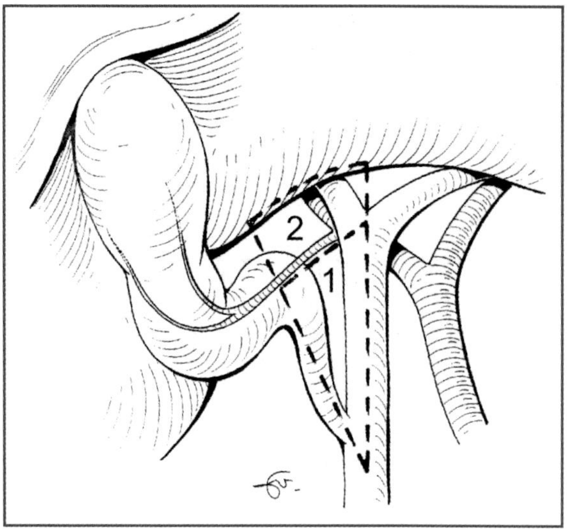

Fig. 21.14 Anatomic limits of Calot's triangle (*1*) are CBD, cystic duct and cystic artery. At present the "hepato-cystic" triangle (*2*) is more frequently reported, its limits are the CBD, cystic duct and inferior surface of the liver. Reproduced with permission from [42]

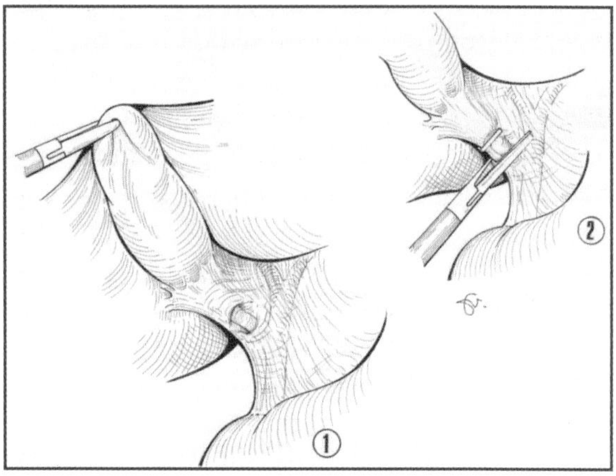

Fig. 21.15 A technical mistake, after dissecting only the anterior peritoneal sheath between the gallbladder and the hepatic pedicle (*1*), is to clip and divide the first visible structure which seems to be the cystic duct, without first complete dissection of the "hepato-cystic" triangle, leading to possible CBD injury (*2*). Reproduced with permission from [42]

ing a BDI; 3) biliary anatomic variations can contribute infrequently to the occurrence of BDI; and 4) only meticulous and correct surgical technique is the best prevention for BDI.

Intraoperative Cholangiography

More than half of BDIs are not recognized at the time of operation. This data is relevant because morbidity and late results of biliary repair are directly related to delay of diagnosis and timing of BDI repair.

According to some authors, the routine use of IOC offers the possibility of always having a complete map of the biliary tree, to discover anatomical variations, and to recognize a biliary injury early, or at least to reduce the severity of the injury [17, 48, 53–57]. Furthermore, routine use of IOC allows the surgeon to get necessary experience in quickly performing the cholangiography, and in correctly reading it. According to authors supporting the routine use of IOC, these arguments suggest that the use and correct interpretation of IOCs decrease the rate of CBD injury and that its broader use will improve patient safety; however, this evidence comes from observational cohort studies rather than randomized trials [56, 57].

Currently, to the best of our knowledge, it is not possible to relate the recognition of biliary anatomic variation with a decrease in the risk of a major BDI [58]. The best way to recognize a biliary variation and to prevent an injury remains anatomic exposure of the hepato-cystic triangle and recognition of all the exposed structures before division of any of these: it is a mistake to think that IOC could replace meticolous anatomical dissection.

The possibility that IOC could avoid or allow minimization of biliary injury should be evaluated in relation to the two steps of the procedure during which an injury can be caused: exposure of the cystic duct, and detachment of the gallbladder from the CBD.

When the CBD misidentified far the cystic duct, cholangiography can be useful because it allows intraoperative diagnosis of the injury and avoids worsening a small lateral injury of the CBD (which can be quickly repaired, often without consequences) in a complete transection, or in resection of a segment of the CBD (Fig. 21.16).

On the contrary, an IOC cannot avoid an injury occurring during detachment of the gallbladder from the CBD because at this point the IOC has already been performed.

Clear demonstration of the role of IOC in preventing BDI is not yet evident [18, 51, 53, 59, 60]. Several prospective trials have tried to evaluate the usefulness of IOC in preventing BDIs, but meaningful conclusions have not been reached because relatively small numbers of patients have been included. In fact, it was recently reconfirmed that BDI is a relatively uncommon event: sample size calculations reveal that in order to show a 50% reduction in the rate of BDI, a trial including more than 30,000 patients would have to be performed to be sufficiently powered [56].

The number of surgeons who use routinely IOC is very small (less than 10% in Italy [14]), but rates of BDI are similar to those that use IOC selectively. This is probably related to a variety of reasons: lack of familiarity with a technique that is more difficult than during open cholecystectomy; frequent unavailability or unreliability of radiological equipment; the time consuming nature of the procedure; its cost; and the risk of causing an injury while attempting to perform the cholangiography [61].

Therefore, the discussion about routine or selective use of IOC is still open because definitive results are not yet available. However, this conclusion does not mean that a surgeon should not have the ability to perform and to correctly read an IOC. Knowledge of biliary anatomy is essential for correct interpretation of a cholangiogram. In fact, in some cases injury is recognizable only because a portion of the biliary tree is lacking, and if there is no capability to recognize all the segmental

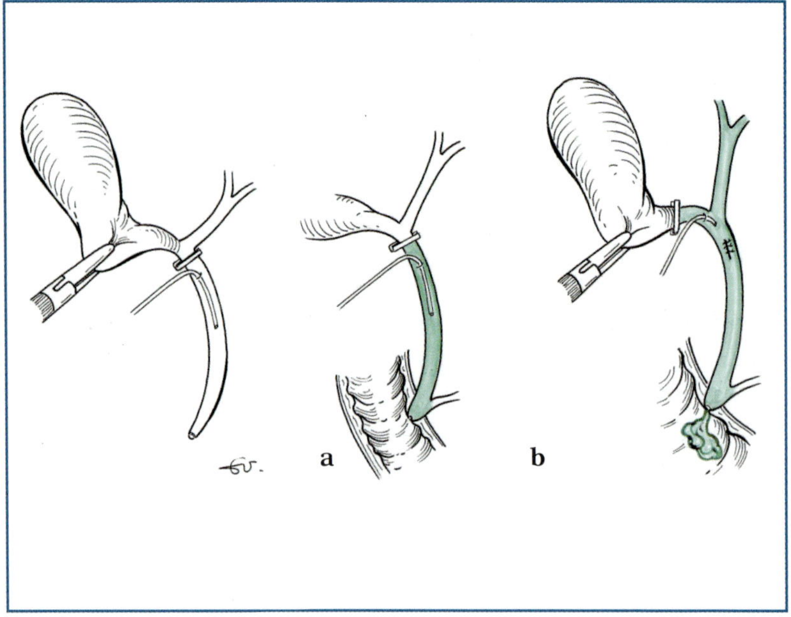

Fig. 21.16 Excessive lateral traction on the gallbladder may laterally pull the CBD, which can be misidentified for the cystic duct and closed with a clip. At this moment, IOC allows recognition of the mistake (absence of CBD visualization above the catheter) (**a**), and avoidance of injury by removing the clip and by correctly placing it on the cystic duct (**b**). The small incision on the CBD for cholangiography is sutured. Reproduced with permission from [42]

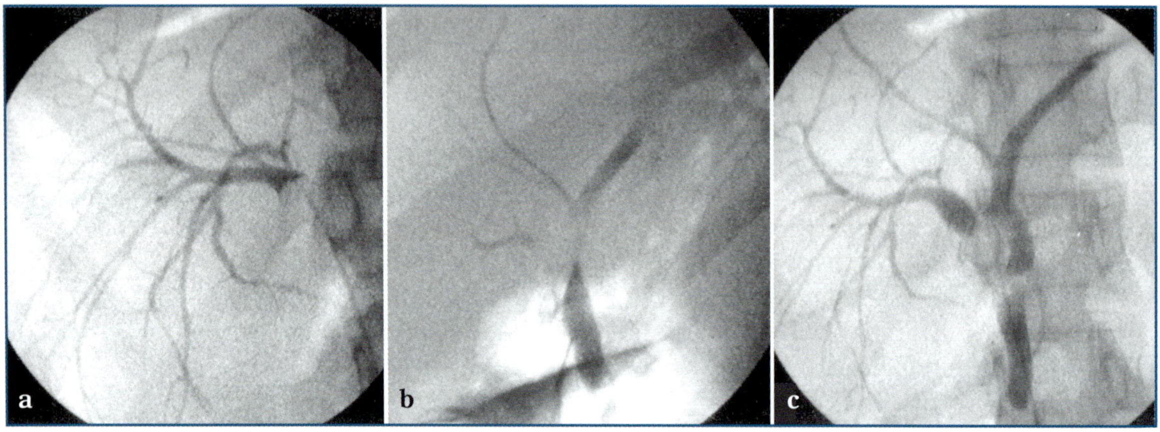

Fig. 21.17 During cholecystectomy in a 40-year-old female patient with previous liver surgery for hydatidosis, occurrence of bile in the operative field. **a** First intraoperative cholangiography: visualization of a portion of right biliary tree. **b** Visualization of the CBD, of the left hepatic duct and of a right bile duct that drains into the left hepatic duct (probably from S 8) is obtained after contrast injection through another catheter. **c** Simultaneous contrast injection through the two catheters allows visualization of the complete biliary tree: incomplete transection of right hepatic duct. Immediate repair by hepatico-jejunostomy was performed. Reproduced with permission from [42]

ducts, the injury will remain undiagnosed, or not completely understood (Fig. 21.17).

Correct interpretation of IOC requires appropriate training. In an analysis of 252 BDIs that occured during cholecystectomy, Way and colleagues [62] reported that 43 IOCs demonstrated a BDI, but only nine (21%) were correctly interpreted at the time of operation. In retrospect, more than half the time, abnormal IOC findings were simply overlooked. Therefore, at the beginning of a surgeon's experience (at least the first 20 cholecystectomies), the routine use of IOC is an important exercise that is initially time consuming, but becomes easy and quick to perform with practice [42].

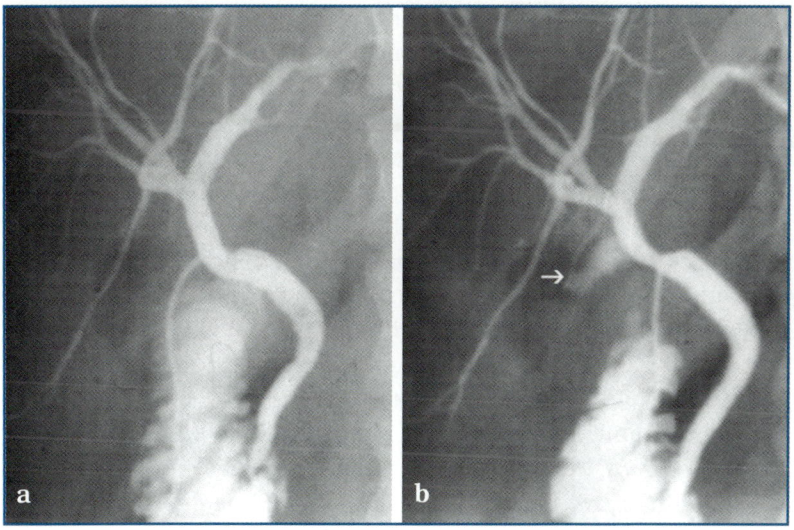

Fig. 21.18 A 37-year-old female. **a** Intraoperative cholangiography after the appearance of bile from the gallbladder bed. Injury to small peripheral bile duct (*white arrow*). **b** Cholangiography after laparoscopic suture showing absence of bile leak and normal CBD. (Published with permission from [42])

However, when there is the suspicion of a BDI, performing an IOC is mandatory: appearance of bile coming from an apparently small opening in the field, can be related to a minor BDI (Fig. 21.18), but complete transection of a thin CBD can be excluded only with IOC. It is important to remember that, if it is true that a randomized trial on the routine use of IOC does not exist, lack of IOC radiogram when BDI has occurred can put the surgeon in a difficult position in case of litigation [63].

In conclusion, discussion on routine or selective use of IOC will continue for a long time: at the moment, as in the past prelaparoscopic era, to perform an IOC remains a matter of surgeon preference according to a case-by-case basis. However, it is clear that IOC should be part of training for laparoscopic cholecystectomy [33].

Causes and Mechanisms of Biliary Injuries

The cause of a BDI is not always identifiable: in around 30% of BDIs the cause remains unrecognized [14]. The most frequently reported cause is misidentification of the anatomy of the hepatic pedicle and almost one third of BDIs are directly related to technical mistakes (Table 21.2).

Table 21.2 Causes and mechanisms of biliary injuries reported in 235 BDIs [14]

	No. (%) of bile duct injuries	
Total	235	(100)
Unrecognized cause	72	(30.6)
Recognized cause	163	(69.4)
Causes and mechanisms of biliary injuries *		
Misidentification of the anatomy of the hepatic pedicle	71	(36.8)
Inflammatory changes in the gallbladder	43	(23.3)
Anatomical anomalies	24	(12.9)
Improper use of monopolar coagulation	23	(12.3)
Unspecified technical mistake	18	(9.8)
Intraoperative bleeding	10	(4.9)

* in 17 cases, more than one cause was reported

In more than half of cases injury occurs during maneuvers aimed at identifying and isolating the cystic duct, and at detaching the gallbladder from the CBD. Misidentification of the CBD for the cystic duct (the classic injury [11]) is reported as the most common cause of BDI and may occur during apparently "simple" cholecystectomy. Excess traction on a soft gallbladder and on a thin hepatic pedicle stretches the CBD, putting the cystic duct and the CBD in the same line (Fig. 21.19). Two possibilities can occur: 1) dissection is continued upward, along the left side of the CBD, then it is turned to the right to begin the detachment of the gallbladder from the liver; here, injury can occur at the level of CBD or of the main biliary confluence; 2) a less severe injury is possible if the distal clip is closed on the CBD and the proximal clip is put on the cystic duct: closure of the distal CBD occurs, with a biliary fistula from the stump of the cystic duct.

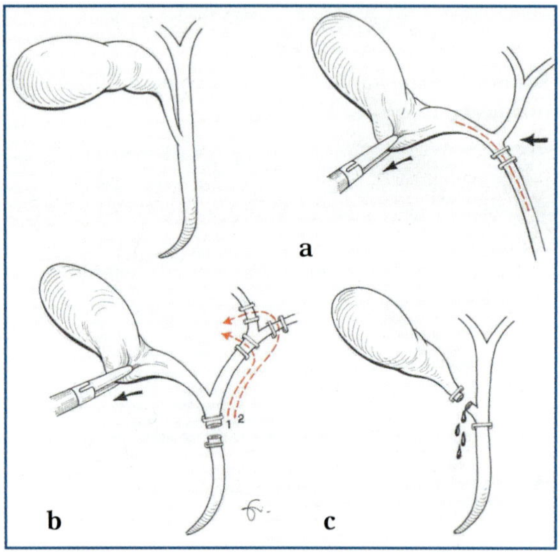

Fig 21.19 Gallbladder with normal wall: apparently "easy" cholecystectomy. Excessive traction on the gallbladder puts the cystic duct and the CBD in the same line; clips are placed on the CBD, which is misidentified for the cystic duct (**a**). Dissection continues along the left side of the CBD and then it turns to the right side: bile duct injury may involve the CBD or both right and left hepatic ducts (**b**). In other cases, the proximal clip is placed on the cystic duct and the distal clip closes the CBD (**c**). In such cases biliary fistula occurs from the stump of the cystic duct above the CBD stricture. Reproduced with permission from [42]

Detachment of the gallbladder from the CBD is the second dangerous step of the procedure when there is not a clear plane for dissection, particularly in chronic cholecystitis [14]. Risk of injuring the CBD is related to dense adhesions between the neck of the gallbladder and the CBD, and to the frequent presence of a stone impacted in the neck, modifying normal anatomy. In these cases, high injuries occur, just below the main biliary confluence, with complete excision of a segment of CBD, or a wide lateral injury can occur (Fig. 21.20).

Other causes can be related to surgical technique. Excess traction of the gallbladder can cause an injury in different ways: the CBD may be tilted and partially or completely closed by the clip on the cystic stump (Fig. 21.21); the cystic artery may be injured and attempts at controlling bleeding may be the cause of either a biliary or a vascular injury (Fig. 21.22); and a thin cystic duct can be torn (Fig. 21.23). Inappropriate use of diathermy, mainly monopolar, may cause a perforation or a late ischemic damage to the CBD either directly or through a clip (Fig. 21.24). Other injuries related to surgical removal of CBD stones are less frequent than in the past because lithiasis of the CBD is more frequently treated by endoscopy [64].

Classification

Introduction of the laparoscopic technique significantly changed the features of BDIs. For example, biliary fistulas from minor BDIs (cystic duct or peripheral bile ducts without the involvement of the CBD) were uncommon in the prelaparoscopic era, but currently represent more than 25% of biliary complications of laparoscopic cholecystectomy [65]. Causes of BDIs and their clin-

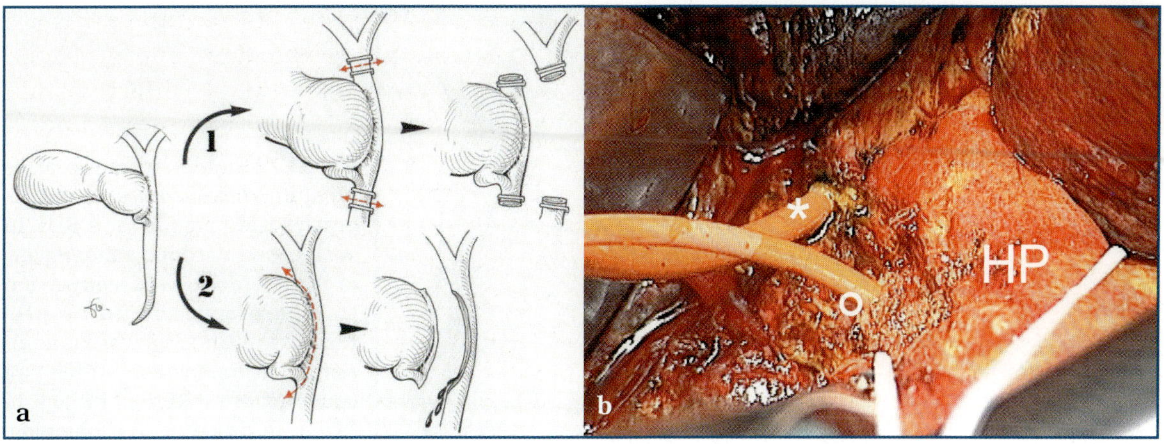

Fig. 21.20 a In case of chronic cholecystitis, inflammatory adhesions or presence of a large stone, join gallbladder wall with CBD. In such cases, two mechanisms of BDI may occur: complete excision of a segment of CBD adjacent to gallbladder (*1*); wide lateral injury of CBD (*2*). **b** Operative field in a patient with loss of a tract of CBD; two catheters are inserted into the proximal (*) and the distal biliary stumps (°). The hepatic pedicle (*HP*) is encircled with a white tape. Fig. 20a reproduced with permission from [42]

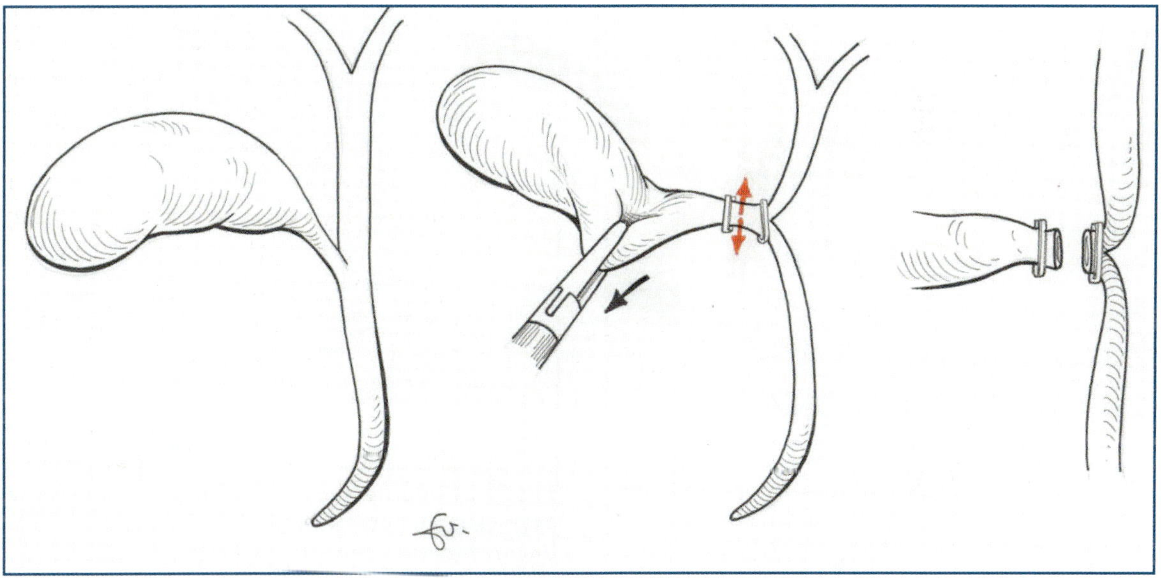

Fig. 21.21 During "easy" cholecystectomies, especially in case of a thin CBD, excessive traction of the gallbladder may tilt the CBD, which can be partially or completely closed. It is important to keep the hepatic pedicle straight in order to avoid this "tenting" injury. Reproduced with permission from [42]

ical manifestations also changed, with biliary fistula and biliary peritonitis more frequent than in the past.

With regard to these changes, several new classifications of BDI during laparoscopic cholecystectomy have been proposed [21, 51, 66–70].

Strasberg's classification [51] is probably the most widely known, even though it is difficult to remember (nine types of injuries are included), and perhaps too detailed: three types for minor injuries are included, another type for partial injuries of CBD, and five types, defined according to same criteria as

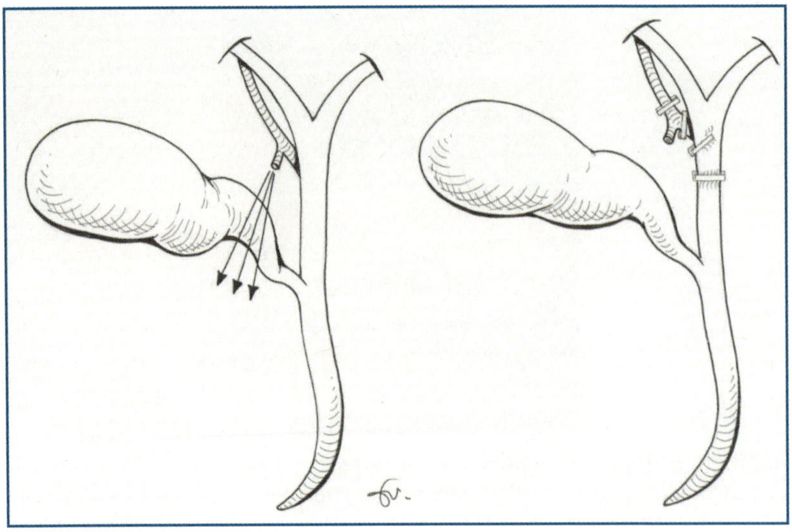

Fig. 21.22 Sudden intraoperative bleeding (*black arrows*) in the operative field may favor a BDI. In such cases, without a clear view of the operative field, conversion to laparotomy should be preferred to blind laparoscopic attempts at hemostasis which can cause different kind of biliary injuries. Intraoperative cholangiography at the end of hemostasis should be performed. Reproduced with permission from [42]

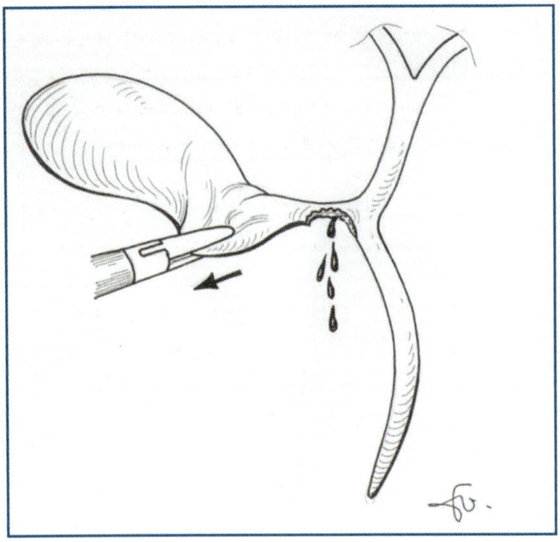

Fig. 21.23 The cystic duct, if thin, can be torn causing a bile duct injury at the level of cystic duct junction with CBD. Reproduced with permission from [42]

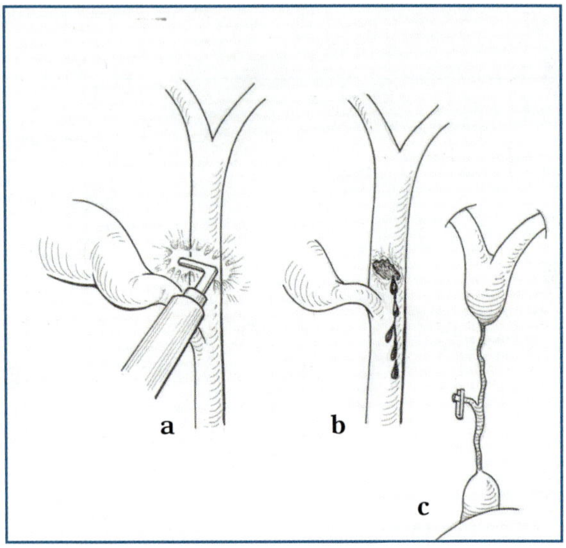

Fig. 21.24 Improper use of diathermy, especially in case of monopolar coagulation, may cause a bile duct injury (**a**): immediate CBD perforation (**b**); ischemic injury with late postoperative stricture (**c**). Reproduced with permission from [42]

Bismuth's classification [43], including complete transection of the CBD in addition to stenosis of the BDI (Fig. 21.25).

An easier classification, frequently used in non-surgical literature, is Bergman's [67], which is based on morphology of the injury, clinical presentation and possible therapeutic choices. Four types of injury are identified: Type A is bile leak from the stump of the cystic duct, or from peripheral ducts (intact CBD); Type B is a bile leak resulting from injury of the CBD, with or without stenosis; Type C is a stenosis of the CBD without bile leak; Type D is a complete transection or excision of a segment of the CBD. In summary, this classification divides BDI into two groups: those injuries with biliary transections (Types A, B and D), and those with biliary stenoses:

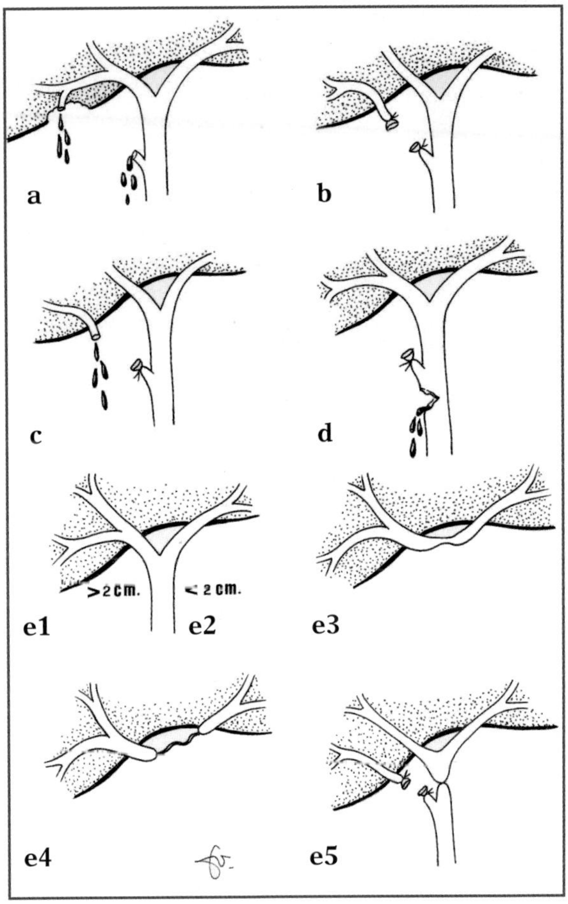

Fig. 21.25 Strasberg's classification. Bile leak from cystic duct stump or minor biliary duct in gallbladder fossa (**a**). Occluded right posterior sectorial duct (**b**). Bile leak from divided right posterior sectorial duct (**c**). Bile leak from lateral injury of main bile duct (**d**). Transected main bile duct with a stricture more than 2 cm from the hilum (**e1**). Transected main bile duct with a stricture less than 2 cm from the hilum (**e2**). Stricture of the hilum with intact main biliary confluence (**e3**). Stricture of the hilum with separated right and left ducts (**e4**). Stricture of the main bile duct and of the right posterior sectoral duct (**e5**). Reproduced with permission from [42]

the difference between the two groups being the presence or absence of bile leak.

Gazzaniga's classification [69] also describes two main biliary injuries: biliary transections and biliary stenoses. Apart from their severity and time of clinical presentation, the most relevant difference is presence or absence of bile leak. This is the most important clinical feature for classification and therefore for treatment decision.

In order to choose the type of treatment in cases of BDI, two pieces of information are necessary. The first, the clinical one, relates to the general condition of patient, and is based on presence or absence of bile in the peritoneal cavity, which can require immediate treatment. The second, the morphological one, is related to the level and extension of the injury, and is essential for deciding the type and technique of repair, after resolution of possible critical phases. In other words, in patients with bile in the peritoneum, the first concern should be to restore acceptable general conditions, and particularly to treat the sepsis that is often present. In these patients biliary repair is not the first goal; it can be evaluated later, after resolution of sepsis and when associated inflammation has subsided.

Several centers, including ours, continue to utilize Bismuth's classification [43, 71], with the addition of a Type 0, which includes minor injuries with an intact CBD (leaks from the cystic stump, liver bed, minor peripheral bile ducts), and of a Type 6, which includes an isolated injury to the right hepatic duct. The other injuries were classified in the classical five types according to the level of injury (stenoses and/or transections) and length of proximal biliary stump (Fig. 21.26).

Apart from different classifications, BDIs are then divided into "major" and "minor" injuries. Major BDIs include all injuries (partial or complete transections, excisions, and partial or complete stenoses, including stenoses of bilio-enteric anastomoses) involving the CBD and bile ducts of the main biliary confluence [72]. Minor BDIs include leak of the cystic stump, transections or stenoses of Luschka's bile duct (small bile ducts draining into the gallbladder), or of a small superficial bile duct of the liver bed [42].

The incidence of minor BDI varies from 0.28% to 1.7% [7, 9, 10, 12, 13], and, as

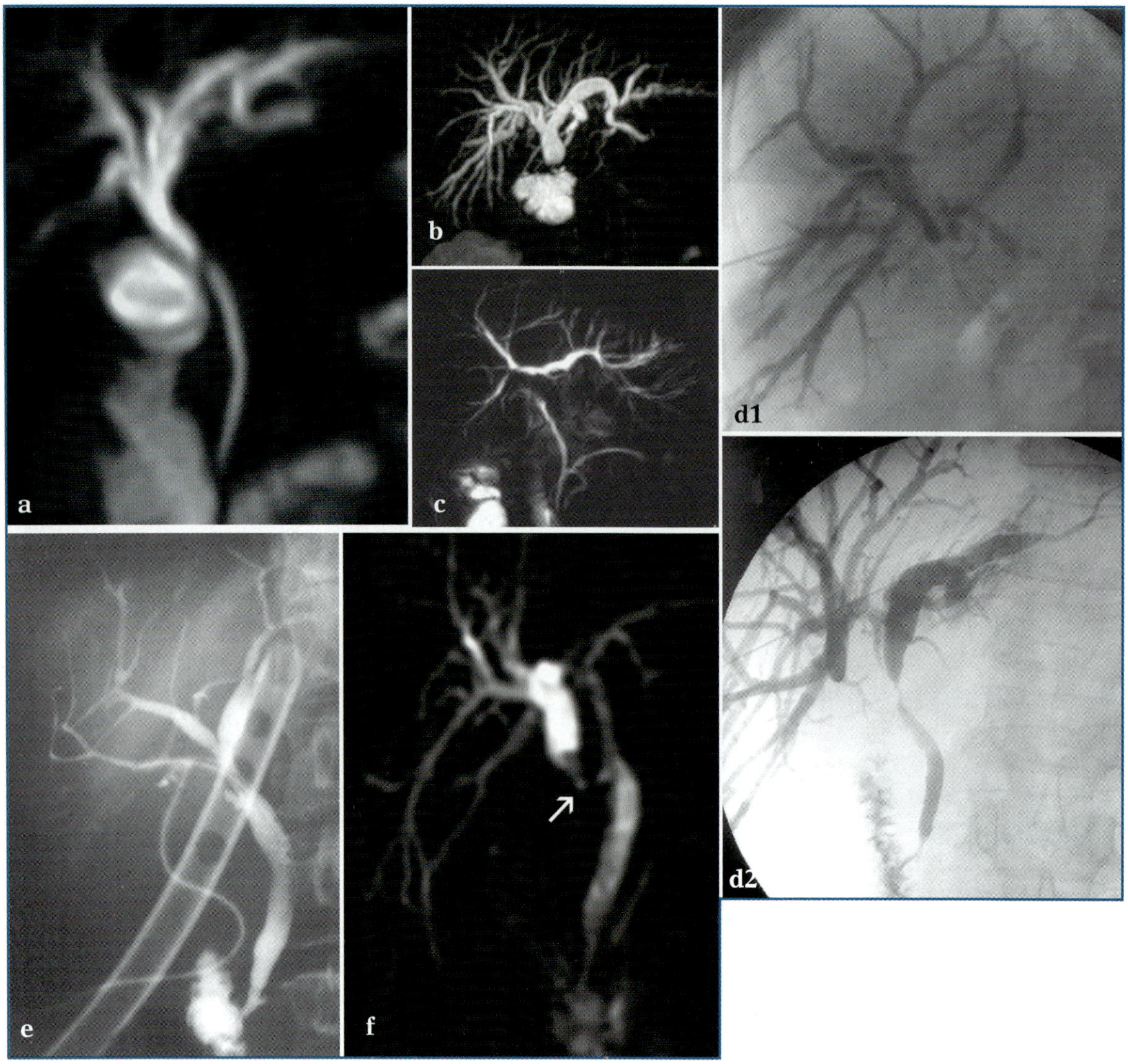

Fig. 21.26 Bismuth's classification. **a** Type 1: stricture of CBD with proximal bile duct stump ≥2 cm. **b** Type 2: stricture of CBD with duct stump < 2 cm. **c** Type 3: proximal injury with intact ceiling of the biliary confluence; right and left ductal systems communicate. Type 4: biliary injury with destroyed confluence; right and left ducts are **d1** less or **d2** more separated. **e** Type 5: bile duct injury involving right posterior sectorial bile duct at its junction with CBD (cholangiography after repair over T-tube). **f** Type 6: isolated injury to the right hepatic duct (*arrow*). Figs. d1, d2 and e reproduced with permission from [42]

already mentioned, accounts for around 25% of biliary complications after laparoscopic cholecystectomy [14, 65].

A leak from the stump of the cystic duct, very infrequent during open cholecystectomy, is one of the most frequent complications of laparoscopic cholecystectomy [42]. The leak is related to a technical mistake occurring during the application of clips; for example, if they are improperly used on a thick and rigid cystic duct, or when clips "scissor" the cystic duct; cautery-induced injuries can also occur during dissection of the cystic duct. In around 25% of cases [73] the leak from the cystic duct is related to the unknown presence of stones in the CBD. In these cases, endoscopic treatment of biliary lithiasis is most frequently used, and drainage of biloma, or of intraperitoneal bile collections can be performed through percutaneous, laparoscopic, or rarely, using a laparotomic approach.

Injury to peripheral ducts in the liver bed can occur when dissection behind the gallbladder is too deep, which sometimes is unavoidable in acute or chronic cholecystitis and in intrahepatic gallbladders [49, 73]. These injuries can cause subhepatic bile collections. The incidence of these ducts is not known [46], and prevention of their injury is based on dissection as close as possible to the wall of gallbladder. Luschka's bile ducts, infrequently present, can also cause subhepatic bile collections, which appear more frequently than during open cholecystectomy [74].

The severity of major BDIs is related to several factors: the level of injury in relation to the main biliary confluence; lateral or complete injury of the CBD; complete excision of a segment of CBD; involvement of main or sectorial biliary confluences; presence of multiple injuries; presence of bile ducts isolated from the biliary tree; and size of the CBD. Most series reported in the literature come from tertiary care centers, which explains why the most severe injuries are more frequently reported. For example, in our center, 85.4% (35/41) of major BDI surgically repaired presented with a high level injury: 27 were classified as Bismuth 3, six as Bismuth 4, and two as Bismuth 6 (isolated injury to the right hepatic duct). It is possible that lateral injuries or sharp transections of the CBD are only apparently less frequently reported because these injuries can be repaired in the hospital where they occur.

Vascular Injury

The incidence rate of vascular injury concomitant to BDI is not clearly defined. In an autopsy series after open cholecystectomy, the incidence was reported as 7% [75]. This is higher in patients with BDIs, ranging between 12% and 61% [76-83]. This wide range can probably be related to different techniques used to detect the vascular injury, or to different groups of patients analyzed.

The higher the biliary injury, the higher the probability of concomitant vascular injury [70]. It has been suggested that because BDIs during laparoscopic cholecystectomy are more proximally located compared to those during open cholecystectomy, a higher incidence of concomitant vascular injury can be expected [51, 67], but other authors do not agree on this presumed higher risk [79].

The most frequent vascular injury is disruption of the right branch of the hepatic artery, or of one of its main branches; arterial pseudoaneurysm of right hepatic artery (Fig. 21.12) and portal vein injury are less frequently observed [79]. Occurrence of these injuries can be detected preoperatively by angiography [79], by computed tomography (CT) with vascular reconstructions, or intraoperatively by surgical exploration and duplex examination [80].

However, the therapeutic implications and clinical impact of these injuries, in particular on long term results of biliary repair, remain controversial, as shown by recent papers. Alves et al. [79] analyzed the outcome of 26 of 55 patients (47%) with concomitant BDI and vascular injury, and concluded that there was no impact on the clinical presentation of BDI, or on the difficulty and the risk of failure of biliary repair. The lack of influence of the arterial injury was explained by the fact that disruption was unilateral, and this allowed free communication between the left and right hepatic arteries through the hilar plate arterial plexus [84]. However, it should be considered that in this series, 43 Hepp-Couinaud biliary repairs and 12 right hepatectomies were performed. On the contrary, Schmidt et al. [80], based on data of 11 patients with BDI and concomitant vascular injury, concluded that the outcome of bile duct recon-

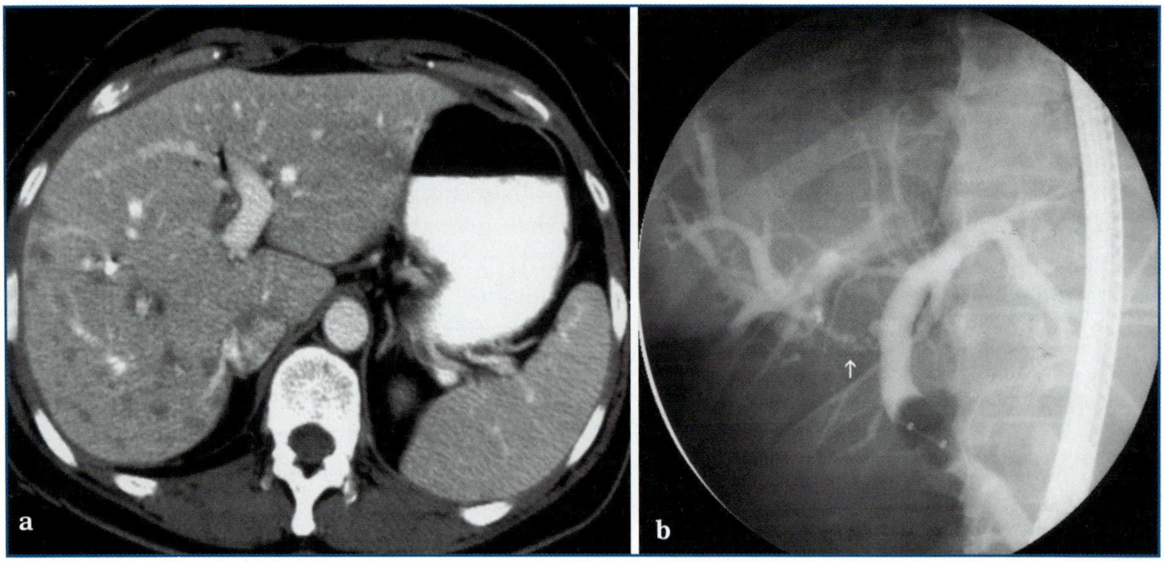

Fig. 21.27 A 52-year-old female who had cholecystectomy 9 years previously, complicated by biliary fistula and sepsis. Recurrent cholangitis for 9 years after cholecystectomy. **a** CT showing right lobe atrophy with multiple abscesses. **b** ERCP showing right hepatic duct stenosis (*white arrow*) with normal CBD and left hepatic duct. The patient underwent right hepatectomy

struction is significantly worse in these patients, and that vascular injury, along with the presence of active peritonitis, was a significant risk factor for postoperative complications. In this series, the most frequent procedure was Roux-en-Y hepaticojejunostomy, both below or at the level of hepatic duct confluence.

It is possible that the different conclusions of these two studies were related to the different types of biliary injuries and to the procedures performed. In fact, in the first example all the repairs were at the hilar plate (Hepp-Couinaud procedure), with a high number of right hepatectomies, and in the second one there were hepaticojejunostomies not only at the hilum: the different level of repair could explain the different results, with the lower repairs at higher risk of late "ischemic" complications.

A late consequence of unrecognized disruption of the right hepatic artery concomitant to stenosis of the right hepatic duct is right lobar hypo-atrophy. In this case, if associated with persistent infection (with cholangitis and hepatic abscesses), right hepatectomy should be performed (Fig. 21.27).

Clinical Manifestations and Treatment

Intraoperative diagnosis

The timing of recognition of BDI is extremely relevant for the choice of treatment and long term outcome. In fact, it has been generally accepted that intraoperative diagnosis of BDI is important because the results of an immediate repair, if performed by an expert surgeon, are better than those of late repair [43, 85]. On the contrary, failure of immediate repair worsens an injury, makes subsequent repairs more difficult, and reduces the possibility of long term success [86].

The rate of intraoperative recognition of BDI is extremely variable, ranging from 27% to 73% (Table 21.3). The chance of getting good results in a biliary repair is related to four factors: 1) the quality of the IOC, 2) the appropriate choice of type of biliary

Table 21.3 Rate of intraoperative recognition of major BDIs

Source	Country	Year	Rate of intraoperative recognition
Wherry DC [7]	USA	1996	73%
Russel JC [8]	USA	1996	55%
Richardson MC [9]	Scotland	1996	48%
Adamsen S [10]	Denmark	1997	33%
Olsen D [87]	USA	1997	27%
Gigot JF [11]	Belgium	1997	45%
MacFadyen BR [12]	USA	1998	66%
Z'graggen K [13]	Switzerland	1998	44%
Archer SB [48]	USA	2001	63%
Francoeur JR [25]	Canada	2003	66%
Nuzzo G [14]	Italy	2005	73%
Bektas H [22]	Germany	2007	36%

repair, 3) the accuracy of the surgical technique, and 4) the experience of the biliary surgeon [54]. Unfortunately, in current practice these four factors are infrequently satisfied. In fact:

1. IOC is routinely performed by a minority of surgeons (less than 10% [14]) and this means that most surgeons are not familiar with this technique; furthermore, when it is performed, often the IOC is not correctly interpreted [62].
2. Surgical repair is no longer the only treatment, as endoscopic and radiological treatments play an essential role. In fact, these techniques, less invasive than surgery, can avoid surgery totally or be a bridge toward the operation: therefore the choice of the treatment is related also to availability of these techniques.
3. Accuracy of surgical technique, necessary to deal with these infrequent and complex situations, is strictly related to the experience of the surgeon in biliary surgery, and experienced biliary surgeons are more likely to be available in high volume centers.

Following these remarks, the question is: what should be done when a biliary injury is recognized? The first step is to understand perfectly what happened by IOC, then it is necessary to evaluate one's own surgical experience and consider the opportunity to consult a more expert colleague, keeping in mind some guidelines: 1) to assume that the present repair could not be the last one [42]; 2) to apply an extremely accurate surgical technique in order to avoid any biliary leak from the anastomosis; and 3) to sacrifice as little healthy bile duct tissue as possible. In other words, a worsening of the injury should be avoided.

The diagnosis in most cases is made after the appearance of bile in the operative field, around the hepatic pedicle (injury of CBD?), or in the liver bed (injury of peripheral bile duct?). This was the case of 108 BDIs (46% of all BDIs) reported by a recent Italian survey [14]. Sometimes injury is revealed, after division of the cystic duct, by the persistent adhesion of the gallbladder to the hepatic pedicle; or by the presence of two biliary openings closed with a clip at the level of the cystic duct stump (Fig. 21.21); or by the presence of two divided bile ducts in the operative field (Fig. 21.19.2); or finally by the presence on the surgical specimen, of a segment of CBD attached to the cystic duct (Fig. 21.20). As mentioned above, in case of suspected injury and before making any further decision, IOC should be mandatory for correct and complete diagnosis of the injury. Typical radiological pictures of major BDI are the presence of bile leakage from the CBD, and absence of more or less extended portions of biliary tree.

Management of Intraoperatively Diagnosed BDI

First of all, the surgeon should decide whether or not to convert the laparoscopic procedure. Two different evaluations could induce the surgeon not to convert the procedure after cholangiography: 1) to choose instead a laparoscopic repair, because of surgical expertise in laparoscopic surgery; 2) to consider the injury too complex and therefore to place only one or more subhepatic drainages, and to send the patient to a referral center for injury repair.

In more than 90% of cases reported in the Italian survey [14], the laparoscopic procedure is converted. After conversion, it is extremely important to limit dissection of the hepatic pedicle as much as possible before performing the IOC. After cholangiography, the surgeon should: 1) judge his/her own experience in biliary surgery, also taking into account his/her own psychological conditions; 2) consider the local availability of endoscopic and radiological treatments, which have the possibility of effectively treating some types of injuries; 3) consider the necessity of not worsening the injury, place only subhepatic drains and refer the patient to a dedicated center.

During immediate repair bile ducts are almost always not dilated [54], but have healthy walls that are not yet changed by inflammation, and therefore offer the best chance of successful repair if performed by a specialist surgeon. In fact, primary biliary reconstruction frequently results in failure if not performed by a specialist surgeon [2, 54]. It has been reported that patients treated by the injuring surgeon have an 11% increased risk of death within 9 years [88]. Furthermore, in a review of 88 patients with BDI, only 17% of repairs of those performed by a non tertiary level hepatobiliary surgeon were successful, compared to 94% of those performed by a specialist. Also, hospital stay was three times longer when managed by a non specialist surgeon (78 days vs. 222 days) [54]. Morbidity and mortality rates of those treated by a non specialist compared with a specialist surgeon were 58% and 1.6% versus 4% and 0%, respectively.

The type of surgical repair depends on the type of injury, but in every case accurate and meticulous surgical technique is extremely important.

Lateral injuries without interruption of the continuity of the CBD, and retaining at least one third of the circumference of bile duct, can be repaired over T-tube.

Complete transections can have different features according to the mechanisms of the injury, and the type of repair depends on features of margins of the biliary stumps. Complete transections of the CBD with sharp and well vascularized margins can be repaired with an end-to-end anastomosis: in these cases, wide mobilization of the duodenum is needed in order to avoid tension on the anastomosis, and a T-tube is usually necessary to protect the anastomosis (Fig. 21.28). Techniques to enlarge the size of the anastomosis are difficult and possibly dangerous because they sacrifice healthy biliary tissue and increase the distance between the two biliary stumps. The failure rate of these anastomoses is very high, more than 50% in recent series [42, 54]. However, nowadays with the possibility of calibrating these anastomoses by postoperative endoscopic stents, this technique can be indicated in selected cases. Complete transections of a CBD with irregular or ischemic margins have to be regularized with resection of the

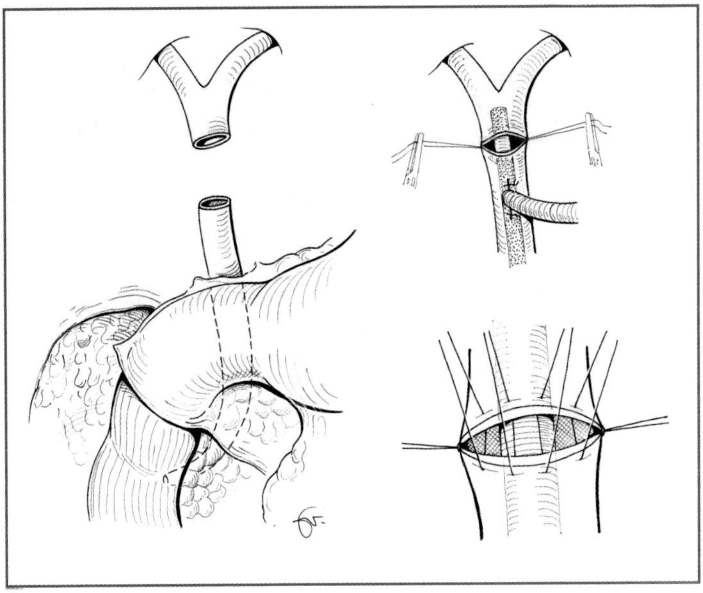

Fig. 21.28 End-to-end single-layer anastomosis of the CBD with interrupted stitches (after wide Kocher maneuver). Upper end of the T-tube is below the main biliary confluence. The long branch of the T-tube comes out from the CBD through a small incision, below the anastomosis. Reproduced with permission from [42]

margins up to reach healthy biliary tissue. It is important not to sacrifice too much biliary tissue, particularly along the proximal biliary stump because it is easy to quickly reach the main biliary confluence: at this level it is difficult to perform an end-to-end anastomosis, and hepaticojejunostomy becomes necessary.

Excisions of segments of the CBD often involve the main biliary confluence, and in some cases also the right sectorial biliary confluence, and these can be repaired only with difficult anastomoses. The entire intrahepatic biliary tree has to be drained, and depending on the type of injury, this can be obtained with multiple biliary anastomoses on the jejunal loop.

Transection of the right sectorial or segmental bile duct with an anomalous course can be of two different types: injuries to the duct alone, and injuries involving the confluence of the duct into the CBD. In both cases IOC is absolutely necessary in order to understand the amount of liver parenchyma isolated from the rest of the biliary tree. The most frequent treatment is repair over a T-tube that can be placed through a choledochotomy in order to protect the suture [89], or as a bridge between the two stumps (Fig. 21.26e). In case of involvement of the CBD, hepaticojejunostomy should be considered.

When the injured bile duct at cholangiography is very small and peripheral, it is better to ligate or suture it with a stitch that is resistant against the postoperative increased biliary pressure in the portion of undrained liver. In these cases it is safer to leave a subhepatic drainage in order to drain the bile out of the abdominal cavity if bile leak occurs.

Transection of the right hepatic duct can be intraoperatively repaired with right hepatic duct-jejunostomy. Placement of a linear catheter through the anastomosis, externalized according to the Volker technique, is recommended. If the right hepatic duct is particularly small, it may be preferable to drain the bile out of the peritoneum for a delayed right hepatic-jejunostomy.

Surgical Technique

After conversion, the best surgical access is a right subcostal incision, enlarged enough to obtain a comfortable exposure of the operative field (Fig. 21.29). In case of necessity (obese patients, hepatomegaly), it is better

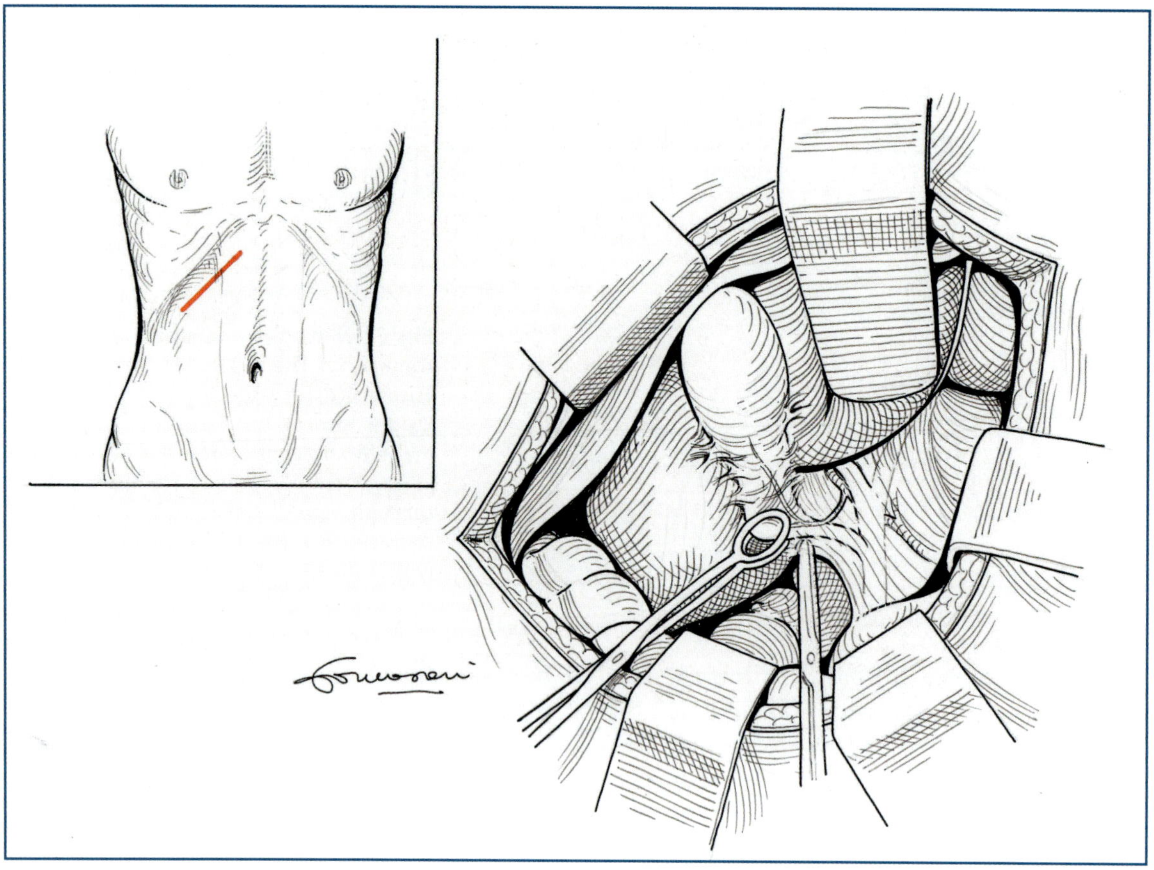

Fig. 21. 29 The right subcostal incision should be enlarged enough to obtain a comfortable exposure of the operative field. Reproduced with permission from [42]

to extend the incision toward the midline, rather than further to the right.

Extreme care should be taken to avoid damaging the margins of the injured bile ducts or to enlarge the size of the injury, to limit exposure of the CBD to avoid possible devascularization, and to avoid blindly applying hemostatic stitches that may cause further injury. In practice, it is extremely important not to worsen the injury with excessive or improper maneuvers. In case of acute inflammation of the hepatic pedicle or when the proximal biliary stump is short, with thin walls and a few millimeters in size, and therefore considered unsafe for a hepaticojejunostomy, or if surgical experience is not sufficient to achieve a good quality anastomosis, the strategy should be to obtain a controlled external biliary fistula, as suggested by many surgeons [42, 43, 54, 72, 86, 90]. One or two large-bore drains should be left close to the biliary injury in order to drain the bile out of the peritoneal cavity and to obtain an external biliary fistula. Thereafter it is necessary to wait for progressive closure of the fistula and to achieve stenosis of the injured bile duct with dilation of proximal bile ducts, and finally to perform a delayed biliary repair on the dilated bile ducts. If this strategy is chosen, it is important not to sacrifice healthy biliary tissue; inserting a drain into the bile duct, or closing the bile duct with a ligature is therefore not recommended, as these maneuvers consume valuable biliary tissue, the level of the injury is moved proximally, as well as the level of the subsequent stenosis wich becomes more difficult to repair (Fig. 21.30).

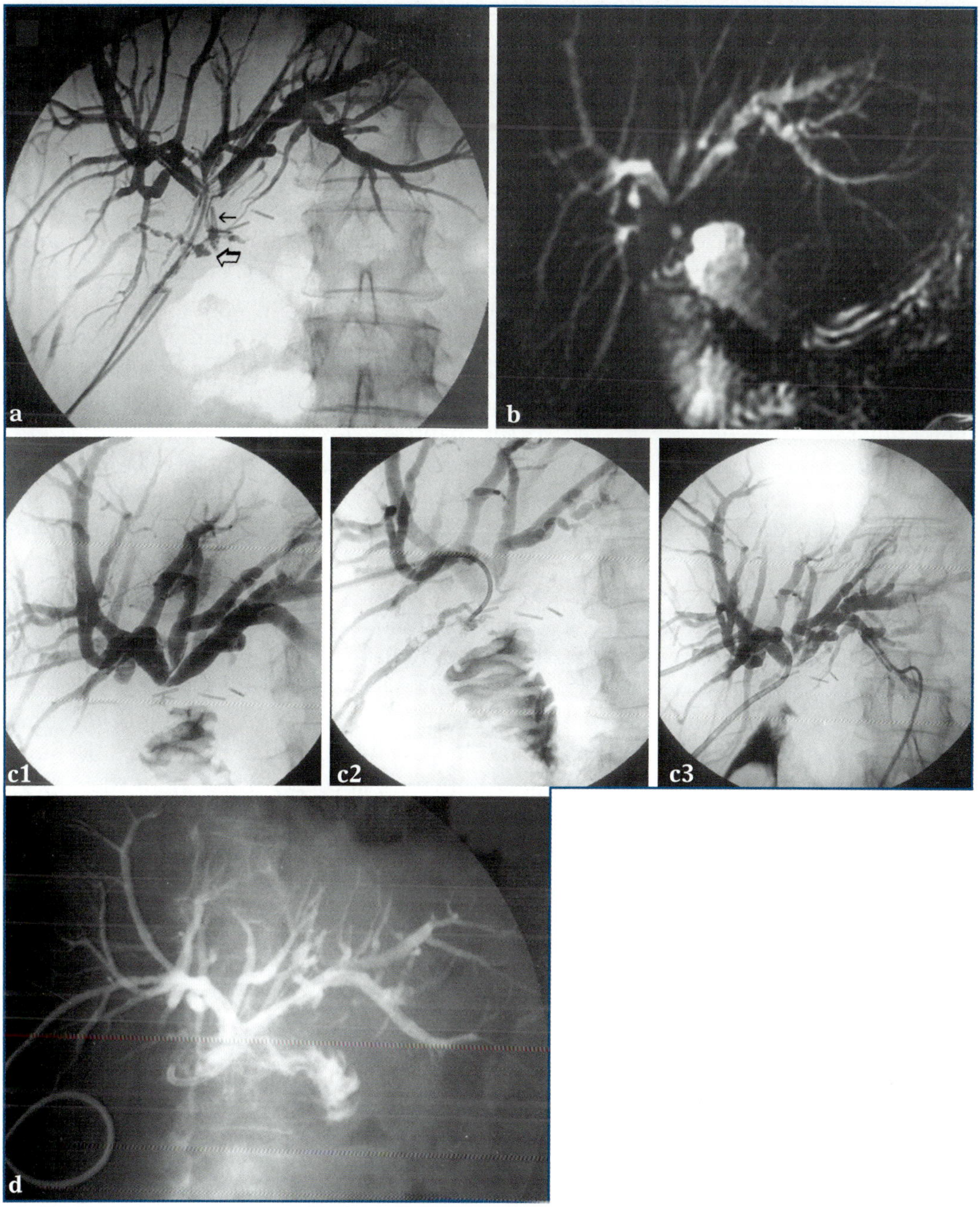

Fig. 21.30 Intraoperative recognition of bile duct injury (CBD transection below the main biliary confluence) in a 53-year-old female. T-tube placement with the two branches inside the two hepatic ducts. Referral to our Unit on postoperative day 6. **a** Cholangiography through the T-tube: visualization of sectioned CBD stump below the main biliary confluence (*black arrow*) with involvement of a right segmental duct that had slipped down (*empty arrow*). Progressive removal of T-tube. **b** Abdominal MR: dilation of intrahepatic biliary tree with stricture at the level of the main biliary confluence. Subsequent increase of levels of cholestasis enzymes. **c** Preoperative PTC showing a stricture that is advanced proximally (type 3 according to Bismuth's classification) with spontaneous bilio-enteric fistula. Two percutaneous biliary drainages are inserted into the right (**c2**) and the left (**c3**) hepatic ducts 2 days before surgery. **d** Postoperative percutaneous cholangiography after hepaticojejunostomy at the hilar plate. Reproduced with permission from [42]

If immediate repair with end-to-end anastomosis is chosen, in order to achieve a perfect muco-mucosal approach between the two biliary stumps, single-layer anastomosis is performed using several, absorbable, fine (5/0), monofilament stitches. The suture should be performed on well vascularized margins, without tension. The use of a T-tube is not mandatory, but can allow the anastomosis to be checked at the end of the procedure with a low pressure injection of chloride solution, to decompress the anastomosis during the first postoperative days, and to perform a cholangiogram after one week. The size of the biliary drain should be smaller than the bile duct, in order to avoid forceful cannulation of the bile duct. In particular, dilation maneuvers of the lumen of bile ducts should not be performed in order to avoid injuries to the mucosa that can cause bile leak and subsequent stricture of the anastomosis.

In case of a very small anastomosis, the drain should be used with the aim of calibrating the anastomosis, and in this case Silastic drainage is preferable because of its low tissue inflammatory reaction. These surgical drains should be removed and replaced with endoscopic stents during the postoperative course.

When a T-tube is inserted, it should emerge from a small vertical incision below the suture line, in order not to hamper the perfect mucosal apposition of the two biliary stumps. The upper end of the T-tube is placed below the main biliary confluence so that both hemilivers can be drained (Fig. 21.28).

When the CBD is extremely small a linear biliary drain, or an endoscopic biliary stent, can be inserted, with the tip passing through the papilla. This can be easily found and replaced endoscopically during the postoperative course.

If bilio-enteric anastomosis is the treatment of choice, hepaticojejunostomy is the best technique, using a 70–80 cm long Roux-en-Y jejunal loop (the technique is described in detail in the Surgical Treatment of Biliary Strictures section). Usually the CBD is very small, and therefore the opening of the jejunal loop should be smaller because the jejunal opening becomes wider than the biliary one: it is enough to make just a hole with the tip of the electro-cautery; excess jejunal

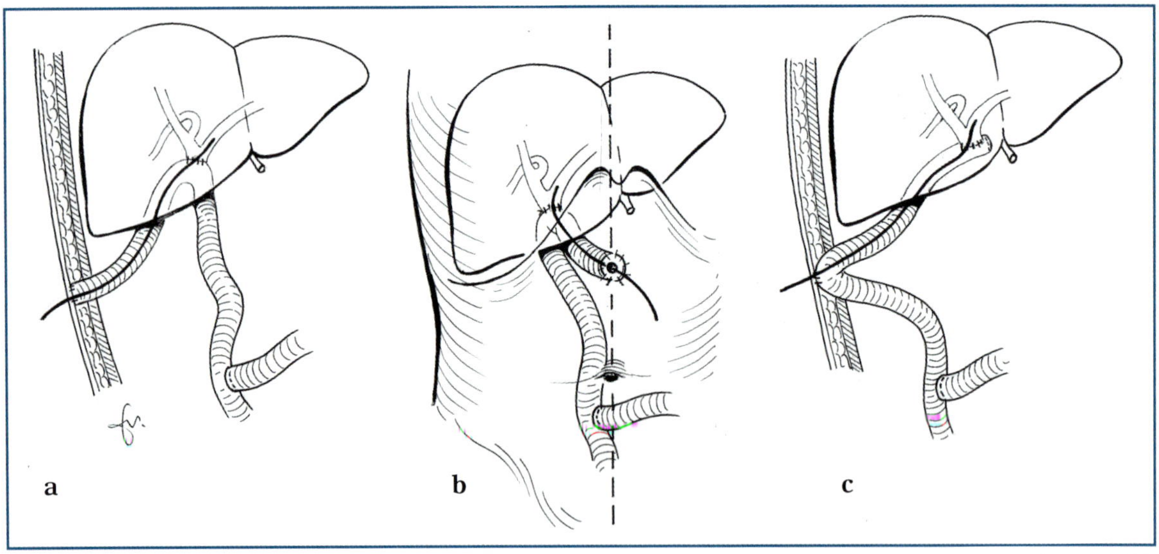

Fig. 21.31 Roux-en-Y hepaticojejunostomy with jejunal loop fixed to the abdominal wall according to different modalities (**a**, **b**, **c**). A metallic ring can be placed on the jejunal loop which is fixed to the skin to help the access to the anastomosis, for endoscopic exploration and possible percutaneous dilatation. Reproduced with permission from [42]

mucosa is resected, according to the Gazzaniga's technique [91].

When a bilio-enteric anastomosis is at particular risk of stricture, techniques of "access loop" can be also considered (Fig. 21.31); i.e., to fix the jejunal loop to the skin, according to different modalities, in order to have easy access to the anastomosis for endoscopic exploration and possible percutaneous dilatation [42, 86].

Early Postoperative Clinical Manifestations

The time of postoperative diagnosis of BDI is extremely relevant because it seriously affects final results. The median delay in diagnosis is 1–2 weeks [92–94], but it can also be several weeks, and for biliary strictures it may be months or years [94].

Inappropriate or untimely decisions on diagnostic workup or therapeutic strategies, or delayed referral of patients to dedicated centers can worsen the injury, increase the complexity of repairs, compromise their long-term results, and worsen the general condition of the patient, who may even risk death [42].

The adverse effects of delayed referral with increased duration of illness warrant further comment. The presence of biliary peritonitis is an independent factor for poor outcome [95], and hepatic fibrosis can occur within 6–12 months of injury without adequate management (Fig. 21.32) [96]. This is particularly concerning, as cirrhosis and portal hypertension significantly increase mortality after BDI [97]. Finally, duration of treatment is also an independent prognostic factor for quality of life after attempts at repair, so delay should be minimized [98].

Biliary fistula, biliary peritonitis and jaundice have been considered classical postoperative clinical manifestations of BDI. After the introduction of laparoscopic cholecystectomy, the occurrence of biliary fistula and biliary peritonitis increased. It has been reported that biliary fistula is the most frequent postoperative clinical manifestation, accounting for 44.1% of 127 postoperatively recognized BDIs [14]. Biliary fistula is caused more frequently by a minor BDI [14, 99]. In the Italian survey [14], it was reported that biliary peritonitis, which accounted for 37.8% of postoperatively recognized BDIs, was more frequently associated with major BDIs. Finally, in the same series, occurrence of jaundice (18.1%) was always due to a major BDI.

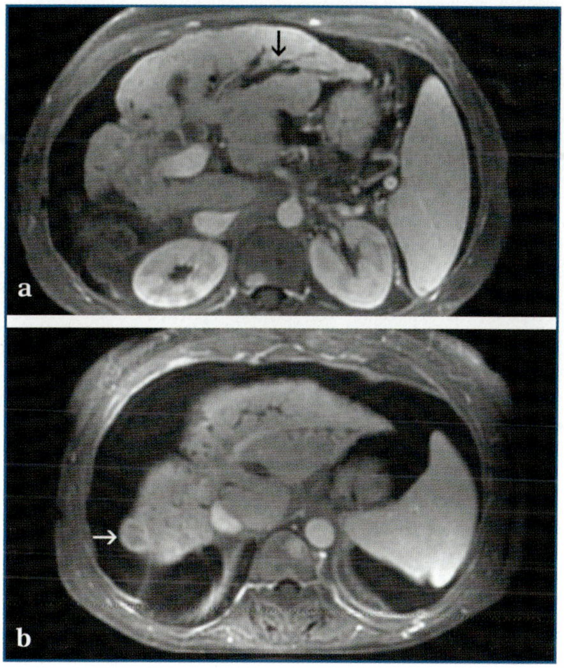

Fig. 21.32 A 54-year-old female. **a** MR showing secondary biliary cirrhosis with right lobe atrophy after untreated injury of main biliary confluence and of right hepatic artery, occurred 12 years after cholecystectomy. Dilation of left biliary tree (*black arrow*). **b** Hepatocellular carcinoma on atrophic right lobe is present (*white arrow*)

Another two possibilities should be added to the classical clinical manifestations. The first possibility is characterized by patients who do not feel well during the early postoperative course (within 48 hours), and complain of unspecific mild abdominal pain, nausea or mild fever. These clinical signs should not be underestimated, but should urge immediate abdominal ultrasonography and blood liver function tests. Indeed, any patient remaining unwell 48 hours after cholecystectomy should be investigated for possible BDI [100].

The second possibility, probably more important, is characterized by patients with more complex clinical manifestations in which biliary fistula, jaundice and biliary peritonitis are all present and associated with sepsis, which is the most frequent cause of death in these patients. These patients should be treated immediately and effectively, as they are at risk of death from BDI.

Biliary Fistula

Cutaneous biliary fistula can be caused by BDIs differing considerably in severity. Therefore, accurate diagnosis of the type of injury is essential, without rushed decisions, especially if the patient does not have other complications. Sometimes a biliary fistula with limited output can spontaneously close within 24–48 hours, without consequences.

The decision of the surgeon to wait or to adopt urgent diagnostic or therapeutic means should depend on the general conditions of the patient and on accurate monitoring of clinical evolution. If general conditions allow, the opportunity of beginning diagnostic workup based on local expertise should be evaluated carefully and possible referral of the patient should be considered.

Investigations usually start with abdominal ultrasonography that should look for adequate outward drainage of the bile leak, presence of ductal dilation, accepting that the absence of such dilation does not exclude an injury, and for fluid collections. After cholecystectomy the incidence of collections in the gallbladder fossa is 10–14% [98]. The presence of fluid outside the gallbladder fossa should not be considered as a normal postoperative finding. Delay in diagnosis of the presence of bile in the peritoneal cavity is associated with an increase in serious complications, and development of infected bile is associated with adverse outcomes [93].

If the ultrasonography results are equivocal in a symptomatic patient, CT should be performed because its sensitivity is higher than that of ultrasonography for diagnosis of abdominal fluid collection (96% vs. 70%) [93]. In addition, CT allows possible concomitant arterial injury to be recognized early.

Further investigations are aimed at obtaining a high quality cholangiogram, and MR is generally preferred [101, 102]: the type and level of injury can be well documented, and presence of undrained bile collections is clearly shown (Fig. 21.33). MR should determine the need for ERCP in case of a minor bile duct leak (small intrahepatic ducts or cystic duct leak) (Fig. 21.34), in case of CBD obstruction due to stones, or in case of major bile duct injuries treatable by endoscopy.

If a biliary drain is present, cholangiography through this drain may be useful for further elucidation of the nature of any injury or leak (Fig. 21.35).

For patients with postoperative external biliary fistula through operatively or postoperatively placed drains, contrast injection through the drainage (sinography) can be performed to define the site of leakage and the anatomy of the biliary tree (Fig. 21.36).

The decision to drain subhepatic collections depends on the general conditions of the patient, and it can be performed via a percutaneous, laparoscopic or laparotomic approach. This can be decided according to the features of the collections and to the time elapsed since cholecystectomy. Right subcostal laparotomy may be the preferred choice in order to achieve a complete drainage of partly organized collections and debridement of surrounding tissue.

A "simple" biliary fistula is a clinical situation less severe and easier to treat than fistula associated with bile peritonitis, which needs more timely treatment. The treatment of "simple" biliary fistula depends on the situation.

A fistula from the cystic duct stump is treated by endoscopic sphincterotomy and placement of a naso-biliary drain, or stent, depending on the case. This kind of fistula is often caused by unknown choledocholithiasis, in particular in patients who have been symptomatic for a long time (Fig. 21.2).

With a fistula from a segmental bile duct, bile leak progressively decreases and spontaneously closes; therefore it is necessary to maintain an abdominal drain and to remove it progressively up to the clo-

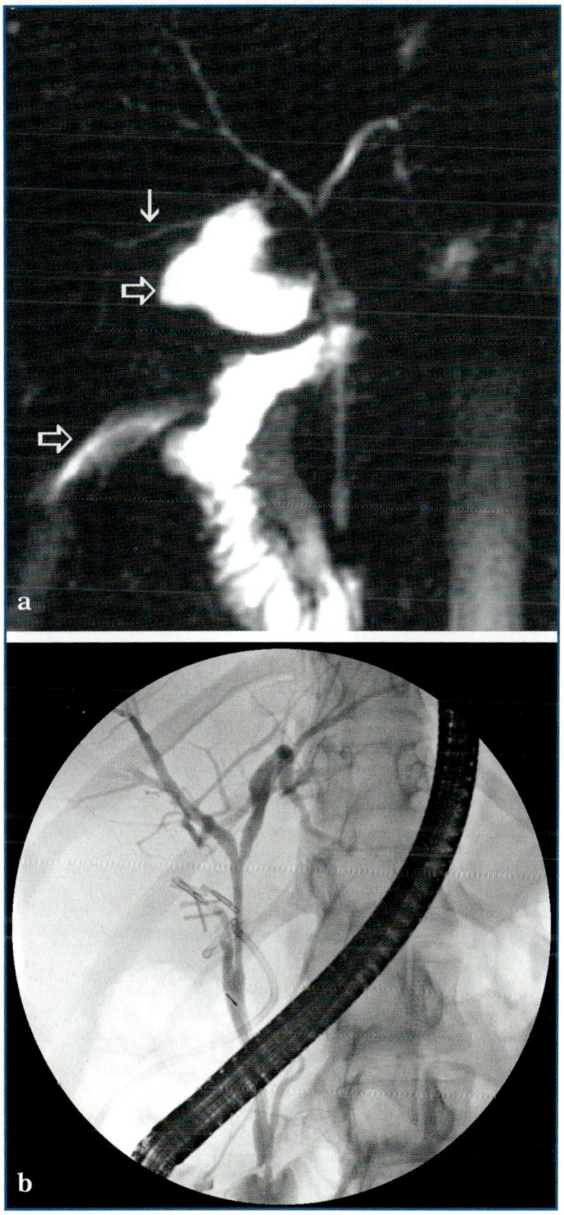

Fig. 21.33 A 20-year-old female. **a** MR-cholangiography: bile leak from injured right posterior sectorial duct (*white arrow*), without continuity with CBD, which is normal. Bile subhepatic collection (*empty arrows*) was percutaneously drained. **b** ERCP shows an intact CBD and absence of right posterior sectoral duct

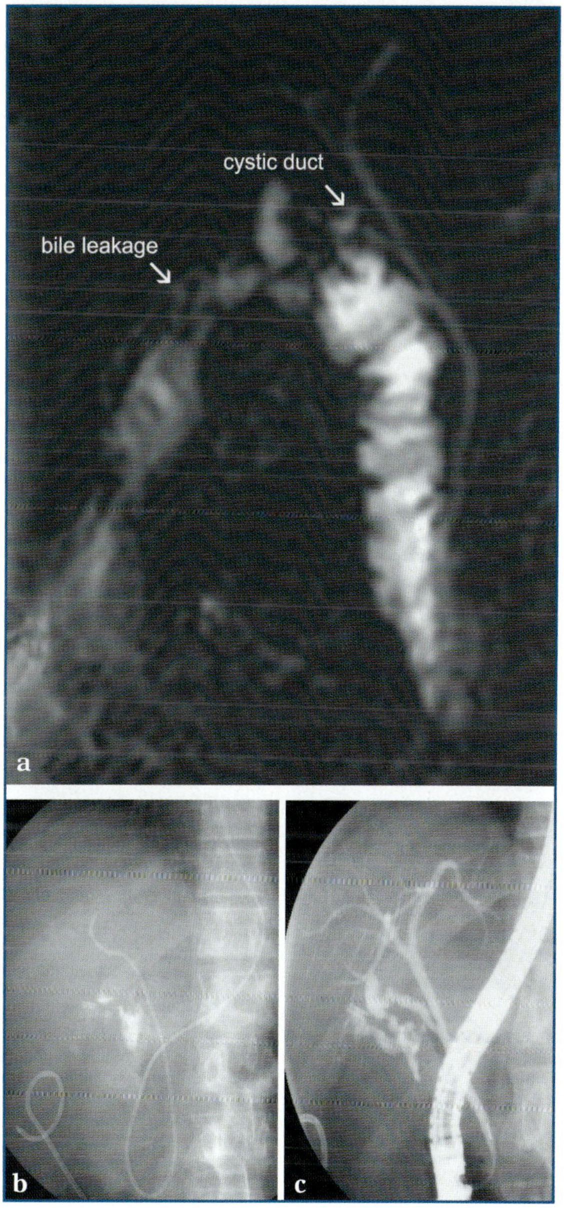

Fig. 21.34 Choleperitoneum and biliary fistula after cholecystectomy. **a** MR-cholangiography: bile leak from cystic duct stump with subhepatic bile collection that was percutaneously drained. **b** ERCP showing bile leak from cystic duct and (**c**) placement of naso-biliary drainage. Subsequent laparoscopic drainage of biliary peritonitis

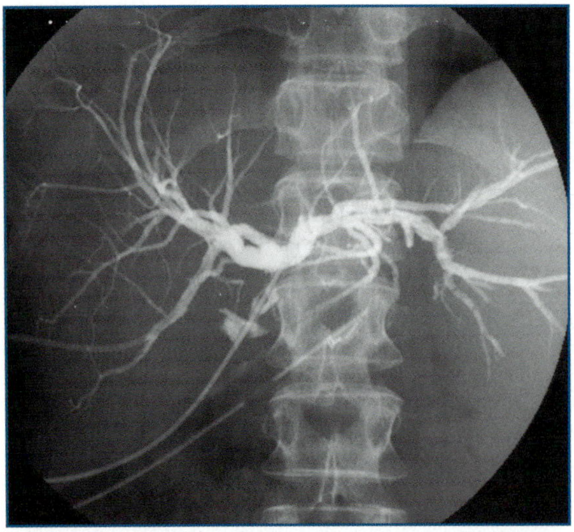

Fig. 21.35 Cholangiography through biliary drain showing Bismuth Type 3 injury

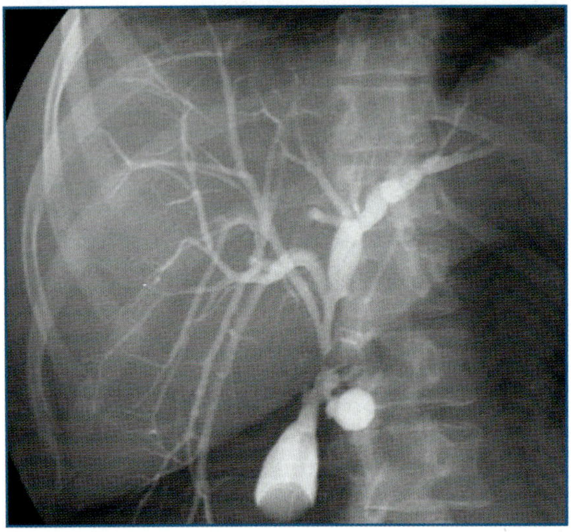

Fig. 21.36 Cholangiography through a Foley catheter inserted in the fistulous tract, 70 days after cholecystectomy: complete CBD transection below the main biliary confluence

sure of bile leak, which generally occurs in a few days.

A fistula from a lateral injury of the CBD can be treated by endoscopic placement of a biliary stent: the wider the biliary injury, the higher the degree of difficulty of treatment.

In case of complete transection of the CBD, at least three therapeutic strategies can be evaluated. The first possibility is immediate surgical repair, with a delay of a few hours if possible, even though the difficulty of dealing with a thin walled bile duct should be considered; according to several surgeons this is not a problem, but the best long term results are reported when anastomosis is performed on dilated bile ducts [26, 43]. However, more frequently, the time interval is several days between diagnosis of the fistula and referral to a dedicated center. As already mentioned, in patients with BDI not recognized at the time of cholecystectomy, the median delay in diagnosis is 1–2 weeks, but it can be also several weeks [98]. In our own experience these "acute" patients were referred after a mean time interval of 15 days (median 8 days), with a range from 4 to 58 days. In this time interval the surrounding tissues become edematous and fragile because of the inflammation caused by the presence of bile and local infection, and this increases the degree of difficulty of the repair.

The second possibility is to wait for some weeks, with a well established and controlled biliary fistula, until the resolution of all accompanying complications (local inflammation, sepsis, malnutrition). This strategy is recommended by Bismuth [43], is used by many surgeons [26, 72, 89] and is also preferred in our center [42]. With this strategy, the abdominal drain is progressively removed from the abdomen. In this way, fibrous tissue and adhesions surrounding the drain avoid spreading bile into the abdomen. Bile comes out through the fistulous tract remaining after complete withdrawal of the drain, but surrounding granulation tissue causes an increase in resistance to outward bile flow, with progressive dilation of proximal bile ducts (Fig. 21.37). Therefore, biliary repair is performed 1–3 months after injury, on dilated bile ducts, without inflamed or scarred tissue, with a well demarcated final level of stricture, and with the patient in good general conditions.

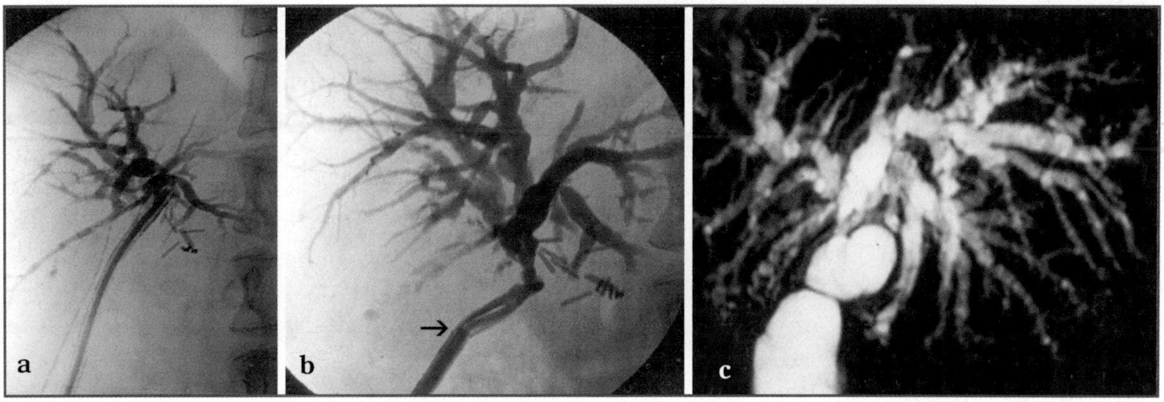

Fig. 21.37 Cholecystectomy in a 70–year-old female. Reoperation on postoperative day 11 for choleperitoneum. Referral to our Unit on postoperative day 15 with sepsis. Intensive care treatment of the sepsis. **a** Cholangiography through the abdominal drain: BDI immediately below the main biliary confluence. Progressive removal of abdominal drain. **b** Cholangiography after partial mobilization of the drain: stricture Bismuth Type 3 (*arrow* showing the upper end of the drain). **c** MRC after complete removal of the drain: evident dilation of biliary tree. Reproduced with permission from [42]

In the most complicated injuries, the day before the operation, a percutaneous biliary drain can be inserted into the hilum, in order to help the surgeon to recognize the biliary stump during dissection, to decompress the anastomosis, and to perform postoperative cholangiogram.

This remains our preferred strategy, even though in some patients the progressive dilation of bile ducts is slower than usual, or episodes of cholangitis occur in the meantime, although these are generally not severe and are easily treated. In the time interval until the repair, a spontaneous bilio-enteric fistula may develop (Fig. 21.30c1, c2), through which the bile drainage is incomplete and may delay the closure of the fistula.

In general, the best results are achieved by end-to-side hepaticojejunostomy [54, 69, 72]. Factors associated with improved outcome of this procedure include the use of several closely placed, absorbable, thin sutured, single-layer anastomoses, on healthy non inflamed or scarred tissue. In order to reduce the stricture rate of hepaticojejunostomy, for ischemic causes or for leak of the anastomosis, the Hepp-Couinaud procedure (left duct approach) should be evaluated [103, 104]. This is the procedure of choice in our center and it will be described in detail in the Surgical Treatment of Biliary Strictures section.

The third possibility is the insertion of biliary stents by endoscopic, percutaneous or combined ("Rendez-vous" technique) approach. Biliary recanalization has been exceptionally reported using this technique, after resection of a tract of CBD up to 2.5 cm long [105]. However, these techniques are available only in highly specialized centers, where very experienced endoscopists and radiologists are available. In these settings, occasionally good results are reported, even though they are not enough to give a definitive evaluation of this treatment.

Another surgical possibility, which should be considered as a possible salvage operation, carried out in one patient in our experience, can occur in a critical phase of the clinical course in a patient with a high-output biliary fistula, when sepsis seems to be controlled and general conditions are improving. A sudden severe worsening of the general conditions of the patient can force the surgeon to operate urgently. After drainage of the abdominal cavity, if absence of a long tract of CBD is found, a T-tube can be inserted as a bridge between the two biliary stumps, in order to drain the bile in the duodenum and to interrupt the biliary fistula, and to get over the critical septic phase. The drawbacks of this choice are the following: in order to fix the T-tube to the proximal biliary stump further biliary tissue is "sacrificed", the main biliary confluence is almost reached, and the level of the injury becomes higher than before. In addition, the presence of the T-tube increases the distance between the two stumps and avoids the dilation of proximal bile ducts. Solutions to this situation can be as follows: 1) after resolution of sepsis, closure of the T-tube and delayed repair (Fig. 21.38); 2) progressive removal of the T-tube in order to obtain a fistulous tract, through which the residual fistula is drained, and to perform a delayed biliary repair; and 3) leaving the T-tube in situ for some months, in order to promote the carrying out of a bilio-duodenal fistula, and subsequently to replace it with endoscopic stents (Fig. 21.39). Instead of placing a T-tube into the CBD as a bridge in such cases, other strategies can be considered: 1) to perform a perfect drainage outward of the bile with large-bore drains, and to wait for closure of the fistula for delayed repair, 2) to insert an external percutaneous drainage through the intrahepatic biliary tree into the proximal biliary stump, and to perform a hepaticojejunostomy immediately.

In case of biliary fistula associated with biliary peritonitis, which can be treated only by percutaneous drainage, the therapeutic strategies are similar to those already mentioned.

In summary, the most important principles for the treatment of patients with biliary fistula that occurred in the immediate postoperative course are: 1) when the fistula is the only manifestation of the injury and it is well drained outward without other complications, it is not necessary to make urgent decisions; 2) immediate reoperation without complete diagnosis of the injury is not indicated for at least three reasons: accurate preoperative definition of the injury may reveal

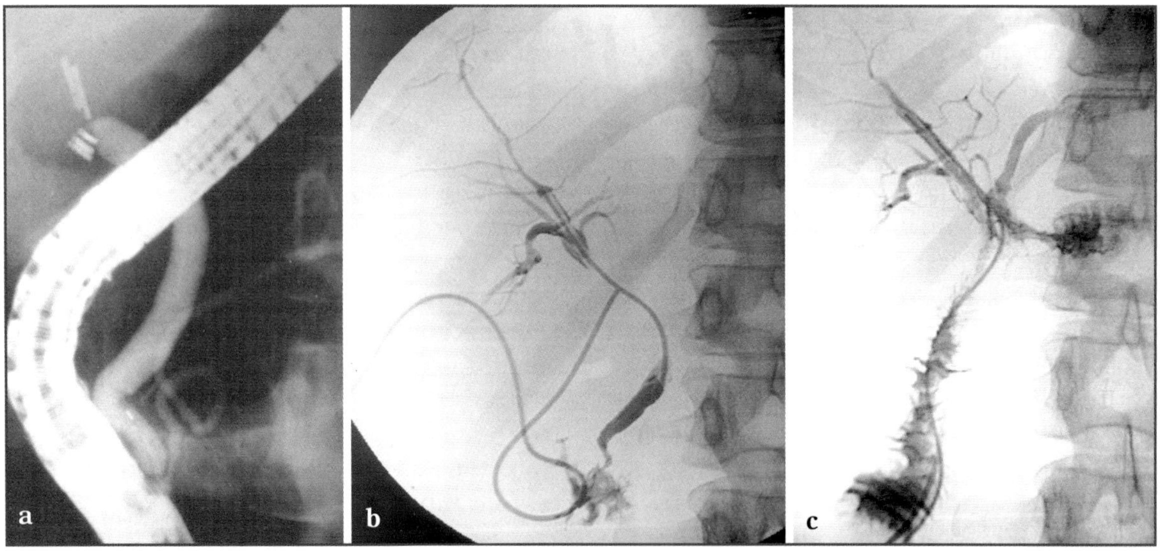

Fig. 21.38 Cholecystectomy in a 28-year-old female. High-output biliary fistula on postoperative day 1. **a** ERCP on postoperative day 7: complete stenosis of the CBD. Referral to our Unit on postoperative day 11 with sepsis and high-output biliary fistula (300–1500 mL/day). Reoperation for biliary peritonitis on postoperative day 12 and recognition of wide CBD excision. Salvage repair over T-tube, placed as a bridge between the two biliary stumps. **b** Postoperative cholangiography showing absence of a long segment of CBD with intact main confluence. Subsequent discharge after closure of the T-tube. Delayed repair by hepaticojejunostomy at the hilar plate. **c** Postoperative cholangiography through transanstomotic drain placed according to Volker technique. Reproduced with permission from [42]

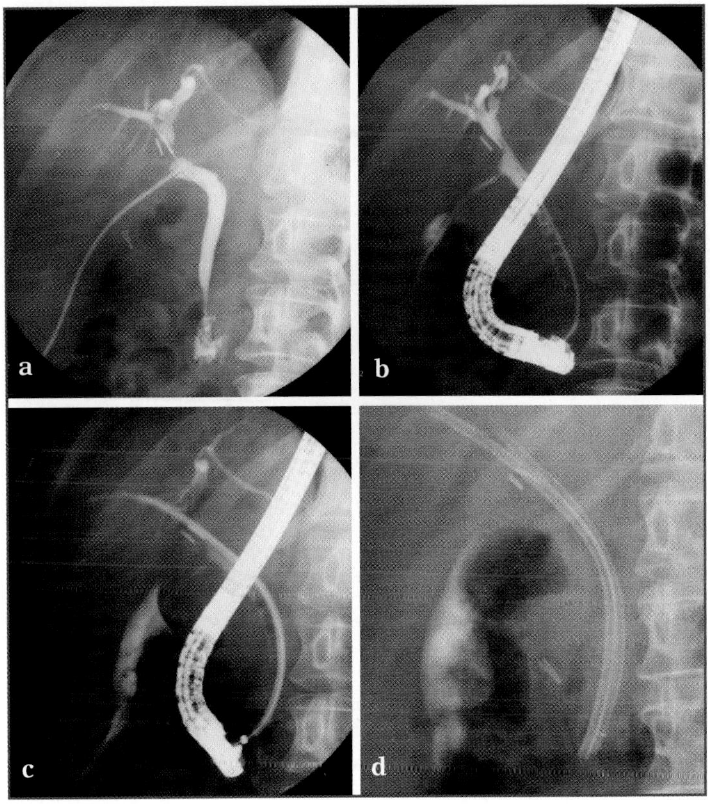

Fig. 21.39 **a** Cholangiography through T-tube showing Bismuth Type 2 injury of CBD. **b** ERCP: insertion of a guide wire through the injury. **c, d** Biliary stents placement and T-tube removal

an injury that can be treated by non surgical procedures, intraoperative diagnosis of the injury can be very difficult, and the type of injury can be too complex for the experience of the surgeon; 3) all the diagnostic and therapeutic options should be available in the hospital, or the referral of the patient to another center where is possible to have a multidisciplinary approach should be carefully evaluated.

Biliary Peritonitis

The most severe injuries are those with bile leak into the peritoneal cavity; these are true emergencies. Presence of bile in the peritoneal cavity can be related to injuries that differ considerably in severity, and can require either very easy or complex treatments, depending on whether they are caused by minor or major injuries. For this reason, when biliary peritonitis is present, it is essential to understand the type of BDI as soon as possible. Biliary peritonitis can be localized in one or more collections (biloma), or it may be diffused within the abdominal cavity: if it is sterile, chemical peritonitis (or "biliary ascites") develops, if it is infected a true biliary peritonitis occurs. The patient may complain of clinical signs of acute abdomen, or less severe symptoms, such as abdominal soreness, minor abdominal distension, slight fever, nausea and dyspeptic signs, to the point that diagnosis can be greatly delayed (Fig. 21.40).

Further remarks should be made on these possible subtle clinical manifestations. Laparoscopic cholecystectomy is a procedure that usually allows the patient to return home quickly and to work a few days after operation. It is important to repeat that the postoperative occurrence of symptoms such as pain, fever, abdominal distension, even if not clearly evident, should suggest particular clinical care and further evaluation by liver function biochemistry and abdominal ultrasonography.

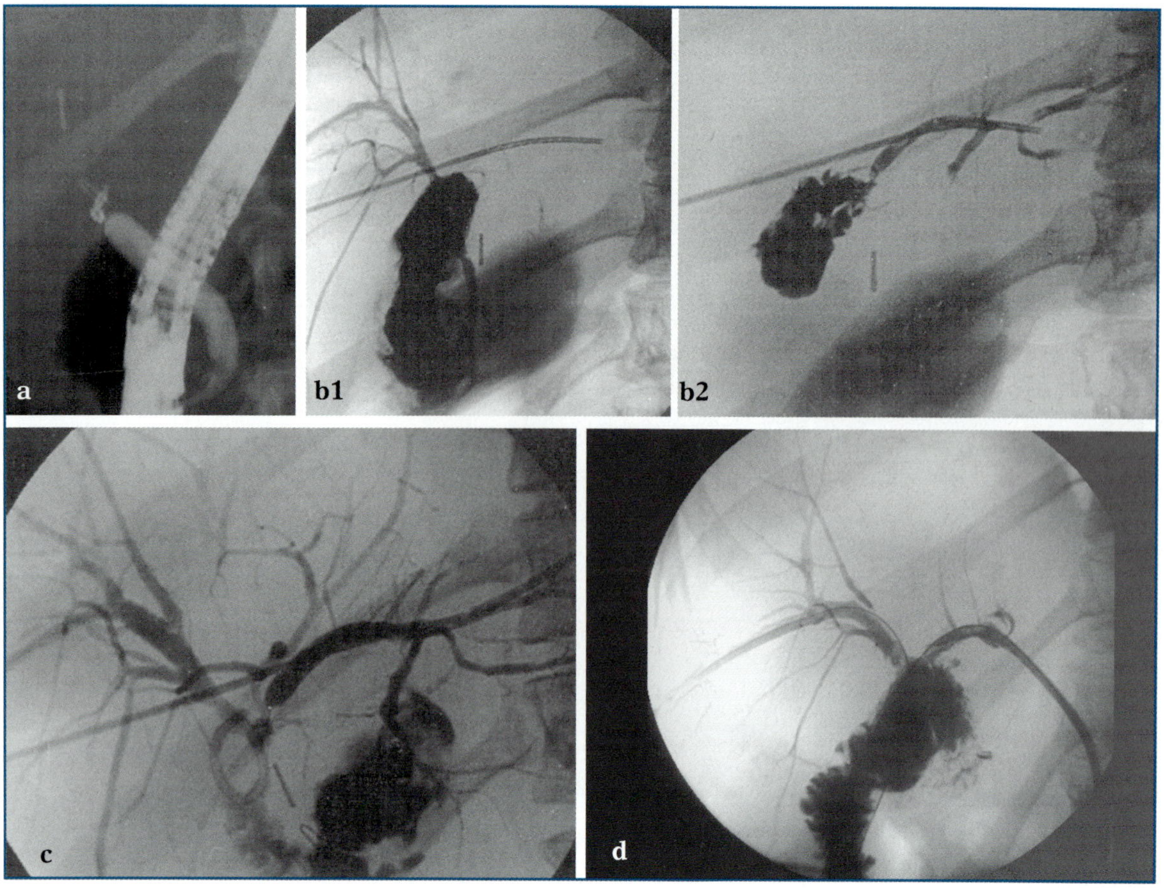

Fig. 21.40 Cholecystectomy in a 22-year-old female. A few days after discharge, light abdominal pain and slight jaundice occurred (total bilirubin: 3.7 mg/dL). Abdominal ultrasound on postoperative day 27: large abdominal collection. Percutaneous drainage of bile (5000 mL). Persistence of abdominal pain and abdominal distension. Reoperation on potoperative day 35 and drainage of diffuse biliary peritonitis. Consequent high-output biliary fistula. **a** ERCP on postoperative day 50: complete stenosis of CBD. PTC with selective injection of **b1** right hepatic duct and **b2** left hepatic duct which drain directly into the abdominal cavity. **c** Simultaneous filling of right and left hepatic ducts with bile leak (Bismuth Type 4b). Referral to our Unit where treatment of sepsis was performed until re-establishment of good general conditions was obtained. On postoperative day 77, two separate right- and left-hepaticojejunostomies were performed. **d** Postoperative cholangiography showing patency of the two anastomoses with transanastomotic percutaneous catheters. The catheters were left in place for 1 year, and changed with catheters of progressively increased size up to 14 Fr. Reproduced with permission from [42]

Clinical suspicion of biliary peritonitis requires four steps: 1) a definitive diagnosis by abdominal ultrasonography and/or CT should be performed, and other complications excluded (Fig. 21.41); 2) the biliary injury that caused the biliary peritonitis should be precisely defined by MR and, according to its results, by ERCP and/or percutaneous transhepatic cholangiography (PTC), which can be the definitive treatment of some injuries; 3) drainage of the biliary peritonitis; and 4) control of the biliary leak that caused the biliary peritonitis.

The drainage of biliary peritonitis can be performed by a simple percutaneous approach, under ultrasound or CT guide, or by a laparoscopic approach. The kind of approach depends on the severity of general conditions, on the site and extension of bile peritonitis, and on the capability to perform

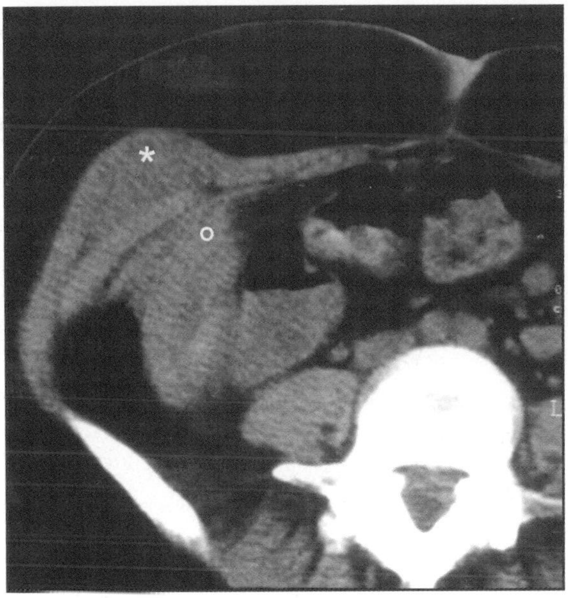

Fig. 21.41 Suspected choleperitoneum 1 week after cholecystectomy because of abdominal pain in right upper quadrant with rebound tenderness in a 37-year-old female. Abdominal CT scan showing hematoma of the abdominal wall probably due to trocar injury of epigastric vessels; hematoma extends through the abdominal muscles either into subcutaneous tissue (*), or into preperitoneal space (°). Spontaneous resolution of symptoms. Reproduced with permission from [42]

a percutaneous or laparoscopic drainage (Fig. 21.34). In many patients a laparotomic approach is necessary, particularly in cases of delayed referral, or of multiple but independent bile collections. It remains controversial whether biliary repair should be performed during this operation. Recently it has been reported that active peritonitis was one of two factors significantly influencing the failure of surgical repair: in fact, the rate of failure was 61.5% in the patients with active peritonitis in whom surgical repair was performed, and 6.1% if peritonitis was not present ($p<0.001$) [80]. It is problematic to perform a biliary repair with inflamed and septic tissues, and with a small bile duct. In addition, as already mentioned, it is necessary to have a complete definition of the injury, which will be more accurate if obtained in a preoperative setting rather than intraoperatively, when it can be often difficult and incomplete. For these reasons, many centers, including our own, prefer to consider the drainage of biliary peritonitis with resolution of sepsis and re-establishment of good general conditions of the patient, as the only and urgent aim of operation in these patients. Biliary repair, through a surgical or non-surgical approach, is delayed until later.

Jaundice

In case of complete stenosis of the CBD, jaundice will occur during the immediate postoperative course, without pain or fever. Usually, bilirubin rapidly increases along with cytolysis and cholestasis enzymes, and after one week pruritus occurs. The patient is in good general condition, and for this reason postoperative occurrence of uncomplicated jaundice is not an emergency, except in case of cholangitis, which is infrequent. In this case a percutaneous biliary drain is indicated, because obstruction of the CBD hampers the endoscopic approach. Except in this case, PTC should be avoided because it decompresses the biliary tree and avoids dilation of bile ducts, increasing the difficulty of the repair. Percutaneous attempts to re-cannulate the distal biliary stump with force can be dangerous, because it may change a jaundiced asymptomatic patient into a patient with biliary peritonitis (Fig. 21.42). The insertion of biliary stents by combined endoscopic and percutaneous approach (“Rendez-vous” technique) is a technique infrequently reported in highly specialized centers, with occasionally good results, needing further clinical evaluation in terms of long term results. Therefore at the moment the technique of biliary recanalization should not be considered as a standard procedure, and should be indicated only in selected cases.

Abdominal ultrasonography can show initial dilation of intrahepatic bile ducts

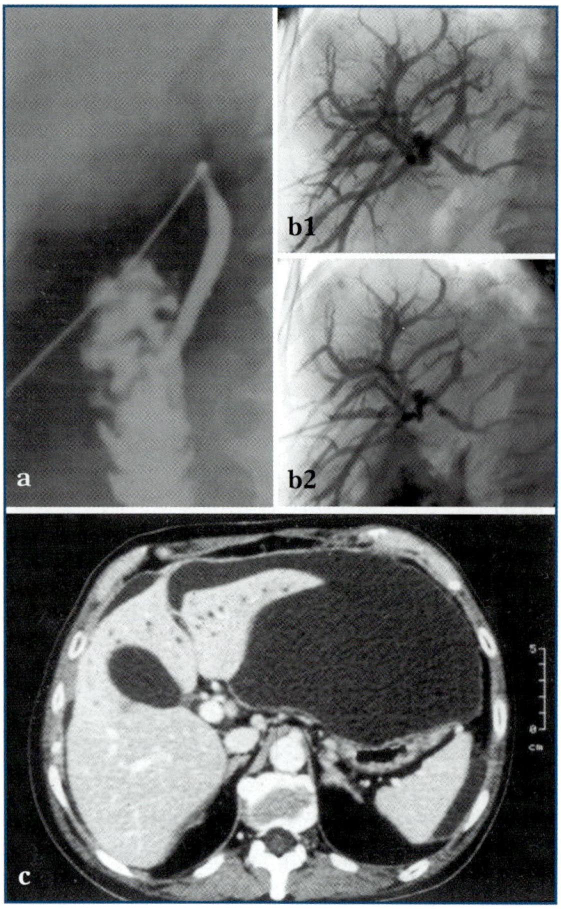

Fig. 21.42 Cholecystectomy with "suture of anomalous bile duct within gallbladder fossa " in a 67-year-old male. **a** Intraoperative cholangiography: complete CBD obstruction. Jaundice during the postoperative course; PTC on postoperative day 7. **b1** Stricture below the main biliary confluence (Bismuth Type 3). **b2** After attempts to forcefully re-cannulate the distal biliary stump, massive choleperitoneum occurs as shown at CT (**c**). Reproduced with permission from [42]

and it can exclude the presence of intra-abdominal fluid collections. MR cholongiography is the preferred imaging technique in these cases; in fact, it offers detailed information on the morphology of biliary tree, the exact level of injury, the distance between the two biliary stumps and the type of injury, without invasiveness (Fig. 21.43).

If ERCP is performed, complete obstruction of the distal CBD is clearly shown,

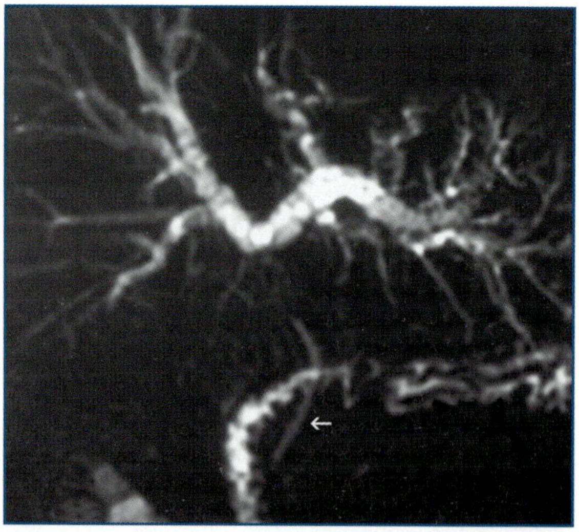

Fig. 21.43 Jaundice after cholecystectomy. MR on postoperative day 15: dilation of biliary tree with bile duct stricture below the main biliary confluence (Bismuth Type 3) and excision of a long tract of CBD. Distal CBD (*arrow*). Hepaticojejunostomy on postoperative day 17. Reproduced with permission from [42]

without visualization of the intrahepatic biliary tree and proximal CBD (Fig. 21.44). After diagnosis of complete closure of the CBD, these patients should be simply followed-up, awaiting dilation of the bile ducts above the stenosis. After around two weeks the proximal biliary stump reaches a size of 10–12 mm. During this time interval, without occurrence of other complications, such as opening of the proximal stump because of high biliary pressure and subsequent biliary peritonitis, an increase in bilirubin is not usually a warning sign. The patient can regularly eat, and renal function with hydroelectrolytic balance should be monitored. In case of changes in coagulation function, Vitamin K should be given to the patient.

After two weeks, the limited inflammatory changes in the operative field that occurred after laparoscopic cholecystectomy are further reduced and the surgeon can perform a Roux-en-Y hepaticojejunostomy in extremely favourable conditions (Fig. 21.45).

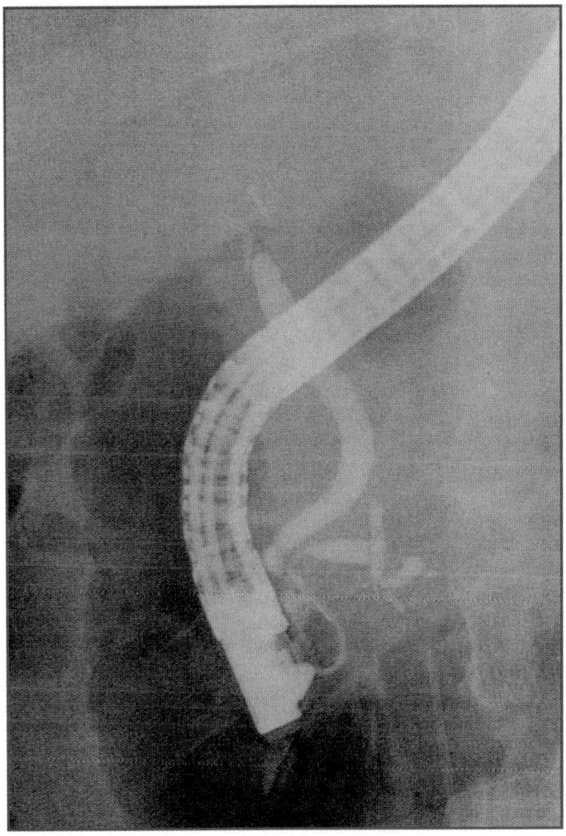

Fig. 21.44 ERCP showing complete obstruction of distal CBD, without visualization of intrahepatic biliary tree and proximal CBD

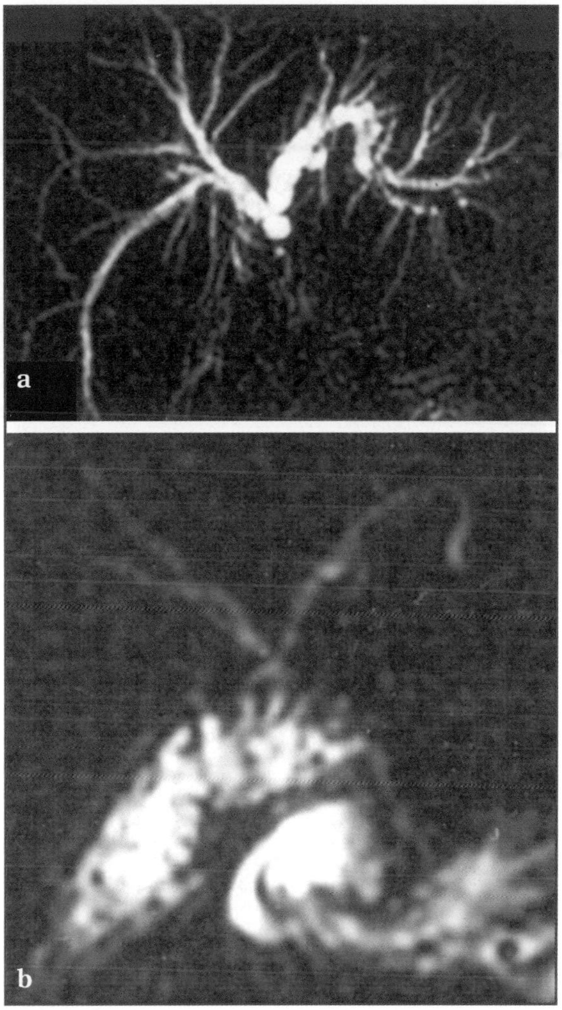

Fig. 21.45 Jaundice after cholecystectomy in a 61-year-old female. Referral to our unit on postoperative day 7 (total bilirubin 10 mg/dL). **a** MR showing bile duct stricture below the main biliary confluence (Bismuth Type 3). Hepaticojejunostomy at the hilar plate on postoperative day 15. **b** MR 2 months after surgical repair showing thin intrahepatic bile ducts. Reproduced with permission from [42]

Subintensive Care in "Complicated" Cases

Biliary fistula, biliary peritonitis and jaundice can be combined in different ways. The main issues are the presence or absence of bile in the peritoneal cavity and the presence of sepsis. If bile is present in the abdomen, drainage is mandatory, and if sepsis occurs it should be vigorously treated with drainage of intraperitoneal bile, of abdominal or hepatic abscesses, of bile ducts in case of cholangitis, and with treatment of possible other causes, e.g., infected biliary or venous catheters.

The subtle face of biliary injuries is that they can appear with only one of the classical manifestations, in patients in good general conditions, and this may lead to an underestimation of the gravity of the situation. Subsequent clinical course can worsen, sometimes also due to inappropriate therapy (Fig. 21.46), and become more complex, sepsis can occur, and may be difficult to treat, and the patient may die. The mortality rate for BDI is difficult to establish, but ranges from 0.9% to 6% [2, 42, 95] and sepsis or its subsequent complications are the main cause. In our experience, out of 65 patients referred to our Unit with major BDI, two (3%) patients died of sepsis after

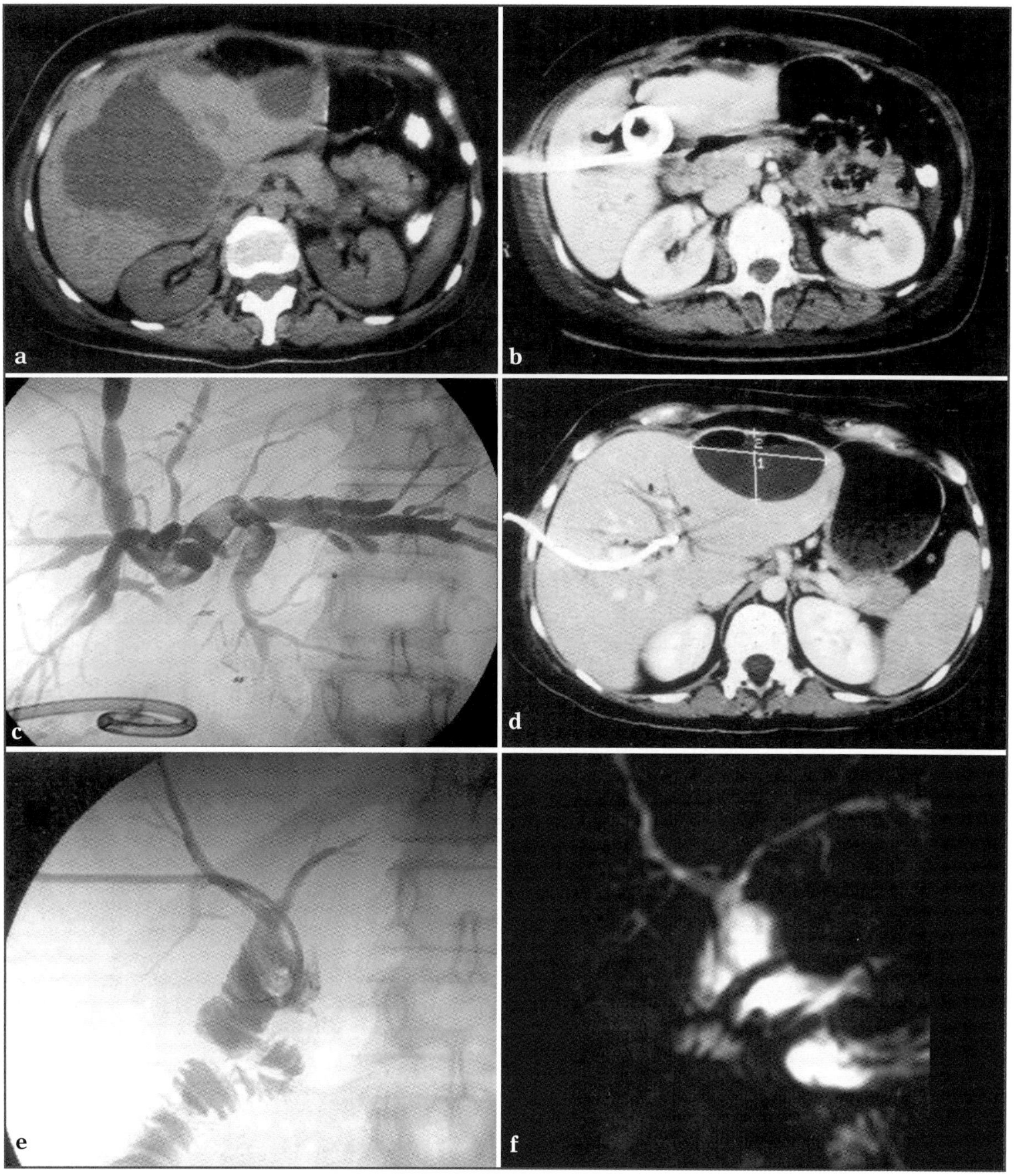

Fig. 21.46 Cholecystectomy converted to laparotomy (bile in the operative field) in a 34-year-old female. Referral at postoperative day 13 with obstructive jaundice, acute abdomen, external biliary fistula and systemic sepsis, after ERCP with diagnosis of interruption of the CBD. **a** CT scan showing choleperitoneum. **b** CT scan-guided percutaneous drainage of choleperitoneum. **c** PTC with biliary drainage (purulent cholangitis, Bismuth Type III stenosis). **d** After transient recovery, recurrence of sepsis and CT scan-guided drainage of residual biloma. Full recovery from sepsis, discharge 36 days after referral with the biliary drainage in place. One month later, readmission in good conditions, elective biliary reconstruction by Hepp-Couinaud hepaticojejunostomy. **e** Cholangiography through percutaneous catheter 45 days after reconstruction and **f** MR after 3 years showing normal intrahepatic bile ducts. Reproduced with permission from [42]

delayed referral, before any attempt at repair.

Prolonged hospital stay may be necessary in order to treat these patients, during which septic episodes can repeatedly occur. Therefore, accurate monitoring of the patient by repeated blood cultures, and cultures of fluids from drains, vascular catheters, and urinary catheters are necessary, not only to modulate antibiotic therapy, but also in order to quickly diagnose the occurrence of mycotic over-infections. At the same time it is essential to maintain other vital functions and to avoid further complications; e.g., the maintenance of sufficient hydration and urinary output is essential in order to avoid toxic renal injury due to prolonged administration of multiple antibiotics.

Nutritional support is essential, as malnutrition is one of the worst complications of sepsis. In these patients malnutrition can be related to the occurrence of events that preclude a normal oral diet (fasting for invasive maneuvers, reoperations, complications such as nausea and vomiting).

Accurate monitoring (renal, respiratory) of these patients is essential for early diagnosis of further complications that are more difficult to treat if recognized later.

In addition to treatment of sepsis, procedures such as ERCP or PTC aimed at defining the type of bile duct injury and can be essential also for the treatment of sepsis causes.

These extremely difficult clinical situations are frequently observed in patients referred late to tertiary care centers, often after more than one attempt at repairing the BDI.

In our series, 21.1% of patients (14/65) had severe sepsis and required intensive care management; four of them underwent surgical drainage of choleperitoneum and ten had multiple percutaneous drainages. As mentioned above, two of these patients died due to septic complications.

Hemobilia

Hemobilia rarely occurs, but it should nevertheless be promptly recognized. It can be caused by a vascular injury accompanying the biliary injury [106].

When intra-operative bleeding occurs during laparoscopic or open cholecystectomy blind attempts at hemostasis can be effective, but may cause injury to the right hepatic artery, or to one of its branches. Subsequently, pseudoaneurysm of the right hepatic artery or its branches can occur with subsequent bleeding into bile ducts.

In patients with a biliary drainage, or with an external biliary fistula, hemobilia can become evident with massive bleeding through the drain, which can induce the surgeon to perform an immediate laparotomy. At laparotomy, recognition of a pseudoaneurysm, which may be intrahepatic, is not easy, and treatment may be difficult. Ligature of the right hepatic artery or one of its branches, or even liver resection should be considered. In one of our cases, the site of bleeding could not be identified at emergency laparotomy; the hepatic artery was encircled with a vascular "tourniquet" that was exteriorized like a drain, with the aim of temporarily closing it in case of further bleeding, awaiting angiography for embolization (Fig. 21.12).

ERCP can show actual bleeding, or presence of clots in the CBD, and attempts at controlling bleeding can be performed by biliary balloon catheters. However, the site of bleeding can be precisely defined by angiography and arterial embolization can be performed.

Late Postoperative Clinical Manifestations

Biliary strictures occurring months or years after cholecystectomy are generally related to failure of previous attempts at repair or, more frequently, are strictures of hepaticojejunostomy. Sometimes a biliary injury is not clearly reported, but it can be suspected in the case of some conditions, such as conversion from laparoscopic to open procedure of an apparently simple cholecystectomy, or the description of an unexplainable choledochotomy, or even the placement of a T-tube.

Episodes of cholangitis are the first clinical manifestations, and often biliary colicky pain is related to intrahepatic stones that occur above the stricture. Concomitant increased levels of cholestasis and of cytolysis enzymes are always present. If these symptoms are not recognized, throughout the years, or even months, chronic cholestasis invariably causes irreversible injuries to the liver parenchyma, up to secondary biliary cirrhosis (Fig. 21.32).

Nowadays, most of these strictures are directly referred to non surgical treatments: endoscopic treatment in case of a stricture after repair of lateral injury or end-to-end repair or percutaneous treatment in case of stricture of hepaticojejunostomy [107, 108]. Surgery is often advocated in case of failure of non surgical treatments (Fig. 21.47), but repeated and prolonged stricture dilations can worsen the situation and move the level of the stricture proximally upwards leading to destruction of the main biliary confluence. Surgical repair in these cases is more difficult and the rate of failure is higher. Sometimes at surgery a greater distance than expected is found between the proximal biliary stump and jejunal loop, and an inflammatory, fibrous cavity between the two sides of the hepaticojejunostomy is discovered. This can be the result of excessively forceful or prolonged percutaneous dilations (Fig. 21.48). In order to limit the occurrence of this traumatic dilation with inflammatory tissue around the anastomosis, when percutaneous dilation of hepaticojejunostomy is indicated it is preferable to progressively dilate it over multiple sessions, using percutaneous stents of increasing size.

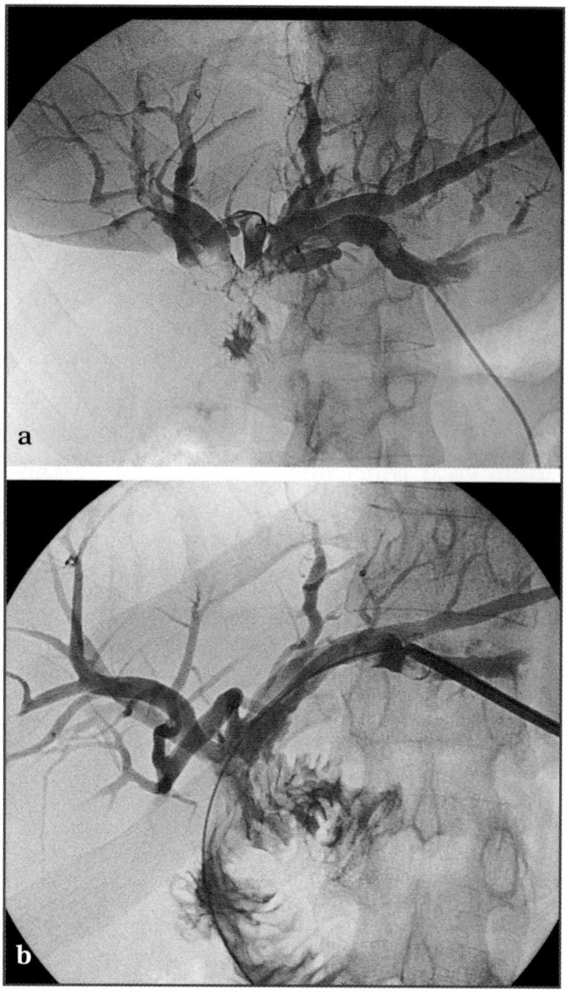

Fig. 21.47 a Stricture of hepaticojejunostomy with stones above the anastomoses, unresolved after percutaneous treatment. **b** Cholangiography 7 days after new hepaticojejunostomy according to Hepp-Couinaud technique: wide anastomosis without stones

Surgical Treatment of Biliary Strictures

Surgical treatment of postoperative bile duct strictures should follow three main goals: 1) to find healthy biliary mucosa above the bile duct stricture; 2) to perform a large hepaticojejunostomy; 3) to obtain an accurate apposition between biliary and jejunal mucosa.

The possibility of realizing a large biliary opening in healthy biliary mucosa depends on the level of the stricture. The biliary stricture is high in most cases and

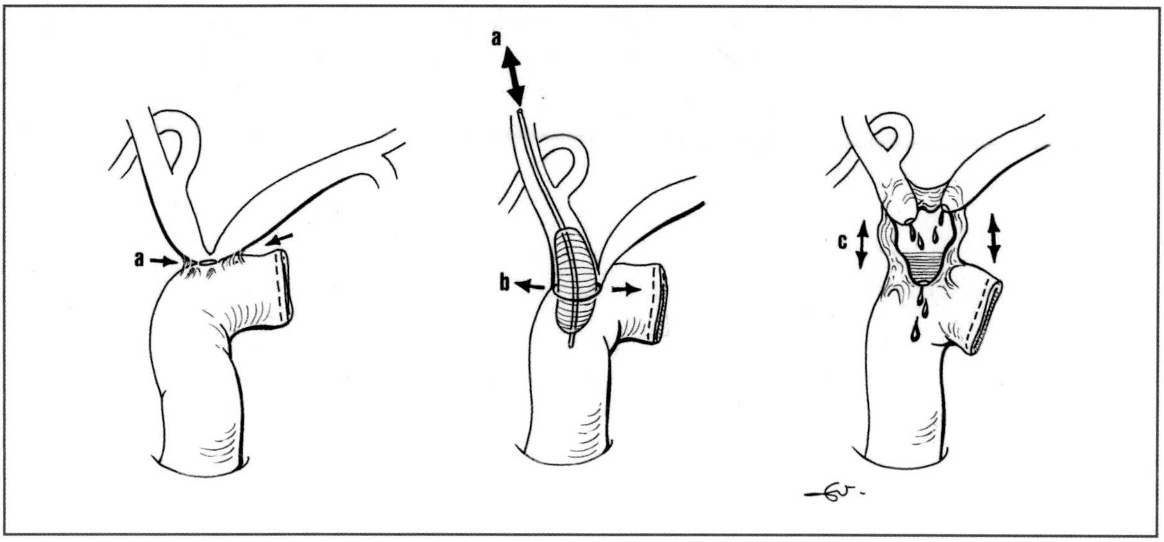

Fig. 21.48 During percutaneous treatment of stricture of hepaticojejunostomy (**a**), forceful and prolonged balloon dilations can cause repeated injuries to the anastomosis (**b**) with consequent occurrence of an inflammatory, fibrous cavity (**c**) between the two sides of the hepaticojejunostomy. Progressive worsening of the biliary stricture and increase of the distance between proximal biliary stump and jejunal loop can progressively occur. Reproduced with permission from [42]

classified as Bismuth Type 3 or Type 4. Biliary stump detection during surgery can be very difficult because of anatomic changes due to the previous injury, to postoperative complications, such as biliary leak, choleperitoneum and abscess, and to previous attempts at repair. Indeed, after every failure of surgical repair the stricture level moves proximally along the CBD, and may eventually involve the main biliary confluence. In these cases, it is our policy to place one or more percutaneous transhepatic drains immediately before surgery (one or two days), to obtain complete and precise cholangiographic mapping of the lesion, to facilitate intraoperative access to the hilar structures, and in the case of complex injuries, to avoid postoperative tension on the anastomoses and to reduce the risk of postoperative strictures. The stent is also useful for postoperative cholangiographic assessment of the anastomoses (Fig. 21.49).

For these reasons, the best surgical choice is not to redissect the hepatic pedicle, but to proceed straight to the hilum in order to lower the hilar plate and to find the main biliary confluence and the left hepatic duct, according to the Hepp-Couinaud technique (left duct approach) [89, 109, 110]. The three goals of surgical repair previously mentioned are accomplished by this technique, which allows a hepaticojejunostomy as large as possible to be performed, on healthy biliary mucosa of the left hepatic duct, with an accurate apposition between biliary and jejunal mucosa.

The hilar plate represents the anatomic principle of Hepp-Couinaud technique. Glisson's capsule covers the base of the quadrate lobe, joins the glissonian sheath of the hilar structures and continues to the hepatic pedicle peritoneum. At the level of the quadrate lobe base, Glisson's capsule becomes thicker and it is called a hilar plate. It extends from the vesicular plate on the right side, to the umbilical plate on the left side. The main biliary confluence is below the hilar plate. Glisson's capsule is opened between the quadrate lobe and the hilum, the avascular plane between the liver and the hilar plate is entered, and the main biliary confluence can be detached from the liver parenchyma. In this way the

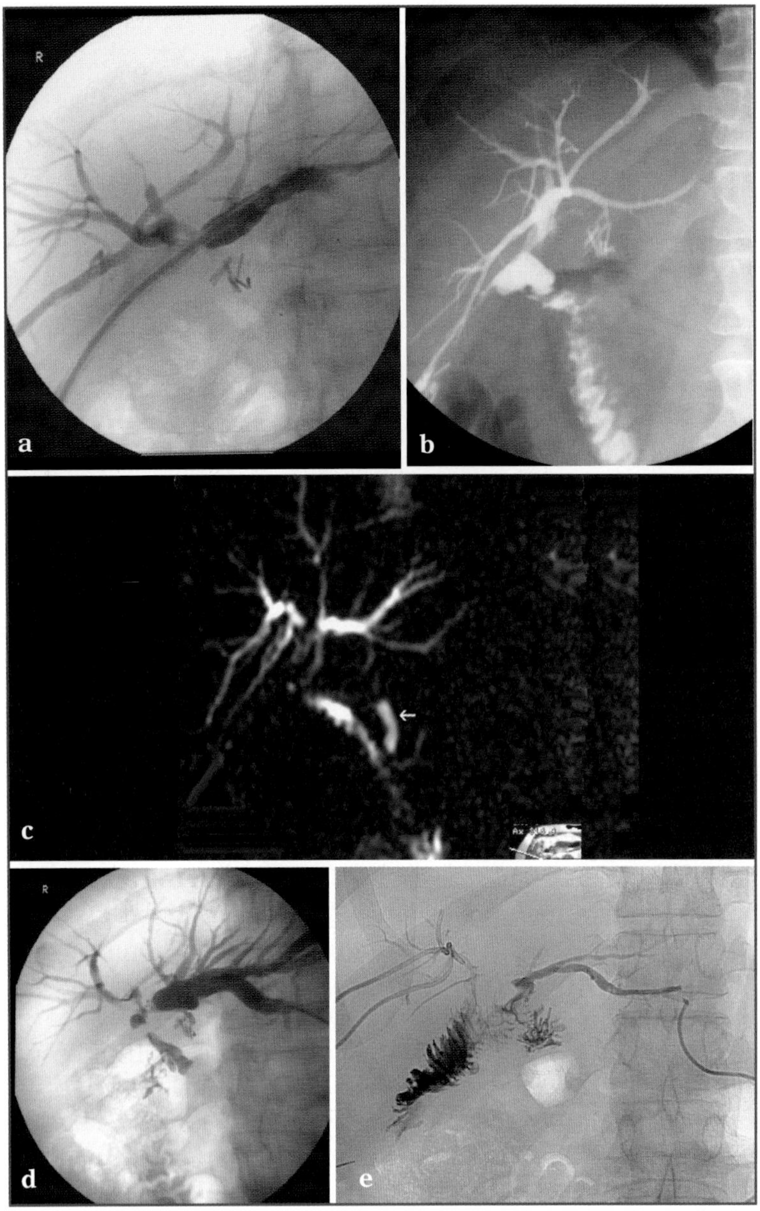

Fig. 21.49 Laparoscopic cholecystectomy converted to open procedure for occurrence of bile in the operative field in a 61-year-old female. Intraoperative diagnosis of biliary injury involving the main biliary confluence and placement of two biliary drains into the right and left hepatic ducts. Referral to our unit on postoperative day 45. **a** Cholangiography through biliary drains showing proximal injury with separation of right and left hepatic ducts (Bismuth Type 4). Subsequent progressive withdrawal of the biliary drains. **b** Sinography 3 months after cholecystectomy, showing right biliary tree with spontaneous bilio-enteric fistula, without visualization of left biliary tree. **c** MR showing excision of a long tract of CBD and of main confluence; right and left intrahepatic biliary trees are mildly dilated (*white arrow*: CBD distal stump). **d** Preoperative cholangiography with placement of percutaneous catheters: dilated left biliary tree and no dilation of right biliary tree for persistent bilio-enteric fistula. **e** postoperative percutaneous cholangiography after separate right- and left-hepaticojejunostomies

hilar plate is lowered and the hilum is rotated forward and inferiorly, and the superior part of the main biliary confluence and of the left hepatic ducts becomes approachable anteriorly, without interposition of vascular structures [71].

Surgical Technique

The liver is exposed through a bilateral subcostal incision.

The first step is to cut down all postoperative adhesions between the liver, the colon and the duodenum, proceeding downward along the inferior surface of the liver. Anatomic limits for this dissection are on the left side the round ligament, which is progressively detached from the liver along the umbilical scissure, and on the right side the fibrous tissue in the gallbladder fossa. Dissection proceeds along the inferior surface of the liver until the plane of the hepatic pedicle is reached. There is often a parenchymal bridge between segments 3 and 4. The hepatic hilum is hidden by adhesions between the inferior surface of the liver and the duodenum. After opening the hepato-gastric ligament, the hepatic pedicle is encircled with a tourniquet and the caudate lobe becomes visible (Fig. 21.50).

The second step is lowering the hilar plate. The last adhesions are divided by retracting the liver upward and the hepatic pedicle and the duodenum downward. The space between the inferior surface of the liver and the hepatic pedicle is freed and the base of the quadrate lobe is completely exposed. Lowering the hilar plate starts at the base of quadrate lobe. Detachment of the hilar plate from the liver parenchyma should be performed bluntly (tip of scissors, small gauzes). Hemostasis is safely controlled by bipolar forceps.

The shape of segment 4b, the so-called quadrate lobe, is often changed by previous operative complications in a triangular fashion. The hilum is completely closed by the fibrous tissue between the umbilical scissure and the gallbladder fossa. The left side the parenchymal bridge previously described is divided in order to enlarge the exposure of the left hepatic duct (Fig. 21.51). On the right side, the right portion of the base of the quadrate lobe is dissected, and the fibrous tissue in the gallbladder fossa is incised, from the anterior margin of the liver to the hepatic pedicle, in order to

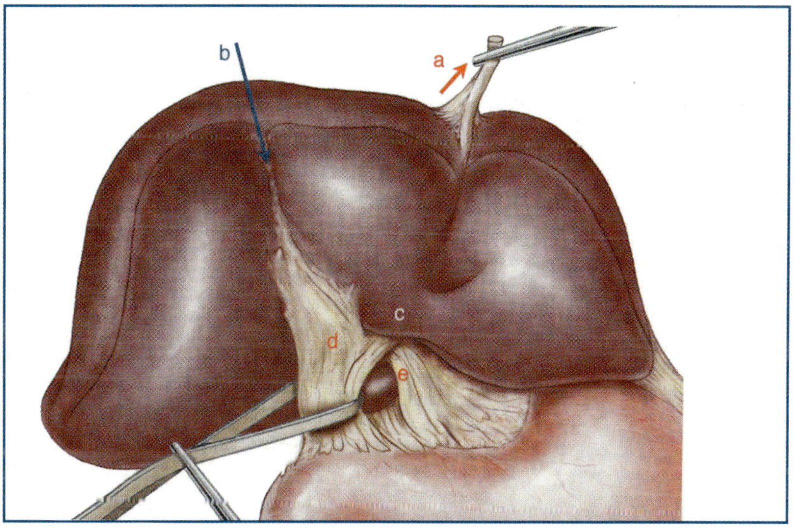

Fig. 21.50 Operative field showing round ligament (*a*), gallbladder fossa (*b*), parenchymal bridge between segments 3 and 4 (*c*) hepatic pedicle encircled with a tape (*d*), caudate lobe (*e*). Reproduced with permission from [110]

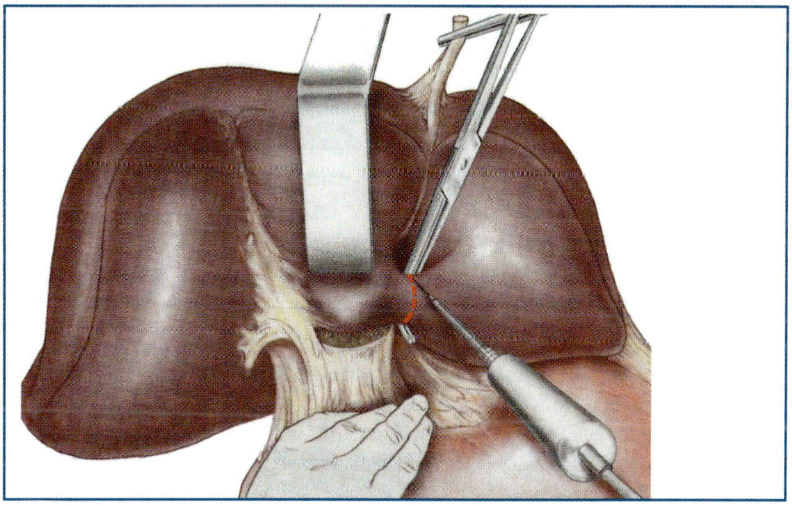

Fig. 21.51 Division of parenchymal bridge between segments 3 and 4. Reproduced with permission from [110]

enlarge the exposure of the main confluence and of the right hepatic duct (Fig. 21.52). On the right side it may be useful to divide the fibrous tissue between the vesicular plate and the hilar plate. After completing the division of the fibrous tissue, the quadrate lobe regains its original quadrate shape between the gallbladder fossa and the umbilical scissure. Finally, complete exposure of the main biliary confluence and of the left hepatic duct is obtained (Fig. 21.53).

In some cases, adhesions between the inferior surface of the liver and duodenum hide a spontaneous bilio-duodenal fistula that could be opened during dissection. In these patients, if preoperative percutaneous biliary drainage has not been placed, a small biliary drain can be inserted through the opening of the fistula and this can be useful to identify the right and the left hepatic ducts and in case an IOC should be performed.

The third step is to open the main biliary confluence. Some absorbable stitches (4/0–5/0) are put on the anterior biliary wall and can help to hold up the main biliary

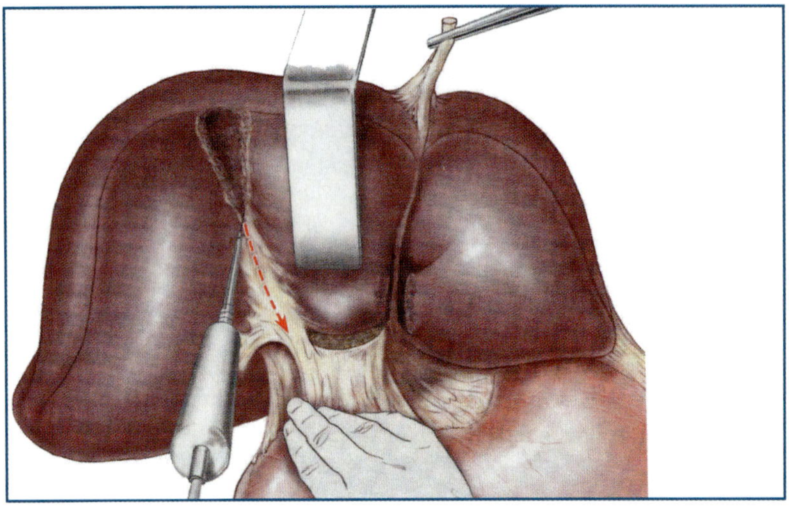

Fig. 21.52 Fibrous tissue of gallbladder fossa is incised from the anterior margin of the liver to the hepatic pedicle. Reproduced with permission from [110]

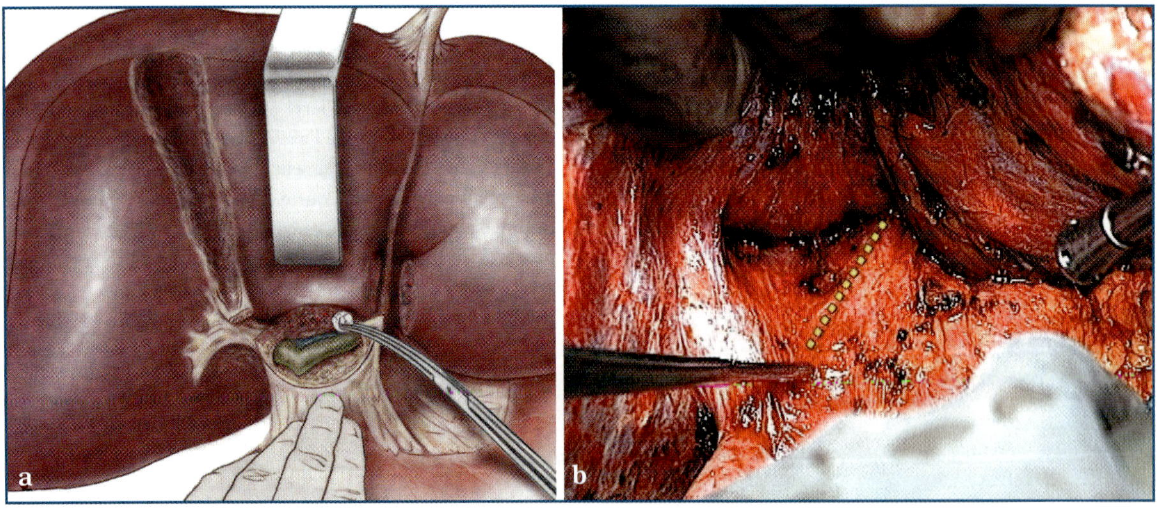

Fig. 21.53 a After lowering the hilar plate, complete exposure of main biliary confluence and of left hepatic duct is obtained. **b** Operative field after lowering the hilar plate: the base of the quadrate lobe is retracted upward and left hepatic duct (*yellow dotted line*) has become approachable anteriorly. Fig. 53a reproduced with permission from [110]

confluence, which is incised by scalpel and opened by right angle forceps along the left hepatic duct. Left hepatic duct opening continues along a horizontal plane in order to obtain a large biliary stump (at least 3 cm). In some cases it can also be useful to open the right hepatic duct partially, so the biliary opening has a "V" shape with a small right vertical branch and a long left horizontal one (Fig. 21.54). Infrequently, in order to increase the size of the right hepatic duct, the posterior aspect of the main biliary confluence can be incised, enlarged and sutured with absorbable 5/0 stitches.

The fourth step is the Roux-en-Y loop of jejunum preparation (Fig. 21.55). The jejunum is divided 20 cm from the Treitz ligament. The jejunal loop should be 70–80 cm in length and should preferably be brought up in a retrocolic fashion. End-to-side jejunojejunal anastomosis is performed by two extramucosal running sutures with absorbable 3/0 stitches.

At the distal end, the jejunal limb is opened on its antimesenteric edge. This incision should be smaller than the biliary opening because it tends to become wider during the anastomosis. The jejunal loop cul-de-sac should be short and usually on the left side.

The fifth step is to perform the hepaticojejunostomy. Good biliary and enteric vascularization is necessary, with no ten-

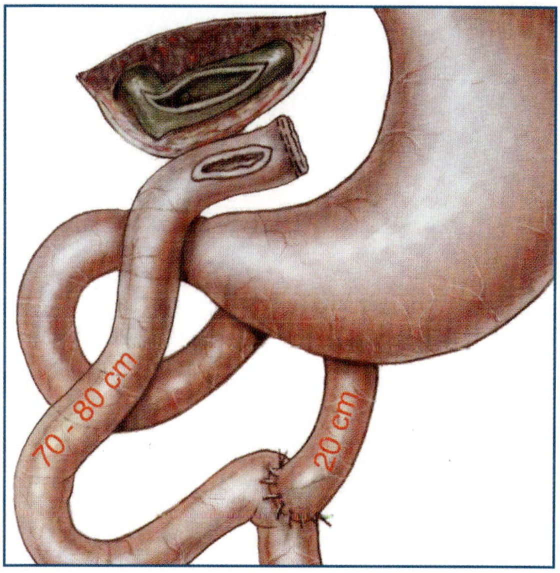

Fig. 21.55 Preparation of Roux-en-Y jejunal loop before the anastomosis. Reproduced with permission from [110]

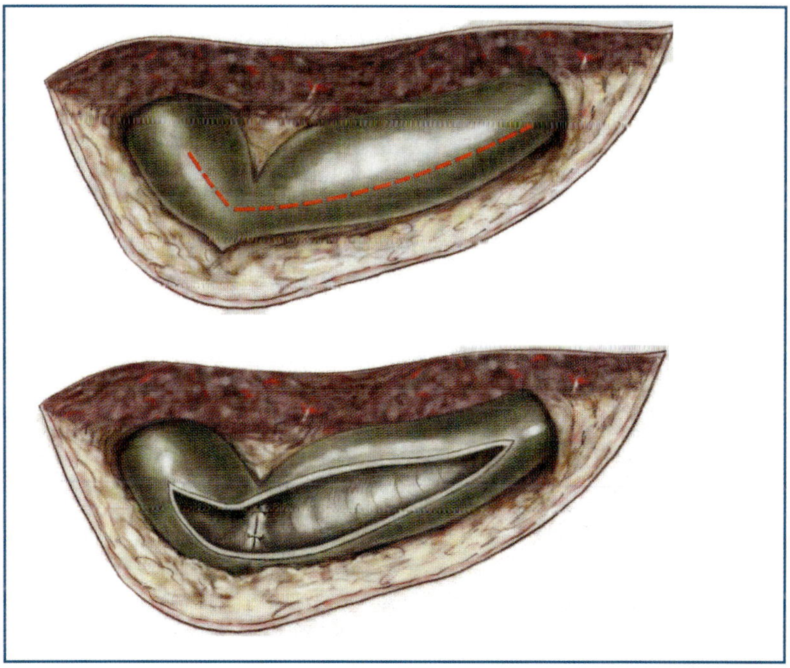

Fig. 21.54 **a** Incision on the main confluence and left hepatic duct: "V" shape biliary opening with a small right vertical branch and a long left horizontal one. **b** Stitches on the posterior wall of the confluence, after incision of the biliary confluence, if necessary, are drawn. Reproduced with permission from [110]

sion of the anastomosis. The first stitch is introduced on the left corner of the biliary and enteric stump, which is tied outside the lumen. End-to-side hepaticojejunostomy is performed with several, close to each other, absorbable, interrupted stitches (4/0 or 5/0), that are full-thickness on the biliary mucosa and extramucosal on the jejunal loop. The posterior layer of sutures is placed first (Fig. 21.56). Sutures are introduced serially starting from the patient's left toward the right, individually held by small Haldstet forceps, and placed progressively into a clamp fixed on the left side of the patient. After introducing all the stitches, knots are tied within the lumen and, if a percutaneous biliary drainage is already in place, it is inserted at this moment into the jejunal loop (Fig. 21.57). Then the anterior layer is started and every stitch is tied as it is introduced (Fig. 21.58). Fixation of Roux-en-Y loop of the jejunum to Glisson's capsule is not necessary.

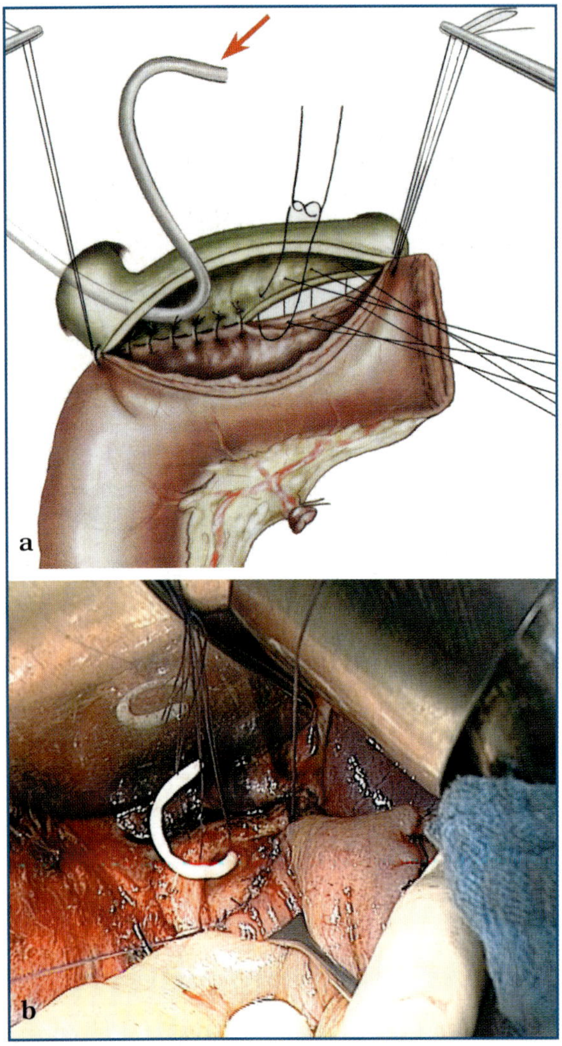

Fig. 21.56 **a** Posterior wall of end-to-side hepaticojejunostomy with percutaneous catheter through the right hepatic duct (*arrow*). **b** Operative field: posterior layer of the anastomosis is completed. Fig. 56a reproduced with permission from [110]

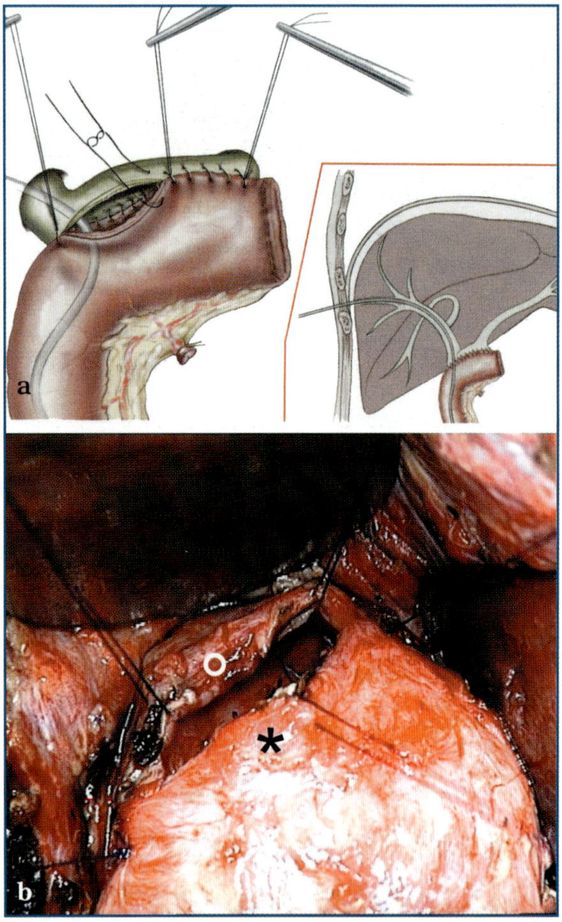

Fig. 21.57 **a** Percutaneous biliary drainage is inserted into the jejunal loop, the anterior layer of hepaticojejunostomy starts and every stitch is tied as it is introduced. **b** Operative field: wide (3 cm) anastomosis, before starting the anterior layer. Jejunal loop (*); left hepatic duct (°). Fig. 57a reproduced with permission from [110]

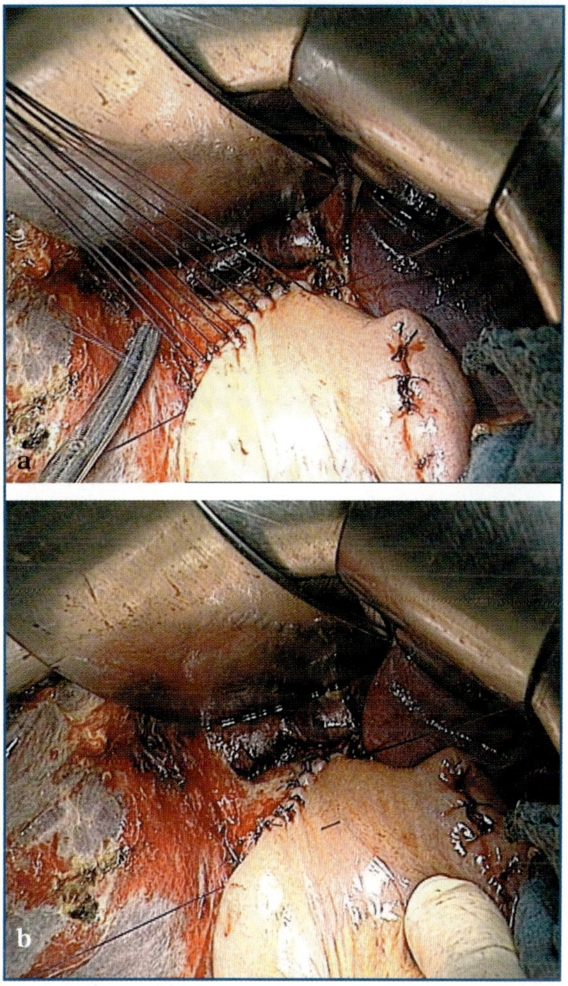

Fig. 21.58 Hepaticojejunostomy according to Hepp-Couinaud technique. **a** All the stitches of the anterior layer are evident. **b** The anastomosis at the end of the procedure: jejunal cul-de-sac on the left side of the patient

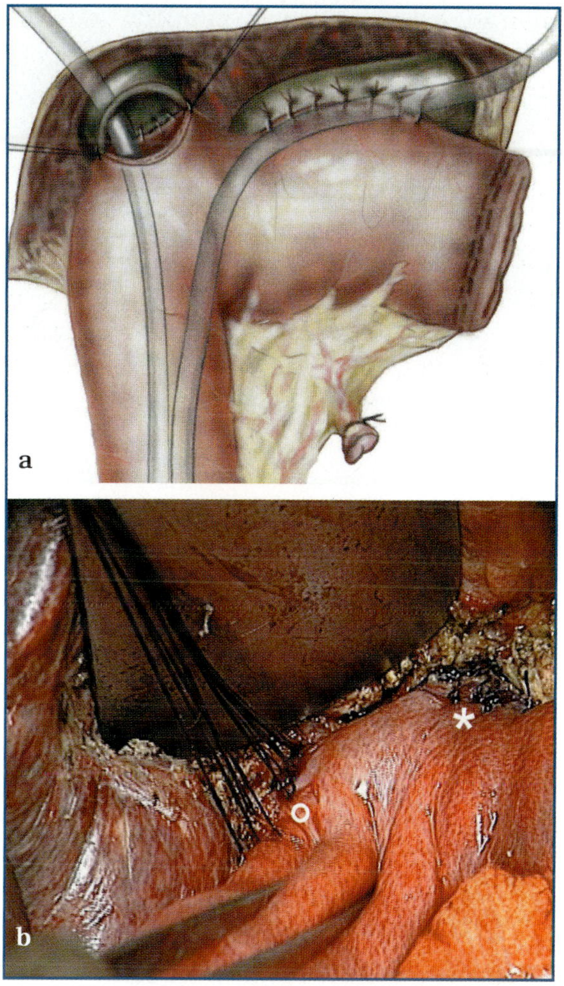

Fig. 21.59 a In case of a destroyed ceiling of the main biliary confluence (Bismuth Type 4), two anastomoses are required: usually, it is easier to perform the left hepaticojejunostomy first; percutaneous catheters are left in place. **b** Operative field: separate anastomoses on the left hepatic duct (*) and on the right hepatic duct (°) are completed. Fig. 59a reproduced with permission from [110]

If the ceiling of the main biliary confluence is destroyed and left and right hepatic ducts are separated (Bismuth Type 4), after lowering the hilar plate two anastomoses are required: it is usually easier to perform the left hepaticojejunostomy first (Fig. 21.59).

In some cases the biliary stricture extends to the main biliary confluence without complete separation of the right and left hepatic ducts. In these cases it is possible to reconstruct the ceiling of the main biliary confluence with interrupted absorbable sutures and to perform a single hepaticojejunostomy (Fig. 21. 60).

After biliary injury, the base of the quadrate lobe may become hypertrophic and cover the hilar structures. Resection of this portion of liver parenchyma is easy and allows a wider approach to the hilar plate, to the left hepatic duct and to the main biliary confluence to be obtained (Fig. 21.61). At the

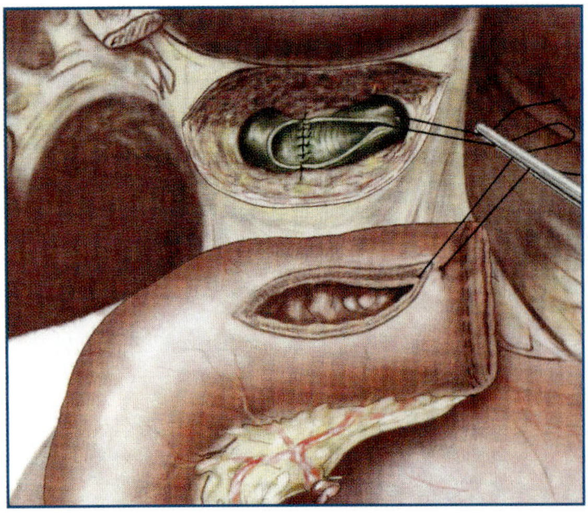

Fig. 21.60 Ceiling of the main biliary confluence is reconstructed with interrupted absorbable sutures and a single hepaticojejunostomy is performed. Reproduced with permission from [110]

end of the procedure, one drain is left close to the anastomosis.

If a percutaneous catheter is placed, ten days after surgical repair cholangiography is performed to check the anastomosis. In case of difficult or multiple anastomoses, percutaneous drainages are left in place for at least 6 months, and possibly up to one year. In this way, the hepaticojejunostomy is dilated by insertion of percutaneous catheters of progressively increasing size, up to 14–16 Fr. The drawbacks of such a strategy are the need for percutaneous multiple sessions, every two or three months, and the prolonged duration of treatment, but best long term results are achieved. Some authors report a similar surgical strategy with prolonged maintenance of biliary stents that are surgically inserted [72, 111, 112].

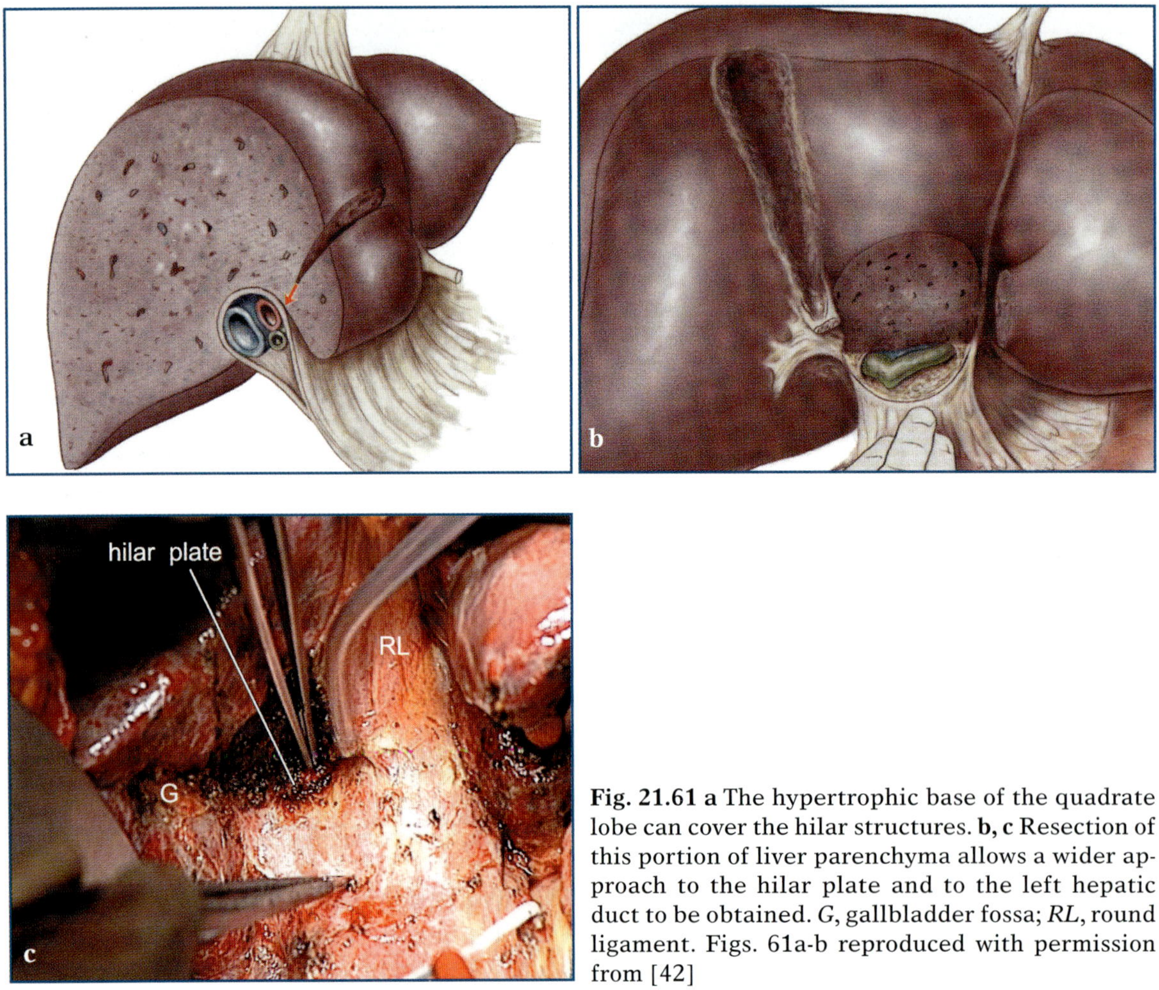

Fig. 21.61 **a** The hypertrophic base of the quadrate lobe can cover the hilar structures. **b, c** Resection of this portion of liver parenchyma allows a wider approach to the hilar plate and to the left hepatic duct to be obtained. *G*, gallbladder fossa; *RL*, round ligament. Figs. 61a-b reproduced with permission from [42]

How to Control Results of Biliary Repair

Immediate evaluation of the results of a biliary repair is not easy, because a good immediate result is not necessarily a sign of final success. Some patients have completely uneventful postoperative courses, and this can induce the surgeon to feel excessive optimism. Actually, the rate of late failure of immediate repairs is high, and these patients should be followed for at least 5 years, even if in most of cases a failed repair is evident within the first 2–3 years [42]. Some patients can be symptom free for a long time, and the appearance of a stricture can become evident only with an increase of cholestasis enzymes (alkaline phosphatase and gamma-glutamyl transpeptidase). Patients at higher risk of stricture are those who have immediate postoperative complications, the most important of which is anastomotic bile leak. The postoperative appearance of a biliary fistula is very often associated with infection around the anastomosis, and this is highly predictive of a stricture. Particular care should be taken in following these patients, because recovery may be only apparent. Also patients with an external fistula after cholecystectomy with spontaneous resolution should be carefully followed. In fact, the fistula can resolve after the occurrence of a spontaneous bilio-duodenal fistula, through wich the bile into the duodenum is only partially drained, and biliary stricture can occur lately. These patients should be strictly followed with clinical checks every 4 or 6 months, looking for the appearance of transitory septic episodes, for an increase in cholestasis enzymes, and for dilation of intrahepatic bile ducts with liver ultrasound. These signs allow a failed repair to be recognized very early, and a delay to be avoided in the treatment of a stricture, which, if untreated, may impair liver parenchyma to the point of cirrhosis development (Fig. 21.32).

Results of repairs of sectorial or segmental bile ducts are difficult to evaluate; very often strictures of these anastomoses do not have clinical manifestations, and their late evolution is atrophy of the undrained portion of the liver. In these cases, levels of cholestasis enzymes may increase only transitorily, usually with almost normal levels: CT or MR of the liver can reveal changes in liver morphology.

In order to evaluate long term results of surgical repairs, different scores have been proposed. One of the most commonly used is that proposed by The Johns Hopkins Medical Institutions, Baltimore [72], which rates the results as *excellent* if there are no symptoms attributable to the biliary tract injury or reconstruction; and *good* if mild symptoms not requiring invasive investigation or treatment are present. Patients classified as either excellent or good are considered to be *treatment successes*. Patients are considered to be *treatment failures* if an invasive investigational or therapeutic procedure, either radiologic or surgical, is necessary to treat ongoing symptoms or stricture recurrence. A successful outcome after surgical repair in tertiary care centers is reported in 88–95% of patients [79, 112–114].

Non-surgical Treatments

The recent advances in endoscopy and interventional radiology should be evaluated for the choices that they offer for BDI therapy. These techniques quite often permit appropriate treatment, especially in the case of minor BDI, partial injuries of the CBD, and strictures of high bilio-enteric anastomoses [14, 24, 52, 67, 105].

Furthermore, it should also be considered that endoscopic and percutaneous procedures can be of paramount importance not only for repair, but also for initial assessment of the injury, treatment of sepsis, contribution to the repair of complex injuries and follow-up. In our experience of 66 cases of major BDI, treated with surgery in 64%

of cases and with non-surgical treatments in 36%, more than 200 ERCPs and PTCs were performed with different aims [114, 115]. Therefore, the need for multidisciplinary care of these patients in specialized centers should be carefully emphasized.

References

1. Thomson BN, Parks RW, Madhavan KK et al (2006) Early specialist repair of biliary injury. Br J Surg 93:216-220
2. Flum DR, Cheadle A, Prela C et al (2003) Bile duct injury during cholecystectomy and survival in medicare beneficiaries. JAMA 290:2168-2173
3. Boerma D, Rauws EA, Keulemans YC et al (2001) Impaired quality of life 5 years after bile duct injury during laparoscopic cholecystectomy: a prospective analysis. Ann Surg 234:750-757
4. Melton GB, Lillemoe KD, Cameron JL et al (2002) Major bile duct injuries associated with laparoscopic cholecystectomy: effect of surgical repair on quality of life. Ann Surg 235:888-895
5. Moore DE, Feurer ID, Holzman MD et al (2004) Long-term detrimental effect of bile duct injury on health-related quality of life. Arch Surg 139:476-481; discussion 481-482
6. Mallon P, White J, McMenamin M et al (2006) Increased cholecystectomy rate in the laparoscopic era: a study of the potential causative factors. Surg Endosc 20:883-886
7. Wherry DC, Marohn MR, Malanoski MP et al (1996) An external audit of laparoscopic cholecystectomy in the Steady State performed in medical treatment facilities of the department of defense. Ann Surg 224:145-154
8. Russell JC, Walsh SJ, Mattie AS, Lynch JT (1996) Bile duct injuries, 1989-1993. A statewide experience. Arch Surg 131:382-388
9. Richardson MC, Bell G, Fullarton GM (1996) Incidence and nature of bile duct injuries following laparoscopic cholecystectomy: an audit of 5913 cases. Br J Surg 83:1356-1360
10. Adamsen S, Hansen OH, Funch-Jensen P et al (1997) Bile duct injury during laparoscopic cholecystectomy: a prospective nationwide series. J Am Coll Surg 184:571-578
11. Gigot JF, Etienne J, Aerts R et al (1997) The dramatic reality of biliary tract injury during laparoscopic cholecystectomy. An anonymous multicenter Belgian survey of 65 patients. Surg Endosc 11:1171-1178
12. MacFadyen BV, Vecchio R, Ricardo AE, Mathis CR (1989) Bile duct injury after laparoscopic cholecystectomy. The United States experience. Surg Endosc 12:315-321
13. Z'graggen K, Wehrli H, Metzger A, Buehler M et al (1998) Complications of laparoscopic cholecystectomy in Switzerland. A prospective 3-year study of 10,174 patients. Swiss Association of Laparoscopic and Thoracoscopic Surgery. Surg Endosc 12:1303-1310
14. Nuzzo G, Giuliante F, Giovannini I et al (2005) Bile duct injury during laparoscopic cholecystectomy: results of an Italian national survey on 56 591 cholecystectomies. Arch Surg:986-992
15. Waage A, Nilsson M (2006) Iatrogenic bile duct injury: a population-based study of 152 776 cholecystectomies in the Swedish inpatient registry. Arch Surg 14:1207-1213
16. Moosa AR, Easter DW, Van Sonnenberg E et al (1992) Laparoscopic injuries to the bile duct: a cause of concern. Ann Surg 215:203-208
17. Fletcher DR (1993) Biliary injury at laparoscopic cholecystectomy: recognition and prevention. Aust N Z Surg 63:673-677
18. Branum G, Schmitt C, Baillie J et al (1993) Management of major biliary complications after laparoscopic cholecystectomy. Ann Surg 217:532-541
19. Roy AF, Passi RB, Lapointe RW et al (1993) Bile duct injury during laparoscopic cholecystectomy. Can J Surg 36:509-517
20. Adams DB, Borowicz MR, Wootton FT et al (1993) Bile duct complications after laparoscopic cholecystectomy. Surg Endosc 7:79-83
21. Mercado MA, Chan C, Orozco H et al (2003) Acute bile duct injury. The need for a high repair. Surg Endosc 17:1351-1355
22. Bektas H, Schrem H, Winny M, Klempnauer J (2007) Surgical treatment and outcome of iatrogenic bile duct lesions after cholecystectomy and the impact of different clinical classification system. Br J Surg 94:1119-1127
23. Khan MH, Howard TJ, Fogel EL et al (2007) Frequency of biliary complications after laparoscopic cholecystectomy detected by ERCP: experience at a large tertiary referral center. Gastrointest Endosc 65:247-252
24. de Reuver PR, Grossmann I, Busch OR et al (2007) Referral pattern and timing of repair are risk factors for complications after reconstructive surgery for bile duct injury. Ann Surg 245:763-770
25. Francoeur JR, Wiseman K, Buczkowski AK et al (2003) Surgeons' anonymous response after bile duct injury during cholecystectomy. Am J Surg 185:468-475
26. Jarnagin WR, Blumgart LH (2000) Benign biliary strictures. In: Blumgart LH, Fong Y (eds) Surgery of the liver and biliary tract. Edinburgh, Harcourt-Saunders, pp 895-933

27. Millat B, Rodier JG (1998) Laparoscopic treatment of common bile duct lithiasis. J Chir 135:279-283
28. Martin FM, Rossi RL (1994) Bile duct injuries. Spectrum, mechanism of injury and their prevention. Surg Clin North Am 74:781-803; discussion 805-807
29. Reinhlod C, Taourel P, Bret PM et al (1998) Choledocholithiasis: evaluation of MR cholangiography for diagnosis. Radiology 209:435-442
30. Taourel P, Bret PM, Reinhlod C et al (1996) Anatomic variants of the biliary tree: diagnosis with MR cholangiopancreatography. Radiology 199:521-527
31. Asbun HJ, Rossi RL (1994) Techniques of laparoscopic cholecystectomy. The difficult operation. Surg Clin North Am 74:755-775; discussion 777-780
32. Gillet M (1993) Chirurgie de voies biliaires chez le cirrhotique. In: La chirurgie digestive chez le cirrhotique. Monographies de l'Association Française de Chirurgie. Rapport présenté au 95e Congrès Français de Chirurgie. Paris, Springer-Verlag, pp 91-99
33. The E.A.E.S. Consensus development Conferences on laparoscopic cholecystectomy, appendectomy, and hernia repair (1994) Consensus statements-September. Surg Endosc 9:550-563
34. Navez B, Mutter D, Ruzier Y et al (2001) Safety of laparoscopic approach for acute cholecystitis: retrospective study of 609 cases. World J Surg 25:1352-1356
35. Habib FA, Kolachalam RB, Khilanani R (2001) Role of laparoscopic cholecystectomy in the management of gangrenous cholecystitis. Am J Surg 181:71-75
36. Yamashita Y, Takada T, Kawarada Y et al (2007) Surgical treatment of patients with acute cholecystitis: Tokyo guidelines. J Hepatobiliary Pancreat Surg 14:91-97
37. Cassone E, Sonzini Austudillo P (1999) Injurias quirurgicas de la via biliar. Congreso Argentino de Cirurgia-Relato Official Rev Argent Cirurg N° extraordinario, pp 47-104
38. Bouchet Y, Passagia JG, Lopez JF (1990) Anatomie voies biliaires extra-hepatiques. Editions techniques, Encycl Méd Chir (Paris-France). Techniques chirugicales-Généralités-Appareil digestif, 40900:16
39. Caputo L, Aitken DR, Mackett MCT et al (1992) Iatrogenic bile duct injuries. The real incidence and contributing factors implications for laparoscopic cholecystectomy. Am J Surg 58:766-771
40. Yoshida J, Chijiiwa K, Yamaguchi K (1996) Practical classification of the branching types of the biliary tree: an analysis of 1,094 consecutive direct cholangiograms. J Am Coll Surg 182:37-40
41. Traverso LW, Hauptmann EM, Lynge DC (1994) Routine intraoperative cholangiography and its contributions to the selective cholangiographer. Am J Surg 167:464-468
42. Nuzzo G, Giuliante F, Giovannini I et al (2002) Le lesioni iatrogene della via biliare principale. Collana monografica n. 18 della Società Italiana di Chirurgia, Relazione biennale al 104° Congresso. Roma, Società Italiana di Chirurgia
43. Bismuth H, Lazorthes F (1981) Les traumatismes opératoires de la voie biliaire principale. Monographies de l'Association Française de Chirurgie. Rapport présenté au 83° Congrès Français de Chirurgie. Paris, Masson
44. Blumgart LH (1988) Benign biliary strictures. In: Blumgart LH (ed) Surgery of the liver and biliary tract. Churchill Livingstone, Vol. 1, pp 721-752
45. Dexter SPL, Miller GV, Davides D et al (2000) Relaparoscopy for the detection and treatment of complication of laparoscopic cholecystectomy. Am J Surg 179:316 319
46. Mc Quillan T, Manolas SG, Hayman JA et al (1989) Surgical significance of the bile duct of Luschka. Br J Surg 76:696-698
47. Meillere D (1968) Variations des artères hépatiques. J Chir 95:5-42
48. Archer SB, Brown DW, Smith CD et al (2001) Bile duct injury during laparoscopic cholecystectomy: results of a national survey. Ann Surg 234:549-559
49. Callery MP (2006) Avoiding biliary injury during laparoscopic cholecystectomy: technical considerations. Surg Endosc 20:1654-1658
50. Windsor JA, Pong J (1998) Laparoscopic biliary injury: more than a learning curve problem. Aust N Z J Surg 68:186-189
51. Strasberg SM, Hertl M, Soper JN (1995) An analysis of the problem of biliary injury during laparoscopic cholecystectomy. J Am Coll Surg 180:101-125
52. Strasberg SM, Eagon CJ, Drebin JA (2000) The "hidden cystic duct" syndrome and the infundibular technique of laparoscopic cholecystectomy: the danger of the false infundibulum. J Am Coll Surg 191:661-667
53. Woods MS, Traverso LW, Kozarek RA et al (1994) Characteristics of biliary tract complications during laparoscopic cholecystectomy. A multi-institutional study. Am J Surg 167:27-33
54. Stewart L, Way LW (1995) Bile duct injuries during laparoscopic cholecystectomy. Factors that influence the results of treatment. Arch Surg 130:1123-1129
55. Fletcher DR, Hobbs MS, Tan P et al (1999) Complications of cholecystectomy: risks of the laparoscopic approach and protective effects of operatic cholangiography: a population-based study.

Ann Surg 229:449-457
56. Massarweh NN, Flum DR (2007) Role of intraoperative cholangiography in avoiding bile duct injury. J Am Coll Surg 204:656-664
57. Traverso LW (2006) Intraoperative cholangiography lowers the risk of bile duct injury during cholecystectomy. Surg Endosc 20:1659-1661
58. Catheline JM, Borie F, Champault G et al (1999) Diagnostic peropératoire de la lithiase de la voie biliaire principale. In: Lithiase de la voie biliaire principale. Monographies de l'Association Française de Chirurgie. Rapport présenté au 101e Congrès Française de Chirurgie. Paris, Masson
59. Soper NJ, Dunnegan DL (1992) Routine versus selective intra-operative cholangiography during laparoscopic cholecystectomy. World J Surg 16:1133-1140
60. Lorimer JW, Fairfull-Smith RJ (1995) Intraoperative cholangiography is not essential to avoid duct injuries during laparoscopic cholecystectomy. Am J Surg 169:344-347
61. White TT, Hart MJ (1985) Cholangiography and small duct injury. Am J Surg 149:640-643
62. Way LW, Stewart L, Gantert W et al (2003) Causes and prevention of laparoscopic bile duct injuries: analysis of 252 cases from a human factors and cognitive psychology perspective. Ann Surg 237:460-469
63. Flum DR, Koepsel T, Heagerty P et al (2001) Common bile duct injury during laparoscopic cholecystectomy and the use of intraoperative cholangiography: adverse outcome or preventable error? Arch Surg 136:1287-1292
64. Csendes A, Navarrete C, Burdiles P et al (2001) Treatment of common bile duct injuries after laparoscopic cholecystectomy: endoscopic and surgical management. World J Surg 25:1346-1351
65. Traverso LW (1994) Commentary-Bile duct injuries: spectrum, mechanism of injury and their prevention. Surg Clin North Am 74:805-807
66. Siewert JR, Ungeheuer A, Feussner H (1994) Bile duct lesions in laparoscopic cholecystectomy. Chirurg 65:748-757
67. Bergman JJ, van den Brink GR, Rauws EA et al (1996) Treatment of bile duct lesions after laparoscopic cholecystectomy. Gut 38:141-147
68. Neuhaus P, Schmidt SC, Hintze RE et al (2000) Classification and treatment of bile duct injuries after laparoscopic cholecystectomy. Chirurg 71:166-173
69. Gazzaniga GM, Filauro M, Mori L (2001) Surgical treatment of iatrogenic lesions of the proximal common bile duct. World J Surg 25:1254-1259
70. Stewart L, Robinson TN, Lee CM et al (2004) Right hepatic artery injury associated with laparoscopic bile duct injury: incidence, mechanism and consequences. J Gastrointest Surg 8:523-530
71. Bismuth H, Majno PE (2001) Biliary strictures: classification based on the principles of surgical treatment. World J Surg 25:1241-1244
72. Lillemoe KD, Melton GB, Cameron JL et al (2000) Postoperative bile duct strictures: management and outcome in the 1990s. Ann Surg 232:430-441
73. Mehta SN, Pavone E, Barkun JS et al (1997) A review of the management of postcholecystectomy biliary leak during the laparoscopic era. Am J Gastroenterol 92:1262-1267
74. Kang EH, Middleton WD, Balfe DM et al (1991) Laparoscopic cholecystectomy: sonographic evaluation. Radiology 181:439-442
75. Halasz NA (1991) Cholecystectomy and hepatic artery injury. Arch Surg 126:137-138
76. Wudel LJ, Wright JK, Pinson CW et al (2001) Bile duct injury following laparoscopic cholecystectomy: a cause for continued concern. Am Surg 67:557-563
77. Davidoff AM, Pappas TN, Murray EA et al (1992) Mechanisms of major biliary injury during laparoscopic cholecystectomy. Ann Surg 215:196-208
78. Bismuth H (1981) How to treat a postoperative stenosis? In: Bismuth H, Lazorthes F (eds) Operative injury of the common bile duct. Paris, Masson, pp 47-107
79. Alves A, Farges O, Nicolet J et al (2003) Incidence and consequence of an hepatic artery injury in patients with postcholecystectomy bile duct strictures. Ann Surg 238:93-96
80. Schmidt SC, Settmacher U, Langrehr JM, Neuhaus P (2004) Management and outcome of patients with combined bile duct and hepatic arterial injuries after laparoscopic cholecystectomy. Surgery 135:613-618
81. Koffron A, Ferrario M, Parsons W et al (2001) Failed primary management of iatrogenic biliary injury: incidence and significance of concomitant hepatic arterial disruption. Surgery 130:772-731
82. Bachellier P, Nakano H, Weber J-C et al (2001) Surgical repair after bile duct and vascular injuries during laparoscopic cholecystectomy: when and how? World J Surg 25:1335-1345
83. Buell JF, Cronin DC, Funaki B et al (2002) Devastating and fatal complications associated with combined vascular and bile duct injuries. Arch Surg 137:703-710
84. Vellar ID (1999) The blood supply of the biliary ductal system and its relevance to vasculobiliary injuries following cholecystectomy. Aust N Z J Surg 69:816-820
85. Savader SJ, Lillemoe KD, Prescott CA et al (1997) Laparoscopic cholecystectomy-related bile duct

injuries: a health and financial disaster. Ann Surg 225:268-273

86. Jarnagin WR, Blumgart LH (1999) Operative repair of bile duct injuries involving the hepatic duct confluence. Arch Surg 134:769-775
87. Olsen D (1997) Bile duct injuries during laparoscopic cholecystectomy. Surg Endosc 11:133-138
88. Hugh TB (2002) New strategies to prevent laparoscopic bile duct injury – surgeons can learn from pilots. Surgery 132:826-835
89. Gigot JF (2005) Chirurgie des voies biliaires. In: Techniques Chirurgicales - Digestif. Paris, Masson
90. Gouma DJ, Go PM (1994) Bile duct injury during laparoscopic and conventional cholecystectomy. J Am Coll Surg 253:229-233
91. Gazzaniga GM, Filauro M, Bagarolo C et al (1997) Tecnica chirurgica nelle neoplasie del tratto prossimale della VBP. In: Le neoplasie delle vie biliari extraepatiche. Relazione biennale al 99° Congresso della Società Italiana di Chirurgia. Padova, Società Italiana di Chirurgia
92. Carroll BJ, Birth M, Phillips EH (1998) Common bile duct injuries during laparoscopic cholecystectomy that result in litigation. Surg Endosc 12:310-314
93. Lee CM, Stewart L, Way LW (2000) Postcholecystectomy abdominal bile collections. Arch Surg 135:538-544
94. Keulemans YC, Bergman JJ, de Wit LT et al (1998) Improvement in the management of bile duct injuries? J Am Coll Surg 187:246-254
95. Schmidt SC, Langrehr JM, Hintze RE, Neuhaus P (2005) Long-term results and risk factors influencing outcome of major bile duct injuries following cholecystectomy. Br J Surg 92:76-82
96. Johnson SR, Koehler A, Pennington LK, Hanto DW (2000) Long-term results of surgical repair of bile duct injuries following laparoscopic cholecystectomy. Surgery 128:668-677
97. Blumgart LH, Kelley CJ, Benjamin IS (1984) Benign bile duct stricture following cholecystectomy: critical factors in management. Br J Surg 71:836-843
98. Connor S, Garden OJ (2006) Bile duct injury in the era of laparoscopic cholecystectomy. Br J Surg 93:158-168
99. Deziel DJ, Millikan KW, Economou SG et al (1993) Complications of laparoscopic cholecystectomy: a national survey of 4,292 hospitals and an analysis of 77,604 cases. Am J Surg 165:9-14
100. De Wit LT, Rauws EA, Gouma DJ (1999) Surgical management of iatrogenic bile duct injury. Scand J Gastroenterol Suppl 230:89-94
101. Khalid TR, Casillas VJ, Montalvo BM et al (2001) Using MR cholangiopancreatography to evaluate iatrogenic bile duct injury. AJR Am J Roentgenol 177:1347-1352
102. Yeh TS, Jan YY, Tseng JH et al (1999) Value of magnetic resonance cholangiopancreatography in demonstrating major bile duct injuries following laparoscopic cholecystectomy. Br J Surg 86:181-184
103. Hepp J, Pernod R, Hautefeuille P (1963) Contribution de la cholangiographie opératoire a la chirurgie réparatrice des traumatismes biliaires. Extrait des Annales De Chirurgie 17:18-36
104. Hepp J, Pernod R, Hautefeuille P (1966) La détection des lésions de la zone de convergence radiculaire en chirurgie biliaire réparatrice. Académie de Chirurgie, pp 246-252
105. Costamagna G, Pandolfi M, Mutignani M et al (2001) Long-term results of endoscopic management of postoperative bile duct strictures with increasing number of stents. Gastrointest Endosc 54:162-168
106. Sandblom JP (2000) Hemobilia and bilhemia. In: Blumgart LH, Fong Y (eds) Surgery of the liver and biliary tract. Edinburgh, Harcourt-Saunders, pp 1319-1339
107. Costamagna G, Familiari P, Tringali A, Mutignani M (2007) Multidisciplinary approach to benign biliary strictures. Cur Treat Options Gastroenterol 10:90-101
108. Misra S, Melton GB, Geschwind JF et al (2004) Percutaneous management of bile duct strictures and injuries associated with laparoscopic cholecystectomy: a decade of experience. J Am Coll Surg 198:218-226
109. Hepp J, Couinaud C (1956) L'abord et l'utilisation du canal hépatique gauche dans les reparations de la voie biliaire principale. Presse Med 64:947-948
110. Nuzzo G, Giuliante F (2006) Surgical approach to common bile duct stricture. J Chir 143:37-43
111. Sicklick JK, Camp MS, Lillemoe KD et al (2005) Surgical management of bile duct injuries sustained during laparoscopic cholecystectomy: perioperative results in 200 patients. Ann Surg 241:786-795
112. Lillemoe KD (2006) Evaluation of suspected bile duct injuries. Surg Endosc 20:1638-1643
113. Sarmiento JM, Farnell MB, Nagorney DM (2004) Quality-of-life assessment of surgical reconstruction after laparoscopic cholecystectomy-induced bile duct injuries: what happens at five years and beyond? Arch Surg 139:483-489
114. Nuzzo G, Giuliante F, Giovannini I (2008) The advantages of the multidisciplinary management of bile duct injuries occurred during cholecystectomy. Am J Surg [Epub ahead of print]
115. De Reuver PR, Rauws EA, Bruno MJ et al (2007) Survival in bile duct injury patients after laparoscopic cholecystectomy: a multidisciplinary approach of gastroenterologists, radiologists, and surgeons. Surgery 142:1-9

Chapter 22

Clinical Pictures of Common Bile Duct Stones

Jürgen Treckmann, Christoph E. Broelsch, Andreas Paul

Introduction

The clinical presentations of common bile duct stones (CBDS) can vary widely: patients with large impacted stones may present as asymptomatic, while other patients may be severely ill with cholangiogenic sepsis or necrotizing biliary pancreatitis due to small stones in the papilla of Vater. Sometimes clinical symptoms of CBDS are residual signs of spontaneous passage with complete clearance of the CBD and without the need for further therapy. In these times of laparoscopic cholecystectomy without routinely performed intraoperative cholangiography, preoperative diagnosis is more important especially because therapeutic splitting with preoperative endoscopic retrograde cholangiopancreatography (ERCP) and clearance of the CBD followed by laparoscopic cholecystectomy is the most frequently applied technique, at least in surveys in Scotland (96.2%) and Germany (94.2%) [1, 2].

As demographics change, an increasing number of older patients with significant comorbidities and more pediatric patients are presenting with symptomatic cholecystolithiasis and CBDS. As less invasive treatment options for CBDS are now well established, it is reported that these groups are being treated more successfully [3, 4]. The complexity of manifestations is illustrated by the different approaches to predict CBDS preoperatively without interventional or expensive examinations like ERCP or magnetic resonance cholangiopancreatography (MRCP).

Clinical evaluation and biochemical tests are often not sufficient to confirm the diagnosis. Serum bilirubin and alkaline phosphatase (AP) are typically elevated in cases of biliary obstruction, but these are neither highly sensitive nor specific for CBDS. Raised gamma glutamyl transpeptidase (GGT) or aspartate aminotransferase (AST) levels have been suggested to be the most sensitive and specific indicator of CBDS, with values of greater than 90 U/L possibly indicating a high risk of biliary duct lithiasis [5]. According to some publications, patients may be classified preoperatively into high, moderate or low risk groups to select for additional diagnostics and interventions. The high risk (> 50% risk) group includes those patients with jaundice or cholangitis, biliary duct stones or a dilated CBD on ultrasound. The moderate risk (10–50%) group includes those patients with a history of pancreatitis or jaundice, elevated preoperative bilirubin and AP levels or multiple small gallstones. It is unlikely that patients with large gallstones, without a history of jaundice or pancreatitis and with normal liver function tests have CBDS (low risk group < 5%) [6–8].

The typical manifestations of CBDS are colic, jaundice, pancreatitis and cholangitis. The frequency of the various manifestations is reported in older publications and books to be very high, with CBDS presenting with colic in 75% and jaundice in 80% of cases. A recent publication analysing the various symptoms showed that only one third of all patients with colic had evidence of CBDS and only 46% (245/532) of patients with CBDS had colic [9]. In this prospective study of 1000 patients with symptomatic gallbladder stones, current or previous evidence for ductal stones was found in 53% of patients according to liver function tests, preoperative measurement of bile duct diameter by ultrasound and intraoperative cholangiography performed only if pre-operative study showed some abnormal finding. CBDS were found in 142 patients at the time of operation. An overall rate of 73% of spontaneous passage of CBDS was concluded from this study. From this and other studies [9–11], the rates of spontaneous passage and spontaneous bile duct clearance in cases of pancreatitis, biliary colic and cholecystitis were 80–93%. The same publication showed that jaundice occurred in 33% (177/532) of patients with choledocholithiasis, with more than 55% of patients passing their stones spontaneously. The four patients who presented with cholangitis in this study had no spontaneous passage before treatment [9].

Cholangitis was a rare manifestation in this study and the prevalence of cholangitis in patients with choledocholithiasis seems to have decreased because of more sensitive diagnostics for CBDS.

Another study analysing the clinical course of patients with symptomatic stones showed that in patients with a diagnosis of impacted CBDS, spontaneous passage occurred in 28% of cases if delayed surgery was performed more than 48 hours after admission compared to immediate surgery in the first 48 hours. Factors being unfavourable for spontaneous passage were age over 70 years, jaundice for more than 7 days and CBDS visible by imaging techniques [12].

There have been no obvious changes in the epidemiology of CBDS over the last 10 years. However, comparing the actual literature with older publications and books gives the impression that in earlier times patients with CBDS presented in most cases with symptoms and complications, and rarely with asymptomatic or unproblematic CBDS, while nowadays CBDS are more and more often diagnosed in the nearly asymptomatic stages.

The exact prevalence of CBDS remains unclear, because potential screening examinations like conventional percutaneous ultrasound can miss up to two-thirds of patients with CBDS and only experienced examiners achieve an accuracy of more than 80% [13]. The gold standard ERCP is too invasive for a screening examination and MRCP is too expensive. Population studies on treatment and clinical course of CBDS are based on patients with symptomatic cholecystolithiasis. It is reported that at the time of cholecystectomy for symptomatic cholecystolithiasis 8–15% of patients younger than 60 years old and 15–60% of patients older than 60 years have CBDS. The incidence has declined in recent years after the widespread acceptance of laparoscopic cholecystectomy, possibly due to earlier presentation in the natural course of symptomatic cholecystolithiasis [6, 14].

When patients with diagnosed CBDS are analysed, 95% have cholecystolithiasis and only 5% have isolated stones in the biliary tree.

The major clinical manifestations of CBDS that will be described are therefore the following:

- asymptomatic stones;
- CBDS and asymptomatic gallbladder stones;
- acute cholangitis;
- biliary pancreatitis;
- recurrent stones after ERCP.

Asymptomatic Common Bile Duct Stones

Of all the clinical manifestations of CBDS “asymptomatic” CBDS are the most difficult to discuss.

First of all we have to answer the question: What are asymptomatic CBDS? Are they stones without clinical symptoms? Are they stones without clinical symptoms and without elevation of laboratory values? Or are they stones without clinical symptoms, without elevation of laboratory values and normal ultrasound? Is dilation of the bile duct already a symptom of choledocholithiasis or is it just a suspicious sign? Is abnormality already illness?

Studies analysing the natural course of asymptomatic CBDS included patients in whom there was at least the suspicion of CBDS at the time of cholecystectomy. Suspicion in case of rare symptoms is raised by laboratory values. In these patients it is sometimes difficult to differentiate symptoms caused by the gallbladder stones or CBDS. When choledocholithiasis is diagnosed, common upper gastrointestinal tract symptoms like nausea, eructation, meteorism and constipation are frequently and coincidently present and thought to be caused by choledocholithiasis. Nevertheless, risk factors disposing to gallbladder stones also favour the development of these symptoms.

CBDS in patients with these unspecific symptoms should not uncritically be categorized as symptomatic biliary duct stones. So, should we discuss patients with asymptomatic CBDS? Is there a consequence on treatment strategy?

While it is well established that asymptomatic cholecystolithiasis is in general no indication for cholecystectomy, surgical or endoscopic treatment for symptomatic as well as for asymptomatic CBDS was, and still seems to be mandatory because of otherwise potentially severe consequences. This treatment increases morbidity and mortality compared to cholecystectomy alone. To counterbalance this increase in morbidity we need reliable data about the clinical course of patients with untreated asymptomatic stones.

So what is the natural history of CBDS? Early epidemiological data result from times when diagnostic tools that do not fit current standards were used and, missing asymptomatic choledocolithiasis, a high rate of symptomatic choledocholithiasis was reported. There is also discussion that introduction of laparoscopic cholecystectomy extended the indication for cholecystectomy and led to earlier operations. This could lead to a reduction of patients presenting with CBDS [6], since prevalence of CBDS increases with the duration of existence of gallbladder stones.

While the prevalence of CBDS is unclear, the prevalence of asymptomatic CBDS is even more so. Assumptions about the rate of patients with asymptomatic choledocholithiasis becoming symptomatic and requiring further interventional treatment in long term range from 15 to 85 % with the lower incidences in recent publications probably also due to more sensitive diagnostics [15].

Without doubt a number of patients stay clinically asymptomatic without abnormalities in laboratory values. All patients with symptomatic or asymptomatic CBDS analysed in studies are patients originally treated for symptomatic gallbladder stones. This could lead to an underestimation of the frequency of asymptomatic CBDS. Few studies deal with the natural history of asymptomatic CBDS. Caddy et al. [16] examined patients who had no preoperative suspicion of CBDS: a group of patients submitted to cholecystectomy without intra-operative cholangiogram were retrospectively reviewed to determine whether post-operative biliary complications had occurred and a control group submitted to cholecystectomy with intra-operative cholangiogram. No biliary complications were found during an observation period of 5 years in the first group, while a prevalence of symptomatic CBDS of 6% was reported in the control group. These results imply that missed stones or untreated stones do not necessarily lead to problems.

There are no other factors that could potentially help us to decide for or against treatment for asymptomatic choledocholithiasis. There is no evidence that size or composition of CBDS have an impact on the patient being symptomatic or asymptomatic. CBDS with a size up to 8 mm seem to pass spontaneously more often, but normally this is not an asymptomatic passage.

While large stones are more often responsible for obstruction with jaundice and cholangitis, small stones and microcalculi are more often the cause of biliary pancreatitis.

In conclusion, asymptomatic CBDS are still an indication for treatment. However, with existing data an individual decision towards observation, especially in high risk patients with asymptomatic stones, can be justified.

Common Bile Duct Stones and Asymptomatic Gallbladder Stones

In most centres, endoscopic sphincterotomy is the treatment of choice for patients with CBDS. Is cholecystectomy mandatory after clearance of the bile duct if the gallbladder stones are asymptomatic? Some studies have compared the results of the wait-and-see policy and prophylactic cholecystectomy to prevent biliary duct stone recurrence and cholecystitis, but results have been controversial [17–19]. While CBDS recurrence could be retreated endoscopically, acute cholecystitis is a definite indication for cholecystectomy. Thus, it still remains controversial as to whether subsequent laparoscopic cholecystectomy is indicated in patients after endoscopic treatment of CBDS. In the study of Lee et al. [19] with observational treatment of patients with ERCP and bile duct clearance, cholecystitis was observed in 17% of patients while recurrence of bile duct stones was a problem for 13% of patients [19].

In most patients with acute cholecystitis, laparoscopic cholecystectomy presents an elevated risk for bile duct injuries. Some prospective data suggest that in selected patients older than 80 years of age an expectant attitude concerning cholecystectomy can be justified, because symptoms and complications are rare (< 15%) and in over one third of patients spontaneous passage of calculi is observed [20, 21].

Cholangitis

The infection of the bile duct system can be clinically diagnosed in most cases through presentation of the trias of pain in right upper quadrant, fever, and jaundice. Normally, the icterus due to CBDS gradually changes, as opposed to in a distal cholangiocellular carcinoma or pancreas head carcinoma. Cholangitis is an indication for immediate therapy usually performed with an ERCP, and rarely with a percutaneous transhepatic cholangiography (PTC). An operative revision is not indicated because of high morbidity and mortality [22].

Cholangitis seems to be a rare manifestation of CBDS. In the well designed study of Tranter et al. [9] only four of 532 patients with CBDS had cholangitis and no spontaneous passage of stones [9].

Biliary Pancreatitis

Beside cholangitis, biliary pancreatitis is the most dangerous complication of CBDS. An impacted stone in the papilla of Vater or small stones penetrating into the pancreatic duct with consecutive obstruction of pancreatic secretion are discussed as main causes. An additional cholangitis can aggravate the situation. Smaller stones (microcalculi < 5 mm diameter) that are more difficult to detect are often responsible for the development of pancreatitis [23]. Improvements in diagnostics have led to classification of more cases of pancreatitis as biliary rather than as idiopathic pancreatitis. Especially in patients 60 years of age or older, biliary stones are the most frequent cause of acute pancreatitis [24, 25]. In some studies up to 75% of patients with acute pancreatitis have biliary pancreatitis. The clinical course of biliary pancreatitis is mild in most cases. In the study of Tranter et al. [9], pancreatitis was the manifestation of CBDS in 14% of patients, with spontaneous passage of CBDS in 80%. Thus, pancreatitis was just the symptom of an already successful bile duct clearance, and in many of these patients besides mild symptoms, only a serologic reaction lasting 3–7 days will be seen.

In the study of Schietroma et al. [26] 30.8% of patients with biliary pancreatitis had a severe pancreatitis according to the Ranson criteria, while 69.2% had a mild pancreatitis without the need for intervention [26].

It is important to differentiate between biliary pancreatitis and other aetiologies because of the therapeutic consequences.

Hints at biliary genesis are the detection of biliary duct stones in diagnostic imaging. If stones are not detected, microlithiasis may be present or stones may have already passed. A temporary increase of AST, alanine aminotransferase bilirubin, AP and GGT is highly predictive for biliary aetiology of pancreatitis.

Biliary pancreatitis with concomitant jaundice and cholangitis is an emergency indication for ERCP in the first 24 hours.

Patients with mild clinical courses and spontaneous improvement of symptoms and laboratory values can be clinically observed and in unclear cases an MRCP should be performed.

Biliary pancreatitis has a high risk of recurrence, because the stones are usually smaller and additional stones will pass from the gallbladder in most of the patients. Therefore an elective cholecystectomy should be performed.

Recurrent Stones after ERCP

Recurrent stones after ERCP and papillotomy occur in 6–24% of patients [27, 28]. Loss of sphincter function leads to duodenobiliary reflux with bacterial colonisation. Many of these patients produce bile that is more lithogenic than normal. Nevertheless, it has been shown that independent of the composition of primary stones, recurrent stones are mainly bilirubin [27, 28]. The development of bilirubin stones is usually induced by β-glucuronidase-producing bacteria. In order to potentially reduce the long term complications of endoscopic sphincterotomy, endoscopic dilatation for stone clearance has been advocated and showed similar clearance rates, less bleeding, and preservation of sphincter function in controlled trials [29, 30].

References

1. Hamouda A, Khan M, Mahmud S et al (2004) Management trends for suspected ductal stones in Scotland (abstract). 9th World Congress of Endoscopic Surgery, Cancun
2. Ludwig K, Lorenz D, Koeckerling F (2002) Surgical strategies in the laparoscopic therapy of cholecystolithiasis and common duct stones. ANZ J Surg 72:547-552
3. Pring CM, Skelding-Millar L, Goodall RJ (2005) Expectant treatment or cholecystectomy after endoscopic retrograde cholangiopancreatography for choledocholithiasis in patients over 80 years old? Surg Endosc 19:357-360
4. Vrochides DV, Sorrells DL Jr, Kurkchubasche AG et al (2005) Is there a role for routine preoperative endoscopic retrograde cholangiopancreatography for suspected choledocholithiasis in children? Arch Surg 140:359-361
5. Peng WK, Sheikh Z, Paterson-Brown S, Nixon SJ (2005) Role of liver function tests in predicting common bile duct stones in acute calculous cholecystitis. Br J Surg 92:1241-1247
6. Sgourakis G, Dedemadi G, Stamatelopoulos A et al (2005) Predictors of common bile duct lithiasis in laparoscopic era. World J Gastroenterol 11:3267-3272
7. Abboud PA, Malet PF, Berlin JA et al (1996) Predictors of common bile duct stones prior to cholecystectomy: a metaanalysis. Gastrointest Endosc 44:450-455
8. Freitas ML, Bell RL, Duffy AJ (2006) Choledocholithiasis: evolving standards for diagnosis and management. World J Gastroenterol 12:3162-3167

9. Tranter SE, Thompson MH (2003) Spontaneous passage of bile duct stones: frequency of occurrence and relation to clinical presentation. Ann R Coll Surg Engl 85:174-177
10. Stone HH, Fabian TC, Dunlop WE (1981) Gallstone pancreatitis: biliary tract pathology in relation to time of operation. Ann Surg 194:305-310
11. Neoptolemus JP, London NJ, Bailey IA et al (1988) Controlled trial of urgent endoscopic retrograde cholangiopancreaticography and sphincterotomy versus conservative management for acute pancreatitis due to gallstones. Lancet 2:979-983
12. Acevedo C, Mandirola F, Teixeira M (2006) Delayed surgery in impacted common bile duct calculi: lower percentage of biliary tract interventions. Cir Esp 79:361-364
13. Rickes S, Treiber G, Mänkemäller K et al (2006) Impact of the operator's experience on value of high-resolution transabdominal ultrasound in the diagnosis of choledocholithiasis: a prospective comparison using endoscopic retrograde cholangiography as the gold standard. Scand J Gastroenterol 41:838-843
14. Scientific Committee of the European Association for Endoscopic Surgery (E.A.E.S.) (1998) Diagnosis and treatment of common bile duct stones (CBDS). Results of a consensus development conference. Surg Endosc 12:856-864
15. Metcalfe MS, Ong T, Bruening MH et al (2004) Is laparoscopic intraoperative cholangiogram a matter of routine? Am J Surg 187:475-481
16. Caddy GR, Kirby J, Kirk SJ et al (2005) Natural history of asymptomatic bile duct stones at time of cholecystectomy. Ulster Med J 74:108-112
17. Boerma D, Rauws EA, Keulemans YC et al (2002) Wait-and-see policy or laparoscopic cholecystectomy after endoscopic sphincterotomy for bile-duct stones: a randomised trial. Lancet 360:761-765
18. Schreurs WH, Vles WJ, Stuifbergen WH, Oostvogel HJ (2004) Endoscopic management of common bile duct stones leaving the gallbladder in situ. A cohort study with long-term follow-up. Dig Surg 21:60-64
19. Lee JK, Ryu JK, Park JK et al (2006) Risk factors of acute cholecystitis after endoscopic common bile duct stone removal. World J Gastroenterol 12(6):956-960
20. Collins C, Maguire D, Ireland A et al (2004) A prospective study of common bile duct calculi in patients undergoing laparoscopic cholecystectomy: natural history of choledocholithiasis revisited. Ann Surg 239:28-33
21. Pring CM, Skelding-Millar L, Goodall RJ (2005) Expectant treatment or cholecystectomy after endoscopic retrogradecholangiopancreatography for choledocholithiasis in patients over 80 years old? Surg Endosc 19:357-360
22. Uhl W, Warshaw A, Imrie C et al (2002) IAP Guidelines for the surgical treatment of acute pancreatitis. Pancreatology 2:565-573
23. Eimiller A, Born P, Berg P et al (1988) Mikrolithen als Verursacher der akuten Pankreatitis. Z Gastroenterol 26:446
24. Appelroos S, Borgström A (1999) Incidence, aetiology and mortalitiy rate of acute pancreatitis over 10 years in a defined urban population in Sweden. Br J Surg 86:465-470
25. Secknus R, Mössner J (2000) Incidenz- und Prävalenzveränderungen der akuten und chronischen Pankreatitis in Deutschland. Chirurg 71:249-252
26. Schietroma M, Carlei F, Lezoche E et al (2001) Acute biliary pancreatitis: staging and management. Hepatogastroenterology 48:988-993
27. Terblanche J, Allison HF, Northover JMA (1983) An ischemic basis for ischemic biliary strictures. Surgery 94:52-57
28. Mercado MA, Chan C, Orozco H (2002) To stent or not to stent bilioenteric anastomosis after iatrogenic injury. A dilemma not answered? Arch Surg 137:60-63
29. Ochi Y, Mukawa K, Kiyosawa K, Akamatsu T (1999) Comparing the treatment outcomes of endoscopic papillary dilation and endoscopic sphincterotomy for removal of bile duct stones. J Gastroenterol Hepatol 14:90-96
30. Tsujino T, Isayama H, Komatsu Y et al (2005) Risk factors for pancreatitis in patients with common bile duct stones managed by endoscopic papillary balloon dilation. Am J Gastroenterol 100:38-42

Chapter 23

Synchronous Treatment of Common Bile Duct Stones by Laparotomy

Olivier Chapuis, Brice Malgras, Anne Bouix

Introduction

When secondary common bile duct (CBD) stones are detected either by preoperative or intraoperative exploration, the method of treatment has to be chosen carefully in order to achieve CBD clearance and cholecystectomy. Biliary surgery has evolved over the last 40 years, with two major milestones: first the advent of endoscopic sphincterotomy at the beginning of the seventies and then the development of a minimally invasive surgical approach (laparoscopy) 20 years later.

Open treatment of CBD stones was the only procedure available until the advent of endoscopic techniques. Before laparoscopic cholecystectomy was developed, randomized trials that compared open surgical treatment for both cholecystectomy and CBD clearance versus endoscopic procedures followed by an elective open cholecystectomy showed that one stage open surgery was superior [1, 2].

Over a long period, most surgeons thought that the laparoscopic approach was inadequate to safely explore the CBD, and the number of endoscopic sphincterotomies increased [3]. More recently, because of skilled surgery and advances in technology, laparoscopic CBD exploration has become a safe alternative to the two-stage treatment, endoscopic sphincterotomy followed by laparoscopic cholecystectomy, with a rate of success as high as 95.6% in expert hands [4].

Open CBD surgery remains, however, the reference surgical treatment of CBD stones and every surgeon should have the skills to perform it. However, the number of such procedures has progressively decreased and it will be difficult to train young surgeons in the coming years [5].

Indications for Synchronous Treatment by Laparotomy

Indications for open surgery could be summarized as contraindications to laparoscopic and endoscopic procedures, failure of endoscopic procedure and conversion of laparoscopy. Absolute contraindications to laparoscopy consist only of lack of appropriate equipment or surgical skills.

Relative contraindications to laparoscopy include medical causes related to pneumoperitoneum, life-threatening conditions (severely burnt or intensive care patients) and surgical causes (patients with a high probability to have multiple and dense peritoneal adhesions because of prior surgery of the upper abdomen, history of peritoneal infection, cholecystitis, and patients with morbid obesity), all of which are associated with high conversion rates.

Endoscopic procedures are not possible if the duodenal papilla cannot be reached because of previous surgery with interruption of the digestive tract between the cardia and the duodenal papilla, of duodenal stenosis and of anatomic abnormalities such as juxta-papillary duodenal diverticulum or variations in duodenal papilla location.

Patients on chronic anticoagulation treatment present a high risk of postoperative bleeding and represent a relative contraindication to an endoscopic procedure. Failure of an endoscopic CBD clearance procedure is an indication for open surgery, particularly when the endoscopic procedure has followed a laparoscopic cholecystectomy. Difficulties in dissection, inability to correctly identify anatomy, intraperitoneal bleeding, unsuspected intraoperative findings or perioperative injury to the CBD are reasons for conversion from a laparoscopic procedure to open surgery [6].

Technique of Synchronous Treatment by Laparotomy

Synchronous treatment by laparotomy consists of both cholecystectomy and CBD clearance.

Anaesthesia

The patient is operated under general anaesthesia. A naso- or oro-gastric tube is placed after induction of anaesthesia.

Perioperative Antibiotics

For antibiotic prophylaxis the recommendations are to inject one dose of cefuroxime before the operation [7]. Fluoroquinolones and metronidazole are administered in case of allergic reaction to penicillin. The dose of antibiotics is repeated if the surgery exceeds 4 hours.

For established infection, such as cholecystitis and acute cholangitis, an adequate antimicrobial spectrum, high diffusion in the blood and in tissues around the biliary tract, rather than within biliary excretion, are the main considerations. Choice of antibiotics is also influenced by patient characteristics and local antibiotic sensitivity patterns [8].

Equipment

The surgeon needs haemostatic devices (monopolar or bipolar electrocauterisation to avoid electrical injury), abdominal retractors, Randall stone forceps, biliary balloon catheters, balloon or plastic dilators, stone baskets and cholangiography catheters. A mobile C-arm with an image intensifier and, if possible, digital capability gives high-definition x-rays during cholangiography. Another advance in biliary surgery is the use of a flexible choledochoscope. If possible, the surgeon would have two different sizes of flexible choledochoscope (3 mm and 5 mm) to allow CBD exploration via the cystic duct or directly in the CBD after choledochotomy. The choledochoscope is ideally connected to a video camera and choledochoscopy can then be seen on a monitor. The most recent advance is intraoperative ultrasonography (IOUS).

Room Setup

The patient is placed on the operating table in a supine position. The arms may be extended, or may be tucked to the sides. The operating table should allow radiological exploration. The surgeon stands generally at the right side of the patient.

Incision, Exposition and Exploration

Various abdominal wall incisions can be used to perform cholecystectomy and exploration of the CBD. The mini-incisions that were used to perform cholecystectomy just before the success of laparoscopic surgery are generally too small to offer a good exposition of the porta hepatis. Moreover, a specific instrumentation is mandatory.

Vertical pararectal or tranversal incisions may be preferred to midline incisions. Midline incisions should be used in emergency, in case of massive hepatomegaly, in case of prior midline scar or if another surgical procedure, such as gastro-esophageal reflux disease surgery, is planned.

The right subcostal incision is the more frequently used. It gives a good exposition of the gallbladder and porta hepatis, as the incision is parallel to the inferior margin of the liver. It is easy to extend towards the left subcostal area if the exposition would not prove to be optimal.

Exposition is improved using abdominal retractors, according to the incision length and the surgeon's preference. To expose the porta hepatis it is essential to elevate the liver and push down the duodeno-pancreatic block. Three abdominal towels are needed to expose and isolate the sub-hepatic area. Kocher's manoeuvre is very useful to allow palpation of the duodenum, head of pancreas and distal part of CBD and to perform perioperative choledochoscopy.

During exploration it is sometimes necessary to liberate adhesions to the liver and the gallbladder and recreate normal anatomic conditions. The surgeon should be able to dissect the porta hepatis and the CBD. When the dissection is hazardous, the risk of perioperative or postoperative complications increases and the surgeon has to decide between performing a surgical approach of the CBD or performing only a cholecystectomy, with the surgery followed by an endoscopic procedure to achieve CBD clearance.

Exposition of Calot's Triangle

The rule is not to divide any anatomical element untill not clearly identified. Obtain exposure of the anterior and posterior layer of peritoneum of Calot's triangle by gentle grasping Hartmann's pouch of the gallbladder. When the gallbladder is tense and difficult to grasp, it should be decompressed using a needle or by opening the gallbladder. Bile should be sent for bacteriological examination. A suture closes the gallbladder. Decompression helps to minimize disruption of the gallbladder wall and peritoneal contamination or stone spillage. Dissection of Calot's triangle should be begun at the gallbladder neck, at the junction between the infundibulum and the cystic duct, by section of the anterior and posterior peritoneal layer. The infundibulo-cystic junction should be carefully delineated, in order to remain distant from the CBD. Clear cystic duct over a 10 mm length. Extract cystic stones after side opening of the cystic duct or by milking them back into gallbladder. Then dissect the cystic artery. At this stage, Calot's triangle is completely released. Do not divide any anatomic structure before the mandatory intraoperative cholangiography has been performed.

In case of severe inflammation, no attempt is made to dissect Calot's triangle and partial cholecystectomy should be considered. Leave the posterior wall of the gallbladder in place, remove the gallbladder's contents and oversew the cystic duct within the gallbladder if possible. A subhepatic drain in such cases is mandatory [9].

In case of moderate inflammation and difficulty in dissecting Calot's triangle, the retrograde "fundus-first" technique is an alternative: first liberate the fundus from the liver, leaving a peritoneal rim. Control bleeding by use of electrocautery, as the cystic artery is not divided. Dissect close to the gallbladder wall until Hartmann's pouch and the junction with the cystic duct are reached. Liberation of the gallbladder from hepatic bed helps in the dissection of Calot's triangle and recognition of the anatomical elements. In this case, a stone is often impacted in the infundibulum. Removing or milking the stone upward into the gallbladder makes the dissection safer.

When the entire circumference of the gallbladder–cystic duct junction is dissected, a clip or a suture is placed as close to the gallbladder as possible.

Intraoperative Cholangiography

Open the cystic duct partially. Introduce the cholangiocatheter, previously purged to avoid any air bubbles, into the cystic duct to a length of several millimetres. Maintain the extremity of the catheter in place using an "integrated" device, a clip, or even by ligature. The cholangiography will necessitate several pictures in order to explore extrahepatic and intrahepatic bile ducts, using if necessary hyperpressure or reverse Trendelenburg position of the patient. Intraoperative cholangiography gives important information about unsuspected stones, characteristics of CBD stones (number, size, location) and anatomy of the biliary tree (width, length, cystic duct junction with the CBD, variations).

Intraoperative Ultrasonography in Open Surgery

Transducers with a frequency of 7.5 MHz are used for screening of the biliary tract and pancreas in open surgery. Transducer probes for IOUS should be small enough to enable easy manipulation within the restricted space of the operative field. Mostly T- or J-shaped transducer probes are used. Experience should be attained before this technique replaces intraoperative cholangiography.

Open CBD Exploration

CBD clearance can be achieved via a cysticotomy, choledochotomy or duodenotomy.

Transcystic Approach

The transcystic approach should be tried whenever possible, even in open surgery. Conditions must be appropriate: the size of the stones must be compatible with the cystic duct diameter. When necessary, the cystic duct can be dilated by means of plastic dilators, or by means of balloon dilators. The number of stones to be extracted is a relative limit, and in case of multiple CBD stones choledochotomy is more appropriate. A choledochotomy is preferred if the location of the stones is above the cystic duct and CBD junction. However, it may be possible to milk the CBD to move the stones down to the distal part of the CBD. The anatomy of the cystic duct must be favourable to the transcystic approach (width, length, type of cystic duct–CBD junction). Dissect the cystic duct to the CBD junction if possible. Transcystic CBD clearance can be achieved using flushing, balloon or basket techniques.

Some authors describe a method of treatment of small CBD stones (< 2 mm diameter) by flushing the CBD with a saline solution. Intravenous administration of glucagon (1–2 mg) may relax the sphincter of Oddi.

Balloon techniques can be ineffective in clearing the CBD when using the transcystic approach, as stones and debris may be withdrawn in the upper biliary tree. Clearance is preferentially achieved by means of a Dormia basket, introduced either freely or under fluoroscopic or choledochoscopic control.

When baskets are used without fluoroscopic or choledochoscopic control, the procedure is dangerous and should be performed by an expert. Fluoroscopic and choledochoscopic control avoids basket transpapillary crossing and accidental perforation of the CBD. However, fluoroscopic control is time-consuming and potentially cumbersome. Extraction under choledochoscopic control is easier when a video camera is connected to the choledochoscope. Introduce the Dormia basket into the operating channel of the choledochoscope or close to it and open it under direct vision beyond the stone. After extraction of a first stone, the procedure is repeated if necessary.

When the stone's diameter is wider than the cystic duct, it may be necessary to perform a short cysticotomy to allow extraction of the stone, rather then the crushing stone maneuver for the risk of cystic duct-CBD junction injury. In case of failure or difficulties, a choledochotomy should be performed. Control of the clearance of CBD is performed by either cholangiography or choledochoscopy. The procedure then ends by closure of the cystic duct or by using external biliary transcystic drainage.

Choledochotomy

Two conditions are required: an accessible CBD according to the inflammatory process of the porta hepatis and a CBD larger than 7–8 mm.

Exposure of the CBD

Continuity of the cystic duct with the gallbladder and CBD may or may not be maintained, but exposure is generally better after gallbladder removal. Send the gallbladder for pathological examination. The CBD is usually easy to identify because of its characteristic blue grey colour, especially if it is large. Dissection is less easy when the pedicle is infiltrated, fat or altered by inflammation. The CBD runs on the right border of the porta hepatis, right up to the hepatic artery. After opening the anterior layer of peritoneum, the CBD is exposed, but only on its anterior wall. If small vessels cross the CBD, a preventive haemostasis is indicated, with gentle electrocautery.

Opening the CBD

Use a sharp scalpel first or cutting electrocautery and then scissors to enlarge the choledochotomy. Opening the CBD under the cystic duct junction is called choledochotomy or hepaticotomy if it is made higher, at the level of or above the cystic duct junction. Hepaticotomy avoids the cystic duct and pancreaticoduodenal vessels wounds, whereas choledochotomy allows choledochoduodenostomy. The choice of opening orientation, vertical or transversal, causes controversy. Tranversal choledochotomy respects the vascular supply of the CBD. It should not exceed more than half of the CBD's circumference and can thus raise problems for large stones extraction. Vertical choledochotomy will interrupt vascular supply. There is also a risk of stenosis in case of a fine CBD. In practice, if the CBD is enlarged, which is often the case, the orientation of the opening probably has no importance. Rules to be applied that guarantee quality of closure and prevention of stenosis are: avoid any wound of the posterior wall of the CBD, do not exceed more than half of the CBD's circumference in case of transversal opening, limit dissection of the CBD's wall to avoid the risk of ischaemia, do not make a vertical choledochotomy if the CBD's diameter is within the limits of normal, and enlarge the choledochotomy according to stone size.

Stone Extraction

Spontaneous issue of one or several stones may occur when opening the CBD. Be careful that they do not spill into the peritoneum. Gently milk the CBD from the head of pancreas toward the choledochotomy. Then wash the biliary tract with a syringe (Soupault's manoeuvre) directly or via a small tube connected to the syringe. Insert the tube's tip into the CBD and inject serum under pressure. These washes are not risky, even in case of biliary infection, provided that the choledochotomy allows the free flow of the serum. The tube is first introduced upward, alternately in the right hepatic duct and then the left. Washes must be repeated at the distal end of the CBD. Passage of the serum in the duodenum, perceived well by the fingers, confirms the permeability of the papilla. If that manoeuvre fails, introduce a biliary balloon catheter through the choledochotomy. This is useful when the stone is impacted. Choledochoscopy would be in such cases the next step: a 3 mm or a 5 mm choledochoscope can be used. Guide the choledochoscope into the CBD to obtain the desired view of the stone. Use a basket in the operating channel to trap the stone. Withdraw both the closed basket and the choledochoscope. A Dormia basket can be introduced blind via the choledochotomy, but this is a dangerous procedure and should be avoided if possible. Instrumental clearance can be another step of the procedure: Randall forceps must be introduced very slowly and gradually with the tips opened so as to avoid pushing the stone into the distal CBD. Fingers are generally necessary to guide the forceps. There is often some difficulty in manipulating the forceps because their opening is limited by the CBD's wall, with a risk of crushing the stone.

Control of Clearance

Choledochoscopy or ultrasonography are effective to control the clearance of the CBD. Cholangiography is feasible through a T-tube.

Closure of the CBD

Primary closure or "ideal choledochotomy": close the choledochotomy with absorbable interrupted sutures or a running suture. The suture should be watertight to avoid shrinking the CBD.

Primitive closure with transcystic drainage avoids hyperpressure and allows postoperative cholangiography.

External drainage: drain with a T-tube (Kehr's drain), the size of which has to be adapted to that of CBD. The horizontal branch should be recut (twice the length of the choledochotomy and split longitudinally). Exteriorize the drain in the right flank and connect it to a non aspirative system. The choledochotomy is usually closed with interrupted sutures so that the T-tube exits from the lower end of the choledochotomy. A control cholangiography should then be performed.

Choledochoduodenostomy: in elderly patients with a large number of CBD stones and a grossly dilated CBD, choledochoduodenostomy, either by side-to-side or by end-to-side anastomosis may prevent postoperative recurrent lithiasis [10].

Duodenotomy

Duodenotomy is used to perform an open surgical sphincterotomy. This technique has to be considered only in patients with CBD stones refractory to endoscopic retrograde procedures.

Special Operative Findings

In the case of a stone enclosed in the lower part of the CBD, if the stone is mobile it can be milked upward. If the stone is blocked in the ampulla, sphincterotomy is preferable, either using an endoscopic or surgical approach.

Intrahepatic stones cannot be extracted using a transcystic approach.

Drainage of the Peritoneal Cavity

A subhepatic drain may be inserted (silicon multitubular flat drain or a silicon tube drain) connected to a close drainage. Some surgeons use suction drains.

Postoperative Management

Perform a cholangiography on the third postoperative day in case of biliary drainage. If there is no residual stone, close the drain and remove the subhepatic drain. If stones are found on the cholangiogram, insert a guide wire into the duodenum under fluoroscopic control. This is helpful during the endoscopic procedure. Biliary drainage (transcystic or T-tube) is removed on an outpatient basis on the twenty-first postoperative day.

Complications

Early Complications

Bile leakage occurs through the subhepatic drain. Otherwise, biloma is found on radiologic imaging. Leakage is usually from the choledochotomy site, rather than from the cystic duct or from the gallbladder bed. Clinical findings, volume of leakage, radiologic investigations (ultrasonography, scanning, cholangiography) and biological findings are helpful when deciding between a percutaneous drainage, or a reintervention.

A retained stone should be removed either by endoscopic stone extraction, via the T-tube tract or by flushing.

Cholangitis after CBD exploration are mainly caused by a retained stone. Management includes drainage of the biliary tract, antibiotics and removal of the retained stone.

Late Complications

Abscess around a spilled stone, recurrent stone or stricture of the CBD are the main late complications. Each of them has a specific management.

References

1. Neoptolemos JP, Carr-Locke DL, Fossard DP (1987) Prospective randomised study of preoperative endoscopic sphincterotomy versus surgery alone for common bile duct stones. BMJ 294:470-474
2. Suc B, Escat J, Cherqui D et al (1998) Surgery vs endoscopy as primary treatment in symptomatic patients with suspected common bile duct stones: a multicenter randomized trial. French associations for surgical research. Arch Surg 133:702-708
3. Lezoche E, Paganini AM (1995) Single-stage laparoscopic treatment of gallstones and common bile duct in 120 unselected, consecutive patients. Surg Endosc 9:1070-1075
4. Paganini AM, Guerrieri M, Sarnari J et al (2007) Thirteen years' experience with laparoscopic transcystic common bile duct exploration for stones. Surg Endosc 21:34-40
5. Shulman CI, Levi J, Sleeman D et al (2007) Are we training our residents to perform open gall bladder and common bile duct explorations? J Surg Res 20(10):1-4
6. Bingener-Casey J, Richards ML, Strodel WE et al (2002) Reasons for conversion from laparoscopic to open cholecystectomy: a 10-year review. J Gastrointest Surg 6:800-805
7. Meijer WS, Schmitz PI, Jeekel J (1990) Meta-analysis of randomised, controlled clinical trials of antibiotic prophylaxis in biliary tract surgery. Br J Surg 77:283-290
8. Van Erpecum KJ (2006) Gallstone disease. Complicatins of bile-duct stones: acute cholangitis and pancreatitis. Best Pract Res Clin Gastroenterol 20:1139-1152
9. Soleimani M, Mehrabi A, Mood ZA et al (2007) Partial cholecystectomy as a safe and viable option in the emergency treatment of complex acute cholecystitis: a case series and review of the literature. Am Surg 73:498-507
10. Li ZF, Chen XP (2007) Recurrent lithiasis after surgical treatment of elderly patients with choledocholithiasis. Hepatobiliary Pancreat Dis Int 6:67-7

Chapter 24

Cholecystocholedocholithiasis: Two-stage Treatment

Mario Morino, Alberto Arezzo

Introduction

Choledocholithiasis, literally the presence of gallstones in the common bile duct (CBD), occurs in 15–20% of patients with cholecystolithiasis. The majority of gallstones are believed to form in the gallbladder where they pass into the CBD via the cystic duct. CBD stones (CBDS) can also be found in patients who have an apparently normal gallbladder; such patients represent about 10% of those with choledocholithiasis. In addition, approximately 5% of patients who have undergone a cholecystectomy have retained or recurrent stones [1].

Endoscopic retrograde cholangiopancreatography (ERCP) and endoscopic sphincterotomy (ES), introduced in the late 1970s, gradually supplanted surgery as the treatment for this condition. This shift was further enhanced by the advent of laparoscopic cholecystectomy (LC) in the early nineties. ERCP was widely used in combination with LC in order to verify CBD patency and sometimes even to obtain a biliary map to identify anatomic variations of the biliary tract. ERCP is not a procedure without risks, and different authors were concerned by the high percentage (20–60%) of negative ERCPs performed before LC. When magnetic resonance cholangiopancreatography (MRCP) was introduced in 1991, patients with suspected CBD obstruction could avoid an invasive procedure like ERCP being used for purely diagnostic reasons. Unlike conventional ERCP, MRCP does not require introduction of a scope or contrast injection into the ductal system and avoids the morbidity associated with endoscopic procedures and contrast materials. Moreover, it provides accurate depiction and measurements of the bile and pancreatic ducts in more than 95% of examinations. MRCP replaced slowly ERCP as a diagnostic tool (see Chapter 6). At present, ERCP should be mainly therapeutic, when CBDS are strongly suspected or confirmed by MRCP: it allows both diagnostic confirmation and stone extraction. Therapeutic ERCP with endoscopic sphincterotomy (ES) thus represents the first step of a two-stage strategy for the treatment of choledocholithiasis associated with cholecystolithiasis, with the second step being LC.

The most frequently used endoscopic techniques for CBDS clearance (including ES, papillary balloon dilatation, stone extraction using baskets and extraction balloons) and mechanical lithotripsy are described here.

Sphincterotomy

Once the bile duct has been cannulated and a retrograde cholangiography has confirmed the presence of stones in the duct (Fig. 24.1) (see Chapter 6), ES is usually performed to allow CBDS clearance. The term sphincterotomy refers to severing of the deep muscle layers of the sphincter of Oddi. In contrast, papillotomy suggests cutting of the superficial papillary sphincter of the main duodenal papilla. However, in practice, these terms are used interchangeably.

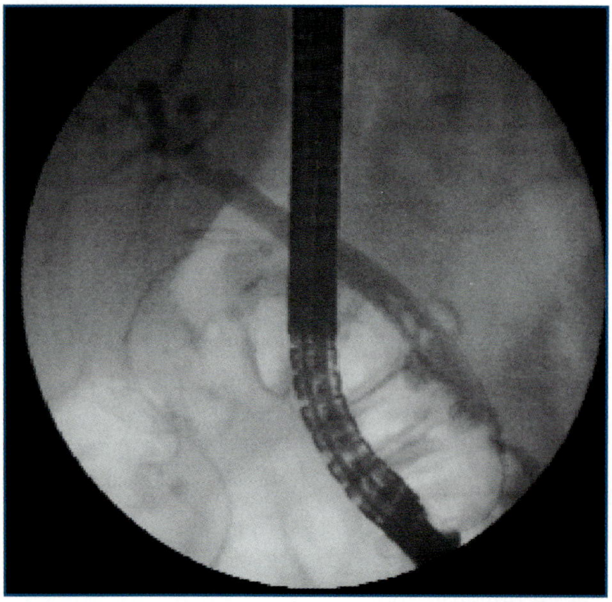

Fig. 24.1 ERCP cannula inserted into the CBD allows performance of a retrograde cholangiography confirming the presence of CBDS

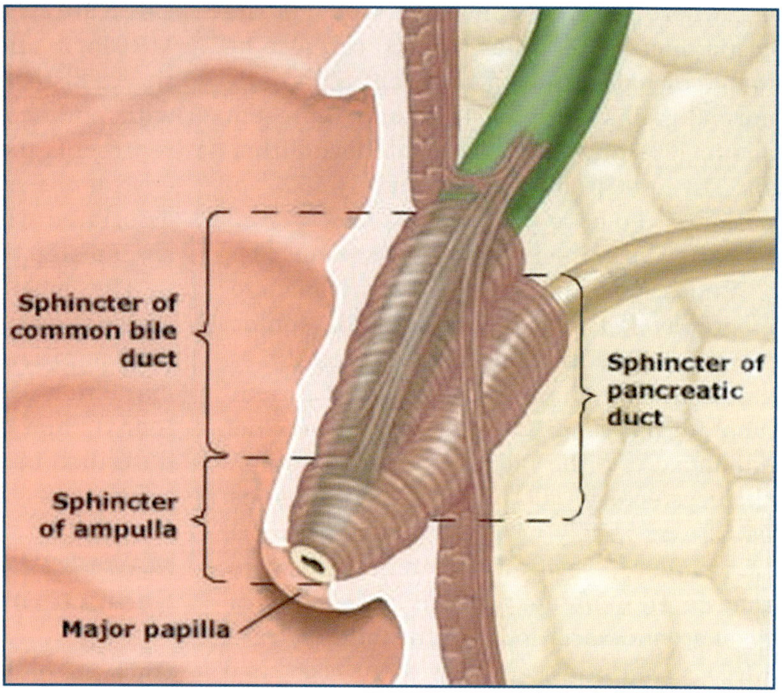

Fig. 24.2 Diagram of the anatomy of the sphincter of Oddi and the ampulla of Vater. The muscle fibers of the spincter of Oddi surround the intraduodenal segment of the CBD and the ampulla of Vater. A circular aggregate of muscle fibers, known as the sphincter of the choledochus (also known as Boyden's sphincter), keeps resistance to bile flow, thereby permitting filling of the gallbladder during fasting and preventing retrograde reflux of duodenal contents into the biliary tree. A separate structure, called the sphincter pancreaticus, encircles the distal pancreatic duct. The muscle fibers of the sphincter pancreaticus are interlocked with those of the sphincter choledochus in a figure eight pattern

ES is the most commonly used therapy for treatment of choledocholithiasis. The goal of ES is to cut the biliary sphincter (Fig. 24.2), thereby eliminating the principal anatomic barrier impeding stone passage and facilitating stone extraction.

Standard ES involves the application of electrocautery to create an incision through the musculature of the biliary portion of the sphincter of Oddi. A number of different devices are available with variations designed to facilitate this procedure, depending upon specific anatomic considerations. In expert hands, ES is possible in up to 95% of patients [2].

Equipment and Technology

The standard technique of ES requires the use of a papillotome, a dedicated high frequency (HF) catheter that is advanced into the biliary sphincter mostly by a guidewire reintroduced into the cannula used for cholangiography. Today multi-lumen sphincterotomes are available, which allow contrast injection and guidewire placement at the same time. Guidewires used must be electrically nonconductive, and preferably Teflon-sheathed rather than Teflon-coated, so that they are less likely to short-circuit as a result of surface imperfections. Papillotomes are available in a number of different configurations, which can be broadly categorized as pull, push, and needle-knife. Several modifications are available within each category, designed for specific clinical settings or anatomic variations. The most commonly used papillotome, the so-called Erlangen or pull-type version, consists of a wire-loop partially enclosed in a Teflon catheter. A wire exits the catheter about 3 cm before its distal end and re-enters the catheter about 3 mm from the tip of the catheter. This way, when the wire is tightened the tip of the catheter is bowed so that the exposed wire is under tension. The exposed wire ranges from 15 to 40 mm. Longer wire devices follow the natural curve of the endoscope and elevator, and are more likely to enter the papilla in the correct orientation. However, the longer wire may not always be an advantage since the ideal transfer of energy occurs when a short segment of cutting wire is applied to sphincter tissue. The diathermy wire can be either braided or monofilament, with monofilament wires preferred since they provide a cleaner incision. Sphincterotomes are usually monopolar. HF electrical current can be applied either as pure-cut, pure coagulation, or a blend of the two. As pure coagulation current during ES may increase the risk of pancreatitis, while pure-cut current appears to be associated with a higher rate of bleeding: most endoscopists prefer blend cutting with coagulation current.

A variety of equipment is available to extract CBDS, although most stones less than 1 cm in diameter pass spontaneously. The most common tools used to extract stones are balloons and baskets. They are available in multiple shapes and sizes and have a variety of characteristics that may be preferentially suited to particular anatomic variations or stone characteristics.

Technique

ES is commonly performed with the endoscope in the so-called short-position along the short curvature of the stomach, although the "long-position" can also be used, along the long curvature. Bowing of the sphincterotome is usually required to force the wire upward toward the roof of the papilla. This maneuver can be facilitated using either the elevator or the up-down deflecting knob, if not both at the same time. It is occasionally desirable to perform ES with the scope in the long-position, since less bowing is needed and the incision can be observed from above.

An ES should be created between the 11 and 1 o'clock position (Fig. 24.3). Following deep cannulation, the endoscopist can withdraw the sphincterotome, tailoring it to the incision length. Generally about one-half to two-thirds of the wire should be visible to prevent retroperitoneal perforation. The incision should be directed along the longitudinal axis of the intramural segment of the CBD and should never be continued beyond the junction of the intramural segment of the bile duct and the duodenal wall. This landmark corresponds to where the superior margin of the bulging impression of the intramural bile duct meets the duodenal wall. A horizontal fold is often present, which can be transected without conse-

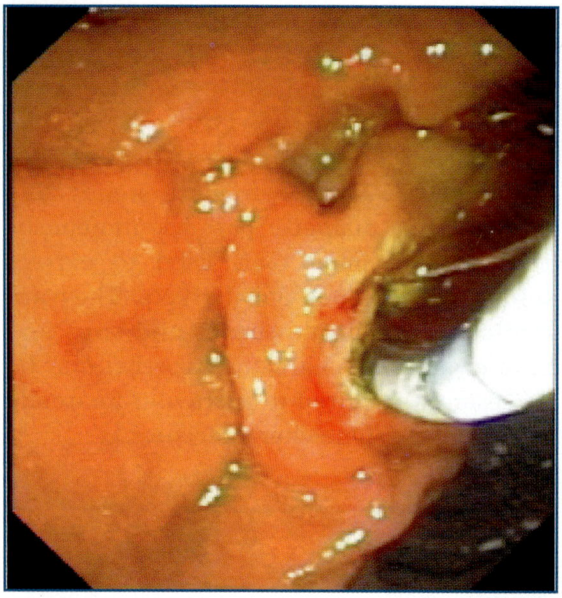

Fig. 24.3 An endoscopic sphincterotomy is performed by means of a sphincterotome. An ES should be created between the 11 and 1 o'clock positions. About one-half to two-thirds of the wire of the sphincterotome should be visible to prevent retroperitoneal perforation

quence. The length of the ES should be tailored to the size of the papilla. It is preferable to create an ES that completely unroofs the papilla since this maximizes access to the CBD and decreases the risk of developing papillary stenosis.

ES in patients who have undergone a partial gastrectomy with Billroth II reconstruction represents a special challenge for the endoscopist. However, in experienced hands, it is often successful. Since the papilla is upside down, the bile duct is cannulated by orienting the catheter downwards in the 6 o'clock position. There are two major techniques for performing ES in this situation. The first requires the use of a needle-knife to cut the sphincter directly through the orifice. This is sometimes performed in a safer way after stenting the bile duct and then cutting over the stent. The incision is continued along the stent towards the junction of the intramural segment and the duodenal wall. Otherwise a reverse sphincterotome is used, with the diathermy wire oriented towards the 6 o'clock rather than the 12 o'clock position.

In all cases of difficult cannulation, a needle-knife fistulotomy can be created, which can then be extended using a conventional sphincterotome, or which can be cannulated with a guide wire across the ampulla and retrieved to advance the sphincterotome safely through it.

ES may be more difficult in the presence of a periampullary diverticulum. In this case, the incision can usually be continued close to the edge of the diverticulum.

As mentioned above, ES is usually performed after deep cannulation of the bile duct has been accomplished. However, in some circumstances, this may not be possible. As an example, impaction of a stone within the papillary sphincter may prohibit advancement of a papillotome or guidewire. In these patients, the use of a needle-knife papillotome in the so called precutting technique is preferable.

Concern regarding the long-term complications related to biliary ES (particularly in young patients) has led to attempts to extract CBDS while preserving the biliary sphincter. One technique involves dilation of the ampulla with a balloon followed by stone extraction. Endoscopic balloon dilation has been evaluated in a number of studies. However, its safety has been questioned. Until more data are available, ES is the method of choice for the treatment of choledocholithiasis.

Once ES or papilla balloon dilatation has been performed, a tool for stone retrieval should be inserted into the CBD. Either a basket or a balloon catheter can be used for the purpose. The choice of a basket seems preferable when the duct is dilated or multiple stones are present (Fig. 24.4), as the balloon may simply squeeze between the stone and the wall, especially in dilated ducts or when the stone is impacted (Fig. 24.5). Once a stone has been grasped within a basket, or a balloon has been advanced proximal to the stone, simple

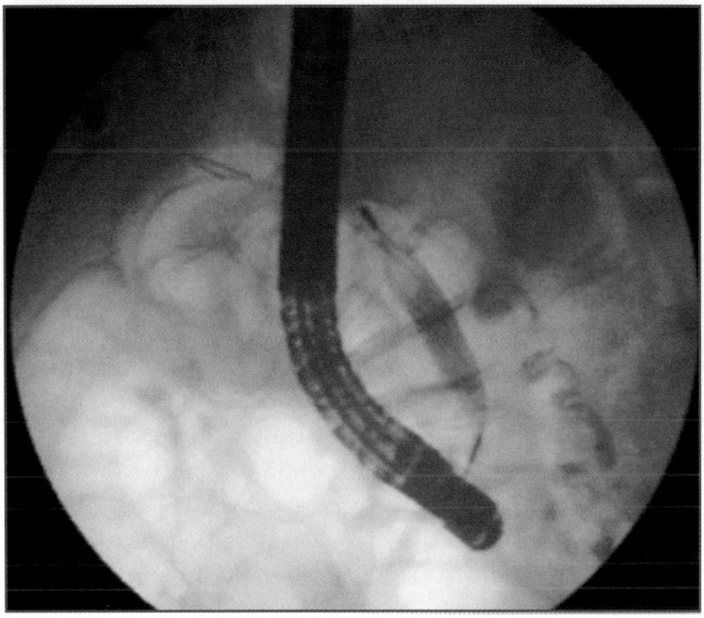

Fig. 24.4 A basket catheter capturing a large stone in the CBD to drag it into the duodenum. The basket is not completely closed to avoid entrapment of the stone in the basket, which would result in a subsequent lithotripsy

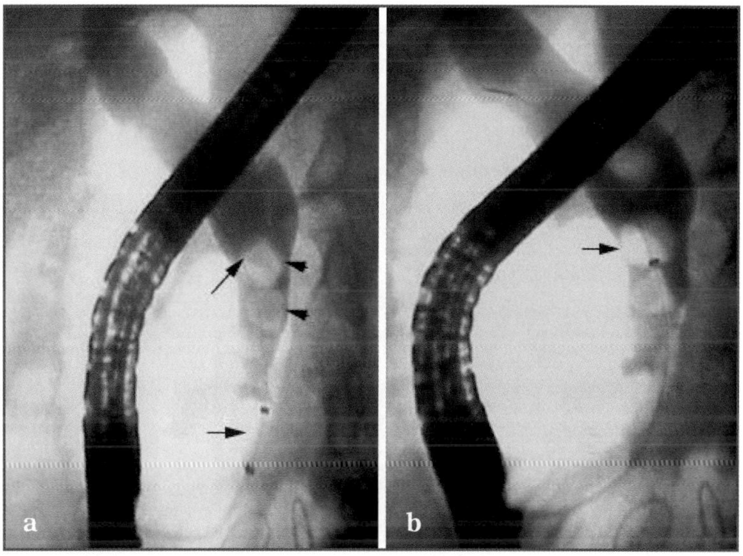

Fig. 24.5 a A balloon catheter being threaded over a guidewire within the CBD (*thin arrows*). At least two gallstones are visible in the distal CBD (*arrowheads*), which is dilated. **b** The balloon has been inflated above a gallstone (*arrow*), which permits the balloon to drag the gallstone out of the duct

pulling of the stone/balloon or stone/basket apparatus is often sufficient to extract the stone. However, in many instances, resistance is encountered when the stone reaches the ampulla, particularly if the ES is smaller than the stone. A force increase in stone retrieval is obtained by deflecting the scope to the right while pushing it further into the stomach, in the so-called "long position", in this way straightening the bile duct axis. One risk of basket extraction is impaction of the basket within the bile duct. When this happens, the basket's wires become impaled within the stone surface and it may not be possible to remove them from the stone. Mechanical lithotripsy with a dedicated lithotriptor is often helpful in these circumstances. In extreme cases, surgery may be required to remove the basket. The risk of impaction can be reduced by extraction of the most distal stone when multiple stones are present, as well as by gently pulling the basket and stone to the preampullary level without closing the basket tightly against the stone (Fig. 24.6). Mechanical lithotripsy is most often used when the standard methods of stone extraction fail.

Mechanical lithotriptors are designed to break stones that are entrapped within a basket. Several devices are available, mostly reusable, including ones that can be passed through the endoscope and others that can be used only after the endoscope has been removed from the patient. These second ones are most common as they are used with standard baskets. The outer sheath of the basket is either cut or disassembled, and the basket wire is then introduced through the metallic sheath of the lithotriptor. Cranking of the lithotriptor forces the metallic sheath to move forward until it reaches the stone, causing tightening; the resulting pressure fragments the stone.

Results

The success rate of ERCP CBDS clearance in the largest series published in the last ten years ranges between 94 and 100% (Table 24.1), decreasing to 80% if lithotripsy is needed. ERCP treatment is nevertheless afflicted by a number of possible complications.

The most common complication associated with ES is biohumoral or clinical pancreatitis, which can also occur during ERCP without ES. Other risks of ES include perforation of the duodenum or bile duct, bleeding, and infection. Short-term complications related to biliary ES occur in less than 10% of patients. In one study that reported data of seven academic medical centres, complications were observed in 112 of 1,921 patients (6%) [2]. Two-thirds of the complications were considered to be mild, i.e., requiring less than 3 days in the hospital. A slightly higher complication rate (10%) was observed in a multicentre study involving 2,347 patients undergoing biliary ES at 17 institutions in the United States and Canada [26]. The most frequent complications included pancreatitis (5%) and bleeding (2%). Most studies have found that the risk of bleeding after ES is increased in patients who have a bleeding diathesis. In addition, the risk of bleeding is probably related to the size of the ES, and may be increased

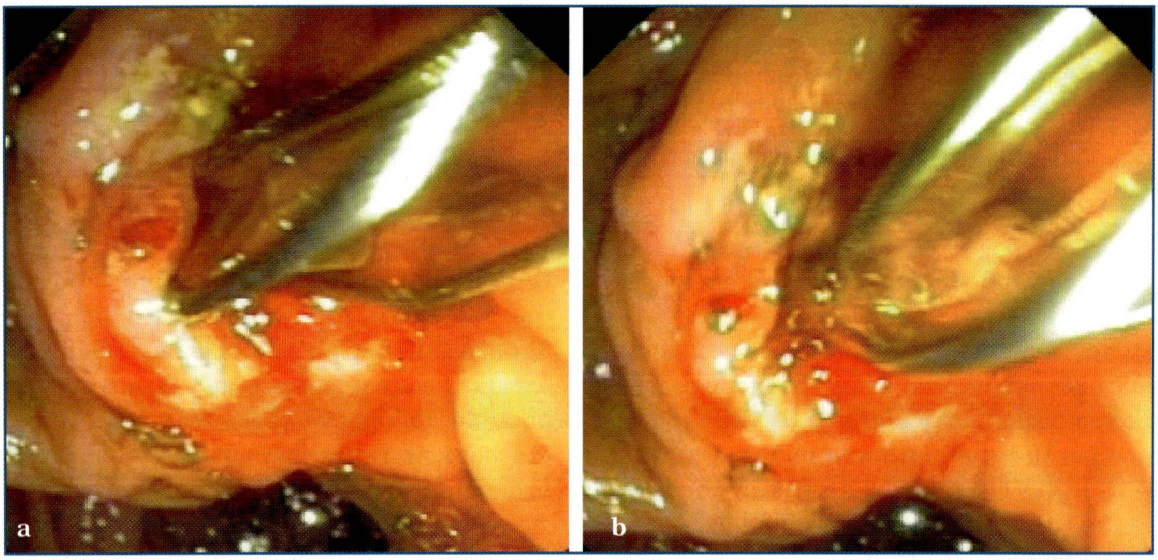

Fig. 24.6 a The risk of impaction can be reduced by extraction of the most distal stone when multiple stones are present, as well as by gently pulling the basket and stone to the preampullary level without closing the basket tightly against the stone. **b** Extraction of a small stone caught in the jaws of a basket

Table 24.1 Results of preoperative ERCP/ES before LC in patients with CBDS – literature review

Author	Year	Number of patients of publication	CBDS suspected	CBDS confirmed at ERCP (%)	Stone clearance (%)	Mortality (%)	Complications (%)	Residual CBDS (%)
Southern [3]	1991	1518	63	10 (16)	9 (90)	0	0	-
Baird [4]	1992	800	11	3 (27)	3 (100)	0	0	-
Larson [5]	1992	1983	65	20 (31)	18 (90)	0	0	6.4
Arregui [6]	1992	622	36	17 (47)	11 (65)	0	7.9	-
Frazee [7]	1993	706	31	18 (62)	18 (100)	0	2	-
Graham [8]	1993	540	36	18 (50)	18 (100)	0	6	-
Leitman [9]	1993	573	45	20 (44)	20 (100)	0	6	-
Barkun [10]	1994	1300	106	50 (47)	45 (90)	0	9	-
Meyer [11]	1994	733	131	58 (44)	55 (95)	0	1	1.8
Salky [12]	1994	822	61	25 (41)	23 (92)	-	-	-
Voyles [13]	1994	1050	51	24 (47)	13 (54)	0	2	2
Rieger [s14]	1994	1140	106	56 (53)	53 (95)	0	1.9	0.7
Rijna [15]	1995	599	119	35 (29)	-	2	14	-
Tanaka [16]	1996	1138	routine	46 (4)	43 (93)	0	6.5	-
Bonatsos [17]	1996	1788	89	54 (61)	53 (98)	0	4.5	-
Kullman [18]	1996	630	84	47 (56)	44 (94)	0	3	6
Masci [19]	1999	841	95	87 (92)	-	0	9.2	-
Bergamaschi [20]	1999	990	155	134 (86)	128 (96)	-	-	-
Coppola [21]	2001	1139	227	121 (53)	117 (97)	0	1.3	-
Romano [22]	2002	1750	193	121 (63)	116 (96)	0	4.1	-
Schreurs [23]	2002	1857	552	273 (49)	271 (99)	0.6	13.5	-
Hamy [24]	2003	-	310	258 (83)	256 (99)	0	1.6	-
Katz [25]	2004	427	41	22 (54)	22 (100)	0	0	0
Average	1991-2004	1003	69*	31 (56)*	28 (91)	0-2	0-13.5	0-6.4

* having excluded data from Tanaka, as ERCP was routinely performed

after repeated procedures, extension of a previous ES and in patients with gallstones impacted in the ampulla.

Long-term complications following ES include stone recurrence, papillary stenosis, and cholangitis, which together occur in approximately 6–24% of patients [27]. Many endoscopists are particularly concerned about these complications in younger patients who will live for many years following ES. This issue was evaluated in two reports [28, 29] with over 10 years of follow-up, and a total of 250 patients. Complications were observed in 38 patients (15%), including 18 patients with papillary stenosis and 13 patients with recurrent CBDS. Most complications were managed endoscopically or conservatively, and only one patient required surgery after failed endoscopic treatment.

In most reports, recurrent CBDS occurs most frequently in patients with concurrent choledocholithiasis and cholecystolithiasis [27]. As a result, it is preferable to perform a cholecystectomy following CBD clearance, except in patients at high risk for surgery from associated co-morbidities. The study of Saito et al. [30] reported the natural history of 371 patients with symptomatic choledocholithiasis and cholecystolithiasis who had a CBD clearance by ERCP with ES without subsequent cholecystectomy. During a mean follow-up of 7.7 years, cholecystitis was observed in 6% of patients, while recurrence of choledocholithiasis was observed in 10% of patients, being successfully treated endoscopically in all but one patient. Two randomised clinical trial (RCT) studies [31, 32] included about 300 patients who underwent ES, and were randomly assigned to immediate LC or to expectant management groups. With a minimum follow-up of 2 years, data showed that recurrent biliary events were significantly more likely in the expectant management group (33% versus 5%).

If mechanical lithotripsy is necessary the overall success rate for ductal clearance is 80–90%, although 20–30% of patients require more than one session [33]. Failure is most often due to impaction of the stone in the bile duct. Complications directly related to the lithotripsy are uncommon.

Laparoscopic Cholecystectomy

The second stage of the treatment consists of LC. As previously discussed, available data suggest that cholecystectomy should be recommended in patients with CBDS. Before LC had gained its current level of reliability, it was justified to leave the gallbladder in situ in patients at high risk for surgery. Today patients with significant comorbidities who present with symptomatic cholecystolithiasis and CBDS are reported to be treated with increasing success [34]. In contrast, some prospective data suggest that in selected patients over 80 years old, an expectant attitude can be justified, because symptoms have been reported in less than 15%, and in over one third of patients spontaneous passage of calculi has been observed [35].

There is concern about the elapsing time between the two stages of the procedures. It seems safe to observe the patient after ERCP at least overnight, and then, after blood test performance the day after the procedure, to schedule LC within 48 hours of the endoscopic bile duct clearance. In case of ERCP complications, LC should be postponed until complete recovery.

ERCP obtains CBD clearance in more than 95% of patients. Possible failures are due to difficult cannulation of the papilla or to bile duct stone impaction. In both cases a Rendez-vous procedure (see Chapter 26) can be proposed, as the insertion of a guidewire through the cystic duct may still be possible, facilitating the further endoluminal approach. In case even a Rendez-vous procedure would not be successful due to impossible passage of the wire into the duodenum or to insufficient clearance of the CBD, patients should undergo a laparoscopic CBD exploration, or, eventually, laparotomy.

The technique of LC after ERCP and ES does not differ from the classical one, as described in Chapter 16, and should be performed according to the surgeon's preferences [36].

Intraoperative cholangiography after ERCP CBD clearance should be performed only in case of failure of preoperative ERCP, anticipating treatment of persisting choledocholithiasis. Otherwise a standard LC should be performed. Hamy et al. [24] demonstrated that routine intraoperative cholangiography performed in 256 patients after ES and CBD clearance detected no residual stones. There is no clear data reported in the literature that supports technical differences in performing LC after ERCP CBDS clearance, compared to standard LC.

Indications and Results of Two-stage Treatment

Two-stage treatment for CBDS and gallbladder stones, including preoperative ERCP, has been used since the beginning of the laparoscopic era by a vast majority of laparoscopic surgeons. At that time it provided an accurate diagnosis and an advisable simplification of surgery [37], compared to laparoscopic CBD exploration.

If we look at the major experiences published in two-stage treatment (Table 24.2), we observe an overall success rate ranging between 60 and 100% of cases, with an overall average of 85%. Morbidity of preoperative ERCP is similar to standard ERCP not combined with subsequent surgical treatment. LC after ERCP shows a similar rate of complications in almost all series. Global morbidity ranges between 3 and 23%, with an average of 8%. Overall mortality is close to nil. In other words, the procedure can be safely performed with a high level of success.

Two technical points should be underlined. First, the risk of ES may be higher in patients with normal-sized ducts. Thus, in these cases, as evidenced by normal or narrow common duct by ultrasound, it may be preferable to proceed directly to a surgical approach. On the other hand, this is controversial since CBD surgical exploration in these patients is associated with even higher risks than ES. Second, systematic clearance of all stones and fragments from the CBD following ES is recommended in all cases. If this cannot be accomplished at the initial endoscopic session due to ES edema, an early repeat ERCP should be performed to complete clearance. In some series ERCP was repeated up to four times to achieve complete CBD clearance before LC. In cases of failed stone removal by preoperative ERCP, it is clear that the CBDS should be removed at the time of cholecystectomy, either endoscopically, or surgically.

In more recent years several different criticisms have been made about performing ERCP prior to LC for symptomatic gallbladder and suspected CBDS. The first criticism regards the rate of unnecessary ERCP. Several prospective studies yielded rates of ERCP negative for duct stones ranging from 38 to 57% [38, 53]. The European Association of Endoscopic Surgeons (EAES) Ductal Stone Cooperative Group reported a rate of 22% [54]. The bottom line of the unnecessary ERCP issue is the selection criteria adopted (see Chapter 12). When the historical predictors are withdrawn, it has been shown that the number of unnecessary ERCPs can be reduced [24]. Although there seems to be consensus that patients with severe biliary pancreatitis, cholangitis, and coexisting major medical diseases should undergo ERCP as a first procedure [55], this is not the case for CBD dilatation in the absence of other risk factors. In this situation, the multivariate analysis-based likelihood of having ductal stones has been shown to be 35% [56]. All patients with symptomatic gallstones and duct dilatation as the only indicator of duct stones could undergo MRCP prior to ERCP

Table 24.2 Results of preoperative ERCP/ES and LC in patients with CBDS and cholelithiasis – literature review

Author	Year of publication	No. of patients	ERCP Success (%)	LC Success (%)	Global Success (%)	Global Morbidity (%)	Global Morbidity (%)	Additional procedure (%)
Rieger [38]	1995	76	96	100	96	6	0	0
Materia [39]	1996	26	85	100	85	14	0	8
Zaninotto [40]	1996	44	84	89	75	n.a.	n.a.	n.a.
Bonatsos [17]	1996	54	96	96	96	3.5	0	0
Valvano [41]	1997	46	86	100	86	14	0	1
Suc [42]	1998	97	69	69	69	13.1	3	28
Solana de Lope [43]	1998	34	100	100	100	7	0	0
Cuschieri [44]	1999	133	62	62	62	12.8	1.5	12.8
Hoyuela [45]	1999	124	93	93	86	6	0	6
Meyer [46]	1999	117	82	100	82	15	0.5	0
Franciosi [47]	2000	93	98	100	98	14	0	2
Coppola [21]	2001	120	97	92	89	4.5	0	0.8
Sgourakis [48]	2002	42	64	64	64	14.3	2.4	11.9
Nardi [49]	2002	41	97	95	93	16	0	0
Sarli [50]	2003	283	89	92	81	4.5	0	n.a.
Hamy [24]	2003	268	95	100	95	3.7	0	0
Rabago [51]	2006	64	97	98	95	23	0	0
Morino [52]	2006	45	80	100	80	8.8	0	0

[57], a technique that has gained more sensitivity during the last years. Endoscopic ultrasound (EUS) has also been proposed for preoperative diagnosis. In most reports, the sensitivity of EUS ranged from 88 to 97% with a specificity of 96–100% [58]. Despite its overall high accuracy, the role of EUS in the diagnosis of CBDS has not been firmly established since EUS is relatively invasive compared to other imaging modalities and does not permit therapeutic intervention.

The second criticism regards failure rates of ERCPs. These rates depend on the definition of attempt, the selection of the patients, and, mainly, the expertise of the operator [59]. Overall failure rates (including both failure at cannulation, ES and CBD clearance) of up to 10% were reported in the late 1980s and mid-1990s. A 20% rate was reported by the EAES Ductal Stone Cooperative Group [54]. However, these data are not representative of community practice. Still, preoperative failure of CBD clearance does not expose the patient to anything more that an intraoperative attempt with a Rendez-vous technique or a laparoscopic CBD exploration, depending on the surgeon's preference and experience.

The third criticism regards ERCP and ES complication rates, which are extremely dependent on the operator experience and range between 0.8–6% with a death rate of up to 0.1% being reported [60]. ES complications have been stratified for importance and risk in the consensus reached by Cotton [61], but vary from 5 to 10% depending on definitions, patient selection, and expertise. Long-term follow-up data showed that late ES complications may occur in 6–24% of patients [27].

The last criticism regards hospital stay and the cost of ERCP prior to LC. The EAES Ductal Stone Cooperative Group trial [54] found a slightly longer stay after ERCP prior to LC compared with that after LC and CBD exploration (9.5 versus 6.5 days). In similar studies, depending on definitions, patient selection, whether or not patients were hospitalized between procedures, and whether or not patients undergoing open surgery were included, hospital stay was reported to be at least 5 days [21, 38, 53].

Nevertheless, data found in the literature regarding selective use of preoperative ERCP and totally laparoscopic treatment are definitely contradictory, with authors on both sides tending to minimize the disadvantages associated with the approach that they prefer. This was recently confirmed by a large meta-analysis study [62], based on 12 randomised trials comparing the two approaches. Despite cholecystectomy being a common operation and with choledocholithiasis complicating up to 10% of cases of symptomatic cholelithiasis, all the trials included were relatively small, introducing a potential bias risk. According to the study, ERCP or surgical common duct exploration were equivalent treatments in terms of duct clearance, mortality and overall morbidity.

It is important to note that although the laparoscopic technique appears to be equivalent to ERCP and may be more cost effective, it has not been widely accepted by the surgical community [63]. A survey of general surgeons practising in the United States showed that although 30 (44%) of 68 confirmed they could perform laparoscopic CBD exploration, only 15 (22%) actually did so routinely. To justify this behaviour, surgeons mostly complained that the procedure was time consuming and that they sometimes lacked specific equipment.

Therefore it seems reasonable to adapt the approach of choledocholithiasis according to local expertise and conditions. In those institutions where access to ERCP is difficult, the preferred approach should be surgery. Where pressure on operating room time is great or the waiting list for cholecystectomy is long, the preferred approach should be simple cholecystectomy after endoscopic clearance.

In an attempt to strike a balance between the two sides and interpret the data coming from different institutions, the Society of Gastrointestinal Endoscopic Surgeons (SAGES) has published guidelines for the treatment of biliary stones (Table 24.3). The SAGES guidelines suggest that the two most important factors to be considered when choosing a treatment modality are the local availability of specific equipment and, more importantly, local expertise. More recently, the combination in a single operation of ERCP and LC has offered a new, more effective, and less invasive treatment modality [46, 52, 65].

Table 24.3 Society of Gastrointestinal Endoscopic Surgeons (SAGES) guidelines for the treatment of biliary stones

1. Clinical suspicion of choledocholithiasis mandates a strategy for assuring short- and long-term biliary tract patency. Diagnosis and management of choledocholithiasis depends on the availability of local resources and consultants.

2. Although endoscopic retrograde cholangiography (ERC) should not be performed in all patients with cholelithiasis, suspicion of common bile duct (CBD) stones may prompt preoperative ERC. If choledocholithiasis is proven, endoscopic extraction is indicated, usually by sphincterotomy. After ERC and sphincterotomy, interval laparoscopic cholecystectomy should usually be performed. Failure to remove CBD stones endoscopically requires surgical removal either by open or laparoscopic CBD exploration (CBDE).

3. In cases where the CBD status is not definitively addressed prior to laparoscopic cholecystectomy and intraoperative cholangiogram or ultrasound confirms choledocholithiasis, options available to the surgeon include, but are not limited to:
   - open CBDE;
   - laparoscopic CBDE via the cystic duct or a choledochotomy;
   - intraoperative ERC/sphincterotomy;
   - postoperative ERC/sphincterotomy;
   - observation (only for very small CBD stones);
   - cystic duct drainage (allows drainage and access to the duct);
   - biliary duct stents;
   - biliary bypass or sphincterotomy.

4. The optimal approach to CBD stones found at laparoscopic operation depends upon the relative skills of the surgeon and the endoscopic experience and resources available.

5. Laparoscopic CBDE is a complex biliary procedure that requires a well-trained operating room team and additional facilities and equipment beyond those required for laparoscopic cholecystectomy. Specialized equipment, including guidewires, balloon catheters, flexible endoscopes and appropriate accessories, is essential.

6. Successful laparoscopic CBDE depends on surgeon experience, hepatic and biliary anatomy, cystic duct size, stone characteristics and CBD diameter. In general, CBD stones less than 8 mm in diameter are amenable to trans-cystic extraction, whereas choledochotomy is required for larger stones. Performance of a choledochotomy requires the surgeon to be adept in laparoscopic suturing techniques.

7. Indications and relative contraindications for laparoscopic CBDE are comparable to those for open CBDE.

References

1. Hermann RE (1989) The spectrum of biliary stone disease. Am J Surg 158:171-173
2. Cotton PB, Geenen JE, Sherman S et al (1998) Endoscopic sphincterotomy for stones by experts is safe, even in younger patients with normal ducts. Ann Surg 227:201-204
3. No authors listed (1991) A prospective analysis of 1518 laparoscopic cholecystectomies. The Southern Surgeons Club. N Engl J Med 324:1073-1078. Erratum in: N Engl J Med 325:1517-1518
4. Baird DR, Wilson JP, Mason EM et al (1992) An early review of 800 laparoscopic cholecystectomies at a university-affiliated community teaching hospital. Am Surg 58:206-210
5. Larson GM, Vitale GC, Casey J et al (1992) Multipractice analysis of laparoscopic cholecystectomy in 1,983 patients. Am J Surg 163:221-226
6. Arregui ME, Davis CJ, Arkush AM, Nagan RF (1992) Laparoscopic cholecystectomy combined with endoscopic sphincterotomy and stone extraction or laparoscopic choledochoscopy and electrohydraulic lithotripsy for management of cholelithiasis with choledocholithiasis. Surg Endosc 6:10-15
7. Frazee RC, Roberts J, Symmonds R et al (1993) Combined laparoscopic and endoscopic management of cholelithiasis and choledocholithiasis. Am J Surg 166:702-705; discussion 705-706
8. Graham SM, Flowers JL, Scott TR et al (1993) Laparoscopic cholecystectomy and common bile duct stones. The utility of planned perioperative endoscopic retrograde cholangiography and sphincterotomy: experience with 63 patients. Ann Surg 218:61-67
9. Leitman IM, Fisher ML, McKinley MJ et al (1993) The evaluation and management of known or suspected stones of the common bile duct in the era of minimal access surgery. Surg Gynecol Obstet 176:527-533
10. Barkun AN, Barkun JS, Fried GM et al (1994) Useful predictors of bile duct stones in patients undergoing laparoscopic cholecystectomy. McGill Gallstone Treatment Group. Ann Surg 220:32-39
11. Meyer C, de Manzini N, Rohr S et al (1994) Treatment of lithiasis of the common bile duct by endoscopic sphincterotomy and laparoscopic cholecystectomy. Ann Chir 48:31-36
12. Salky BA (1994) Laparoscopic management of common bile duct stones. Surg Endosc 8:1161-1162
13. Voyles CR, Sanders DL, Hogan R (1994) Common bile duct evaluation in the era of laparoscopic cholecystectomy. 1050 cases later. Ann Surg 219:744-750; discussion 750-752
14. Rieger R, Sulzbacher H, Woisetschläger R et al (1994) Selective use of ERCP in patients undergoing laparoscopic cholecystectomy. World J Surg 18:900-904; discussion 904-905
15. Rijna H, Borgstein PJ, Meuwissen SG et al (1995) Selective preoperative endoscopic retrograde cholangiopancreatography in laparoscopic biliary surgery. Br J Surg 82:1130-1133
16. Tanaka M, Sada M, Eguchi T et al (1996) Comparison of routine and selective endoscopic retrograde cholangiography before laparoscopic cholecystectomy. World J Surg 20:267-70; discussion 271
17. Bonatsos G, Leandros E, Polydorou et al (1996) ERCP in association with laparoscopic cholecystectomy. A strategy to minimize the number of unnecessary ERCPs. Surg Endosc 10:37-40
18. Kullman E, Borch K, Lindström E et al (1996) Management of bile duct stones in the era of laparoscopic cholecystectomy: appraisal of routine operative cholangiography and endoscopic treatment. Eur J Surg 162:873-880
19. Masci E, Fanti L, Mariani A et al (1999) Selection criteria for pre-operative endoscopic retrograde cholangiography and endoscopic-laparoscopic treatment of biliary stones. Eur J Gastroenterol Hepatol 11:781-784
20. Bergamaschi R, Tuech JJ, Braconier L et al (1999) Selective endoscopic retrograde cholangiography prior to laparoscopic cholecystectomy for gallstones. Am J Surg 178:46-49
21. Coppola R, Riccioni ME, Ciletti S et al (2001) Selective use of endoscopic retrograde cholangiopancreatography to facilitate laparoscopic cholecystectomy without cholangiography. A review of 1139 consecutive cases. Surg Endosc 15:1213-1216
22. Romano F, Franciosi CM, Caprotti R et al (2002) Preoperative selective endoscopic retrograde cholangiopancreatography and laparoscopic cholecystectomy without cholangiography. Surg Laparosc Endosc Percutan Tech 12:408-411
23. Schreurs WH, Juttmann JR, Stuifbergen WN et al (2002) Management of common bile duct stones: selective endoscopic retrograde cholangiography and endoscopic sphincterotomy: short- and long-term results. Surg Endosc 16:1068-1072
24. Hamy A, Hennekinne S, Pessaux P et al (2003) Endoscopic sphincterotomy prior to laparoscopic cholecystectomy for the treatment of cholelithiasis. Surg Endosc 17:872-875
25. Katz D, Nikfarjam M, Sfakiotaki A, Christophi C (2004) Selective endoscopic cholangiography for the detection of common bile duct stones in patients with cholelithiasis. Endoscopy 36:1045-1049
26. Freeman ML, Nelson DB, Sherman S et al (1996) Complications of endoscopic biliary sphincterotomy. N Engl J Med 335:909-918

27. Wojtun S, Gil J, Gietka W, Gil M (1997) Endoscopic sphincterotomy for choledocholithiasis: a prospective single-center study on the short-term and long-term treatment results in 483 patients. Endoscopy 29:258-265
28. Bergman JJ, van der Mey S, Rauws EA et al (1996) Long-term follow-up after endoscopic sphincterotomy for bile duct stones in patients younger than 60 years of age. Gastrointest Endosc 44:643-649
29. Prat F, Malak NA, Pelletier G et al (1996) Biliary symptoms and complications more than 8 years after endoscopic sphincterotomy for choledocholithiasis. Gastroenterology 110:894-899
30. Saito M, Tsuyuguchi T,Yamaguchi T et al (2000) Long-term outcome of endoscopic papillotomy for choledocholithiasis with cholecystolithiasis. Gastrointest Endosc 51:540-545
31. Lau JY, Leow CK, Fung TM et al (2006) Cholecystectomy or gallbladder in situ after endoscopic sphincterotomy and bile duct stone removal in Chinese patients. Gastroenterology 130:96-103
32. Boerma D, Rauws EA,Keulemans YC et al (2002) Wait-and-see policy or laparoscopic cholecystectomy after endoscopic sphincterotomy for bileduct stones: a randomised trial. Lancet 360:761-765
33. Shaw MJ, Mackie RD, Moore JP et al (1993) Results of a multicenter trial using a mechanical lithotripter for the treatment of large common bile duct stones. Am J Gastroenterol 88:730-733
34. Pring CM, Skelding-Millar L, Goodall RJ (2005) Expectant treatment of cholecystectomy after endoscopic retrograde cholangiopancreatography for choledocholithiasis in patients over 80 years old? Surg Endosc 19:357-360
35. Collins C, Maguire D, Ireland A et al (2004) A prospective study of common bile duct calculi in patients undergoing laparoscopic cholecystectomy: natural history of choledocholithiasis revisited. Ann Surg 239:28-33
36. Cuschieri A, Dubois F, Mouiel J et al (1991) The European experience with laparoscopic cholecystectomy. Am J Surg 161:385-387
37. Tham TC, Lichtenstein DR, Vandervoort J et al (1998) Role of endoscopic retrograde cholangiopancreatography for suspected choledocholithiasis in patients undergoing laparoscopic cholecystectomy. Gastrointest Endosc 47:50-56
38. Rieger R,Wayand W (1995) Yield of prospective, noninvasive evaluation of the common bile duct combined with selective ERCP/sphincterotomy in 1390 consecutive laparoscopic cholecystectomy patients. Gastrointest Endosc 42:6-12
39. Materia A, Pizzuto G, Silecchia G et al (1996) Sequential endoscopic-laparoscopic treatment of cholecystocholedocholithiasis. Surg Laparosc Endosc 6:273-277
40. Zaninotto G, Costantini M, Rossi M et al (1996) Sequential intraluminal endoscopic and laparoscopic treatment for bile duct stones associated with gallstones. Surg Endosc 10:644-648
41. Valvano L, Tassetti V, Vix M et al (1997) Sequential treatment of lithiasis of the common bile duct. Ann Ital Chir 68:315-319; discussion 319-320
42. Suc B, Escat J, Cherqui D et al (1998) Surgery vs endoscopy as primary treatment in symptomatic patients with suspected common bile duct stones: a multicenter randomized trial. French Associations for Surgical Research. Arch Surg 133:702-708
43. Solana de Lope J, Aguilera E et al (1998) Endoscopic retrograde cholangiopancreatography prior to laparoscopic cholecystectomy in patients with suspected choledocholithiasis. Rev Gastroenterol Mex 63:77-81
44. Cuschieri A, Lezoche E, Morino M et al (1999) EAES multicenter prospective randomized trial comparing two-stage vs single-stage management of patients with gallstone disease and ductal calculi. Surg Endosc 13:952-957
45. Hoyuela C, Cugat E, Bretcha P et al (1999) Must ERCP Be routinely performed if choledocholithiasis is suspected? Dig Surg 16:411-444
46. Meyer C, Le JV, Rohr S et al (1999) Management of common bile duct stones by laparoscopic cholecystectomy and endoscopic sphincterotomy: pre, per- or postoperative sphincterotomy? Dig Surg 16:26-31
47. Franciosi C, Caprotti R, De Fina S et al (2000) Sequential endo-laparoscopic treatment in patients with common bile calculi. Minerva Chir ;55:665-671
48. Sgourakis G, Karaliotas K (2002) Laparoscopic common bile duct exploration and cholecystectomy versus endoscopic stone extraction and laparoscopic cholecystectomy for choledocholithiasis. A prospective randomized study. Minerva Chir 57:467-474
49. Nardi M Jr, Perri SG, Pietrangeli F et al (2002) "Sequential" treatment: is it the best alternative in cholecysto-choledochal lithiasis? Chir Ital 54:785-798
50. Sarli L, Iusco DR, Roncoroni L (2003) Preoperative endoscopic sphincterotomy and laparoscopic cholecystectomy for the management of cholecystocholedocholithiasis: 10-year experience. World J Surg 27:180-186
51. Rábago LR, Vicente C, Soler F (2006) Two-stage treatment with preoperative endoscopic retrograde cholangiopancreatography (ERCP) compared with single-stage treatment with intraoperative ERCP for patients with symptomatic cholelithiasis with possible choledocholithiasis. Endoscopy 8:779-786
52. Morino M, Baracchi F, Miglietta C et al (2006) Pre-

operative endoscopic sphincterotomy versus laparoendoscopic Rendez-vous in patients with gallbladder and bile duct stones. Ann Surg 244:889-896; discussion 893-896
53. Widdison AL, Longstaff AJ, Armstrong CP (1994) Combined laparoscopic and endoscopic treatment of gallstones and bile duct stones. Br J Surg 81:595-597
54. Cuschieri A, Croce E, Faggioni A et al (1996) EAES ductal stone study. Preliminary finding of multi-center prospective randomized trial comparing two-stage versus single-stage management. Surg Endosc 10:1130-1135
55. Cuschieri A (1996) Of stones and bile ducts: single versus two-stage management. Surg Endosc 10:1124
56. Alponat A, Kum CK, Rajnakova A et al (1997) Predictive factors for synchronous common bile duct stones in patients with choledocholithiasis. Surg Endosc 11:928-982
57. Soto JA, Barish MA, Yucel EK et al (1996) Magnetic resonance cholangiography: comparison with endoscopic retrograde cholangiopancreatography. Gastroenterology 110:589-597
58. Buscarini E, Tansini P, Vallisa D et al (2003) EUS for suspected choledocholithiasis: Do benefits outweigh costs? A prospective, controlled study. Gastrointest Endosc 57:510
59. Cotton PB, Lehman G, Vennes J et al (1991) Endoscopic sphincterotomy, complications and their management. An attempt at consensus. Gastrointest Endosc 37:383-393
60. Reiertsen O, Skjoto J, Jacobsen CD, Rosseland AR (1987) Complications of fibroptic gastrointestinal endoscopic. Five years experience in a central hospital. Endoscopy 19:1-6
61. Cotton PB (1993) Endoscopic retrograde cholangiopancreatography and laparoscopic cholecystectomy. Am J Surg 165:474-478
62. Clayton ESJ, Connor S, Alexakis N and Leandros E (2006) Meta-analysis of endoscopy and surgery versus surgery alone for common bile duct stones with the gallbladder in situ. Br J Surg 93:1185-1191
63. Poulose BK, Arbogast PG, Holzman MD (2006) National analysis of in-hospital resource utilization in choledocholithiasis management using propensity scores. Surg Endosc 20:186-190
64. Basso N, Pizzuto G, Surgo D et al (1999) Laparoscopic cholecystectomy and intraoperative endoscopic sphincterotomy in the treatment of cholecysto- choledocholithiasis. Gastrointest Endosc 50:532-535
65. Meyer C, Le JV, Rohr S et al (1999) Management of common bile duct stones in a single operation combining laparoscopic cholecystectomy and perioperative endoscopic sphincterotomy. Surg Endosc 13:874-877

Chapter 25

Synchronous Treatment of Common Bile Duct Stones by Laparoscopy

Alessandro M. Paganini, Adriana Rotundo, Emanuele Lezoche

Introduction

Single-stage laparoscopic treatment of gallstones and common bile duct (CBD) stones in elective patients is an alternative treatment option to two-stage endo-laparoscopic treatment and to open choledocholithotomy with cholecystectomy [1]. In some centers it has been performed for more than 10 years and several reports have demonstrated its feasibility, safety, efficacy and cost-effectiveness [2–7].

Laparoscopic CBD exploration in the course of laparoscopic cholecystectomy (LC) was introduced to overcome some of the problems related to the two-stage approach, such as the need for preoperative screening of ductal stones, which is burdened by a high rate of negative and therefore useless examinations, a longer hospital stay and higher costs, as well as by the morbidity/mortality of endoscopic sphincterotomy (ES). In a clinical trial set up by the European Association for Endoscopic Surgery (EAES), the single-stage laparoscopic approach proved to be superior to the two-stage approach [5]. This finding was confirmed by a systematic literature review comparing laparoscopic exploration with ES [8] and by a meta-analysis published by the Cochrane Collaboration comparing surgical versus endoscopic treatment of bile duct stones [9].

Surgical Technique

There is no single uniform approach to treat CBD stones. Treatment should be tailored to the individual patient's condition according to information from intraoperative cholangiography (IOC), to the technology available in the operating room and to the surgeon's experience.

Patient preparation includes antibiotic prophylaxis to reduce contamination from intraperitoneal spillage of bile and stones, and prophylaxis for deep vein thrombosis (DVT) because the reverse Trendelenburg position and pneumoperitoneum lead to venous pooling in the lower limbs. DVT prophylaxis includes anti-embolic stockings, pneumatic compression devices and postoperative low molecular weight heparins. Intraoperatively, a naso-gastric tube is positioned and is removed before the end of anesthesia. The use of a Foley catheter may be required in complex cases and, if employed, it is also removed before the patient is awakened.

The surgical instruments for CBDS clearance, beyond those that are usually employed for a standard LC, include:

- Olsen cholangiogram clamp (5 mm) with 4 Fr ureteral catheter;
- choledocoscope, 2.7 mm or 3.5 mm in external diameter;
- second camera, light source and cable

- mixer for "picture in picture" on a single monitor or a second monitor;
- irrigation system for choledochoscopy;
- needle holder;
- four-wire Dormia baskets;
- T-tube (3 or 4 mm in external diameter);
- PDS II 4-0 suture (PDS II; Ethicon, Johnson & Johnson Intl., Brussels, Belgium);
- ureteral balloon dilator;
- lithotriptor (electrohydraulic lithotriptor or pulsed-dye laser);
- irrigation catheters.

The procedure begins with the patient placed on the operating table under general anesthesia in the supine position and with the right arm abducted on an arm holder. The surgeon stands on the left side of the patient with the first assistant standing on the right side of the patient and the assistant holding the camera standing to the left of the surgeon.

The cart containing the laparoscopic instruments (insufflator, camera, light source, monitor, and video recorder) is positioned to the right of the patient at the level of the patient's right shoulder. The second light source and camera, together with the mixer connected to both cameras and TV monitor, are placed on the same cart.

Trocar Position

LC is initiated after establishing pneumoperitoneum in the supra-umbilical site with open or closed technique, according to the surgeon's preference and to the presence of scars from previous abdominal operations. Trocar position is most important for the success of cholangiography and it should be the same for both LC and laparoscopic CBD exploration because any single LC may become a CBD exploration if routine IOC is performed. In our experience, 47% of CBD stones were unsuspected and were discovered at routine IOC. The first 10 mm trocar (trocar A) is placed in the supraumbilical position to accommodate the 30-degree or 45-degree telescope with the 3CCD camera (Fig. 25.1). Before inserting the other trocars the surgeon explores the abdominal cavity to check for the absence of any complication from the Veress needle insertion, if this was used. Three more trocars are then positioned under direct vision with the table tilted in the reverse Trendelenburg position and to the left (right side up). The second 10 mm trocar (trocar B) is introduced two fingerbreadths left of the midline in the epigastrium (Fig. 25.1) so the instruments introduced from the epigastric trocar and those introduced from the midclavicular trocar meet at an angle of approximately 90-degrees. This angle with respect to the choledochal axis makes suture of the CBD easier. The third trocar (trocar C) (5 mm) is inserted into the right hypochondrium on the midclavicular line perpendicular

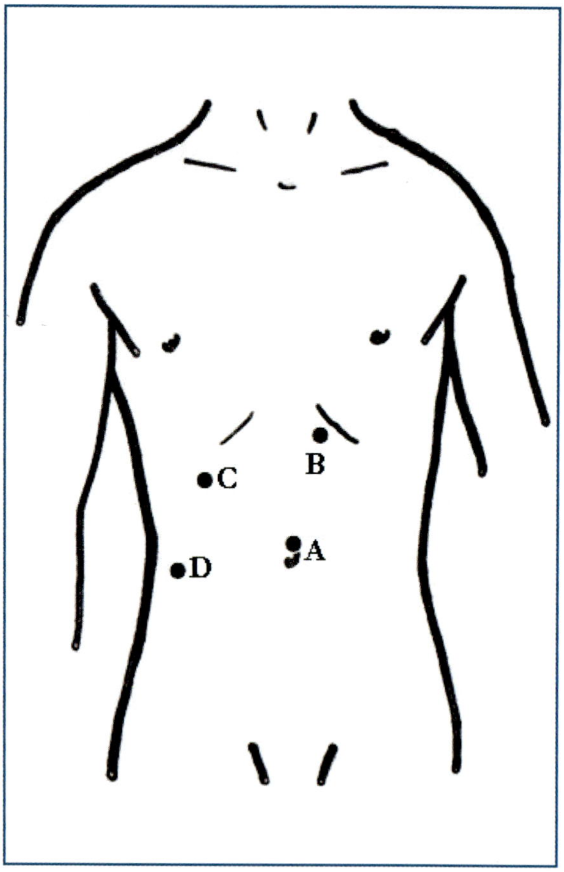

Fig. 25.1 Trocar position

to the cystic duct–CBD junction (Fig. 25.1), in order to obtain the most convenient *vis a tergo* (push) and therefore to facilitate progression of the cholangiogram and Dormia catheters through the cystic duct. The fourth trocar (trocar D) (5 mm) is placed in the right flank region along the right anterior axillary line (Fig. 25.1) and the instrument introduced through this trocar will apply cephalic traction on the gallbladder fundus to expose the cystic duct and to eliminate redundancy on the gallbladder body. Care is taken to avoid tenting the cystic duct, which may place the CBD at risk of injury. Any existing adhesions between the gallbladder and omentum are divided. A second grasper entering the abdomen from the right midclavicular trocar grasps the gallbladder infundibulum and displaces it laterally to the right, thereby opening up Calot's triangle, and providing countertraction for the dissector entering from the epigastric port. Blunt division of the serosal layer covering the body of the gallbladder near its reflection on the liver parenchyma is performed, beginning on the anterior-left side of the gallbladder and dissecting this from the liver bed. Dissection is then continued at the same level of the gallbladder body on its posterior-right side after displacing the infundibulum towards the left side of the patient ("flag" movement of the infundibulum), creating a window behind the gallbladder body, which is dissected off the liver bed. Blunt dissection of the body of the gallbladder from its liver bed proceeds alternatively on its anterior-left and posterior-right sides in an antegrade direction towards the cystic duct, until a "critical view of safety", as described by Strasberg et al. [10] is obtained. Electrocautery and other energy sources should not be used at all, to avoid causing any thermal damage to the extrahepatic bile ducts or to their blood supply. No structure is divided before the cystic duct and artery are conclusively identified [10].

Blunt dissection is continued down the cystic duct to its junction with the common hepatic duct and the CBD, unless this is very low and intrapancreatic or if the cystic duct spirals around the CBD and joins it on its medial side. This preparation, which is essentially aimed at freeing the cystic duct from fat, fibrous and areolar tissue, will facilitate the subsequent maneuvers of cystic duct cannulation because it allows the cystic duct to be straightened up along the same axis of the instruments (cholangiogram clamp and catheter, choledochoscope, baskets), which will be introduced into the abdomen from the mid-clavicular port. Alignment of the cystic duct along the same axis as the instruments entering from the right mid-clavicular trocar will facilitate cystic duct cannulation. After conclusive identification of the cystic duct and artery, a titanium clip is applied on the cystic duct close to the infundibulum of the gallbladder and three clips are applied on the cystic artery close to the gallbladder. A short cystic duct anterior incision is then performed with scissors entering from the right mid-clavicular trocar.

IOC provides essential information on the anatomy of the cystic duct and the CBD (direction and dilatation of the cystic duct, dilatation of the CBD) as well as about the number, size, and location of the ductal stones. The decision between trans-cystic duct CBD exploration (TC-CBDE) and choledochotomy is usually taken on the basis of this information, so it is important that the IOC is performed correctly.

The type of cholangiogram catheter that is commonly used is a 4 French ureteral catheter (Laboratoires Pharmaceutiques, Rüsch France, 67660 Betschdorf, France), passed through the Olsen cholangiogram clamp (Karl Storz GmbH & Co. KG, Tuttlingen, Germany). The catheter is introduced through the cholangiogram clamp inside the cystic duct opening and it is gently pushed to negotiate continent Heister valves until the side hole of the catheter is inside the cystic duct, upon which the prongs of the clamp are closed onto the cystic duct. The C-arm of the fluorocholangiographer (GE Medical Systems S.A., Buc Cedex, France) is then positioned over the patient and dynamic fluorocholangiography is obtained by injecting a solution of contrast medium (Bracco S.p.A., Milan, Italy) and sterile normal saline (concentration of the solution approximately 125 mg of iodine/ml) into the ductal system. A higher concentration of the contrast solution may mask smaller stones. The following five radiologic details are examined in every case:

1. absence of CBD injuries;
2. both intra- and extrahepatic bile ducts must be visualized, checking that the clips placed on the cystic artery are not too close to the common hepatic duct;
3. presence of biliary anomalies suggested by opacification of an aberrant duct or, in very rare cases, of the gallbladder;
4. presence of ductal images suggestive of ductal stones;
5. regular passage of dye through the papilla and into the duodenum.

When ductal images suggestive of ductal stones are identified on IOC they must be distinguished from artifacts, particularly from air bubbles, although a correct technique should avoid the presence of air bubbles. This is accomplished considering: 1) the size (air bubbles are usually small); 2) the shape (air bubbles are usually round); and 3) the fact that air bubbles are very sensitive to the flow of contrast medium and to the movements of the plunger of the syringe.

Once the surgeon is reasonably confident that the ductal filling defects are not air bubbles, the following details are considered:

1. number, size, and location of the stones;
2. presence of extrahepatic bile duct dilatation, including dilatation of the cystic duct;
3. anatomy of the cystic duct–CBD junction.

Based on these elements the surgeon should be able to decide whether a trans-cystic duct approach is feasible or if a choledochotomy is required.

Trans-cystic Duct CBD Exploration

Trans-cystic duct CBD exploration was developed initially to treat unsuspected ductal stones found at routine IOC [2]. It is preferable to a choledochotomy because it is less invasive, therefore it should be the first option to be considered in every case. The indications are the following:

1. small size CBD stones (< 8 mm);
2. no more than 5–6 CBD stones, in order not to prolong the operative time;
3. no stones in the common hepatic duct;
4. favorable cystic duct–CBD junction: i.e., the cystic duct joins the common hepatic duct on its right lateral or right posterior-lateral aspect.

When these conditions are present, the manual dexterity that is required is essentially the same that is required for IOC; it is therefore readily accomplished. The procedure is performed through the mid-clavicular port (trocar C) after repositioning the right lateral grasper to hold the infundibulum rather than the fundus of the gallbladder. Cannulation of the cystic duct is facilitated by the fact that the cystic duct is frequently patent and dilated because of the increased pressure inside the biliary tree, if CBD stones are present. If a non-dilated cystic duct is present, however, this can be dilated up to a diameter of 6 mm with a balloon ureteral dilator catheter (W. Cook Europe APS, Bjaeverskov, Denmark).

For a safe technique, a choledochoscope (Karl Storz GmbH, Tuttlingen, Germany) is used to perform CBD exploration. No guidewire is used. The choledochoscope is introduced inside a 5 mm cannula from the mid-clavicular port. The use of a cannula prevents the scope from being damaged by the trocar valve and it helps to prevent kinking of the shaft while the tip is being introduced through the cystic duct incision. After initiating high-pressure saline irrigation through its working channel, the scope is introduced through the cystic duct incision into the CBD and is guided down the CBD to visualize the ductal stones. It is important:

1. to keep the flexible part of the instrument that is outside the abdomen straight, so that the rotation movements of the handle will be transmitted to the tip of the scope;
2. to maintain constant flow of sterile saline through the choledochoscope for adequate ductal distention;
3. to keep the tip of the instrument at the center of the ductal lumen by rotating the handle of the instrument with the left hand and by applying torsion movements on the flexible part of the scope with the right hand. These movements must be gentle to avoid rupture of the fragile instruments' fibers.

To avoid dislodging any stone from the CBD into the common hepatic duct due to the effect of irrigation, it is recommended to exert a mild extrinsic pressure on the common hepatic duct with a blunt instrument introduced through the epigastric trocar. After the CBD stone has been visualized, a 3 Fr flat wire basket (W. Cook Europe APS) is passed through the working channel of the scope. When the tip of the basket is seen exiting the distal tip of the scope, it is guided down below the level of the stone and it is opened under vision. The opened basket is then pulled slightly backwards until the stone is seen passing inside the wires of the basket. This is then closed to hold the stone in place and the scope with the basket and stone is then withdrawn though the cystic duct incision into the peritoneal cavity, where it is subsequently collected with 10 mm spoon forceps.

Some authors suggest that the CBD be explored under fluoroscopic control with a basket, using choledochoscopy only to check for complete clearance of the CBD (completion choledochoscopy). As more experience is gained with TC-CBDE, this maneuver may even be performed without radiologic control to reduce X-ray exposure ("blind basketing"). However, the advantage of using the choledochoscope is to confirm that the images seen on the cholangiogram are in fact stones, therefore avoiding unnecessary basketing of the CBD, and it makes the procedure safer because every step is performed under direct vision.

Lithotripsy

Sometimes a stone may be impacted at the level of the papilla and it may not be possible to mobilize it with a basket. In these cases, having an alternative energy source for lithotripsy, such as the electrohydraulic (Circon Acmi, Stamford, CT; Karl Storz GmbH & Co. KG, Tuttlingen, Germany) or the Alexandrite pulsed-dye laser lithotriptor (Medecom, Tettnang, Switzerland) is very useful in order to break the stone. The lithotripsy probe is passed through the working channel of the choledochoscope. The electrohydraulic lithotriptor, which is less expensive and more efficient, is also more dangerous than the pulsed-dye laser lithotriptor because the electric spark that is generated at its tip may injure the ductal wall if the instrument is activated with the tip in contact with the wall. For this reason, the instrument should always be activated under vision. The Alexandrite pulsed-dye laser, on the other hand, is safer because the emitted light does not damage the CBD wall, but it is somewhat slower in obtaining stone fragmentation and it is also more expensive. When several stone fragments are present after lithotripsy, the papilla may be gently dilated using the same balloon ureteral dilator catheter used to dilate the cystic duct at the beginning of CBD exploration (W. Cook Europe APS). The CBD is then flushed with saline, thus allowing stone fragments to be more easily washed out of the CBD and into the duodenum.

After all the stones that were identified on the cholangiogram have been retrieved, completion trans-cystic choledochoscopy and IOC are performed to check for complete clearance and for its documentation.

Biliary Drainage after Trans-cystic Exploration

On completion of the procedure, the decision to place trans-cystic duct biliary drainage is taken according to the following indications, as previously described [3]:

1. presence of fibrin debris adherent to the inside walls of the CBD, which may subsequently obstruct the papilla, possibly causing postoperative biliary colics and/or cholangitis;
2. whether any instrumental maneuver on the papilla has been performed, such as trans-papillary passage of a basket or papillary balloon dilation, which may be followed by postoperative edema of the papilla, increasing the risk of postoperative cholangitis;
3. presence of any retained CBD stone, demonstrated on completion of IOC, which is impossible to remove. In this case biliary drainage provides access for postoperative percutaneous trans-cystic duct stone removal (Burhenne technique) and it may also aid in performing postoperative ES, should the postoperative percutaneous approach fail.

The type of biliary drainage that is used is soft rubber one (Willy Ruesch AG, Kerner, Germany) obtained after trimming away the transverse branches of a T-tube and cutting a small extra side-hole near the distal tip of the drainage. The diameter is usually 3 mm if the tube is positioned only for biliary drainage or 4 mm if a residual stone is present. After introducing the biliary drainage completely inside the peritoneal cavity through the epigastric port, its tapered end with side hole is introduced through the cystic duct opening and it is advanced 1.5–2 cm inside the CBD. The biliary drainage is then secured in place with a 4-0 transfixing absorbable suture on a straight needle (PDS II mounted on ST-4 black needle; code number Z620E, Ethicon™, Johnson & Johnson Intl., Edinburgh, Scotland, UK), according to a previously published original technique [11]. The suture is passed through both the cystic duct wall and the biliary drainage, then looped on both sides around the cystic duct before knotting it, to prevent subsequent bile leakage. When trans-cystic duct biliary drainage is not deemed necessary, the cystic duct is closed with a medium-large absorbable clip (Absolok APS 300, Ethicon GmbH, Norderstedt, Germany). If the cystic duct wall is thickened by inflammation and the absorbable clip is not large enough to close it, the cystic duct must be closed with a 4-0 transfixing absorbable suture on a straight needle (PDS II mounted on a ST-4 black needle, code number Z620E, Ethicon™, Johnson & Johnson Intl., Edinburgh, Scotland, UK). The procedure continues with retrograde laparoscopic cholecystectomy and the positioning of subhepatic drainage, which exits the abdomen from the right lateral incision. The biliary drainage, on the other hand, exits the abdomen through the right mid-clavicular incision, taking care to avoid kinking of the biliary drainage. After checking for trocar site bleeding, the peritoneum and fascia of the 10 mm epigastric and periumbelical trocars are closed with an absorbable suture.

Laparoscopic Choledochotomy

This technique was developed to treat large and multiple ductal stones not amenable to TC-CBD removal [11]. It is more challenging than the trans-cystic duct approach because it requires laparoscopic suturing expertise, but the ductal exploration maneuver itself is somewhat easier. A prerequisite for a safe choledochotomy is the presence of a dilated CBD (> 8 mm in diameter).

The indications for a choledochotomy are the following:

1. the presence of multiple CBD stones (> 6);
2. larger ductal stones (> 8 mm);
3. stones in the common hepatic duct, proximal to the cystic duct–CBD junction;
4. medial junction of cystic duct with CBD (unfavorable for TC-CBDE);
5. failure of trans-cystic duct approach because of tight Heister valves or of cystic duct rupture during the exploration maneuvers.

When trans-cystic duct exploration is not feasible because of the presence of any of the above conditions, a direct CBD exploration is performed by means of a transverse choledochotomy.

The advantages of a transverse versus a longitudinal choledochotomy are that a transverse choledochotomy prevents the surgeon from extending the incision, because it is limited by the diameter of the CBD. A short and transverse choledochotomy incision interrupts less ductal arterioles and its suture results in less ischemia than the suture of a long and longitudinal choledochotomy. These tiny vessels follow a transverse course on the anterior and posterior ductal wall [11] and they are terminal arterioles of the two major arteries originating from the hepatic and pancreaticoduodenal arteries, supplying the extrahepatic ducts and running along their medial and lateral aspects. Their course on the anterior aspect of the major bile duct is readily visible due to the magnifying effect of laparoscopy and the choledochotomy incision should be carried out with attention paid in order to not interrupt them. This greater respect for the CBD vasculature provides the theoretical basis for the absence of any ischemic stricture at long-term follow-up after laparoscopic transverse choledochotomy, as reported in prior publications [12, 14].

After dividing the serosa covering the major bile duct, it is exposed both above and below the junction with the cystic duct. The major bile duct is then opened up transversely on its anterior surface with scissors entering the abdomen from the epigastric port. Due to the above-mentioned considerations, bleeding from the choledochotomy incision is usually very limited. Occasionally it may be required to stop the bleeding from one tiny vessel. This is done by electrocautery, decreasing the power of the energy source to avoid extensive electrocoagulation.

After choledochotomy is completed, the maneuvers for direct CBD exploration follow the same steps as described for the trans-cystic duct approach. Larger baskets (W. Cook Europe APS) can also be used in parallel with the choledochoscope and saline irrigation facilitates the escape of stone fragments through the choledochotomy incision and into the peritoneal cavity.

After ductal exploration is completed, both below and above the level of the choledochotomy incision, the decision of whether or not to place biliary drainage is taken according to the indications mentioned earlier. Briefly, the presence of extensive fibrin clots on the walls of the bile ducts, the presence of residual stones or the performance of exploration maneuvers through the papilla are indications for biliary drainage, in order to prevent postoperative bile stasis and cholangitis. This may be accomplished with trans-cystic duct biliary drainage, according to the technique described above, or with a T-tube.

Biliary Drainage after Choledochotomy

If a T-tube is used, the type of biliary drainage that is preferred again is a soft rubber one (Willy Ruesch AG, Kerner, Germany). The diameter of the T-tube is usually

3 mm, if it is positioned only for biliary drainage, or 4 mm if a residual stone is demonstrated on completion IOC. This may have to be left for postoperative percutaneous management if it cannot be removed at surgery. The transverse branches of the T-tube are cut short and tapered to facilitate their introduction through the choledochotomy. An extra hole is cut on the transverse part of the tube opposite the long branch to facilitate postoperative T-tube extraction.

The T-tube is then introduced entirely inside the peritoneal cavity from the epigastric port, and the transverse branches are placed inside the CBD through the ductal incision. This maneuver may be difficult if the choledochotomy is too short. The transverse choledochotomy is then closed with one continuous suture on one side of the T-tube. Laparoscopic suturing with extracorporeal or intracorporeal knot-tying may be time-consuming, particularly if the surgeon is not experienced. A technique of suture of the choledochus that avoids the use of knots and avoids placing metal clips in contact with the CBD was thus developed and published [13]. The suture is a PDS 4-0 (Ethicon Inc. Somerville, NJ, USA) on a straight atraumatic needle. The thread carries a LAPRA-TY® absorbable suture clip of violet Poly-P-Dioxanone (Johnson & Johnson Gateway, LLC 2000-2007), placed 7 cm from the needle, and stopped by a knot. After two or three stitches have been applied to approximate the edges of the choledochotomy, the suture is completed and requires a second knot. At this point, a second LAPRA-TY® absorbable suture clip is placed on the suture, which is kept under tension by the needle-holder.

After the suture is completed, the suture line is tested with a T-tube cholangiogram to exclude leakage. Should leakage occur, the continuous suture may be tightened by pulling at one end and applying one more absorbable clip on the suture.

If T-tube drainage is not used, the incision is closed with a single continuous suture and the completion cholangiogram is done through the cystic duct. Laparoscopic cholecystectomy is completed in the usual manner, and a drain is placed in the subhepatic space.

Postoperative Evaluation and Follow-up

Patients who have undergone laparoscopic CBD exploration without biliary drainage are dismissed on the first or second postoperative day. When a trans-cystic biliary drainage is present the patient undergoes direct cholangiography through the biliary drainage on the second postoperative day. If this is negative for bile leakage and for residual stones, the biliary drainage is closed, placed under a wound dressing and the patient is dismissed after subhepatic drainage removal on third or fourth postoperative day.

In the occasional patient with a residual CBD stone or stone fragment demonstrated at postoperative direct cholangiography, the biliary drainage is used to flush the CBD with saline, to aid in clearance of the residual stone. If there is free flow of contrast medium through the papilla the patient is discharged with the biliary drainage closed and placed under a wound dressing. Four weeks after the operation, a direct cholangiogram through the biliary drainage is repeated. If this is negative for residual stones, the biliary drainage is removed in the radiology suite immediately after cholangiography as a day-hospital procedure.

The 4 week interval is required for the development of a mature sinus tract around the biliary drain. If a residual stone is identified at control cholangiography, the presence of a mature sinus tract allows the surgeon to access the CBD percutaneously through the biliary drainage sinus tract, in the radiology suite under fluoroscopic vision and local anesthesia, using the 2.7 mm choledochoscope (Burhenne technique). Under fluoroscopy, a soft-tipped guidewire is introduced through the biliary drainage into the CBD and through the papilla into the duodenum. The biliary drainage is then removed leaving the guidewire in place. Next, the guidewire is introduced into the working channel of the choledochoscope and this is advanced through the sinus tract into the CBD. The guidewire is then removed, saline irrigation is initiated and the CBD is explored with a 3 Fr basket to grasp the residual stone under choledochoscopic vision. The electrohydraulic lithotriptor should be available at this time to deal with any residual stone that is difficult to remove with a basket and that can be fragmented by lithotripsy. When the percutaneous approach fails, or in patients with suspected residual stones in the absence of a biliary drain, endoscopic retrograde cholangiopancreatography (ERCP) and ES are employed. Very rarely, a residual stone may be impacted inside a pre-papillary pseudodiverticulum preventing success with any of the above techniques. In this case, with a very difficult CBD stone, extracorporeal shockwave lithotripsy may be a useful adjunct to fragment the stone.

Conclusion

Single-stage laparoscopic treatment of gallstones and CBD stones has proven to be feasible and safe. The short and long-term results of laparoscopic trans-cystic duct and of direct CBD exploration in large series of consecutive, unselected patients have been published [14, 15]. It allows extensive preoperative screening of ductal stones to be avoided, reducing the diagnostic and therapeutic burden for the patient. In the era of open cholecystectomy, open bile duct exploration was superior to ERCP/ES in achieving CBD stone clearance, as reported by the Cochrane Collaboration review [9]. In the laparoscopic era, the available evidence demonstrates no significant benefit to ERCP clearance of CBD stones, which requires an increased number of procedures per patient [9], with increased hospital stay and increased costs.

References

1. Berci G, Morgenstern L (1994) Laparoscopic management of common bile duct stones. A multi-institutional SAGES study. Society of American Gastrointestinal Endoscopic Surgeons. Surg Endosc 8:1168-1174; discussion 1174-1175
2. Phillips EH, Rosenthal RJ, Carroll BJ, Fallas MJ (1994) Laparoscopic trans-cystic-duct common bile duct exploration. Surg Endosc 8:1389-1394
3. Lezoche E, Paganini AM (1995) Single-stage laparoscopic treatment of gallstones and common bile duct stones in 120 unselected, consecutive patients. Surg Endosc 9:1070-1075
4. Rhodes M, Sussman L, Cohen L, Lewis MP (1998) Randomised trial of laparoscopic exploration of common bile duct versus postoperative endoscopic retrograde cholangiography for common bile duct stones. Lancet 351:159-161
5. Cuschieri A, Lezoche E, Morino M et al (1999) E.A.E.S. multicenter prospective randomized trial comparing two-stage vs single-stage management of patients with gallstone disease and ductal calculi. Surg Endosc 13:952-957
6. Millat B, Borie F, Fingerhut A (2000) Prospective trials in laparoscopic bile duct exploration. Semin Laparosc Surg 7:279-287
7. Urbach DR, Khajanchee YS, Jobe BA et al (2001) Cost-effective management of common bile duct stones: a decision analysis of the use of endoscopic retrograde cholangiopancreatography (ERCP), intraoperative cholangiography, and laparoscopic bile duct exploration. Surg Endosc 15:4-13
8. Tranter SE, Thompson MH (2002) Comparison of endoscopic sphincterotomy and laparoscopic exploration of the common bile duct. Br J Surg 89:1495-1504
9. Martin DJ, Vernon DR, Toouli J (2006) Surgical versus endoscopic treatment of bile duct stones. Cochrane Database Syst Rev 2:CD003327
10. Strasberg SM, Eagon CJ, Drebin JA (2000) The "hidden cystic duct" syndrome and the infundibular technique of laparoscopic cholecystectomy –

the danger of the false infundibulum. J Am Coll Surg 191:661-667
11. Lezoche E, Paganini AM, Carlei F (1996) Laparoscopic treatment of gallbladder and common bile duct stones: a prospective study. World J Surg 20:535-541; discussion 542
12. Paganini AM, Lezoche E (1998) Follow-up of 161 unselected consecutive patients treated laparoscopically for common bile duct stones. Surg Endosc 12:23-29
13. Lezoche E, Paganini A, Feliciotti F, Chan R (1993) Laparoscopic suture technique after common bile duct exploration. Surg Laparosc Endosc 3:209-212
14. Paganini AM, Guerrieri M, Sarnari J et al (2005) Long-term results after laparoscopic transverse choledochotomy for common bile duct stones. Surg Endosc 19:705-709
15. Paganini AM, Guerrieri M, Sarnari J et al (2007) Thirteen years' experience with laparoscopic transcystic common bile duct exploration for stones. Effectiveness and long-term results. Surg Endosc 21:34-40

Chapter 26

Rendez-vous Technique

Giuseppe Borzellino, Edoardo Saladino, Francesco Lombardo, Claudio Cordiano

Definition

The so-called Rendez-vous technique refers to a combined surgical, either laparoscopic or open, endoscopic approach to common bile duct stone treatment. The term Rendez-vous (a French word meaning appointment) was adopted when the surgeon and the endoscopist met one other at the level of the duodenum, the former by the way of a trans-cystic guidewire and the latter with his lateral view endoscope for biliary procedures, as originally ideated by radiologists through percutaneous trans-hepatic access.

Historical Evolution of Common Bile Duct Stone Treatment

The first successful exploration of the common bile duct was performed by Thornton in 1889, followed shortly by the work of Courvoisier and Kehr, who were the first to insert a T-tube into the main bile duct [1]. The first intra-operative cholangiography was reported in 1931 by Mirizzi and a common bile duct exploration with a rigid choledocoscope by McIver in 1941 [2, 3]. Endoscopic cannulation of the papilla for diagnostic purposes was reported in 1968 [4] and for treatment of common bile duct stones some years later [5]. After the introduction of laparoscopic cholecystectomy, with the aim of avoiding conversion for retrieved common bile duct stones due to the early limited experience, the two stage approach was generally used. However, with increasing laparoscopic experience and with pre-operative diagnostic uncertainty of common bile duct stones resulting in unnecessary pre-operative or hazardous post-operative endoscopic retrograde cholangiopancreatography (ERCP), minimally invasive one-stage treatment of cholecysto-choledocal stones has been investigated.

Overview of One-Stage Treatment of Common Bile Duct Stones

Minimally invasive one-stage treatment of common bile duct stones includes different options. The less invasive option is the trans-cystic approach, although this is strongly conditioned by the cystic duct diameter and by stone diameter that needs to be removed through the cystic duct. In a recent series of 505 patients approached by laparoscopy, the trans-cystic approach was attempted in only 50% of cases with a 75% success rate [6].

The second approach is trans-choledocal, by way of a laparoscopic choledocotomy with primary closure or T-tube closure of the main bile duct. Although this procedure has been favorably compared with the trans-papillary approach as reported in a review [7], and confirmed in a more recent randomized study [8], it is still technically demanding and has some limitations in relation to main bile duct diameters and a potential risk of post-operative bile leakage and late stenosis [9].

The third option that has been reported is an intra-operative endoscopic sphincterotomy [8, 10, 11]. This trans-papillary approach may be more difficult due to the supine position of the patients and may increase the risk of complications since difficult cannulation, injection of contrast into the pancreatic duct and pre-cut sphincterotomy have been found to correlate with post-ERCP pancreatitis [12, 13].

With the Rendez-vous technique, cannulation of the papilla under the guidance of a wire may allow these complications to be avoided even when patients are in the supine position.

Rendez-vous Technique

Two different Rendez-vous techniques have been described: we report our own technique that was performed on 90 patients from 2001 to 2006.

Specific Materials

A 150 cm double channel balloon catheter of 6 French diameter and a 450 cm Teflon-coated guidewire of 0.035 in. are used. Introduction of the guidewire through one channel of the catheter makes handling much easier, while cholangiography or flushing with saline solution may be performed whenever necessary through the other one channel. Moreover, the balloon allows the catheter to be anchored without trauma on the common bile duct and it avoids the rising of insufflated air from the duodenal endoscopy into the peritoneum through a patent cystic duct.

Surgical Technique

A four trocar technique is used as for a traditional laparoscopic cholecystectomy. After dissection of Calot's triangle and section of the cystic artery, a small incision is performed in the upper part of the cystic duct just under the gallbladder neck. A 5 French catheter is introduced for intra-operative cholangiography. If positive for common bile duct stones, the endoscopic team is invited to prepare their instrumentation for the biliary endoscopy. Awaiting endoscopy arrangement, the surgeon introduces the double lumen balloon catheter with tips positioned via the cystic duct at the level of the middle to distal part of the common bile duct under radioscopic guidance. The balloon is filled with 2 ml of air to make it more visible under radioscopy. This position facilitates guidewire passage through the papilla after it has been introduced through the dedicated channel of the catheter and allows it to run beyond the duct stones (Fig 26.1).

At this stage, the endoscopist reaches the duodenum with his lateral view endoscope and catches the flexible extremity of the guidewire with a polypectomy snare (Fig. 26.2), and with combined cautious maneuvers assisted by the surgeon he pulls the guidewire out of the mouth of the patient. A traditional sphincterotome is

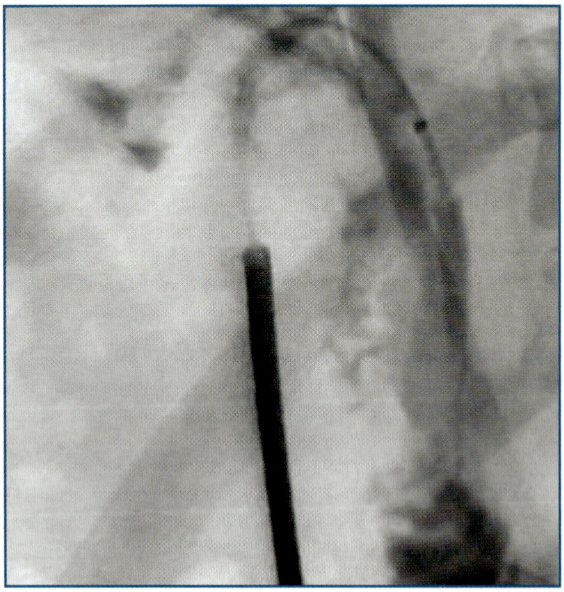

Fig. 26.1 Guidewire pulled through the papilla under radioscopic guidance

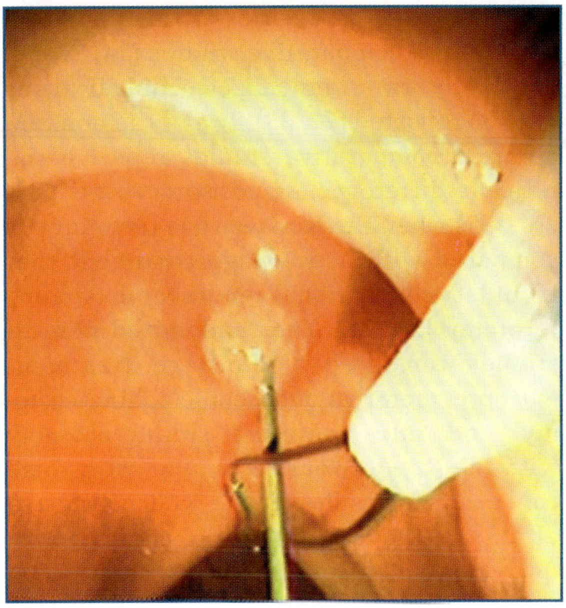

Fig. 26.2 Guidewire caught by endoscopy with a polypectomy snare

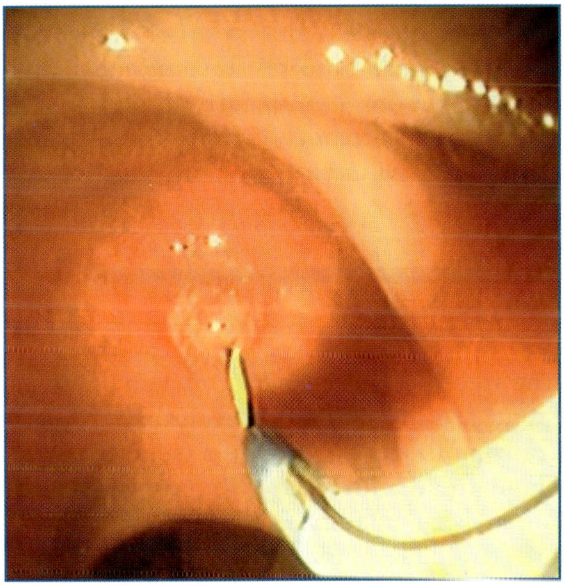

Fig. 26.3 Cannulation of the papilla with the sphincterotome under wire guidance

introduced along the guidewire, a gentle traction from the surgical field allows the papilla to be cannulated easily and sphincterotomy is performed (Figs. 26.3 and 26.4).

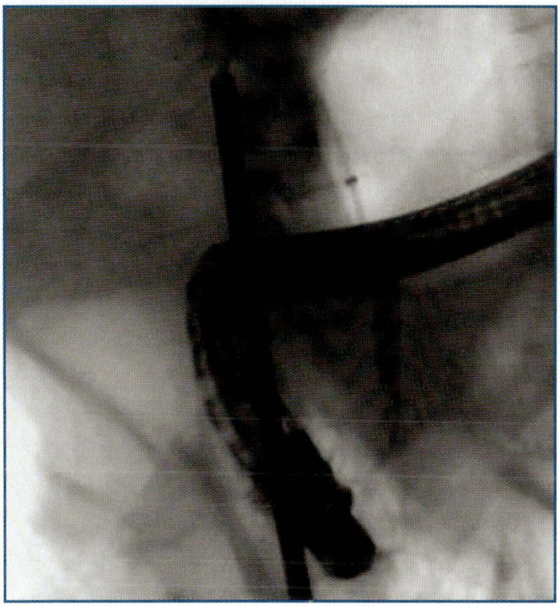

Fig. 26.4 Radioscopic control of papilla cannulation

Further maneuvers for common bile duct clearance are also performed under the guidance of the wire, a similar balloon catheter to that used for cystic cannulation is inserted through the papilla for stone extraction (Figs. 26.5, 26.6) as well as a Dormia basket, when necessary. A cholangiographic control by contrast injection may be performed through the second lumen of the trans-cystic or trans-papillary catheter when required. At the end of the procedure, a naso-biliary catheter is positioned under the guidance of the wire after it has been withdrawn into the main bile duct and the cystic stump has been clipped by the surgeon. After aspiration of insufflated air in the stomach, cholecystectomy is carried out in the usual manner.

While some minor variations of the technique have been described, a substantially different technique has been reported by Cavina [14]. In his technique, the Rendez-vous is performed by way of a Dormia basket inserted through the cystic duct into the duodenum in order to grasp the endoscopically-placed guidewire.

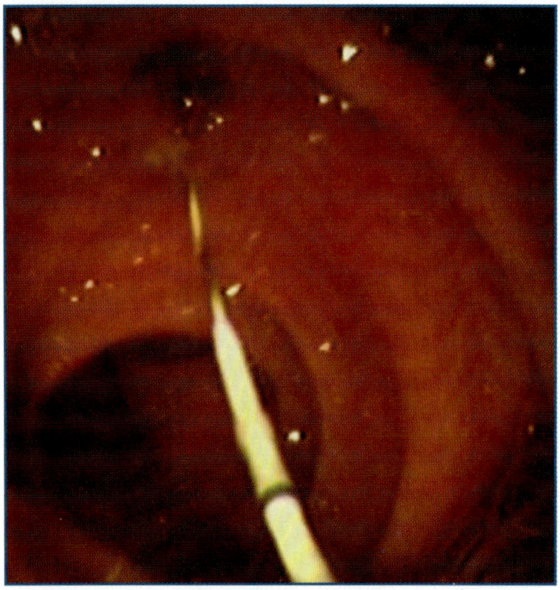

Fig. 26.5 Balloon catheter inserted in the common bile duct under wire guidance

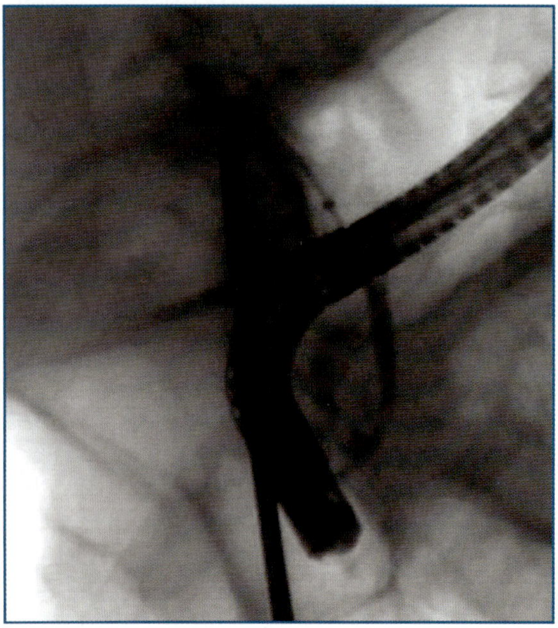

Fig. 26.6 Radioscopic control during stone extraction with a balloon catheter

Surgical Outcomes of the Rendez-vous Technique

Several studies have reported results of the Rendez-vous technique; the literature reveals mainly case series [15, 16] and non randomized comparative studies [14, 17–21] with only two randomized clinical trials (RCTs) reported [22, 23]. Two of the non randomized comparative studies report a significant difference in post-procedure pancreatitis when the Rendez-vous technique is compared with a two-stage treatment that includes conventional endoscopic sphincterotomy [20, 21]. The randomized clinical studies compared a two-stage treatment with pre-operative endoscopic sphincterotomy, and intra-operative sphincterotomy with the Rendez-vous technique, with some controversial results. In the RCT of Rabago et al. [22] the success rate of common bile duct clearance was not different between the two approaches, while Morino et al. [23] showed a significant difference favoring the Rendez-vous approach (80 vs. 95.6%; p = 0.06). Post-ERCP pancreatitis was higher in the two-stage treatment (12.7 vs. 1.7%; p = 0.03) in one RCT [22], while such a difference was not seen in the other RCT [23]. However, mean hospital stay and mean hospital cost were significantly higher in the two-stage treatment than in the Rendez-vous approach in both studies.

Conclusion

The treatment options for common bile duct stone are in continuous evolution. When a transpapillary approach is selected, one stage treatment with a Rendez-vous technique is mandatory in those patients who are candidates for surgery. Laparoscopic choledocotomy has been proposed but may suffer from some limitations. Moreover, this approach may be questionable in the setting of acute cholecystitis since the inflammatory process involving the hepatico-duodenal ligament and the gallbladder may increase the risk of bile leakage.

In our experience, among 90 patients treated for a common bile duct stones with a Rendez-vous technique, 38 suffered an acute cholecystitis. This approach was also adopted for the treatment of common bile duct stones in 17 patients in the early stages of an acute biliary pancreatitis, four of whom also had cholecystitis. The treatment of common bile duct stones with the Rendez-vous technique has been performed without major procedure-related complications in all our cases of acute cholecystitis and acute biliary pancreatitis (unpublished data).

References

1. Cervantes J (2000) Common bile duct stones revisited after the first operation 110 years ago. World J Surg 24:1278-1281
2. Mirizzi PL (1937) Operative cholangiography. Surg Gynecol Obstet 65:702
3. McIver MA (1941) An instrument for visualizing the interior of the common duct at operation. Surgery 9:112-114
4. McCune WS, Shorb PE, Moscovitz H (1968) Endoscopic cannulation of the ampulla of vater: a preliminary report. Ann Surg 167:752-756
5. Classen M, Demling L (1974) Endoskopische sphikterotomie der papilla vateri und steinextraktion aus dem ductus choledocus. Dtsch Med Wochenschr 99:496
6. Berthou JC, Dron B, Charbonneau P et al (2007) Evaluation of laparoscopic treatment of common bile duct stones in a prospective series of 505 patients: indications and results. Surg Endosc 21:1970–1974
7. Tranter SE, Thompson MH (2002) Comparison of endoscopic sphincterotomy and laparoscopic exploration of the common bile duct. Br J Surg 89:1495-1504
8. Hong DF, Xin Y, Chen DW (2006) Comparison of laparoscopic cholecystectomy combined with intraoperative endoscopic sphincterotomy and laparoscopic exploration of the common bile duct for cholecystocholedocholithiasis. Surg Endosc 20:424-427
9. Moore KB, Adrales GL, Mastrangelo MJ Jr (2004) Laparoscopic common bile duct exploration. Curr Surg 61:294-296
10. Wei Q, Wang JG, Li LB, Li JD (2003) Management of choledocholithiasis: comparison between laparoscopic common bile duct exploration and intraoperative endoscopic sphincterotomy. World J Gastroenterol 9:2856-2858
11. Wright BE, Freeman ML, Cumming JK et al (2002) Current management of common bile duct stones: is there a role for laparoscopic cholecystectomy and intraoperative endoscopic retrograde cholangiopancreatography as a single-stage procedure? Surgery 132:729-735
12. Freeman ML, DiSario JA, Nelson DB et al (2001) Risk factors for post-ERCP pancreatitis: a prospective, multicenter study. Gastrointest Endosc 54:425-434
13. Masci E, Mariani A, Curioni S, Testoni PA (2003) Risk factors for pancreatitis following endoscopic retrograde cholangiopancreatography: a meta-analysis. Endoscopi 35:830-834
14. Cavina E, Franceschi M, Sidoti F et al (1998) Laparo-endoscopic "Rendez-vous": a new technique in the choledocholithiasis treatment. Hepatogastroenterology 45:1430-1435
15. Tricarico A, Cione G, Sozio M et al (2002) Endolaparoscopic Rendez-vous treatment: a satisfying therapeutic choice for cholecystocholedocolithiasis. Surg Endosc 16:585-588
16. Iodice G, Giardiello C, Francica G et al (2001) Single-step treatment of gallbladder and bile duct stones: a combined endoscopic-laparoscopic technique. Gastrointest Endosc 53:336-338
17. Filauro M, Comes P, De Conca V et al (2000) Combined laparoendoscopic approach for biliary lithiasis treatment. Hepatogastroenterology 47:922-926
18. Saccomani G, Durante V, Magnolia MR et al (2005) Combined endoscopic treatment for cholelithiasis associated with choledocholithiasis. Surg Endosc 19:910-914
19. Enochsson L, Lindberg B, Swahn F, Arnelo U (2004) Intraoperative endoscopic retrograde cholangiopancreatography (ERCP) to remove common bile duct stones during routine laparoscopic cholecystectomy does not prolong hospitalization: a 2-year experience. Surg Endosc 18:367-371
20. Lella F, Bagnolo F, Rebuffat C et al (2006) Use of the laparoscopic endoscopic approach, the so-called "Rendez-vous" technique, in cholecystocholedocholithiasis: a valid method in cases with patient-related risk factors for post-ERCP pancreatitis. Surg Endosc 20:419-423
21. La Greca G, Barbagallo F, Di Blasi M et al (2007) Rendez-vous technique versus endoscopic retrograde cholangiopancreatography to treat bile duct stones reduces endoscopic time and pancreatic damage. J Laparoendosc Adv Surg Tech A 17:167-171
22. Rabago LR, Vicente C, Soler F et al (2006) Two-stage treatment with preoperative endoscopic

retrograde cholangiopancreatography (ERCP) compared with single-stage treatment with intraoperative ERCP for patients with symptomatic cholelithiasis with possible choledocholithiasis. Endoscopy 38:779-786

23. Morino M, Baracchi F, Miglietta C et al (2006) Preoperative endoscopic sphincterotomy versus laparoendoscopic Rendez-vous in patients with gallbladder and bile duct stones. Ann Surg. 244:889-893

Chapter 27

Flow Chart for the Treatment of CBDS and Critical Comparison of Techniques

David Martin, Ian Martin

Introduction

The most common techniques for the treatment of common bile duct (CBD) stones have been outlined in detail in the preceding four chapters. In this chapter we evaluate the published evidence for these techniques and provide conclusions with clinical validity for practicing physicians. We have summarised these findings with the use of a flow diagram (Fig. 27.1) for quick reference to help guide evidence- and expertise-based management.

Gallstone disease is the most common gastrointestinal cause for hospital admission in Western countries: surgery for this ailment is one of the most common abdominal procedures performed. Occurring in 15% of the population, asymptomatic gallstones are reported to cause either symptoms or complications in 10–50% of patients within 10–20 years of diagnosis [1, 2]. Large longitudinal studies of patients with symptomatic gallstones show that 58–72% will have ongoing symptoms and complications [3, 4] and as such, patients with symptomatic gallstones are recommended to undergo cholecystectomy to alleviate symptoms and to prevent complications.

Approximately 10–18% of patients undergoing cholecystectomy for gallbladder stones will also have CBD stones [5–7]. These may be suspected pre-operatively by symptoms or signs of jaundice, pancreatitis or cholangitis, by derangement in liver function tests, or on imaging showing duct dilation or actual ductal stones. However, up to 25% of CBD stones are discovered unexpectedly at surgery [1, 5]. The natural history of CBD stones is not known, though complications appear to be more frequent and severe than with asymptomatic gallstones [1], with optimal care required for their detection and removal either before, during, or after planned cholecystectomy.

Treatment Options for Common Bile Duct Stones

Treatment options for CBD stones include pre- or post-operative endoscopic retrograde cholangiopancreatography (ERCP) or open or laparoscopic surgery. These techniques have been widely reported in numerous large cohort series, compared in several randomised controlled trials (RCTs) and critically analysed in a contemporary Cochrane Review meta-analysis [1]. More recent cohorts and several RCTs have also published outcomes for a hybrid or "Rendezvous" technique, as outlined in Chapter 26, which utilises laparoscopic guidewire cannulation of the CBD to facilitate intra-operative ERCP.

Below we have summarised the outcomes and internal and external validity of comparisons of techniques evaluated in relevant RCTs. This is followed by a brief summary of the efficacy and safety of the individual techniques as gained from the individual arms of these trials and from large cohort

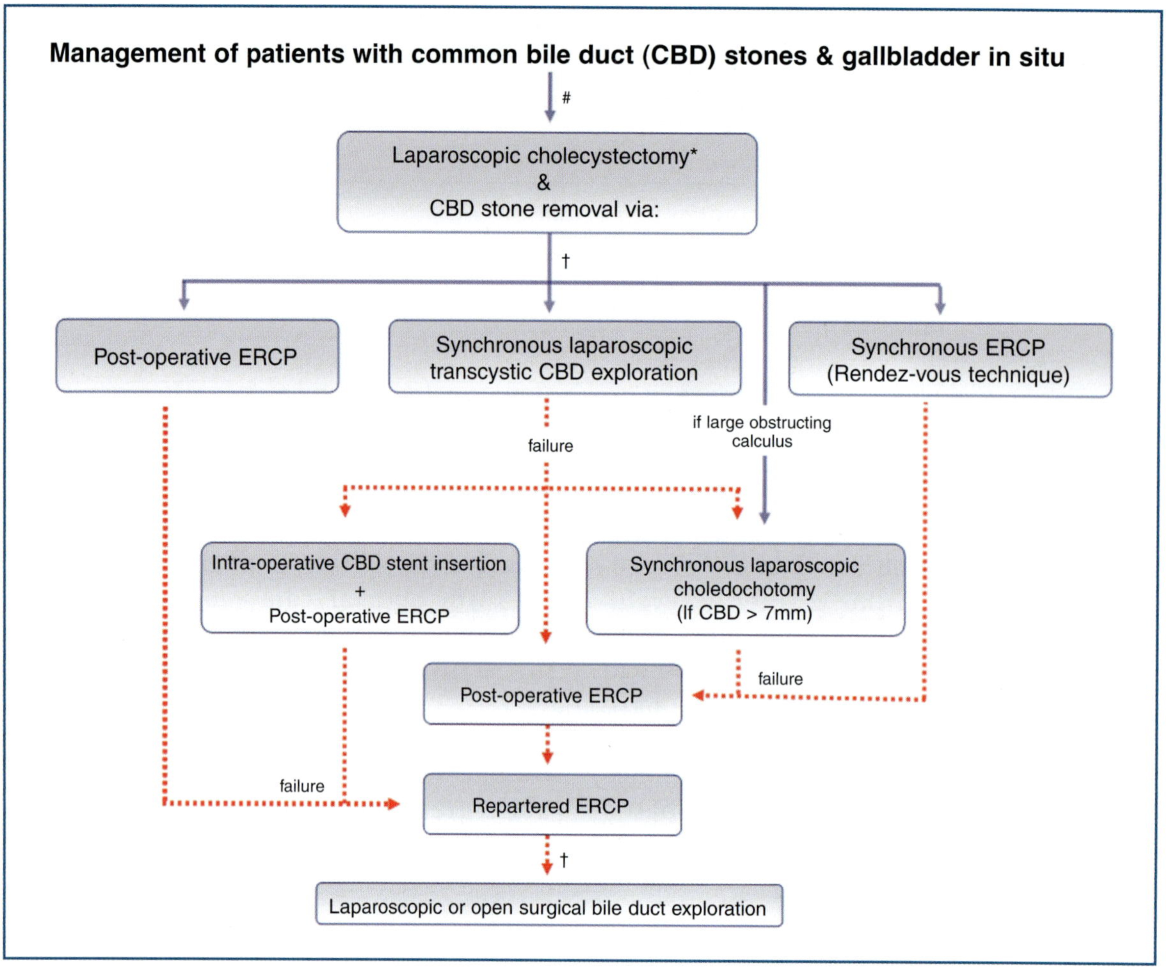

Fig. 27.1 Management of patients with common bile duct (CBD) stones and gallbladder in situ. Patients with established cholangitis, frail and high risk patients, and those with persistent jaundice and ambiguous diagnosis should proceed directly to ERCP (#). Confirmation or diagnosis of CBD calculi during laparoscopic cholecystectomy is typically made with an on-table cholangiogram (*). Choice between therapeutic techniques is often dependent upon local experience – see text for comparison of techniques and caveats (†)

studies. It is hoped that this will provide a reference not only for decision-making between therapeutic options, but also for the expected outcomes of individual techniques, which can then be used to guide individual patient management.

The following RCTs apply to patients with cholelithiasis and choledocholithiasis. The outcomes do not apply to patients with established cholangitis or severe pancreatitis complicated by biliary obstruction: for these patients ERCP remains the appropriate treatment [8].

Summary of Outcomes of Randomised Controlled Trials

ERCP plus Open Cholecystectomy versus Open Cholecystectomy plus Bile Duct Exploration

Evidence from eight RCTs involving 760 patients showed that open bile duct exploration at the time of open cholecystectomy was more effective (93% efficiency) than pre-operative ERCP (80% efficiency) in clearing bile duct stones, with no difference in morbidity, mortality or hospital stay [1]. No difference resulted from subgroup analysis of morbidity for the three trials in the group that had cholecystectomy performed only selectively in the ERCP arm. Assessment of this evidence found it to be internally valid but dated, with median trial dates for these studies ranging from 1983 to 1992 [1]. While both endoscopic and surgical outcomes have improved, this data would suggest that a surgeon should have no misgivings about proceeding with a surgical bile duct clearance for CBD stones at the time of open cholecystectomy. Surgical training with this technique is, however, rapidly decreasing as completion rates for laparoscopic cholecystectomy approach 100% [9].

Pre-operative ERCP plus Laparoscopic Cholecystectomy (Two-stage) Versus Laparoscopic Cholecystectomy plus Laparoscopic Common Bile Duct Exploration (LCBDE)

Evidence from three trials involving over 400 patients found no difference in primary treatment success (88% for both arms), morbidity or mortality [10–12]. The routine use of pre-operative ERCP entailed an extra procedure resulting in prolonged patient stay and costs in that arm [1]. Arguments that pre-operative ERCP is important to establish diagnosis and knowledge of ERCP-refractory CBD stones prior to surgery are not supported by meta-analysis in terms of procedure numbers, morbidity, mortality, and hospital stay [1]. This is further supported by the small randomised trial that compared pre- versus post-operative ERCP below.

Laparoscopic Cholecystectomy plus Post-operative ERCP (Two-stage) Versus Laparoscopic Cholecystectomy plus LCBDE

Two trials involving 166 patients found no difference in primary clearance success (75% ERCP, 84% LCBDE), morbidity or mortality [13, 14]. Again, the use of ERCP in the endoscopy arm entailed an extra procedure resulting in increased patient hospital stay with respect to the LCBDE arm. Subgroup analysis of our own trial in this group comparing laparoscopic choledochotomy versus post-operative ERCP, randomised at surgery after failed transcystic laparoscopic clearance, found no difference in outcome except again for longer hospital stay in the ERCP arm [1, 13]. Primary duct clearance rate was 95% for the laparoscopic choledochotomy arm.

On-table 'synchronous' ERCP at the time of laparoscopic cholecystectomy (without Rendez-vous type guidewire facilitation) has also been compared to LCBDE in one randomised trial that found equivalence in all outcomes but which was floored by an inadequate randomisation method [15]. A large cohort comparison of these techniques found reduced morbidity and costs favouring LCBDE [16].

Pre-operative ERCP plus Laparoscopic Cholecystectomy (Two-stage) Versus Rendez-vous Technique

Three trials involving a total of 334 patients found reduced hospital stay and costs for the Rendez-vous technique [17–19]. Two of these trials found equivalent efficacy between techniques (96% pre-operative

ERCP, 90% Rendez-vous) but increased morbidity in the two-stage group [17, 18]. The lower morbidity in the intra-operative ERCP (Rendez-vous) arms resulted from lower rates of post-ERCP pancreatitis and cholecystitis. Another trial in this comparison found equal morbidity between arms but reduced clearance in the pre-operative ERCP group (80% ERCP versus 96% Rendez-vous) that was probably due to a less aggressive approach to sphincterotomy in these patients [19].

Pre-operative ERCP plus Laparoscopic Cholecystectomy (Two-stage) Versus Laparoscopic Cholecystectomy plus Post-operative ERCP

A single trial of 60 patients with mild gallstone pancreatitis found selective post-operative ERCP and CBD stone extraction is associated with a shorter hospital stay, less cost, no increase in combined treatment failure rate (10% both arms), and significant reduction in ERCP use compared with routine pre-operative ERCP [20]. This was largely due to an increased number of unnecessary ERCPs in the pre-operative arm (60%) despite relatively high yield indicators including a CBD greater than 8 mm in diameter on ultrasound and persisting elevation of bilirubin and liver enzymes.

Specific Outcomes of Common Techniques

Further to the RCT and meta-analysis above, brief cohort evidence (including arms from the above RCTs) from the best quality and most relevant publications is outlined below. Data are presented as either a consistent result or a range of results from representative trials.

Rendez-vous Technique [17–19, 21]

Primary duct clearance success: 85–100%. Morbidity: 3–10%; Mortality: < 1%. Operative time: 70–120 min. Hospital stay: 4 days.

The Rendez-vous technique requires availability of both laparoscopic and ERCP equipment and the appropriate specialist or specialists able to perform both techniques. An equivalent but two-stage technique with low morbidity that uses laparoscopic insertion of a biliary stent at the time of LC facilitating subsequent post-operative ERCP has also been reported [22]. This latter variant does not require an endoscopist or ERCP to be present during laparoscopic cholecystectomy and could potentially be combined with LCBDE and preserved for patients who fail a relatively quick transcystic basket technique at the time of guidewire placement.

Laparoscopic Common Bile Duct Exploration (LCBDE) [1, 5, 6, 12–16, 23, 24]

Primary duct clearance success: 80–96%. Morbidity: 5–19%. Mortality: < 1%. Operative time: 90–130 min for various combined procedures (105–150 min for choledochotomy subset). Hospital stay: 2 days (6 days for choledochotomy subset).

LCBDE exploration is usually initiated by diagnostic intra-operative cholangiogram or choledochoscopy with subsequent removal of CBD calculi using catheter or choledochoscopy guided baskets. It is our experience that up to 75% of stones can be removed with transcystic techniques with more a technically demanding choledochotomy preserved for larger stones (mean 1.1 mm) that are unable to be removed via the cystic duct [5, 6, 13]. LCBDE in the setting of acute cholecystitis is also a potentially challenging procedure.

ERCP Clearance of Bile Duct Stones [8, 18, 25, 26]

Primary duct clearance success: 80–96%. Morbidity: 5–12% (5–18% for combined laparoscopic cholecystectomy and ERCP). Mortality: < 1%.

ERCP is an effective method for stone removal, is the treatment of choice in patients with previous cholecystectomy and established cholangitis and is an important adjunct to surgical bile duct exploration.

*Open Surgery for Clearance of Bile Duct Stones [27, 28, 29]**

Primary duct clearance: 90–94%. Morbidity: 12–23%. Mortality: 0–3%. Procedure time: 210 min. Hospital stay: 6–22 days

*trials published 1995–1998

Conclusion

For patients with a gallbladder in situ and undergoing cholecystectomy, all contemporary methods of stone removal are efficacious, offering primary duct clearance in 80–95% of patients and a relatively low morbidity of 6–15%. The routine use of either pre- or post-operative ERCP is inferior to LCBDE in terms of hospital stay and costs, while pre-operative ERCP is also inferior on the same counts to post-operative ERCP and Rendez-vous techniques. Somewhat more technically demanding laparoscopic choledochotomy, as a subset of LCBDE, is probably equivalent to post-operative ERCP in terms of efficacy and morbidity and superior in terms of hospital stay, while more recent experience with the Rendez-vous techniques may demonstrate improved safety over aggressive pre-operative ERCP. There appears to be no advantage of on-table non-guidewire facilitated ERCP during laparoscopic cholecystectomy over LCBDE. Thus for most patients, excluding those with severe cholangitis, initial laparoscopic cholecystectomy will form the basis of treatment with employment of appropriate adjuncts such as LCBDE, Rendez-vous techniques or post-operative ERCP as dictated by local experience and pathology. Open CBD exploration, whilst no longer considered first line management, still has a role to play with dated but substantial data supporting the use of this procedure when necessary.

Caveats – Application of Evidence to Minority Cases

There is no RCT evidence for patients with CBD stones who have had a previous cholecystectomy, though the standard treatment is first to employ ERCP with surgical intervention in refractory cases. It is our experience and that of the published literature that given the high success rates of current techniques it is not common for patients to fail repeated ERCP for residual stones after cholecystectomy. The surgeon or referring practitioner should feel reassured by the prevailing evidence that a return to theatre to remove recalcitrant CBD calculi is a rare but possible outcome after evidence based, safe, and cost-effective initial management strategies. There is little more than anecdotal evidence for correct management of such CBD stones, and whilst several options exist, the most pragmatic approach is usually surgical, via either laparoscopic or open means and dependent upon patient status, tissue status and surgical experience.

One criticism of evidence-based medicine is that it is generalised for patient populations rather than addressing the needs of an individual patient. This may be the case for pre-operative ERCP, the routine use of which in RCTs for suspected CBD stones has been shown to be inferior on cost and hospital stay outcomes. This is in part due to patients undergoing unnecessary intervention. Whilst routine use appears difficult to justify, the selective use of pre-operative ERCP still has a role in cases with ambiguous diagnosis and persistent jaundice.

In high risk or frail patients with a gallbladder in situ and symptomatic CBD stones, an ERCP and sphincterotomy alone may be performed with no cholecystectomy undertaken. At 6 years the risk of recurrent biliary symptoms in these patients is approximately 20%, double the 10% for those in whom the gallbladder is removed [30].

For patients with CBD stones with no endoscopic access to the CBD, such as after previous gastrectomy or as seen with growing frequency following bypass procedures for obesity, the options are numerous. Published techniques include laparoscopic and open surgical exploration, percutaneous transhepatic cholangiography, and transgastric laparoscopic-guided ERCP. There is not enough data to provide meaningful comparisons between techniques in this scenario though available surgical, radiological and endoscopic expertise would no doubt affect management. For those with a gallbladder in situ, laparoscopic or open surgery remain key options and would be expected to approach success rates of 90–95%. Indeed, younger surgeons may have more experience with laparoscopic rather than open biliary surgery, with one study reporting success rates of 94% and low morbidity for LCBDE in patients with recurrent stones with a past history of open cholecystectomy [31].

References

1. Martin DJ, Vernon DR, Toouli J (2006) Surgical versus endoscopic treatment of bile duct stones. Cochrane Database Syst Rev Apr 19:2
2. Ko CW, Lee SP (2002) Epidemiology and natural history of common bile duct stones and prediction of disease. Review. Gastrointest Endosc 56:S165-S169
3. Lund J (1960) Surgical indications in cholelithiasis: prophylactic cholecystectomy elucidated on the basis of long-term follow up on 526 nonoperated cases. Ann Surg 151:153-162
4. Wenckert A, Robertson B (1996) The natural course of gallstone disease: eleven-year review of 781 nonoperated cases. Gastroenterology 50:376-381
5. Martin IJ, Bailey IS, Rhodes M et al (1998) Towards T-tube free laparoscopic bile duct exploration: a methodologic evolution during 300 consecutive procedures. Ann Surg 228:29-34
6. Hammett I, Martin IJ, Martin DJ et al (2008) Long term outcomes following laparoscopic bile duct exploration: A consecutive 5 year follow-up of 150 patients. ANZ J Surg (in press)
7. Courvoisier L (1890) Statististische Beitrage zur Pathologie und Chirurgie der Gallenwege [Statistical article on the pathology and surgery of the biliary system]. Leipzig: Vogel 387:57-58
8. Vitale GC (2007) Early management of acute gallstone pancreatitis. Ann Surg 245:18-19
9. Schulman CI, Levi J, Sleeman D et al (2007) Are we training our residents to perform open gall bladder and common bile duct operations? J Surg Res 142:246-249
10. Sgourakis G, Karaliotas K (2002) Laparoscopic common bile duct exploration and cholecystectomy versus endoscopic stone extraction and laparoscopic cholecystectomy for choledocholithiasis. A prospective randomized study. Minerva Chirurgica 57:467-474
11. Lella F, Bagnolo F, Rebuffat C et al (1999) E.A.E.S. multicenter prospective randomized trial comparing two-stage vs single-stage mangement of patients with gallstone disease and ductal calculi. Surg Endosc 13:952-957
12. Rogers S, Cello JP, Horn JK et al (1999) Randomized controlled clinical trial of laparascopic cholecystectomy plus laparoscopic common bile duct exploration (LC+LCBDE) vs ERCP sphincterotomy plus laparascopic cholecystectomy (ERCP/S+LC) for common bile duct stone disease [abstract]. J Gastroenterol Hepato 14(Suppl):S110
13. Nathanson LK, O'Rourke NA, Martin IJ et al (2005). Postoperative ERCP versus laparoscopic choledochotomy for clearance of selected bile duct calculi: a randomized trial. Ann Surg 242:188-192
14. Rhodes M, Sussman L, Cohen et al (1998) Randomised trial of laparoscopic exploration of common bile duct versus postoperative endoscopic retrograde cholangiography for common bile duct stones. Lancet 351:159-161

15. Hong DF, Xin Y, Chen DW (2006) Comparison of laparoscopic cholecystectomy combined with intraoperative endoscopic sphincterotomy and laparoscopic exploration of the common bile duct for cholecystocholedocholithiasis. Surg Endosc 20:424-427
16. Wei Q, Wang JG, Li LB, Li JD (2003) Management of choledo-cholithiasis: comparison between laparoscopic common bile duct exploration and intraoperative endoscopic sphincterotomy. World J Gastroenterol 9:2856-2858
17. Rabago LR, Vicente C, Soler F et al (2006) Two-stage treatment with preoperative endoscopic retrograde cholangiopancreatography (ERCP) compared with single-stage treatment with intraoperative ERCP for patients with symptomatic cholelithiasis with possible choledocholithiasis. Endoscopy 38:779-786
18. Lella F, Bagnolo F, Rebuffat C et al (2006). Use of the laparoscopic-endoscopic approach, the so-called "Rendez-vous" technique, in cholecystocholedocholithiasis: a valid method in cases with patient-related risk factors for post-ERCP pancreatitis. Surg Endosc 20:419-423
19. Morino M, Baracchi F, Miglietta C et al (2006) Preoperative endoscopic sphincterotomy versus laparoendoscopic Rendez-vous in patients with gallbladder and bile duct stones. Ann Surg 244:889-893
20. Chang L, Lo S, Stabile BE et al (2000) Preoperative versus postoperative endoscopic retrograde cholangiopancreatography in mild to moderate gallstone pancreatitis: a prospective randomized trial. Ann Surg 231:82-87
21. Tricarico A, Cione G, Sczio M et al (2002) Endolaparoscopic Rendez-vous treatment: a satisfying therapeutic choice for cholecysterctocholedocholithiasis. Surg Endosc 16:585-588
22. Martin CJ, Cox MR, Vaccaro L (2002) Laparoscopic transcystic bile duct stenting in the management of common bile duct stones. ANZ J Surg 72:258-264
23. Rojas-Ortega S, Arizpe-Bravo D, Marin Lopez ER et al (2003) Transcystic common bile duct exploration in the management of patients with choledocholithiasis. J Gastrointest Surg 7:492-496
24. Topal B, Aerts R, Penninckx F (2007) Laparoscopic common bile duct stone clearance with flexible choledochoscopy. Surg Endosc 21:2317-2321
25. Bergman JG, Rauws EA, Fockens P et al (1997) Randomised trial of endoscopic balloon dilation versus endoscopic sphincterotomy for removal of bile duct stones. Lancet 349:1124-1129
26. Freeman ML, Nelson DB, Sherman S et al (1996) Complications of endoscopic biliary sphincterotomy. N Engl J Med 335:909-918
27. Hammarstrom LE, Holmin T, Stridbeck H et al (1995) Long-term follow-up of a prospective randomized study of endoscopic versus surgical treatment of bile duct calculi in patients with gallbladder in situ. Br J Surg 82:1516-1521
28. Suc B, Escat J, Cherqui et al (1998) Surgery vs endoscopy as primary treatment in symptomatic patients with suspected common bile duct stones: a multicenter randomized trial. French Associations for Surgical Research. Arch Surg 133:702-708
29. Targarona EM, Perez Ayuso RM, Bordas JM et al (1996) Randomised trial of endoscopic sphincterotomy with gall bladder left in situ versus open surgery for common bile duct calculi in high risk patients. Lancet 347:926-929
30. Pereira-Lima JC, Jakobs R, Winter UH et al (1998) Long-term results (7 to 10 years) of endoscopic papillotomy for choledocholithiasis. Multivariate analysis of prognostic factors for the recurrence of biliary symptoms. Gastrointest Endosc 48:457-464
31. Chen B, Hu SY, Wang L et al (2007) Reoperation of biliary tract by laparoscopy: a consecutive series of 26 cases. Acta Chir Belg. 107:292-296

Chapter 28

Common Bile Duct Stones in Cholecystectomized Patients

Carmelo Sciumè, Girolamo Geraci, Franco Pisello, Tiziana Facella, Francesco Li Volsi, Giuseppe Modica

Introduction

The incidence of retained or primary stones is approximately 2–5% after conventional and laparoscopic cholecystectomy (LC) and 5–15% after common bile duct exploration (CBDE) [1]: in principle these patients are in need of further intervention [2–3].

Residual common bile duct stones (CBDS) are called secondary when they originate in the gallbladder and later pass down through the cystic duct into the CBD. On the other hand, they are called primary when the stones originally form in the CBD.

Reported cases of CBDS found in patients with a congenital absence of the gallbladder provide proof of their origin [4]. In the United States, up to 85% of all CBDS are secondary [5].

The identification of primary CBDS by gross morphology at the time of surgery can be difficult. If the gallbladder is still in place, or has only recently been removed, the origin of the stones in the CBD is impossible to prove.

The real incidence of primary CBDS is controversial and varies widely from 4% [6] to 56% [7], according to the different methods of identification or definition (the amount of time since cholecystectomy and CBD size, morphology, color and texture of the stone).

Saharia and coworkers [6–7] classified patients as having primary stones if they met all the following criteria, subsequently revisited by Kim and coworkers [8]:

1. previous cholecystectomy with or without CBDE;
2. at least a 2-year asymptomatic period after the original biliary tract surgery;
3. presence of solitary, ovoid, soft, friable, light brown stones or sludge in the CBD [7];
4. absence of a long cystic duct remnant or biliary stricture due to previous surgery;
5. bile duct diameter of 13 mm or greater at the time of cholecystectomy [8].

Although most cholecystectomized patients with retained or primary CBDS can be managed by nonoperative and nonsurgical techniques, stone retention remains a potentially serious complication that can considerably prolong hospitalization and convalescence. Inappropriate intervention may aggravate the situation and lead to complications.

The increasing popularity of minimally invasive procedures has resulted in an increased demand for endoscopic retrograde cholangiopancreatography (ERCP) for CBDS extraction [9].

Accordingly, it would be reasonable to affirm that the problem of retained stones would be proportionately less after LC. Instead, the true incidence of CBDS and retained stones may actually be higher, as silent stones can be overlooked in centers where operative cholangiography is not routinely performed. The reasons for the apparent lower incidence of retained CBDS are threefold [3]:

1. the incidence of retained CBDS increases with duration of symptoms and patient's age;
2. elderly patients and those who present

with obstructive jaundice, cholangitis and severe acute pancreatitis are now being treated endoscopically;
3. experience in endoscopic extraction has increased due to the relative inexperience in laparoscopic bile duct exploration, even if this technique has not been shown to produce better results than surgical bile duct exploration in the open cholecystectomy era.

After surgical or endoscopic treatment, the long-term recurrence of choledocholithiasis is 2.8–5.2% in secondary and 12.2–21.3% in primary disease [10].

Conceivably, the large dilated duct may represent an abnormal functional dilatation following cholecystectomy, rather than arising secondary to mechanical obstruction by ampullary stenosis or duodenal periampullary diverticula, or being produced by the common duct stasis and the stone itself. This abnormal functional dilatation could then result in stasis and stone formation.

Juxtapapillary duodenal diverticula (JDD) is an important causative factor in the formation of bile duct stones. Duodenal diverticula are usually acquired lesions. The prevalence of JDD in the general population ranges between 10 and 23%; there is a strong association between the frequency of JDD and age. The presence of JDD increases with age, being rare in patients younger than 40 years old [11]. This relationship with advancing age suggests a degenerative process involving local supporting structures as an additional factor in the pathogenesis of JDD. This dynamic process may interfere with biliary drainage and promote lithiasis, either by establishing an unfavorable pressure gradient across the biliary outflow tract or by direct obstruction of flow caused by contraction of the duodenal wall and bile duct sphincter. Bile duct obstruction may also result from bolus impaction of food in the diverticulum with secondary inflammation. In turn this may contribute to stasis in both the biliary and pancreatic ductal systems and thereby promote infection and increase the lithogenicity of bile [12].

Although there are various theories, the exact pathogenesis of primary CBDS remains unclear. A number of factors, including associated sphincter of Oddi dysfunction and mechanical obstruction may be involved. It seems likely, however, that the initial step is bile deconjugation, which results in the precipitation of calcium bilirubinate and formation of pigment stones.

In Asian populations, infestation with *A. lumbricoides* and *C. sinensis* may promote stasis by either blocking the biliary ducts or by damaging the duct walls, resulting in stricture formation. Bactobilia is also common in these instances, probably secondary to episodic portal bacteremia [5].

Clinical Presentation of Retained CBDS

Clinical presentation of retained CBDS can range from being completely asymptomatic (7%) to jaundice with/without pain, biliary colic, pancreatitis, and abnormal cholestatic and liver test function [13].

Approximately 25–50% of asymptomatic CBDS eventually cause symptoms and require treatment. Symptoms occur when the stones obstruct the CBD. The clinical presentation varies depending on the degree and level of obstruction and on the presence or absence of biliary infection [5].

If a stone obstructs the CBD in the absence of infected bile, asymptomatic jaundice, often fluctuating, ensues and in many patients spontaneous complete resolution occurs. Spontaneous resolution of jaundice occurs if a ductal dilation develops, and the stone floats back up the CBD and away from the narrow distal end as edema subsides; it should not be assumed that the CBD is free of stones when jaundice clears. Occasionally, jaundice is relieved, however, because the stone is passed [1].

About 50% of patients present with acute cholangitis: abdominal upper right pain, jaundice, fever ("Charcot triad"), from a few day to many years after cholecystectomy [6].

Diagnostic Tests

Laboratory tests are helpful, but results are nonspecific for the diagnosis of choledocholithiasis. Patients with choledocholithiasis are often asymptomatic, and, in such patients, laboratory test results can be completely normal. White blood cell count elevations indicate the presence of infection or inflammation, but this finding is nonspecific. Alkaline phosphatase and gamma-glutamyl transpeptidase levels are elevated in patients with obstructive choledocholithiasis. These tests have a good predictive value for the presence of CBDS. Serum bilirubin level elevations indicate obstruction of the CBD; the higher the bilirubin level, the greater the predictive value. CBDS are present in approximately 60% of patients with serum bilirubin levels greater than 3 mg/dL. Aminotransferases are elevated in patients with complicated choledocholithiasis. Transabdominal ultrasound (TUS) exhibits only modest test performance at detecting CBDS, with sensitivities in the range of 25 to 58% and specificities of 68–91%, but the sensitivity of TUS in detecting common bile duct dilatation is 96% [13,14].

Besides, an authoritative meta-analysis of 67 published controlled trials shows that magnetic resonance cholangiopancreatography (MRCP) has excellent overall sensitivity (95%) and specificity (97%) for demonstrating the level and the presence of biliary obstruction [15]. However, MRCP is less sensitive for detecting stones (91%) and differentiating malignant from benign obstruction (88%) [16]. Moreover, the sensitivity of MRCP for detecting stones seems to decrease according to stone size: 67–100% for stones greater than 10 mm in size, 89–94% for stones measuring 6–10 mm, and 33–71% for bile duct stones less than 6 mm in size. However, its ability to diagnose small stones in nondilated ducts may be limited [14].

The sensitivity of endoscopic ultrasound (EUS) is 93–100%, the specificity is 95%, the positive predictive value is 91%, the negative predictive value is 100%, and the overall accuracy is 97% [17]. EUS is not particularly invasive and very able to detect small stones in nondilated ducts [18].

In patients with dilated ducts, EUS and MRCP have high diagnostic performance overall, without statistically significant differences between them. In choosing between EUS and MRCP, other factors need to be taken into account, such as resource availability, experience, and cost considerations. [18]

Helical computed tomography cholangiography (hCTC) achieves a sensitivity of 87%, a specificity of 97% and an overall accuracy of 95% for the diagnosis of CBDS [19]. The major advantages of hCTC are its low level of invasiveness, operator independence, and low technical failure rate (1%), as well as provision of a three-dimensional understanding of the biliary tree. The major drawback of hCTC is a risk of adverse reaction to the iodinated contrast agents (1%), while its main limitation is in high-grade obstructions in which cases, partially impaired contrast elimination does not allow a complete visualization of the biliary tree. The artifacts produced by patient's movement or intolerance to apnea might also limit the diagnostic value of this test [14].

Controversy persists in choosing between the different diagnostic managements because of the variety of approaches, the difficulty of comparing all strategies in all-encompassing prospective trials, regional variation in expertise and availability of technologies.

Management

The management strategy for retained CBDS is related to the timing of presentation and the mode of detection [3].

Retained CBDS in the Early Postoperative Period

Patients with a retained CBDS in the immediate or early postoperative period can be classified into two categories: those with a T-tube in place after surgical CBDE, and those without a T-tube.

Patient with a T-tube in Place after Surgical CBDE

In the era of LC, the use of the T-tube has increased the possibility of accessing the CBD without further invasive procedures [1]. With a T-tube in place, there are three possible management options:

1. observation ("wait and see"): in the absence of signs and symptoms of infection, an observation time of 4–6 weeks is necessary; during this period, 10–25% of stones pass spontaneously into the duodenum [20], especially if the stone is less than 10 mm in diameter [1]. If a stone passes spontaneously in the duodenum, no further treatment is required. If, after 4–6 weeks, the stone persists, the choice of treatment is either a radiological or an endoscopic approach.
2. Mechanical extraction: because of a high success rate (95%) and low morbidity (4%) and mortality (no deaths reported), this is an attractive treatment option. When complications occur (sepsis, biliary leakage), they can be treated in a conservative way and only 0.2% of cases require surgery [21]. Alternative techniques include T-tube irrigation with or without pharmacologic relaxation of the sphincter of Oddi with glucagon or nitrates, T-tube infusion of

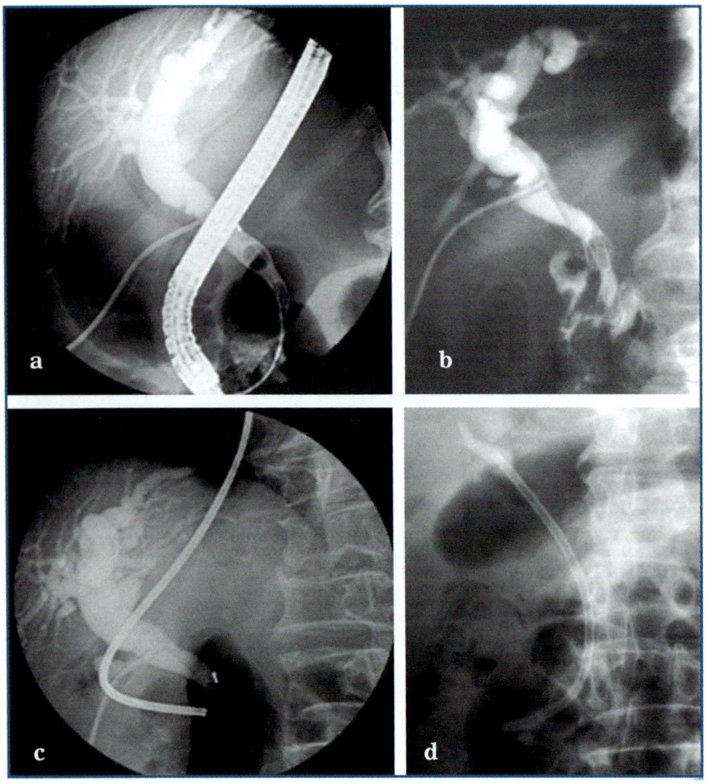

Fig. 28.1 "Difficult residual stone" with T-tube in situ and intradiverticular ampulla: endoscopic removal after Dormia impaction [25]. **a** Stone impaction; **b** broken Dormia in CBD; **c** Dormia extraction; **d** cholangiography after T-tube removal and stent placement

cholesterol solvents [22] (currently obsolete due to toxicity), T-tube tract choledochoscopy and lithotripsy [23], and percutaneous extraction of stones through a mature T-tube sinus tract. The success rate with the latter techniques ranges from 77–96%, but multiple sessions are often required [1].

3. Endoscopic sphincterotomy (ES): ES today is the most effective method for the management of retained stones with the T-tube in situ (if necessary, a guide-wire should pass through the T-tube to penetrate the ampulla) and it should be carried out soon after cholecystectomy (Fig. 28.1), to reduce complications related to the presence of stones and/or the T-tube [24]. Altogether, ES has the advantage that if retained stones are discovered, further treatment may be unnecessary since stones may pass spontaneously. ES may be best employed when the patient is critically ill, or when mechanical extraction has failed (Table 28.1) [1].

Patients without T-tube In Situ

After a cholecystectomy, ERCP is the modality of choice to treat retained stones that were undetected or were left behind to be dealt with endoscopically (Figs. 28.2–28.4). The success rate of stone extraction by ERCP in cases of choledocholithiasis is 85–90% in experienced hands [5].

Endoscopic treatment is indicated in young, fit, post-cholecystectomy patients even with ducts of normal diameter [42].

Moreover, ERCP has also been used for postoperative evaluation of an abnormal intraoperative cholangiogram (IOC). Although a normal IOC is very suggestive of a disease-free

Table 28.1 Results of endoscopic treatment of retained stones with T-tube in situ [3, 20, 43–45]

Reference	Patient No.	Clearance rate	Complication rate	Mortality (%)
Cotton [26]	34	33 (97)	NS	NS
Soehendra [27]	75	72 (90)	0	0
Escorrou [28]	28	26 (93)	NS	NS
Simpson [29]	16	16 (100)	0	0
O'Doherthy [30]	39	37 (95)	3	0
Lambert [31]	73	63 (86)	19	3
Bickerstaff [32]	14	14 (100)	0	0
Askew [33]	30	27 (90)	1	3
Danilewitz [34]	20	20 (100)	6	0
Tandon [35]	28	26 (93)	3	0
Nussinson [36]	68	52 (76)	4	0
Ovartlarnporn B [37]	15	13 (87)	1	1
Abu-Khalaf [38]	27	22 (88)	1	0
Cheung [39]	NR	(100)	4	0
Gamal [40]	17	17 (100)	2	0
Christoforidis [20]	45	41 (100)	1	0
Total / mean	529	479 (90)	0–19	0–3

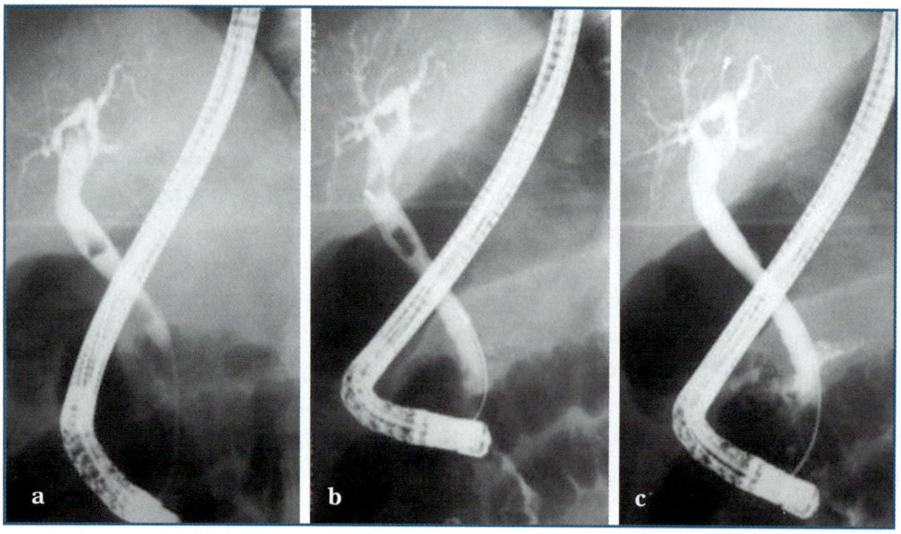

Fig. 28.2 **a** Residual choledocholithiasis 12 years after open cholecystectomy. **b** Stone trapped in Dormia basket. **c** Cholangiography after endoscopic stone removal [41]

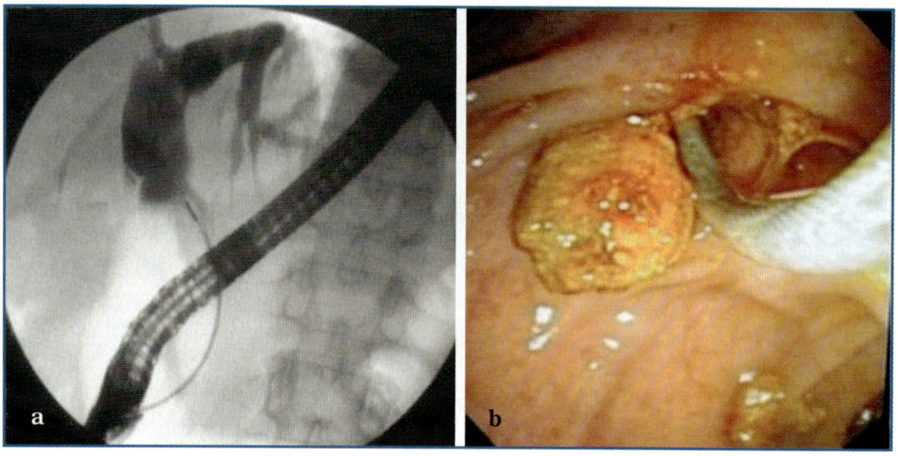

Fig. 28.3 **a** Residual choledocholithiasis 1 year after videolaparoscopic cholecystectomy. **b** Endoscopic treatment and stone morphology

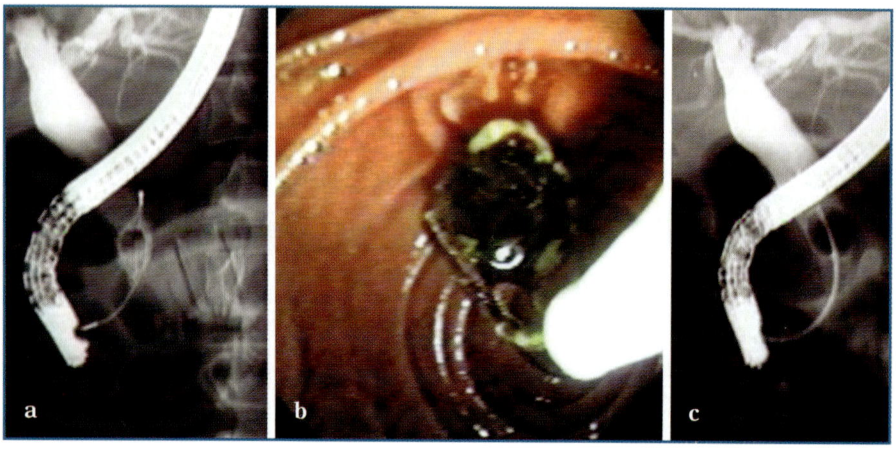

Fig. 28.4 **a** Residual choledocholithiasis 3 years after videolaparoscopic cholecystectomy; **b, c** endoscopic treatment and stone morphology

CBD, abnormal studies are associated with high false-positive rates. A prospective study investigated 51 patients with abnormal IOC at LC who underwent postoperative ERCP at two tertiary referral centers over a 3 year period. The study concluded that one-third of patients with an abnormal IOC have normal postoperative ERCPs. Elevated liver function tests can help to identify patients who merit further evaluation by ERCP. The use of less invasive methods such as EUS or MRCP should be considered for patients with normal liver function tests in order to minimize unnecessary ERCPs [43].

When ERCP is difficult to perform (retained intrahepatic stones or patients with previous gastric surgery), percutaneous transhepatic cholangiography (PTC) is indicated. Other factors, such as the patient's age, operative risk, American Society of Anesthesiologists' (ASA) class, stone size, associated biliary stenosis and the technical skill of the team should also be considered when selecting the appropriate treatment.

The choice of best treatment is influenced by:

1. general condition of the patient;
2. clinical pictures;
3. clinical expertise and multidisciplinary approach (gastroenterologist, surgeon, and operative radiologist);
4. availability of technology, instruments and tools,
5. presence/absence of T-tube or trans-cystic drainage.

Today the surgical approach is limited to the relatively rare case of failure of ERCP and/or PTC [1].

Late CBDS after Cholecystectomy

Retained stones in the CBD postoperatively are usually dealt with endoscopically or by interventional radiology. If both methods fail, surgical management is contemplated.

Endoscopic Management

In patients who present after cholecystectomy with recurrent biliary symptoms, ERCP with ES is the procedure of choice [3] and should be attempted first, with a success rate of more than 85% in achieving overall clearance of stones from the CBD [1, 44]. Although early complication rates for ES are 5–10%, emergency surgery is required only in 1–2% of cases and most complications can be managed conservatively [45]; mortality is mostly reported in fragile and elderly patients (Table 28.2 and 28.3).

CBD clearance with the Dormia basket or Fogarty balloon is effective in 76–98% of cases [67], but these classic accessories do not perform well in cases of difficult choledocholithiasis. If extraction with routine baskets seems difficult, many endoscopists will use mechanical lithotripsy (crushing baskets), with success rates for stone clearance of approximately 90% [1, 68]. Use of mechanical lithotripsy avoids the potential embarrassment of an entrapped basket within the bile duct [69]. For stones where endoscopic techniques of mechanical lithotripsy have been unsuccessful, defined as difficult stones, [70] suitable adjuvant procedures exist, such as nasobiliary drain for chemical contact dissolution therapy and/or extracorporeal shock waves lithotripsy (ESWL), intracorporeal electrohydraulic and laser lithotripsy, percutaneous transhepatic therapy or stent. These usually increase the success rate of stone clearance to 95–99% [67].

Difficult stones can depend on stone factors, including size, number (Fig. 28.5), texture, shape and location of stone; on ductal factors, such a contour, diameter at the level of and distal to the stones, and presence of a coexisting stricture with the stone located proximal to a stricture; or on the anatomic alterations from postsurgical treatments (Table 28.4) [1].

A mechanical lithotriptor consists of a wire basket, a metal sheath and a handle,

Table 28.2 Complications of ERCP [45]

Authors	Patient no.	Pancreatitis				Bleeding			Perforation		Infection		
		Mild	Moderate	Severe	Death	Moderate	Severe	Death	All	Death	Mild	Severe	Death
Barthet [46]	1,159	5	7	9	3	7	1	0	12	2	6	2	1
Boender [47]	242	0	3	1	1	13	2	0	4	0	9	2	0
Chen [48]	210	4	5	2	0	1	1	0	2	0	1	1	1
Choudari [49]	562	35	8	6	1	1	1	0	4	0	4	0	0
Christensen [50]	1,177	30	10	5	3	7	4	1	13	1	52	7	3
Christoforidis [51]	516	12	3	2	0	3	0	0	0	0	2	0	0
Deans [52]	958	0	8	2	2	2	2	0	3	0	0	7	0
Dickinson [53]	328	0	11	1	1	1	0	0	1	0	0	0	0
Freeman [54]	2,347	53	65	9	1	36	12	2	8	1	30	5	2
Koklu [55]	299	7	0	0	0	8	4	0	4	0	2	2	0
Leese [56]	394	6	0	2	1	12	7	1	3	1	4	3	0
Loperfido [57]	2,769	0	33	3	1	17	4	2	16	4	20	4	4
Lal [58]	210	0	10	0	0	5	0	0	0	0	1	0	0
Masci [59]	2,103	0	41	3	1	19	11	0	16	0	17	2	2
Ong [60]	336	15	2	1	0	3	0	0	1	0	4	4	1
Rabenstein [61]	438	0	16	3	0	3	7	2	0	0	4	0	0
Sherman [62]	423	11	4	2	0	4	2	0	2	0	3	1	1
Suissa [63]	534	20	8	2	1	8	2	0	9	1	20	6	3
Tanner [64]	255	0	0	7	0	0	5	0	0	0	0	1	0
Tzovaras [65]	372	4	0	1	0	1	0	0	2	0	6	1	1
Vandervoolt [66]	1,223	60	22	6	2	9	1	0	1	0	9	0	0
Total	16,855	262	256	67	18	160	66	8	101	10	194	48	19
%		1.55	1.52	0.40	0.11	0.95	0.39	0.05	0.60	0.06	1.15	0.28	0.11

Table 28.3 Post-ERCP morbidity and mortality rates [45]

Authors	Patient no.	ERCP-specific complications	Severe complications	ERCP-related fatalities	Miscellaneous	All death (%)
Barthet [46]	1159	49 (4.2%)	24 (2.1%)	6 (0.52%)	–	–
Boender [47]	242	34 (14%)	9 (3.7%)	1 (0.4%)	–	–
Chen [48]	210	17 (8.1%)	6 (2.9%)	1 (0.5%)	–	
Choudari [49]	562	59 (10.5%)	11 (2.0%)	1 (0.2%)	–	–
Christensen [50]	1177	128 (10.9%)	29 (2.5%)	8 (0.7%)	69 (5.9%)	4% (0.34)
Christoforidis [51]	516	22 (4.3%)	2 (0.39%)	0	2 (0.4%)	0%
Deans [52]	958	24 (2.5%)	14 (1.5%)	2 (0.2%)	–	–
Dickinson [53]	328	14 (4.3%)	2 (0.6%)	1 (0.3%)	–	–
Freeman [54]	2347	218 (9.3%)	34 (1.5%)	6 (0.3%)	25 (1.1%)	4% (0.17)
Koklu [55]	299	27 (9.0%)	10 (3.3%)	0	1 (0.33)	0%
Lal [56]	210	16 (7.6%)	0	0	1 (0.5%)	0%
Leese [57]	394	37 (9.4%)	15 (3.8%)	3 (0.8%)	4 (1%)	0%
Loperfido [58]	2759	97 (3.5%)	27 (1.0%)	11 (0.4%)	14 (0.5%)	0%
Masci [59]	2103	109 (5.2%)	32 (1.5%)	3 (0.1%)	9 (0.4%)	0%
Ong [60]	336	30 (8.9%)	6 (1.8%)	1 (0.3%)	4 (1.2%)	0%
Rabenstein [61]	438	33 (7.5%)	10 (2.3%)	2 (0.5%)	1 (0.2%)	0%
Sherman [62]	423	29 (6.9%)	7 (1.7%)	1 (0.2%)	0	0%
Suissa [63]	534	75 (14.0%)	19 (3.6%)	5 (0.9%)	1 (0.19)	0%
Tanner [64]	255	13 (5.1%)	13 (5.1%)	0	0	1% (0.39)
Tzovaras [65]	372	15 (4.0%)	4 (1.1%)	1 (0.27%)	1 (0.27)	0%
Vandervoort [66]	1,223	108 (8.8%)	8 (0.7%)	2 (0.2%)	41 (3.4%)	0%
Total	16855	1,154 (6.85%)	282 (1.67%)	55 (0.33%)	173 (1.33%)	9% (0.07%)

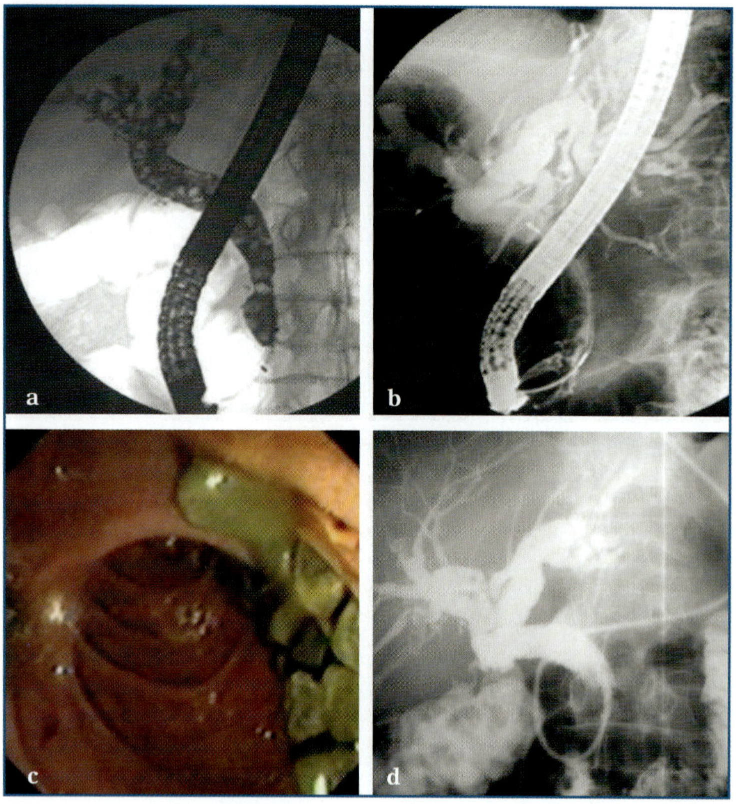

Fig. 28.5 a Multiple residual difficult choledocholithiasis; **b, c** endoscopic removal and control with nasobiliary tube (**d**)

Table 28.4 Criteria for definition of difficult stones [1]

Anatomic alteration*	Stone factors*	Duct factors
Periampullary diverticula	> 15 mm in diameter	Contour (sigmoid-shaped) duct, kinking)
Billroth II	> 10 in number	Diameter distal to stone
Roux-en-Y reconstruction	Hard in consistency	Stones proximal to a stricture or a tumor
	Square, "piston" or faceted in shape	
	Stones tightly fit the bile duct	
	Stones packed against each other	
	Intrahepatic stones	
	Impacted stones [72]	

* Common factor is the discrepancy between the stone dimension and papillotomy size

which provides mechanical retraction of the basket into the metal sheath, directing a crushing force to the stone [71].

Laser lithotripsy is based on pulsed-dye laser technology. The application leads to rapid expansion and collapse of plasma on the stone-surface, resulting in a mechanical shock wave. However, this technique has a high complication rate (10%) and low rate of mortality (1%), due to ductal lesions, with a success rate from 67–88% [70].

Recently, laser lithotripsy has been possible under fluoroscopic guidance with the use of devices that recognize the difference between stone and tissue.

With ESWL, direct contact with a stone is unnecessary. Stones are localized by fluoroscopic focusing during cholangiography through a trans-nasobiliary catheter previously placed at time of ERCP, or through a percutaneous drain. Several studies report success rates for ESWL stone fragmentation of 53–91% and duct-clearance of 58–90%. On the negative side, it is less effective when multiple stones are present [1].

Electrohydraulic lithotripsy (EHL) is a recent technique that utilizes a flexible catheter with two coaxially isolated electrodes at the tip, capable of delivering electric sparks in short, rapid pulses leading to expansion of the surrounding liquid environment, generating pressure that induces stone fragmentation. In comparison with the other techniques of lithotripsy, EHL minimizes the risk of CBD injury and perforation, and has a high rate of complete stone clearance after multiple sessions, reported from 76% [70] to 86% [1], comparable to the ESWL success rate.

With the use of endoscopic techniques such a mechanical lithotripsy, EHL, laser lithotripsy and ESWL, successful stone removal is reported in 98% of cases [73].

If treatment by endoscopy and lithotripsy fails, an endoscopic biliary endoprosthesis can be placed to provide biliary decompression and prevent stone impaction in the distal CBD.

Stenting

Plastic stent insertion as a definitive treatment for CBDS, without any further subsequent intervention, may be considered but should be limited to patients with severe comorbid illnesses or in case of incomplete or impossible stone extraction due to stone size, local anatomy, bleeding, or technical difficulty (Figs. 28.6, 28.7) [13]. Studies have shown

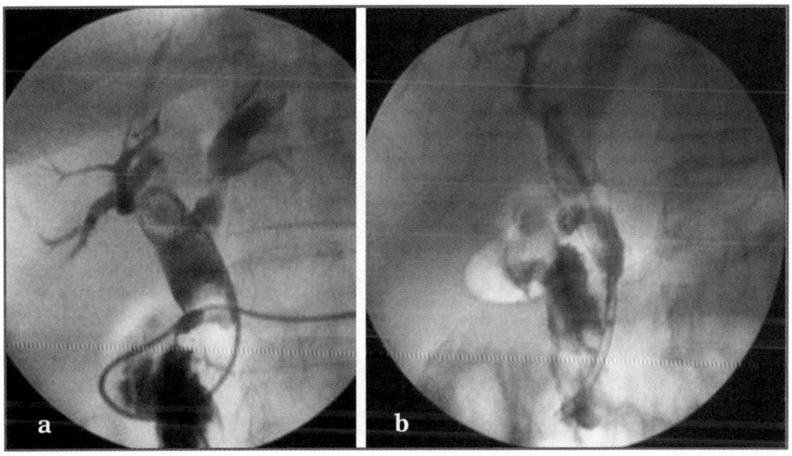

Fig. 28.6 a "Difficult" multiple choledocholithiasis 21 years after open cholecystectomy: stent placement (**b**)

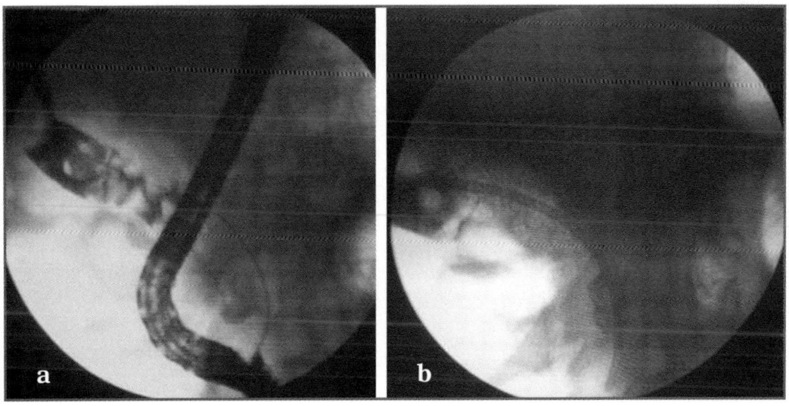

Fig. 28.7 a "Difficult" multiple choledocholithiasis 18 years after open cholecystectomy: stent placement after naso-biliary tube placement (**b**)

that the majority of CBDS reduce in size following stenting and therefore should be easier to remove at repeat ERCP [74].

There have been several studies investigating the role of stent insertion as the sole treatment of CBDS that could not be removed at ERCP. In the study of Bergman and coworkers [75], 58 of 117 (49%) patients had permanent biliary stent insertion as their treatment for CBDS (stent exchange only if complications occurred). At 2 years follow up, 60% of these patients were alive and of these, 70% were symptom free. However, overall the complication rate was 40% and the mortality rate related to complications of the biliary stent was 16%. Cholangitis and jaundice were felt to be the cause of the death in these patients, occurring after a median time of 42 months [75]. These results are similar to a study by De Palma and coworkers [76], who followed up 49 patients with stent insertion for irretrievable CBDS, with a 40% late complication rate and 6% mortality related to biliary sepsis over a 3 year follow-up period. Jain and coworkers [77] carried out a prospective study on 20 patients with difficult CBDS (the mean stone diameter was 1.7 cm). In each case a 7F pigtail stent was inserted and ERCP was repeated at 6 months. In 20% of patients the stones had fragmented and allowed balloon clearance of the duct. However, in 35% of patients the duct had cleared spontaneously. There is a potential advantage of pigtail stents over straight stents in that the duodenal portion of the stent comes out angulated and may keep the biliary orifice open more effectively. If the stent becomes occluded after several months, it still has the potential to keep the CBDS from impacting. Pigtail stents also have a lower rate of stent migration [70].

PTC Management

Percutaneous extraction is performed after diagnostic PTC findings have confirmed the presence of CBDS. An external biliary catheter is placed, and the tract is dilated over 2–6 weeks up to 16F in size by the placement of progressively larger catheters. The CBDS are then extracted using a Dormia basket or a choledochoscope. Stones or their fragments can be trapped inside a basket and passed through the sphincter of Oddi into the duodenum. The procedure may need to be repeated for complete clearance. The morbidity rate is approximately 10%, and the mortality rate is 1% [5].

Surgical Management

Surgery should be considered only when combined ERCP and ES fail, either for technical reasons or when an additional drainage procedure is required, because of its high mean mortality rate of 1.6% (range 0–4%) (Table 28.5) [1, 78].

Table 25.5 Mortality of biliary reoperation for retained or recurrent bile duct stones. Modified from [1, 78–81]

Reference	Mortality (%)
Saharia et al. [6]	0
Jones [82]	0
McSherry et al. [83]	2
Allen et al. [84]	2
Choi et al. [85]	3
Lygidakis [86]	1.7
De Almeida et al. [87]	4
Broughan et al. [88]	0.8
Den Besten et al. [89]	2.3
McSherry [78]	4
Girard [90]	0
Pejovic [79]	1
Nathanson et al. [80]	0
Bratucu et al. [81]	0
Range (mean)	0–4 (1.6)

The surgical techniques for patients reoperated upon for retained or recurrent CBDS are:

1. choledocholithotomy with T-tube placement followed by cholangiography. T-tube drainage is not necessary if prior ERCP and ES were attempted;
2. choledocholitotomy with side-to-side choledochoduodenostomy or choledochojejunostomy.

Choledochotomy is performed by placing two traction sutures on either side of the intended choledochotomy incision on the CBD distal to the cystic duct. The anterior wall of the CBD is opened longitudinally for a distance of approximately 1–1.5 cm, while traction is applied to the sutures. Stone forceps, scoops, Fogarty balloon catheters, and irrigating catheters can be used for the removal of stones. A choledochoscope can be used to confirm that the CBD is clear and to remove any retained stones. A Dormia basket can be helpful at this point. Once the CBD is cleared, it is closed over a 16F T-tube using 4-0 monofilament absorbable suture. A closed suction drain is placed in the foramen of Winslow. A T-tube cholangiogram is performed 10–14 days postoperatively, and the T-tube is removed if no retained stones are seen. Although this procedure carries a low morbidity and mortality rate in young patients (< 1%), the mortality rate is as high as 4% in elderly populations [5]. Moreover, it is associated with greater postoperative pain and discomfort, and a longer recovery period is needed compared to the laparoscopic or endoscopic methods. A small-caliber duct (< 6 mm in diameter) is a relative contraindication to choledochotomy [5].

Biliary-enteric drainage is the recommended procedure to prevent further problems in patients with previous choledocholithotomy or if any of following occur [1]:

1. stricture or stenosis of distal bile duct or sphincter of Oddi;
2. marked dilation of the duct (> 2 cm);
3. multiple (> 4) or primary bile duct stones [5];
4. inability to remove all stones from the duct;
5. a third operation.

Choledochoduodenostomy is the most commonly employed drainage procedure and can be performed either side-to-side or end-to-side. In the side-to-side procedure, sump syndrome is a feared complication, in which food particles reflux into the CBD, resulting in obstruction, cholangitis, and/or pancreatitis. This complication can be diminished if the size of the anastomosis is limited to 14 mm [5].

Recent reports on choledochoenterostomy have recommended "side-to-side" anastomosis [91]. Using this type of anastomosis, the longitudinal incision in the anterior wall of the bile duct can be anastomosed with the incision in the anterior wall of the duodenal bulbus on the side of the lesser curvature of the stomach without having to completely ablate the bile duct. The procedure is also easy to perform and can be used for high-risk patients, especially elderly patients [92]. However, side-to-side anastomosis of the bile duct and the duodenum can also cause foreign bodies to enter the residual bile duct after surgery, triggering the onset of intractable and recurrent cholangitis and liver abscess, which is defined as sump syndrome. End-to-side anastomosis should be performed to prevent this intractable syndrome. The worst complication is bile duct cancer developing after choledochoduodenostomy [93].

Choledochojejunostomy is performed either in continuity or preferably as a Roux-en-Y loop that is passed in a retrocolic fashion. The preferred anastomotic size is 2.5 cm. It has the disadvantage of an added anastomotic line, but the advantage that it is not associated with reflux of food particles [5].

A recent report examined recurrent lithiasis after surgical treatment of elderly patients with choledocholithiasis; the recurrence rate was significantly higher in patients with choledocholithiasis who had undergone T-tube drainage or choledochojejunostomy than in those who had undergone choledochoduodenostomy, especially in those with primary CBDS. The results indicate that choledochoduodenostomy is superior to T-tube drainage and is recommended for elderly patients with primary bile duct stones to prevent postoperative recurrent lithiasis [92].

Choledocholithotomy with transduodenal sphincteroplasty is a retrograde approach to the clearance of the CBD, indicated in patients with a stone impacted at the ampulla, or Billroth II gastrectomy. It is rarely necessary because ES suffices in many cases. In transduodenal sphincteroplasty a Fogarty balloon catheter is passed through the choledochotomy or transcystic route into the CBD and through the sphincter of Oddi. The duodenum is then mobilized by performing the Kocher maneuver. The ampulla is identified by palpating the balloon catheter, and a small transverse duodenotomy is performed on the anterior duodenal wall just above the ampulla. A sphincterotomy is performed at the 11 o'clock mark (to avoid the pancreatic duct, which is located between the 4 and 5 o'clock positions). The sphincterotomy is carried for a distance of approximately 1 cm. The edges of the incision are sutured at the beginning of the incision and at its apex using an absorbable suture. The balloon catheter is withdrawn from the CBD and inserted through the ampulla in a retrograde fashion to extract the stones. A choledochoscope can also be used. Finally, duodenotomy is closed in a transverse fashion, a completion cholangiogram is performed and choledochotomy or the cystic stump is closed. There is no need to insert a T-tube, which lengthens the hospital stay and may predispose the patient to stenosis and infection of the CBD. The advantages of this procedure are that it is good for small-caliber CBDs (< 15 mm), and it facilitates drainage. The drawbacks are that it requires open surgery and opening of the duodenum. The success rate in an earlier series was reported as 90–100% [5], but the method carries a greater risk of postoperative pancreatitis. Transduodenal sphincteroplasty is contraindicated in the presence of large CBD (> 2 cm) or where there is a long suprasphincterial stricture; it should not be attempted in the presence of a duodenal diverticulum or where there is severe periampullary inflammation [1]. A retrospective study of Sellner [94] in 1988 found that the factors affecting mortality are age > 70 years, bilirubin level > 85 mmol/L, diabetes, renal failure and coagulopathy. The mortality rate of choledochoduodenostomy is lower than that attending transduodenal sphincteroplasty, and it has been shown to be a safe and simple operation with low morbidity and mortality, especially in elderly patients. The overall mortality rate after reoperation for recurrent bile duct stones is less than 2%.

Long term follow-up data after surgical treatment of the CBD revealed that complications had been treated in 3% of the choledochoduodenostomy group, and 6% of the transduodenal sphincteroplasty group (mainly cholangitis), with additional symptoms on interview in 8% of the choledochoduodenostomy and 5% of the transduodenal sphincteroplasty group [1].

Conclusion

In the era of LC, the incidence of retained or primary CBDS is lower than at the time of conventional cholecystectomy because of better preoperative imaging and of endoscopic treatments.

Today, many options are available to treat retained or primary CBDS by multidisciplinary approach: gastroenterologists, radiologists and surgeons need to work in close cooperation to evaluate and treat the patient in the best way.

The treatment chosen (open or laparoscopic surgery, endoscopy or operative radiology) should be related to the team's expertise, but also to the general condition of the patients, local availability and efficacy of different techniques. In summary, a tailored approach and treatment are desired.

The procedure of choice in primary or retained CBDS, with universal agreement, should be ES, which has a high success rate and low morbidity and mortality rates. In case of ES failure or its contraindications, surgical re-operation is a rational option, with satisfactory outcome.

Finally, the availability of nonoperative methods of stone extraction should not reduce the vigilance towards pre- and intraoperative tests and techniques used during the LC to prevent retained CBDS.

References

1. Blumgart LH (2007) Surgery of the liver, biliary tract and pancreas, IV edn, vol 1. Saunders Elsevier
2. Roslyn JJ, Binns GS, Hughes EF et al (1993) Open cholecystectomy. A contemporary analysis of 42,474 patients. Ann Surg 218:129-137
3. Berci G, Cuschieri A (1997) Bile duct and bile duct stones. Philadelphia, WB Saunders Company
4. Gerwig WH jr, Countriman LK, Gomez AC (1961) Congenital absence of gallbladder and cystic duct: report of 6 cases. Ann Surg 153:113-125
5. Dandan IS, Soweid AM, Abiad F (2003) Choledocholithiasis. In: Plantz SH (ed) eMedicine (web based reference textbook)
6. Saharia PC, Zuidema G, Cameron JL (1977) Primary common duct stones. Ann Surg 185:598-602
7. Madden JL (1973) Common duct stones; their origin and surgical management. Surg Clin North Am 53:1095-1113
8. Kim DI, Kim MH, Lee SK et al (2001) Risk factors for recurrence of primary bile duct stones after endoscopic sphincterotomy. Gastrointest Endosc 54:42-48
9. Legorreta A, Brooks RJ, Staroscik RN et al (1995) Increased ERCP rate following the introduction of LC. J Laparaendosc Surg 5:271-278
10. Uchiyama K, Honishi H, Tani M (2003) Long-term prognosis after treatment of patients with choledocholithiasis. Ann Surg 238:97-102
11. Christoforidis E, Goulimaris I, Kanellos I et al (2002) The role of juxtapapillary duodenal diverticula in biliary stone disease. Gastrointest Endosc 55:543-547
12. Chandy G, Hart WJ, Roberts-Thomson IC (1997) An analysis of the relationship between bile duct stones and periampullary duodenal diverticula. J Gastroenterol Hepatol 12:29-33
13. Caddy GR, Tham TC (2006). Symptoms, diagnosis and endoscopic management of common bile duct stones. Best Pract Res Clin Gastroenterol 20:1085-1101
14. Tse F, Barkun JS, Barkun AN (2004) The elective evaluation of patients with suspected choledocholithiasis undergoing LC. Gastrointest Endosc 60:437-448
15. Romagnuolo J, Bardou M, Rahme E et al (2003) Magnetic resonance cholangiopancreato-graphy: a meta-analysis of test performance in suspected biliary disease. Ann Intern Med 139:547-557
16. David V, Reinhold C, Hochman M et al (1998) Pitfalls in the interpretation of MR cholangiopancreatography. AJR Am J Roentgenol 170:1055-1059
17. de Ledinghen V, Lecesne R, Raymond JM et al (1999). Diagnosis of choledocholithiasis: EUS or magnetic resonance cholangiography? A prospective controlled study. Gastrointest Endosc 49:26-31
18. Verma D, Kapadia A, Eisen GM et al (2006) EUS vs MRCP for detection of choledocholithiasis. Gastrointest Endosc 64:248-254
19. Maniatis P, Triantopoulou C, Sofianu E et al (2003) Virtual CT cholangiography in patients with choledocholithiasis. Abdom Imaging 28:536-544
20. Christoforidis E, Vasiliadis K, Goulimaris I et al (2004) Endoscopic management of retained bile stones with an indwelling T-tube. Surg Endosc 18:1582-1586
21. Mazzariello RM (1978) A fourteen-year experience with nonoperative instrument extraction of retained bile duct stones. World J Surg 2:447-455
22. Tritapepe R, Caspani P, Pozzi C (1988) Postoperative trans-T-tube cholangiography: possibilities of false-negatives in residual calculi. Minerva Chir 43:867-870
23. Josephs LG, Birkett DH (1992) Laser lithotripsy for the management of retained stones. Arch Surg 127:603-604
24. Hammarström LE, Stridbeck H, Ihse I (1996) Long-term follow-up after endoscopic treatment of bile duct calculi in cholecystectomized patients. World J Surg 20:272-276
25. Sciumè C, Pisello F, Geraci G et al (2001) Multiple choledocholithiasis. Ann Ital Chir 72:473-476
26. Cotton PB, Vallon AG (1980) Post-cholecystectomy ERCP. Lancet 29:1-710
27. Soehendra N, Kempeneers I, Eichfuss HP et al (1981) Early post-operative endoscopy after biliary tract surgery. Endoscopy 13:113-117

28. Escourrou J, Cordova JA, Lazorthes F et al (1984) Early and late complications after endoscopic sphincterotomy for biliary lithiasis with and without the gall bladder 'in situ'. Gut 25:598-602
29. Simpson CJ, Gray GR, Gillespie G (1985) Early endoscopic sphincterotomy for retained common bile duct stones. J R Coll Surg Edinb 30:288-289
30. O'Doherty DP, Neoptolemos JP, Carr-Locke DL (1986) Endoscopic sphincterotomy for retained common bile duct stones in patients with T-tube in situ in the early postoperative period. Br J Surg 73:454-456
31. Lambert ME, Martin DF, Tweedle DE (1988) Endoscopic removal of retained stones after biliary surgery. Br J Surg 75:896-898
32. Bickerstaff KI, Berry AR, Chapman RW, Britton J (1988) Early postoperative endoscopic sphincterotomy for retained biliary stones. Ann R Coll Surg Engl 70:350-351
33. Askew AR, Ward M, Cowen AE (1989) Early postoperative endoscopic sphincterotomy for retained common duct stones. Ann R Coll Surg Engl 71:359-360
34. Danilewitz MD (1989) Early postoperative endoscopic sphincterotomy for retained common bile duct stones. Gastrointest Endosc 35:298-299
35. Tandon RK, Nijhawan S, Arora A (1990) Management of retained common bile duct stones in patients with T-tube in situ: role of endoscopic sphincterotomy. Am J Gastroenterol 85:1126-1131
36. Nussinson E, Cairns SR, Vaira D et al (1991) A 10 year single centre experience of percutaneous and endoscopic extraction of bile duct stones with T tube in situ. Gut 32:1040-1043
37. Ovartlarnporn B, Piratvisuth T, Wacharasin R et al (1992) Endoscopic removal of stone in patients with retained common bile duct stone and T-tube after cholecystectomy. Is it justified? J Med Assoc Thai 75:524-528
38. Abu-Khalaf A (1995) Endoscopic removal of retained common bile duct stones in patients with T tube in situ. Surg Laparosc Endosc 5:17-20
39. Cheung MT (1997) Postoperative choledochoscopic removal of intrahepatic stones via a T tube tract. Br J Surg 84:1224-1228
40. Gamal EM, Szabò A, Szule E et al (2001) Choledochoscopic treatment of retained biliary stones via dilated T-tube tract. Surg Endosc 15:473-476
41. Sciumè C, Geraci G, Pisello F et al (2003) Endoscopic removal of a Dormia basket impacted in the biliary tract during treatment of a difficult residual choledocholithiasis. Report of a case. Ann Ital Chir 74:209-212
42. Cotton PB (1984) Endoscopic management of bile duct stones (apples and oranges). Gut 25:587-597
43. Varadarajulu S, Eloubeidi MA, Wilcox CM et al (2006) Do all patients with abnormal intraoperative cholangiogram merit endoscopic retrograde cholangiopancreatography? Surg Endosc 20:801-805
44. Baron TH, Petersen BT, Mergener K et al (2006) Quality indicators for endoscopic retrograde cholangiopancreatography. Am J Gastroenterol 101:892-897
45. Andriulli A, Lo Perfido S, Napolitano G et al (2007) Incidence Rates of Post-ERCP Complications: a systematic survey of prospective studies. Am J Gastroenterol 102:1-8
46. Barthet M, Lesavre N, Desjeux A et al (2002) Complications of endoscopic sphincterotomy: results from a single tertiary referral center. Endoscopy 34:991-997
47. Boender J, Nix GA, de Ridder MA et al (1994) Endoscopic papillotomy for common bile duct stones: factors influencing the complication rate. Endoscopy 26:209-216
48. Chen YK, Foliente RL, Santoro MJ (1994) Endoscopic sphincterotomy-induced pancreatitis: increased risk associated with nondilated bile ducts and sphincter of Oddi dysfunction. Am J Gastroenterol 89:327-333
49. Choudari CP, Fogel E, Kalayci C et al (1999) Therapeutic biliary endoscopy. Endoscopy 31:80-87
50. Christensen M, Matzen P, Schulze S, Rosenberg J (2004) Complications of ERCP: a prospective study. Gastrointest Endosc 60:721-731
51. Christoforidis E, Goulimaris I, Kanellos I et al (2002). Post-ERCP pancreatitis and hyperamylasemia: patient-related and operative risk factors. Endoscopy 34:286-292
52. Deans GT, Sedman P, Martin DF et al (1997) Are complications of endoscopic sphincterotomy age related? Gut 41:545-548
53. Dickinson RJ, Davies S (1998) Post-ERCP pancreatitis and hyperamylasaemia: the role of operative and patient factors. Eur J Gastroenterol Hepatol 10:423-428. Erratum in: Eur J Gastroenterol Hepatol (1998) 10:731
54. Freeman ML, Nelson DB, Sherman S et al (1996) Complications of endoscopic biliary sphincterotomy. N Engl J Med 335:909-918
55. Köklü S, Parlak E, Yüksel O, Sahin B (2005) Endoscopic retrograde cholangiopancreatography in the elderly: a prospective and comparative study. Age Ageing 34:572-577
56. Leese T, Neoptolemos JP, Carr-Locke DL (1985) Successes, failures, early complications and their management following endoscopic sphincterotomy: results in 394 consecutive patients from a single centre. Br J Surg 72:215-219

57. Loperfido S, Angelini G, Benedetti G et al (1998) Major early complications from diagnostic and therapeutic ERCP: a prospective multicenter study. Gastrointest Endosc 48:1-10
58. Lal D, Lane M, Wong P (2003) Complications of endoscopic retrograde cholangiopancreatography. N Z Med J 116(1177):U496
59. Masci E, Mariani A, Curioni S, Testoni PA (2003) Risk factors for pancreatitis following endoscopic retrograde cholangiopancreatography: a meta-analysis. Endoscopi 35:830-834
60. Ong TZ, Khor JL, Selamat DS et al (2005) Complications of endoscopic retrograde cholangiography in the post-MRCP era: a tertiary center experience. World J Gastroenterol 11:5209-5212
61. Rabenstein T, Hahn EG (2002) Post-ERCP pancreatitis: is the endoscopist's experience the major risk factor? JOP 3:177-187
62. Sherman S, Ruffolo TA, Hawes RH, Lehman GA (1991) Complications of endoscopic sphincterotomy. A prospective series with emphasis on the increased risk associated with sphincter of Oddi dysfunction and nondilated bile ducts. Gastroenterology 101:1068-1075
63. Suissa A, Yassin K, Lavy A, Lachter J (2005) Outcome and early complications of ERCP: a prospective single center study. Hepatogastroenterology 52:352-355
64. Tanner AR (1996) ERCP: present practice in a single region. Suggested standards for monitoring performance. Eur J Gastroenterol Hepatol 8:145-148
65. Tzovaras G, Shukla P, Kow L et al (2000) What are the risks of diagnostic and therapeutic endoscopic retrograde cholangiopancreatography? Aust N Z J Surg 70:778-782
66. Vandervoort J, Soetikno RM, Tham TC et al (2002) Risk factors for complications after performance of ERCP. Gastrointest Endosc 56:652 626
67. Esber EJ, Sherman S (1996) The interface of endoscopic retrograde cholangiopancreatography and laparoscopic cholecystectomy. Gastrointest Endosc N Am 6.57-80
68. Chang WH, Chu CH, Wang TE et al (2005) Outcome of simple use of mechanical lithotripsy of difficult common bile duct stones. World J Gastroenterol 11:593-596
69. Roberts-Thomson IC (2004) The management of bile duct stones. Indian J Gastroenterol 23:102-106
70. Hui CK, Lai KC, Ng M et al (2003) Retained CBDS: a comparison between biliary stenting and complete clearance of stones by electrohydraulic lithotripsy. Aliment Pharmacol Ther 17:289-296
71. Di Sario J, Chuttani R, Croffie J et al (2007) Biliary and pancreatic lithotripsy devices. Gastrointest Endosc 65:750-756
72. Katsinelos P, Galanis I, Pilpilidis I et al (2003) The effect of indwelling endoprosthesis on stone size or fragmentation after long-term treatment with biliary stenting for large stones. Surg Endosc 17:1552-1555
73. Schumacher B, Frieling T, Haussinger D et al (1998) Endoscopic treatment of symptomatic choledocholithiasis . Hepatogastroebterology 45:672-676
74. Chan AC, Ng EK, Chung SC et al (1998). CBDS become smaller after endoscopic biliary stenting. Endoscopy 30:356-359
75. Bergman JJ, Rauws EA, Tijssen JG et al (1995) Biliary endoprostheses in elderly patients with endoscopically irretrievable CBDS: report on 117 patients. Gastrointest Endosc 42:195-201
76. De Palma GD, Galloro G, Siciliano S et al (2001) Endoscopic stenting for definitive treatment of irretrievable common bile duct calculi. A long-term follow-up study of 49 patients. Hepatogastroenterology 48:56-58
77. Jain SK, Stein R, Bhuva M et al (2000) Pigtail stents: an alternative in the treatment of difficult bile duct stones. Gastrointest Endosc 52:490-493
78. McSherry CK (1989) Cholecystectomy: the gold standard. Am J Surg 158:174-178
79. Pejovic T (2001) Residual choledocholithiasis in elective cholecystectomy and choledocholithotomy. Acta Chir Iugosl 48:37-39
80. Nathanson LK, O'Rourke NA, Martin IJ et al (2005) Postoperative ERCP versus laparoscopic choledochotomy for clearance of selected bile duct calculi: a randomized trial. Ann Surg 242:188-192
81. Bratucu E, Straja D, Marincas M et al (2006) Late choledochal pathology after cholecystectomy for choledocholithiasis. Chirurgia (Bucur) 101:289-295
82. Jones SA (1978) The prevention and treatment of recurrent bile duct stones by transduodenal sphincteroplasty. World J Surg 2:473-485
83. McSherry CK, Glenn F (1980) The incidence and causes of death following surgery for nonmalignant biliary tract disease. Ann Surg 191:271-275
84. Allen B, Shapiro H, Way LW (1981) Management of recurrent and residual common duct stones. Am J Surg 142:41-47
85. Choi TK, Wong J, Ong GB (1982) Choledochojejunostomy in the treatment of primary cholangitis. Surg Gynecol Obstet 155:43-45
86. Lygidakis NJ (1982) Infective complications after choledochotomy. Incidence after T-tube drainage of the common bile duct or after choledochoduodenostomy. J R Coll Surg Edinb 27:233-237

87. De Almeida AM, Cruz AG, Aldeia FJ (1984) Side-to-side choledochoduodenostomy in the management of choledocholithiasis and associated disease. Facts and fiction. Am J Surg 147:253-259
88. Broughan TA, Sivak MV, Hermann RE (1985) The management of retained and recurrent bile duct stones. Surgery 98:746-751
89. Den Besten L, Berci G. (1986) The current status of biliary tract surgery: an international study of 107 consecutive patients. World J Surg 10:116-122
90. Girard RM (2000) Stones in common bile duct: surgical approaches. In Blumgart LH, Fong Y (eds): Surgery of the liver and biliary tract , 3rd ed Philadelphia, Saunders, p. 737
91. Srivengadesh G, Kate V, Ananthakrishnan N (2003) Evaluation of long-term results of choledochoduodenostomy for benign biliary obstruction. Trop Gastroenterol 24:205-207
92. Zhe-Fu Li, Xiao-Ping Chen (2007) Recurrent lithiasis after surgical treatment of elderly patients with choledocholithiasis. Hepatobiliary Pancreat Dis Int 6:67-71
93. Maeda A, Yokoi S, Kunou T et al (2003) Bile duct cancer developing 21 years after choledochoduodenostomy. Dig Surg 20:331-334
94. Sellner FJ, Wimberger M, Jelinek R (1988) Factors affecting mortality in transduodenal sphincteroplasty Surg Gynecol Obstet 167:23-27

Chapter 29

Acute Biliary Pancreatitis

Giuseppe Borzellino, Edoardo Saladino, Anna M. Minicozzi, Claudio Cordiano

Historical Survey

The aetiology of acute pancreatitis has been reported as biliary in 60% and idiopathic in 21% of cases in a recent Italian survey [1]. New diagnostic approaches have, however, implicated micro-lithiasis and biliary crystals in the pathogenesis of acute pancreatitis and have allowed a better definition of pancreatitis aetiological epidemiology, with the frequency of biliary pancreatitis reported to be up to 80% [2–5].

The relationship between lithiasis obstruction and pancreatic damage has been known since Opie's observations in 1901 [6]. In the seventies Acosta and Stone [7, 8] hypothesized a relationship between the duration of obstruction and pancreatic damage, since the comparative studies they published reported better outcomes with early surgical removal of stones versus delayed intervention. However, further studies on timing of surgery, both prospective observational and randomised clinical trials (RCTs), reported different results with a higher morbidity and mortality when early surgery was performed [9–11]. Since then, early surgery in acute pancreatitis has been contraindicated.

Progress in intensive care and in the physiopathological understanding of acute pancreatitis have made it possible to reduce mortality rates to 7.5–9%, but mortality in early severe pancreatitis has remained unchanged and is still reported in 40–60% of cases of overall mortality [12–15]. Moreover, due to an increased incidence in pancreatitis in the population, and to a higher mortality incidence in older patients, the overall population mortality per 100,000 patients has remained unchanged [16].

New data on physiopathology confirm the theory of biliary obstruction and the role of micro-lithiasis and biliary sludge in the initiating process of pancreatitis [17–20], while in a recent study Acosta et al. [21] confirmed that duration of the obstruction influences pancreatitis course.

The feasibility of the endoscopic approach reported by some authors in the early eighties [22, 23], even for the early stages of pancreatitis without the risks feared by the pioneers of the method [24], along with associated laparoscopic cholecystectomy in the nineties [25–27], initiated the minimally invasive era and opened up new perspectives for the treatment of acute pancreatitis.

Minimally Invasive Treatment of Acute Biliary Pancreatitis

Urgent Treatment

Since a higher morbidity and mortality were found with an urgent surgical approach, further studies on urgent treatment of acute biliary pancreatitis have been limited to the endoscopic approach. A meta-analytic review from the Cochrane Library [28] included

511 patients from three selected RCTs, comparing urgent endoscopic retrograde cholangiography (ERC) with selective sphincterotomy versus conservative treatment [29–31].

No differences were reported in mortality rates nor in mild pancreatitis (OR = 4.64; 95% CI = 0.22–98.12), neither in predictive severe pancreatitis (OR = 0.62; 95% CI = 0.27–1.41). No differences were found in morbidity for mild pancreatitis (OR = 0.89; 95% CI = 0.53–1.59), while urgent endoscopy reduced morbidity in severe pancreatitis (OR = 0.27; 95% CI = 0.14–0.53). A more recent evidence-based review [32] reports a meta-analytic study based on the same randomised trials but the conclusions were slightly different since no differences were found in mortality (0.7% vs. 0.7%, $p = 0.99$) or morbidity (14.5% vs. 14.7%, $p = 0.97$) in mild acute pancreatitis, while significant differences favouring the endoscopic approach were found for severe pancreatitis both for mortality (17.9% vs. 3.6%, $p = 0.03$) and for morbidity (57.1% vs. 18.2%, $p = 0.0001$). However, these results related to the sub-groups of mild and severe pancreatitis were extracted from only two of the three RCTs since the analysis was not performed in the third RCT.

Based on one RCT, cholangitis has been identified as a determinant factor for complications in severe acute pancreatitis. Although possibly confounding related to cholangitis was taken into account, different timing was adopted in the included studies with endoscopic treatment performed within 24 hours of admission [30], within 72 hours of onset of symptoms [31] and within 72 hours of admission [29]. One study was multicentre with a mean of two patients per year per centre [31]. Furthermore, endoscopic sphincterotomy was not systematically performed, but only if lithiasis was found during retrograde cholangiography.

A third meta-analysis [33] included the RCT of Nowak [34], whose methodology was different from the other three trials. Pooled data highlighted better results in the treatment group both for complications (25% vs. 38.2%, $p < 0.001$) and for mortality (5.2% vs. 9.1%, $p < 0.05$). However, no differentiation of results between mild and severe pancreatitis was reported.

Besides those reported in the meta-analysis, two further RCTs have been published on the urgent endoscopic approach with selective sphincterotomy for acute biliary pancreatitis. One study [35] randomised 45 patients (20 approached by urgent endoscopy and 25 by conservative treatment) and reported significant differences favouring the endoscopic approach when comparing cost, morbidity and hospital stay for severe acute pancreatitis ($p < 0.05$), while no differences were found for mild pancreatitis. This study included a small number of patients and conservative treatment referred to traditional Chinese medicine. A more recent randomised study [36] seems to confirm the results of the other RCTs on the endoscopic approach with selective sphincterotomy, in patients in whom there was a pre-operative suspicion of biliary obstruction. Patients admitted within 48 hours of symptoms were included and randomised to receive conservative treatment or to be approached by urgent endoscopy. No differences were found in the evolution of pancreatitis based on organ failure score and computed tomography (CT) severity index, in local complications (6% vs. 6%, $p = 0.99$) overall morbidity (21% vs. 18%, $p = 0.8$) and mortality (6% vs. 2%, $p = 1$).

Elective Treatment

Indications

Only one randomised study [37] has been published on the comparison of pre-operative ERCP with laparoscopic cholecystectomy and selective post-operative ERCP if required on the basis of intra-operative cholangiography. A longer hospital stay (11.7 vs. 9 days, $p = 0.042$) and higher costs (10.210 vs. 8.586 USD, $p = 0.049$) were found in the pre-operative ERCP group, but no differences were found in the length of the intensive care unit stay, failure of cholangiographies, morbidity, or prevalence of common bile duct stones. Patients with cholangitis and necrotising pancreatitis were however excluded.

Recurrence of pancreatitis has been reported as 0% and 0.7% in two prospective studies [38, 39] with a median follow up of 39 and 29.6 months, respectively, in patients treated with endoscopic sphincterotomy and no further cholecystectomy. However, in the first study [38], failed endoscopic procedures were excluded. Furthermore, symptoms related to lithiasis occurred in 34.5% of patients, 45% of whom required cholecystectomy. In the other study [39] a relapse of pancreatitis was observed in two of three failed endoscopic approaches. The risk of recurrence of pancreatitis was evaluated in a prospective study to be higher in patients in whom cholecystectomy was not performed after selective endoscopy, with an OR of 31.5% (95% CI: 7.22–137.84). In the group of patients that was not operated upon, the risk of recurrence was much higher in those not treated by sphincterotomy (37% vs. 0%, $p = 0.019$) [40]. A prospective study [41] reported controversial results, since no differences were observed in biliary lithiasis-related symptoms whether or not cholecystectomy was performed after the endoscopic approach with selective sphincterotomy at a follow up of 33 months. The number of patients in the two groups was different, with 83 patients operated upon and 34 not operated upon, with no indications about the characteristics of gallbladder lithiasis.

There were no differences in morbidity (8% vs. 13.7%) or mortality (1.9% vs. 1.8%) reported in an historical comparative study [42] of laparoscopic and open cholecystectomy, but a longer hospital stay was shown for the latter (1.5 vs. 7.5 days, $p < 0.05$).

Timing

A retrospective comparison between early (within a week) and delayed (after a week) laparoscopic cholecystectomy did not show significant differences for mild pancreatitis, while a higher conversion rate (67% vs. 18%, $p = 0.08$) and a longer post-operative stay (5.4 vs. 2.7 days, $p < 0.03$) in the early intervention were shown for severe cases [43]. A study including patients with peri-pancreatic fluid collection confirms these results [44], with a higher morbidity (44% vs. 5%, $p < 0.05$) and a longer post-operative hospital stay (9.2 vs. 20.1 days, $p < 0.05$) in the cases operated on early, compared with a delayed cholecystectomy. Resolution of peri-pancreatic fluid collection was registered in 40% of patients in the delayed group and in 21% of the patients in the early group.

A retrospective study [45] reported that patients operated on during the same admission have no increase in conversion rate (4% vs. 7.1%), less morbidity (11% vs. 43%, $p = 0.023$) and a shorter hospital stay (15.3 vs. 36.6 days, $p = 0.006$) when compared with patients operated upon during a delayed second admission. Furthermore, unprogrammed readmission due to pancreatitis was registered in 61.5% of these patients. A more recent study [46] reports the feasibility of laparoscopic cholecystectomy during the same admission, within two weeks of admission, for mild pancreatitis with intra-operative cholangiography and laparoscopic common bile duct exploration when required. A comparison with a delayed cholecystectomy group did not show differences in terms of operative time, morbidity or post-operative hospital stay, but the number of patients was limited and a common bile duct stone was retrieved in 14% of cases.

Recommendations and Guidelines

A number of guidelines on the treatment of acute biliary pancreatitis have been published [47–50]. Recommendations based on the highest level of evidence stated that urgent ERC with endoscopic sphincterotomy is indicated within 72 hours of symptom onset in severe acute pancreatitis, in the presence of jaundice or with evidence of cholangitis and common bile duct stones. Patients should undergo definitive management of gallstones during the same admission within 2 weeks in mild pancreatitis, while severe cases should be operated on for the biliary lithiasis after an improvement in general condition. The common bile duct should be investigated to ensure that it is clear of stones (intraoperative cholangiography, magnetic resonance cholangiopancreatography (MRCP), or endoscopic ultrasound) but there are no recommendations even in the more recent guidelines on the treatment of retrieved common bile duct stones in the setting of laparoscopic cholecystectomy. The choice between pre- or post-operative ERCP and intra-operative choledocotomy either by laparoscopy or by open surgery should be made depending on endoscopic or imaging availability and surgical expertise.

The Other Side of the Evidence

Treatment options are selected on the basis of the severity of pancreatitis. When local or systemic complications are present and clearly define the course of pancreatitis, recommendations for treatment are well stated. However, local or systemic complications cannot be confirmed in the early stages of pancreatitis. In this phase, severity may only be predicted by clinico-biological scores. However, such parameters are markedly influenced by the general condition of the patient and may be altered by associated diseases. CT severity index cannot be considered as predictive in the early stages, since the score is based on the presence of necrosis, which is not always evident within 72 hours of symptom onset [51].

Selected RCTs are based on selective sphincterotomy in the endoscopic approach groups. The confounding nature of a retrograde cholangiography that fails to diagnose microlithiasis or biliary sludge and the role of cannulation of the papilla without sphincterotomy in the evolution of pancreatitis were not taken into account. However, United Kingdom guidelines recommend sphincterotomy in all patients approached by. These results confirm that ERC whether or not retrograde cholangiography shows biliary stones [48].

In a prospective study [52], microlithiasis and biliary sludge were retrieved in 88.2% at 24 hours and in 68.6% between the fourth and the seventh day in the collected bile of patients with acute pancreatitis and a negative retrograde cholangiography. These results confirm that ERC without sphincterotomy may not be suitable for the evaluation of the common bile duct when retrograde cholangiography looks normal.

The randomised study of Nowak et al. [34], although published only in abstract form, shows a significant reduction in morbidity and mortality either in mild or severe pancreatitis with systematic sphincterotomy. A more recent abstract published by the same author [53] reports that the sooner sphincterotomy is performed after symptom onset, the lower the rates of morbidity and mortality are observed. A case control study has confirmed these results since evolution of pancreatitis to a more severe form was significantly reduced when early sphincterotomy was performed with a rate of 4.7% vs. 33.3% in the control group ($p < 0.02$) [54].

Low rates of severe evolving pancreatitis of 2.1% and 7% were found in two prospective studies with endoscopic sphincterotomy [38, 55]. A prospective study on acute biliary and idiopathic pancreatitis was initially comparative, but was interrupted due to better results with systematic sphincterotomy [56]. We based our own study on a prospective series of 129 acute pancreatitis treated by urgent endoscopic sphincterotomy [25, 57–59]. No mortality was observed in 99 patients treated within 48 hours of onset of symptoms, but three of 23 patients treated between 48 and 72 hours and one of seven of those treated after 72 hours of symptom onset evolved to severe pancreatitis. Two deaths were registered in patients in whom a failed endoscopic approach was attempted at 48 and 72 hours.

Comparative and prospective observational studies [35, 38, 53-56, 59] seem to show better outcomes of pancreatitis when sphincterotomy is systematically performed, while in studies on selective sphincterotomy such results are limited to severe pancreatitis. Although results of the endoscopic approach may be biased by selective sphincterotomy, the result of major concern is that in the control group up to 80% of pancreatitis cases have a benign course [29–31] as confirmed by other randomised and observational studies [60–62].

In a more recent RCT published by Acosta et al. [63] endoscopic sphincterotomy was performed in the study group in cases of failed spontaneous disobstruction of the common bile duct. This study confirms that early patency of the main bile duct, within 48 hours of onset of symptoms, reduces complications rate, since a risk difference of 70% was retrieved with the control group. However, only nine patients in the control group did not disobstruct spontaneously and these were compared to 52 patients in whom disobstruction was spontaneous or therapeutically achieved.

Early disobstruction of the common bile duct may reduce morbidity and mortality due to ongoing severe acute pancreatitis. Randomised studies with endoscopic systematic rather than selective sphincterotomy would have to be performed in order to confirm this hypothesis. However, such an approach is not suitable since a very high number of endoscopic procedures would be unprofitable due to the natural history of acute pancreatitis.

The group of patients for whom early patency of the main bile duct would prevent ongoing severe acute pancreatitis remain to be identified and the timing definition of early patency remains to be assessed.

New Hypotheses on Acute Biliary Pancreatitis

The data in the literature and our own experience allow us to advance some new hypotheses on acute biliary pancreatitis. A first hypothesis is that correct early diagnosis would help to select patients for therapeutic endoscopic sphineterotomy. An observation that may condition such a strategy is the effective relationship between detectable biliary obstruction and the course of pancreatitis. A second question is whether, as for cholangitis, other biliary complications, such as cholecystitis, may change or alter the course of pancreatitis. Some suggestions may finally be advanced on how early the patency of the main bile duct has to be checked in order to prevent, if possible, the evolution of severe pancreatitis.

Detectable Common Bile Duct, Choledocal Clearing, and the Course of Pancreatitis

Experimental and clinical studies [21, 53, 64] show that the course of acute biliary pancreatitis may be influenced by the duration of biliary obstruction. Data in the literature do not allow confirmation of such a correlation, since timing starts from admission rather than from onset of symptoms in a majority of publications, and since different criteria to evaluate the severity of pancreatitis and different diagnostics and treatment modalities were also reported.

Some observations may, however, be considered. In the study of Neoptolemos et al. [29], 25% of the cases of mild acute pancreatitis proved to have a common bile duct stone at 72 hours from admission. In our experience, biliary lithiasis was retrieved in 72.9% of patients within 48 hours of symptom onset and 45.4% after 48 hours of the predicted mild pancreatitis [59]. Other epidemiological data appear significant: the finding of common bile duct stones during intra-operative cholangiography in patients submitted to cholecystectomy in the course of a mild pancreatitis has been reported in 4.6% and 11% of cases [65, 66] between 4 and 7 days, respectively, of the acute episode. Only one study did not find common bile duct stones in patients operated 4 days after the acute episode of mild pancreatitis; however, a selection bias has to be taken into account since the sample was extracted from a series of laparoscopic cholecystectomies and criteria for inclusion were hyperamylasemia 2N and cholelithiasis [67]. In the study of Fan et al. [30] nine of 58 cases approached with a conservative treatment evolved to a severe pancreatitis, in eight of these cases pancreatitis was of biliary origin and only four of them proved to have a choledcolithiasis at ERCP. In his study, Oria [36] reported five cases of new onset of organ failure in patients successfully treated by endoscopic sphincterotomy within 48 hours of symptom onset; however, evolution of pancreatitis was evaluated only on the basis of organ failure and a correlation with pancreatic necrosis was not reported.

A correlation between persistent obstruction and severity of pancreatitis has not been proven in all cases. Finding of common bile duct stones in 25% of patients at 72 hours and 11% at 4 days in mild acute pancreatitis implies that not all patients with persistent biliary obstruction have severe acute pancreatitis. Other factors, such as genetic predisposition, different combinations of anatomical varieties of the sphincter of Oddi and stone dimension [19] may have to be taken into account. Other hypotheses may be considered, such as that the duration of obstruction necessary to induce severe pancreatitis could be different among patients, or the hypothesis that succeeding gallbladder stone migration may play a role [68]. The greater rate of retrieved common bile duct stones in severe acute pancreatitis may be explained by the distribution of probability of all the required factors necessary to induce severity rather than the expression of a direct physiopathologically proven correlation. Based on this hypothesis, the probability that a patient with acute pancreatitis has a persistent obstruction is a priori 50%. Based on epidemiological data, this value may be adjusted to 40% at 48 hours from symptom onset. The distribution of the probability of a second factor necessary to induced severe pancreatitis would be a priori 50% in patients with and 50% in patients without obstruction; as a result persistent obstruction and a second factor would be found in 25% of patients, or more precisely in 20%, if a 48 hour timing is considered. The reported 20% prevalence of severe acute pancreatitis seems to confirm this theory.

Furthermore, patients with confirmed mild pancreatitis may have an undetectable biliary lithiasis, although the percentage decreases during the first days of pancreatitis, probably due to early spontaneous clearing of the main bile duct. The negative retrograde cholangiography in severe pancreatitis in the study of Fan [30] may be explained by microlithiasis or biliary sludge; these may be considered as non-detectable biliary lithiasis, which may reduce bile flow through the papilla. Based on the physiopathological theory of the biliary obstruction and on results of experimental and clinical studies such as those of Acosta [63], it can be hypothesised that it is the early restored patency of the common bile duct that helps to prevent severe evolution of pancreatitis. This concept is slightly different from that of negative diagnostic investigations by ERC for the common bile duct: as it has been proven by a randomised study [36], early diagnosis of common bile duct stones as a selection of patients to treat in the early stage of pancreatitis is not effective for the prevention of severe evolution of pancreatitis.

Acute Biliary Pancreatitis and Acute Cholecystitis

There are no specific studies, but only isolated reports on associated cholecystitis during acute biliary pancreatitis. Fan et al. [30] reported a case of sepsis due to gangrenous cholecystitis, Oria et al. [36] reported five case of phlegmonous or perforated cholecystitis and in our experience, of 217 cases of acute biliary pancreatitis, 26 acute cholecystitis were suspected and pathological examination showed that five of them were phlegmonous and one was gangrenous (data not published). Acute cholecystitis, as well as acute cholangitis, may influence the course of pancreatitis due to possible ongoing sepsis. The prevalence of severe acute cholecystitis is estimated to be less than 5% based on data in the literature [30, 36, 59]: it is slightly less frequent than that of cholangitis, which is reported to be 3–10% [29, 69, 70]. While cholangitis has been highlighted due to the benefit of early endoscopic treatment, acute cholecystitis has remained in the shadows of the failed conservative or endoscopic treatment.

Timing of Early Biliary Patency

Based on physiopathology, it can be considered that once pancreatic necrosis has developed, it will dictate the course of the pancreatitis. An intervention that would prevent such a severe evolution of the pancreatitis would therefore have to be performed before necrosis developed. Physiopathological studies have reported that the enzymatic cascade is activated within 24 hours; however, the peak of mediators in the bloodstream is reached at 48 hours, inducing the known systemic manifestations and local evolution of the pancreatitis [18, 20]. Clinical studies on early biliary disobstruction report very low complications and mortality, with a benign course of the pancreatitis when patency of the common bile duct is granted within 24 and no more than 48 hours from symptom onset [53, 63]. Based on these observations, patency of the common bile duct would ideally be performed within 48 hours. However, since no evidence has yet been found, it may be considered that untill necrosis is not detectable, restored patency of the common bile duct may play a role in the evolution of the pancreatitis.

Conclusion

Until there is other evidence, new onset of acute pancreatitis should be considered as an emergency even in patients who are not critically ill. When the course of pancreatitis is demarcated, treatment strategies are well defined. Although the exact relationship between common bile duct lithiasis and the course of pancreatitis is not well understood, early restored patency of the main bile duct, spontaneous or therapeutic, may prevent a severe evolution of the pancreatitis. The endoscopic approach has proven to be effective, but sphincterotomy has to be systematically performed. Due to the high rate of pancreatitis with a benign course, without treatment such an invasive procedure cannot be proposed routinely.

Intra-operative cholangiography represents a way to check early patency of the main bile duct without an invasive procedure on the papilla. Such an early trans-cystic cholangiographic approach allows the patency of the common bile duct to be determined, since bile flow through the papilla can be assessed without uncertainty. In the cases of stone obstruction, a less traumatic procedure on the papilla than traditional endoscopic sphincterotomy should be performed by way of a laparoscopic and endoscopic approach with a Rendez-vous technique.

Since cholecystectomy is necessary to complete acute biliary pancreatitis treatment, a prospective trial to verify the feasibility of such an approach in the very early stage of pancreatitis has been performed in our institution. Preliminary results show that it is feasible without the increase in septic complications reported by some authors, since the laparoscopic cholecystectomy is performed in the early stage of pancreatitis when necrosis has not still developed. A randomised multicentre study would verify the efficacy of such an approach on the evolution of pancreatitis and correlated morbidity and mortality.

References

1. Cavallini G, Frulloni L, Bassi C et al; ProInf-AISP Study Group (2004) Prospective multicentre survey on acute pancreatitis in Italy (ProInf-AISP): results on 1005 patients. Dig Liver Dis 36:205-211
2. Neoptolemos JP, Davison BR, Winder AF, Vallance D (1988) Role of duodenal bile crystal analysis in the investigation of "idiopathic"pancreatitis. Br J Surg 79:450-453
3. Ross E, Navarro S, Bru C et al (1991) Occult microlithiasis in "idiopathic" acute pancreatitis: prevention of relapses by cholecystectomy or ursodesoxycholic acid therapy. Gastroenterology 101:1071-1079
4. Lee SP, Nicholls JF, Park HZ (1992) Biliary sludge as a cause of acute pancreatitis. N Engl J Med 326:589-593
5. Acosta JM, Pellegrini CA, Skinner DB (1990) Etiology and pathogenesis of acute biliary pancreatitis. Surgery 88:118-125
6. Opie EL (1901) The etiology of acute hemorrhagic pancreatitis. Bull Johns Hopkins 12:182-188
7. Acosta JM, Rossi R, Galli OM et al (1978) Early surgery for acute gallstone pancreatitis: evaluation of a systematic approach. Surgery 83:367-370
8. Stone HH, Fabian TC, Dunlop WE (1981) Gallstone pancreatitis: biliary tract pathology in relation to time of operation. Ann Surg 194:305-312
9. Kelly TR, Wagner DS (1988) Gallstone pancreatitis: a prospective randomized trial of the timing of surgery. Surgery 104:600-605
10. Frei GJ, Frei VT, Thirlby RC, McClelland RN (1986) Biliary pancreatitis: clinical presentation and surgical management. Am J Surg 151:170-175
11. Ranson JH (1979) The timing of biliary surgery in acute pancreatitis. Ann Surg 189:654-663
12. McKay CJ, Evans S, Sinclair M et al (1999) High early mortality rate from acute pancreatitis in Scotland, 1984-1995. Br J Surg 86:1302-1305
13. Isenmann R, Rau B, Beger HG (2001) Early severe acute pancreatitis: characteristics of a new subgroup. Pancreas 22:274-278
14. Toh SK, Phillips S, Johnson CD (2000) A prospective audit against national standards of the presentation and management of acute pancreatitis in the South of England. Gut 46:239-243
15. de Beaux AC, Palmer KR, Carter DC (1995) Factors influencing morbidity and mortality in acute pancreatitis; an analysis of 279 cases. Gut 37:121-126
16. Yadav D, Lowenfels AB (2006) Trends in the epidemiology of the first attack of acute pancreatitis: a systematic review. Pancreas 33:323-330
17. Mofidi R, Duff MD, Wigmore SJ et al (2006) Association between early systemic inflammatory response, severity of multiorgan dysfunction and death in acute pancreatitis. Br J Surg 93:738-744
18. Zyromski N, Murr MM (2003) Evolving concepts in the pathophysiology of acute pancreatitis. Surgery 133:235-237
19. van Brummelen SE, Venneman NG, van Erpecum KJ, VanBerge-Henegouwen GP (2003) Acute idiopathic pancreatitis: does it really exist or is it a myth? Scand J Gastroenterol Suppl (239):117-122
20. Frossard JL, Hadengue A (2001) Acute pancreatitis: new physiopathological concepts. Gastroenterol Clin Biol 25:164-176
21. Acosta JM, Ronzano GD, Pellegrini CA (2000) Ampullary obstruction monitoring in acute gallstone pancreatitis: a safe, accurate, and reliable method to detect pancreatic ductal obstruction. Am J Gastroenterol 95:122-127
22. Safrany L, Cotton PB (1981) A preliminary report: urgent duodenoscopic sphincterotomy for acute gallstone pancreatitis. Surgery 89:424-428

23. Rosseland AR, Solhaug JH (1984) Early or delayed endoscopic papillotomy (EPT) in gallstone pancreatitis. Ann Surg 199:165-167
24. McCune WS, Shorb PE, Moscovitz H (1968) Endoscopic cannulation of the ampulla of vater: a preliminary report. Ann Surg 167:752-756
25. Borzellino G, Ricci F, Veraldi D, Cordiano C (1994) Role of endolaparoscopic surgery in acute biliary pancreatitis. In: Lezoche E, Paganini AM, Berci G. Thoraco-laparoscopic and minimally invasive surgery. Edizione Documento Editoriale, pp 145-148
26. Rhodes M, Armstrong CP, Longstaff A, Cawthorn S (1193) Laparoscopic cholecystectomy with endoscopic retrograde cholangiopancreatography for acute gallstone pancreatitis. Br J Surg 80:247
27. Pellegrini CA (1993) Surgery for gallstone pancreatitis. Am J Surg 165:515-518
28. Ayub K, Imada R, Slavin J (2004) Endoscopic retrograde cholangiopancreatography in gallstone-associated acute pancreatitis. Cochrane Database Syst Rev 18(4):CD003630
29. Neoptolemos JP, Carr Locke DL, London NJ et al (1988) Controlled trial of urgent endoscopic retrograde cholangiopancreatography and endoscopic sphincterothomy versus conservative treatment for acute pancreatitis due to gallstones. Lancet 2:979-983
30. Fan St, Lai E, Mak F et al (1993) Early treatment of acute biliary pancreatitis by endoscopic papillotomy. N Engl J Med 328:228-232
31. Folsch UR, Nitsche R, Ludtke R et al (1997) Early ERCP and papillotomy compared with conservative treatment for acute biliary pancreatitis. The German study group on acute biliary pancreatitis. N Engl J Med 336:237-242
32. Heinrich S, Schäfer M, Rousson V, Clavien PA (2006) Evidence-based treatment of acute pancreatitis: a look at established paradigms. Ann Surg 243:154-168
33. Sharma VK, Howden CW (1999) Metaanalysis of randomized controlled trials of endoscopic retrograde cholangiography and endoscopic sphincterotomy for the treatment of acute biliary pancreatitis. Am J Gastroenterol 94:3211-3214
34. Nowak A, Nowakowska-Dulawa E, Marek TA, Rubicka J (1995) Final results of the prospective randomized, controlled study of endoscopic sphincterotomy versus conventional management in acute biliary pancreatitis. Gastroenterology 108(Suppl):A380
35. Zhou MQ, Li NP, Lu RD (2002) Duodenoscopy in treatment of acute gallstone pancreatitis. Hepatobiliary Pancreat Dis Int 1:608-610
36. Oría A, Cimmino D, Ocampo C et al (2007) Early endoscopic intervention versus early conservative management in patients with acute gallstone pancreatitis and biliopancreatic obstruction: a randomized clinical trial. Ann Surg 245:10-17
37. Chang L, Lo S, Stabile BE et al (2000) Preoperative versus postoperative endoscopic retrograde cholangiopancreatography in mild to moderate gallstone pancreatitis: a prospective randomized trial. Ann Surg 231:82-87
38. Gislason H, Vetrhus M, Horn A et al (2001) Endoscopic sphincterotomy in acute gallstone pancreatitis: a prospective study of the late outcome. Eur J Surg 167:204-208
39. Welbourn CR, Beckly DE, Eyre-Brook IA (1995) Endoscopic sphincterotomy without cholecystectomy for gall stone pancreatitis. Gut 37:119-120
40. Hernandez V, Pascual I, Almela P et al (2004) Recurrence of acute gallstone pancreatitis and relationship with cholecystectomy or endoscopic sphincterotomy. Am J Gastroenterol 99:2417-2423
41. Kaw M, Al-Antably Y, Kaw P (2002) Management of gallstone pancreatitis: cholecystectomy or ERCP and endoscopic sphincterotomy. Gastrointest Endosc 56:61-65
42. Schwesinger WH, Page CP, Gross GW et al (1998) Biliary pancreatitis: the era of laparoscopic cholecystectomy. Arch Surg 133:1103-1106
43. Tang E, Stain SC, Tang G et al (1995) Timing of laparoscopic surgery in gallstone pancreatitis. Arch Surg 130:496-500
44. Nealon WH, Bawduniak J, Walser EM (2004) Appropriate timing of cholecystectomy in patients who present with moderate to severe gallstone-associated acute pancreatitis with peripancreatic fluid collections. Ann Surg 239:741-751
45. Alimoglu O, Ozkan OV, Sahin M et al (2003) Timing of cholecystectomy for acute biliary pancreatitis: outcomes of cholecystectomy on first admission and after recurrent biliary pancreatitis. World J Surg 27:256-259
46. Griniatsos J, Karvounis E, Isla A (2005) Early versus delayed single-stage laparoscopic eradication for both gallstones and common bile duct stones in mild acute biliary pancreatitis. Am Surg 7:682-686
47. Uhl W, Warshaw A, Imrie C et al; International Association of Pancreatology (2002) IAP Guidelines for the Surgical Management of Acute Pancreatitis. Pancreatology 2:565-573
48. Working Party of the British Society of Gastroenterology; Association of Surgeons of Great Britain and Ireland; Pancreatic Society of Great Britain and Ireland; Association of Upper GI Surgeons of Great Britain and Ireland (2005) UK guidelines for the management of acute pancreatitis. Gut 54 Suppl 3:1-9
49. Sauerland S, Agresta F, Bergamaschi R et al (2006) Laparoscopy for abdominal emergencies: evidence-based guidelines of the European Asso-

ciation for Endoscopic Surgery. Surg Endosc 20:14-29
50. Kimura Y, Takada T, Kawarada Y et al (2006) JPN Guidelines for the management of acute pancreatitis: treatment of gallstone-induced acute pancreatitis. J Hepatobiliary Pancreat Surg 13:56-60
51. Toosie K, Chang L, Renslo R et al (1997) Early computed tomography is rarely necessary in gallstone pancreatitis. Am Surg 63:904-907
52. Kohut M, Nowak A, Nowakowska-Duiawa E, Marek T (2002) Presence and density of common bile duct microlithiasis in acute biliary pancreatitis. World J Gastroenterol 8:558-561
53. Nowak A, Nowakowska-Dulawa E, Marek TA, Kaczor R (1996) Timing of endoscopic sphincterotomy for acute biliary pancreatitis. Gastrointest Endosc 143:401 (Abstract)
54. Pezzilli R, Billi P, Barakat B et al (1998) Effects of early ductal decompression in human biliary acute pancreatitis. Pancreas 16:165-168
55. Billi P, Barakat B, D'Imperio N, Pezzilli R (2003) Relapses of biliary acute pancreatitis in patients with previous attack of biliary pancreatitis and gallbladder in situ. Dig Liver Dis 35:653-655
56. Cuilleret J, Balique JG, Barthelemy C et al (1998) What place for endoscopic sphincterotomy in treatment of acute pancreatitis? Chirurgie 123:131-137
57. Ricci F, Castaldini G, de Manzoni G et al (1997) Minimally invasive treatment of acute biliary pancreatitis. Surg Endosc 11:1179-1182
58. Ricci F, Castaldini G, de Manzoni G et al (2002) Treatment of gallstone pancreatitis:six-year experience in a single center. World J Surg 26:85-90
59. Borzellino G, De Manzoni G, Castaldini G et al (2002) Endoscopic, percutaneous and laparoscopic treatment for acute biliary pancreatitis. Ann Chir 127:461-466
60. Anglade D, Letoublon C, Russier Y et al (2000) Is it useful to maintain specific scores for the early determination of the severity of acute pancreatitis? Ann Chir 125:325-333
61. Blum T, Maisonneuve P, Lowenfels AB, Lankisch PG (2001) Fatal outcome in acute pancreatitis: its occurrence and early prediction. Pancreatology 1:237-241
62. Johnson CD, Abu-Hilal M (2004) Persistent organ failure during the first week as a marker of fatal outcome in acute pancreatitis. Gut 53:1340-1344
63. Acosta JM, Katkhouda N, Debian KA et al (2006) Early ductal decompression versus conservative management for gallstone pancreatitis with ampullary obstruction: a prospective randomized clinical trial. Ann Surg 243:33-40
64. Runzi M, Saluja A, Lerch MM et al (1993) Early ductal decompression prevents the progression of biliary pancreatitis: an experimental study in the opossum. Gastroenterology 105:157-164
65. Shayan H, Kopac D, Sample CB (2007) The role of intraoperative cholangiogram in the management of patients recovering from acute biliary pancreatitis. Surg Endosc 21:1549-1552
66. Isla A, Griniatsos J, Rodway A (2003) Single-stage definitive laparoscopic management in mild acute biliary pancreatitis. J Laparoendosc Adv Surg Tech A 13:77-81
67. Himal HS (1999) Preoperative endoscopic retrograde cholangiopancreatography (ERCP) is not necessary in mild gallstone pancreatitis. Surg Endosc 13:782-783
68. Arendt T, Monig H, Stuber E et al (2000) Gallstones, the choledochoduodenal junction and initiation of acute pancreatitis: are two stones the culprits rather than one stone? Med Hypotheses 54:570-573
69. Shimizu S, Chijiiwa K, Yamaguchi K, Tanaka M (1997) Gallstone pancreatitis: Sixteen years of clinical management. J Hepatobiliary Pancreat Surg 4:436-440
70. Chang L, Lo SK, Stabile BE et al (1998) Gallstone pancreatitis: a prospective study on the incidence of cholangitis and clinical predictors of retained common bile duct stones. Am J Gastroenterol 93:527-531

Chapter 30

Incidence and Management of Mirizzi Syndrome

Markus K. Müller, Frauke Löhlein, Markus Schäfer

Introduction

Mirizzi syndrome is a rare clinical entity that is defined as a benign mechanical obstruction of the hepatic duct caused by an impacted gallstone in the gallbladder neck or cystic duct. It includes a wide spectrum of anatomical changes, ranging from simple gallstone impaction with biliary obstruction to complete erosion of the gallbladder wall and hepatic duct with consecutive cholecysto-choledochal fistula formation.

The reported incidence of Mirizzi syndrome in patients undergoing cholecystectomy ranges from 0.3% to 1.4% [1, 2]. Yet, some Native Americans (those of Navajo and Zuni heritage) reveal an increased incidence of up to 2.7% [3]. The true incidence of Mirizzi syndrome is unknown, since most cases occur in symptomatic patients undergoing biliary surgery, while all others remain undetected.

Since laparoscopic cholecystectomy has almost completely replaced open cholecystectomy for the treatment of symptomatic gallstone disease and new imaging modalities, e.g., magnetic resonance cholangiopancreatography (MRCP), have become widely available, Mirizzi syndrome has attracted some clinical interest again. Its association with gallbladder cancer further impacts on its management.

History and Classification

The first descriptions of bile duct obstruction as a sequela of an impacted gallstone and its local inflammatory changes were published at the beginning of the twentieth century by Kehr and Ruge, respectively [4, 5].

In 1948, Pablo Mirizzi (1893–1964, a surgeon in Argentina) reported a "functional hepatic syndrome" in patients with compression of the common hepatic duct related to an impacted gallstone in the gallbladder neck or cystic duct [6]. He erroneously assumed that different local factors, such as impacted gallstones, inflammatory changes in the hepatoduodenal ligament, recurrent cholangitis, or aberrant vessels, might trigger a spasm in a circular muscular sphincter in the hepatic duct. Although it had long been obvious that there was no sphincter in the extrahepatic bile ducts, the name coined for the clinical entity of recurrent cholangitis and obstructive jaundice caused by external compression of the common hepatic duct by an impacted gallstone in the gallbladder neck was 'Mirizzi syndrome'.

The clinical feature of a cholecystobiliary fistula was first described by Puestow in 1942, and during the 1950s some additional cases were reported by Mirizzi and others [7]. A first classification of different types of cholecystobiliary fistulas based on 24 cases was then proposed by Corlette and Bismuth in 1975 [8].

With the advent of endoscopic retrograde cholangiopancreatography (ERCP) during the early 1980s, new insights into the anatomical features of Mirizzi syndrome were possible. In 1982 McSherry et al. proposed a novel classification of two different types of Mirizzi syndrome based on the ERCP findings [9]. Type I is defined as simple external compression of the hepatic or common bile duct by an impacted large gallstone in the cystic duct or Hartmann's pouch while the gallbladder and the common hepatic duct remain free of any lesion. Type II is characterized by the presence of a cholecystobiliary fistula. It is assumed that the long-standing local inflammation makes partial or complete penetration of an impacted gallstone into the extrahepatic bile duct system easier by erosion of the gallbladder wall and bile duct wall, respectively. Some years later, Csendes et al. proposed a more detailed classification with four different types of Mirizzi syndrome [10]. Type I is defined in a similar way to McSherry's type I, external compression of the extrahepatic bile ducts by an impacted gallstone being the main criterion. Type II lesions reveal a limited partial defect affecting up to one third of the circumference of the common bile duct, while type III lesions have a more extensive defect (up to two thirds of the circumference of the common bile duct). In type IV, the entire wall of the common bile duct is destroyed, with a consequent correspondingly large communication between the gallbladder and common

McSherry classification	Type I	Type II		
Csendes classification	Type I	Type II	Type III	Type IV
Morphology	External compression by an impacted stone	Presence of cholecystobiliary fistula, subtype depend on size of tissue defect		
	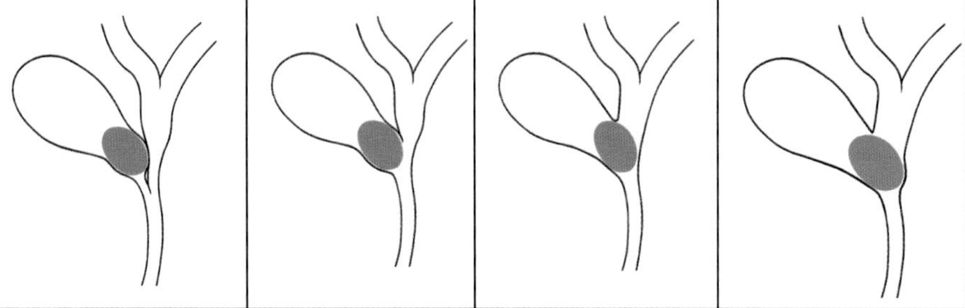			
Surgical therapy	Tootal cholecystectomy; if not possible, partial to subtotal resection	Partial cholecystectomy, repair of bile duct lesion by suturing, T-tube insertion, or choledochoplasty; if not possible, Roux-en-Y hepaticojejunostomy		Roux-en-Y hepaticojejunost omy

Fig. 30.1. Classification systems and type-related surgical treatment

bile duct (Fig. 30.1). Although more classification systems for Mirizzi syndrome have been proposed during the last three decades, the McSherry and Csendes classifications are the ones currently used in clinical practice and publications [11]. The ultimate goal of all these classification systems is to enable surgeons to tailor the surgical treatment to the individual case.

Even though precise classification systems are available, preoperative recognition of Mirizzi syndrome remains difficult, and the majority of cases are detected intraoperatively. Particularly if jaundice is lacking as a warning clinical symptom, ERCP and MRCP are not routinely used before cholecystectomy.

Clinical Symptoms

The two predominant clinical symptoms are right upper quadrant pain and jaundice [3, 11–15]. Pain is generally reported by most patients, and there is no association with any particular subtype of Mirizzi syndrome. In contrast, jaundice is less common in type I (<40%) than in types II–IV (>60–80%) [12, 13]. Jaundice can occur in recurrent episodes rather than being present constantly. Fever, as the third symptom in the Charcot triad indicating cholangitis, is reported to occur with a frequency ranging from 15% to 50% [11, 12]. A long-standing history of recurrent biliary symptoms is frequently reported by the patients. Common laboratory findings are elevated transaminases, alkaline phosphatase, and hyperbilirubinemia [16].

Owing to the lack of pathognomonic symptoms and clear indications in the history, Mirizzi syndrome can only be suspected on the grounds of a clinical examination, and further investigations are necessary to establish an accurate diagnosis.

Diagnosis

It has been stressed by several authors that a precise preoperative diagnosis of Mirizzi syndrome is of crucial importance, both for the surgical planning and to prevent complications [11, 16, 17]. However, even though quite a number of imaging studies can now be performed, Mirizzi syndrome is diagnosed preoperatively in only 8–62% of patients [3, 10, 12, 16].

Ultrasonography (US) of the abdomen is widely used as a noninvasive screening test for the assessment of biliary disease [18]. A shrunken gallbladder together with a large gallstone in the gallbladder neck, dilatation of the proximal bile duct and intrahepatic bile ducts, and a common bile duct with a normal diameter below the obstruction are the typical radiological features suggesting Mirizzi syndrome.

Computed tomography (CT) shows similar findings to US regarding the biliary anatomy. However, CT provides additional valuable information on the area of the porta hepatis, making it possible to differentiate between Mirizzi syndrome and malignancy of the extrahepatic biliary system and gallbladder [11, 16, 19].

Magnetic resonance imaging (MRI) and MRCP are recently established noninvasive imaging techniques that provide an accurate delineation of the biliary anatomy [20–22]. MRCP can show the typical features of Mirizzi syndrome, such as external compression of the hepatic ducts by an impacted gall stone, and dilatation of the proximal biliary system (Fig. 30.2). Nonetheless, the precise role of MRCP in the detection of Mirizzi syndrome remains to be elucidated. In a similar way to CT, MRI can provide additional useful information on the surrounding tissue of the gallbladder and porta hepatis.

ERCP is still our mainstay in the diagnosis of Mirizzi syndrome [11, 16]. ERCP

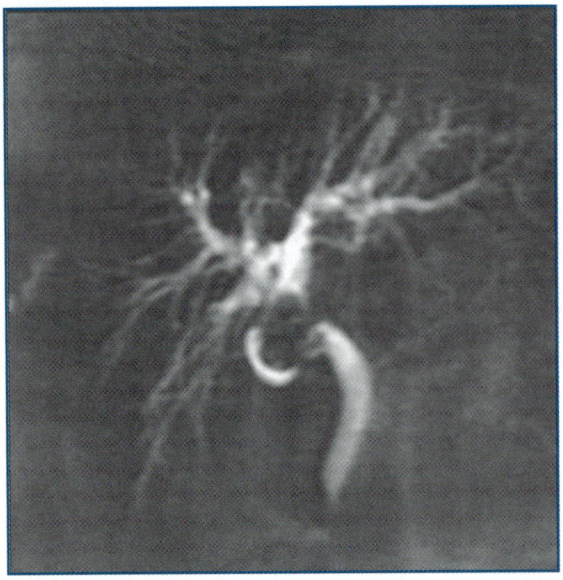

Fig. 30.2. Magnetic resonance cholangiopancreatography (MRCP) showing Mirizzi syndrome type II

sharply depicts all anatomical changes that arise in Mirizzi syndrome, such as the curvilinear impression of an impacted gallstone on the common hepatic duct by extrinsic compression from the gallstone, dilatation of the proximal biliary system, cholecystobiliary fistula, and additional bile duct stones. In addition, ERCP offers several diagnostic options and therapeutic interventions, e.g., endoscopic US, brush cytology, stone extraction, and biliary stent placement. In a few cases, if ERCP is not possible, percutaneous transhepatic drainage (PTC) may be a technical alternative. The main disadvantages of PTC are that it is difficult to visualize the distal biliary system because of proximal bile duct obstruction and a low-lying cystic duct, and that fewer therapeutic options are available than with ERCP.

Treatment

Since preoperative diagnosis of Mirizzi syndrome is difficult, both intraoperative recognition and surgical experience in biliary surgery remain critical to the achievement of a good surgical result with no complications. The presence of chronic inflammatory changes with dense adhesion formation in the triangle of Calot, a shrunken gallbladder with an immobile gallstone in Hartmann's pouch, and a distorted anatomy of the porta hepatis are clinically highly suggestive of Mirizzi syndrome. While open surgical treatment represents the gold standard in management for Mirizzi syndrome, providing good short-term and long-term results, the role of laparoscopic surgery is still under debate. Regardless of whether or not the diagnosis is known preoperatively, surgical treatment strategies should be stratified according to the presence of a cholecystobiliary fistula.

Without Cholecystobiliary Fistula (McSherry Type I, Csendes Type I)

There is a wide range of local inflammatory changes in the triangle of Calot that may cause type I Mirizzi syndrome, so that different surgical approaches may be possible. Basically, any lesion of the biliary tract should be avoided. If there is only moderate inflammation, total cholecystectomy can be performed. In the case of major local inflammation severely hampering safe dissection of the cystic duct, the common hepatic duct, and the vascular structures of the porta hepatis, retrograde fundus-first cholecystectomy is the preferred approach. In many cases, complete cholecystectomy is not possible without injuring the common hepatic duct. Bornman and Terblanche proposed subtotal cholecystectomy for these cases, with the neck of the gallbladder left in place [23]. This procedure has been shown to be effective and safe for type I Mirizzi syndrome [1, 10, 24, 25]. The gallbladder is opened at a convenient point, and bile and gallstones are removed. The opening of the cystic duct is then identified from inside the gallbladder, followed by an attempt to remove impacted gallstones. The gallbladder is partially or even subtotally resected with a clear safety margin at the gallbladder neck. The cystic duct is secured, or if this seems to be too risky, a drain is placed until the cystic duct has closed spontaneously. The common bile duct should be explored by either intraoperative cholangiography or surgical dissection to exclude further causes of obstruction. A T-tube may be needed for temporary biliary decompression.

Cholecystobiliary Fistula (McSherry Type II, Csendes Types II–IV)

Jaundice is a very common clinical symptom in McSherry type II (Csendes type II–IV) Mirizzi syndrome; ERCP is often performed when it is observed, and in this way the presence of a cholecystobiliary fistula can be confirmed preoperatively. During operative dissection of the biliary system, a cholecystobiliary fistula must be strongly suspected if bile flows back from the common hepatic duct after removal of a previously impacted gallstone in the cystic duct.

The recommendations for surgical repair of a cholecystobiliary fistula are based solely on small series and the personal experience of distinguished experts [1, 8, 10–17]. The extent of the circumferential defect of the biliary tree, the local quality of the inflamed tissue and, finally, the surgeon's experience are the crucial factors that impact on the type of surgical repair. Partial cholecystectomy leaving a remnant of the gallbladder around the area of the fistula is the most popular surgical approach [8, 11]. Small defects of the common hepatic duct (Csendes type II) can be closed by suturing the fistula opening, a T-tube that is inserted distally to the fistula being used as temporary stenting in order to prevent leakage and stenosis attributable to circumferential scar formation. Larger defects of the biliary wall require a choledochoplasty to restore the circumference and tissue lost from the bile duct. Choledochoplasty can be performed by using either a gallbladder flap or the cystic duct as a pedunculated graft [26, 27]. The biliary tree is first explored through a choledochotomy distal to the fistula, after which a T-tube is inserted through the fistula and secured by the gallbladder remnant, which is closed around the T-tube. The use of vein patches and ligamentum teres as substitutes to cover large fistula defects has been described in case reports [28, 29].

For Csendes type IV Mirizzi syndrome, and for all cases in which a choledochoplasty is not feasible owing to extensive destruction of the common bile duct, a bilioenteric anastomosis represents the final option [1, 11, 16]. From a technical point of view, an anastomosis of the cholecysto-choledochal defect to a Roux-en-Y jejunal loop is constructed. Otherwise, complete transection of the bile duct proximal to the fistula is needed, and a hepaticojejunostomy must be performed. During recent years, hepaticojejunostomy has increasingly been preferred by most hepaticopancraticobiliary (HPB) surgeons, since it has a high success rate, also in long-term follow-up.

Mirizzi Syndrome and Gallbladder Cancer

Gallbladder cancer is a rare disease in most Western countries, while its incidence is higher in Eastern countries. Its development is fostered by long-standing gallstone disease and chronic cholecystitis, which are also predisposing risk factors for Mirizzi syndrome [30–33]. It may be difficult to differentiate between gallbladder cancer and Mirizzi syndrome preoperatively, since both have similar radiological features. Nevertheless, CT and MRI should be performed if there is any suspicion of a malignant bile duct obstruction.

The reported incidence of gallbladder cancer and Mirizzi syndrome occurring together ranges from 5% to 28% [12, 34–37]. Redaelli et al. found an alarmingly high rate of 27.8% of gallbladder cancer among patients with Mirizzi syndrome, while in most other series much lower coincidences were reported, ranging from 5% to 11% [12, 34–37]. These incidences are still several times as high as the reported incidences of gallbladder cancer in patients undergoing cholecystectomy for uncomplicated gallstone disease. The incidence of incidental gallbladder cancer is reported to range from 0.3% to 1.8% [34, 38, 39]. The wide differences in the incidence of gallbladder cancer between patients with Mirizzi syndrome and those with uncomplicated gallstone disease support the hypothesis of common risk factors predisposing for both conditions. Long-standing complicated gallstone disease with recurrent inflammatory episodes might cause Mirizzi syndrome first and then cancerous changes [34]. This idea is further supported by the clinical finding that patients with Mirizzi syndrome have a prolonged history of gallstone disease and are 10–20 years older than patients with uncomplicated gallstone disease [34].

The mainstay of surgical treatment of gallbladder cancer is still radical open cholecystectomy with removal of lymph nodes in the porta hepatis, and if necessary, bile duct resection with Roux-en-Y hepaticojejunostomy. Advanced tumor stages require additional liver resection to achieve R0 resection. Therefore, if there is any preoperative suspicion of malignancy, surgery should be performed by an open approach. A frozen section should be obtained in all cases in which gallbladder cancer is detected intraoperatively. Conversion from laparoscopy to an open approach is recommended, since reoperation after laparoscopic cholecystectomy has a less favorable long-term survival than one-stage open radical resection [11, 40]. Moreover, gallbladder perforation must be avoided to prevent local recurrence. Whether port-site metastases do occur more frequently, as was reported in the 1990s, is still under debate [41].

Laparoscopic Surgery in Treatment

The successful advent of minimally invasive surgery has induced major changes in the management of many gastrointestinal diseases during the last two decades. Laparoscopic cholecystectomy has almost completely replaced open cholecystectomy for the treatment of symptomatic gallstone disease and acute cholecystitis, which was previously considered to be a contraindication. Even laparoscopic bile duct exploration can be safely performed in centers dedicated to laparoscopy, although laparoscopic bile duct clearance has not been adopted as standard treatment by most laparoscopic surgeons. The overall incidence of bile duct injuries remains higher after laparoscopic than after open cholecystectomy, making a laparoscopic approach more hazardous particularly in difficult anatomical situations.

Since the diagnosis is often not known preoperatively, laparoscopic surgeons must be aware that they could be faced with Mirizzi syndrome intraoperatively. Careful dissection of the triangle of Calot, early recognition, and a low threshold for conversion are of utmost importance in order to prevent any bile duct injury and damage of the arterial supply of the liver. Whereas type I Mirizzi syndrome can be managed by a laparoscopic approach, conversion to open surgery is always mandatory in type II (Csendes type II-IV) Mirizzi syndrome [11, 12]. Laparoscopic (sub)total cholecystectomy and stone removal is most often possible, while thorough bile duct evaluation and repair are generally too complicated for a minimally invasive approach. In most series, laparoscopic treatment of Mirizzi syndrome is associated with higher morbidity, ranging from 9% to 60% [11–14, 17]. Therefore, if it is already known before surgery that Mirizzi syndrome is present and a cholecysto-choledochal fistula is either strongly suspected or even known to be present, a primary open approach for open bile duct revision should be preferred; this is still the gold standard.

Endoscopic Treatment

Nonsurgical management of Mirizzi syndrome should be limited to patients with multiple co-morbidities who are at increased risk for surgery. Endoscopic treatment can also be used as an adjunct, to restore biliary flow before surgery. Removal of gallstones and stent placement are the most common endoscopic procedures. Standard gallstone extraction is performed by using either a balloon or a basket. Impacted or large stones may need further interventional treatment before removal. Mechanical, electrohydraulic, or extracorporeal lithotripsy or dissolution therapy is used to crush gallstones into small pieces that can be removed afterwards [42–46].

Endoscopic treatment has several limitations. Multiple sessions are often needed to achieve complete bile duct clearance, which cannot be accomplished even then in all patients. Patients who undergo repeated ERCP sessions are at increased risk of complications, e.g., bile leak and cholangitis with consecutive biliary sepsis. Only experienced gastroenterologists are qualified to perform such advanced procedures. Considerable technical equipment is necessary (e.g., endoscopic lithotripters). As a consequence, multiple sessions and the use of the sophisticated technical equipment mean higher costs. Percutaneous transhepatic management is used as a technical alternative only in patients who have not been helped by ERCP [47, 48]. There are few reports on it in the literature, and no standard is yet defined.

References

1. Baer HU, Matthews JB, Schweizer WP et al (1990) Management of Mirizzi syndrome and the surgical implications of cholecystocholedochal fistula. Br J Surg 77:743-745
2. Bower TC, Nagorney DM (1988) Mirizzi syndrome. HPB Surg 1:67-74
3. Curet MJ, Rosendale DE, Congilosi S (1994) Mirizzi syndrome in a Native American population. Am J Surg 168:616-621
4. Kehr H (1905) Die in meiner Klinik geübte Technik der Gallensteinoperationen, mit einem Hinweis auf die Indikationen und die Dauererfolge. Munich: JF Lehmann
5. Ruge E (1908) Beiträge zur Chirurgie der grossen Gallenwege (Ductus hepaticus, choledochus, und pancreaticus). Arch Clin Chir 78:47
6. Mirizzi P (1948) Syndrome del conducto epatico. J Int Chir 1948; 8:731-777
7. Puestow CB (1942) Spontaneous internal biliary fistula. Ann Surg 115:1053-1054
8. Corlette MB, Bismuth H (1975) Biliobiliary fistula. A trap in the surgery of cholelithiasis. Arch Surg 110:377-383
9. McSherry CK (1982) The Mirizzi syndrome: suggested classification and surgical therapy. Surg Gastroenterol 1:219-225
10. Csendes A, Diaz JC, Burdiles P et al (1989) Mirizzi syndrome and cholecystobiliary fistula: a unifying classification. Br J Surg 76:1139-1143
11. Lai ECH, Lau WY (2006) Mirizzi syndrome: history, present and future development. A NZ J Surg 76:251-257
12. Schäfer M, Schneiter R, Krähenbühl L (2003) Incidence and management of Mirizzi syndrome during laparoscopic cholecystectomy. Surg Endosc 17:1186-1190
13. Kok KY, Goh PY, Ngoi SS (1998) Management of Mirizzi's syndrome in the laparoscopic era. Surg Endosc 12:1242-1244
14. Yeh CN, Jan YY, Chen MF (2003) Laparoscopic treatment for Mirizzi syndrome. Surg Endosc 17:1573-1578
15. Al-Akeely MHA, Alam MK, Bismar HA et al (2005) Mirizzi syndrome: ten years experience from a teaching hospital. World J Surg 29:1687-1692
16. Ahlawat SK, Singhania R, Al-Kawas FH (2007) Mirizzi syndrome. Curr Treat Opt Gastroenterol 10:102-110
17. Tan KY, Ching HC, Chen CYY et al (2004) Mirizzi syndrome: noteworthy aspects of a retrospective study in one study. A NZ J Surg 74:833-837
18. Baron RL, Tublin ME, Petterson MS (2002) Imaging the spectrum of biliary tract disease. Radiol Clin N Am 40:1325-1354

19. Salloum RM, Koniaris L (2004) Image of the month. Mirizzi syndrome. Arch Surg 28:54-57
20. Becker CD, Grossholz M, Mentha G et al (1997) MR cholangiopancreatography:technique, potential indications, and diagnostic features of benign, postoperative, and malignant conditions. Eur J Radiol 7:865-874
21. Kim PN, Outwater EK, Mitchell DG (1999) Mirizzi syndrome: evaluation by MRI imaging. Am J Gastroenterol 94:2546-2550
22. Kaya D, Karcaaltincaba M, Akhan O et al (2006) MRCP diagnosis of Mirizzi syndrome in a pediatric patient: importance of T1-weighed gradient echo images for diagnosis. Pediatr Radiol 36:980-982
23. Bornmann PC, Terblanche J (1985) Subtotal cholecystectomy: for the difficult gallbladder in portal hypertension and cholecystitis. Surgery 98:1-6
24. Douglas PR, Ham JM (1990) Partial cholecystectomy. A NZ J Surg 60:595-597
25. Cottier DJ, McKay C. Anderson JR (1991) Subtotal cholecystectomy. Br J Surg 78:1326-1328
26. Chourdakis CN, Androulakakis PA, Lekakos NL (1976) Repair of the cholecystocholedochal fistulas using gallbladder patching. Arch Surg 111:197-199
27. Stugnell NA, Sali A (1995) Choledochoplasty for cholecystocholedochal fistula (Mirizzi syndrome type II): a case report and literature review. A NZ J Surg 65:285-288
28. Settaf A, Balafreij S (1993) Biliary surgery using the ligamentum teres. Technique for repairing loss of substance in the common bile duct. Ann Chir 47:529-533
29. Rutledge RH (1983) Methods of repair of noncircumferential bile duct defects. Surgery 93:333-342
30. Frauenschuh D, Greim R, Kraas E (2000) How to proceed in patients with carcinoma detected after laparoscopic cholecystectomy. Langenbecks Arch Surg 385:594-500
31. Lazcano-Ponce EC, Miquel JF, Munoz N et al (2001) Epidemiology and molecular pathology of gallbladder cancer. CA Cancer J Clin 2001; 51:349-364
32. Hsing AW, Bai Y, Andreotti G et al (2007) Family history of gallstones and the risk of biliary tract cancer and gallstones: A population-based study in Shanghai, China. Int J Cancer 121:832-838
33. Chow WH, Johansen C, Gridley G et al (1999) Gallstones, cholecystectomy and risk of cancers of the liver, biliary tract and pancreas. Br J Cancer 79:640-644
34. Prasad TLVD, Kumar A, Sikora SS et al (2006) Mirizzi syndrome and gallbladder cancer. J HBP Surg 13:323-326
35. Redaelli CA, Buchler MW, Schilling MK et al (1997) High coincidence of Mirizzi syndrome and gallbladder cancer. Surgery 121:58-63
36. Miller FH, Sica GT (1996) Mirizzi syndrome associated with gallbladder cancer and biliary-enteric fistulas. Am J Radiol 167:95-97
37. Nishio H, Kamiya J, Nagino M et al (2000) Biliobiliary fistula associated with gallbladder cancer. Br J Surg 87:1656-1657
38. Darmas B, Mahmud S, Abbas A, Baker AL (2007) Is there any justification for the routine histological examination of straightforward cholecystectomy specimens? Ann R Coll Surg Engl 89:238-241
39. Zgraggen K, Birrer S, Maurer CA et al (1998) Incidence of port site recurrence after laparoscopic cholecystectomy for preoperatively unsuspected gallbladder carcinoma. Surgery 124:831-835
40. Misra MC, Guleria S (2006) Management of cancer gallbladder found as a surprise on a resected gallbladder specimen. J Surg Oncol 93:690-698
41. Steinert R, Nestler G, Sagynaliev E et al (2006) Laparoscopic cholecystectomy and gallbladder cancer. J Surg Oncol 93:682-689
42. England RE, Martin DF (1997) Endoscopic management of Mirizzi's syndrome. Gut 40:272-276
43. Tsuyugucchi T, Saisho H, Ishihara T et al (2000) Long-term follow-up after treatment of Mirizzi syndrome by peroral cholangioscopy. Gastrointest Endosc 52:639-644
44. Benninger J, Rabenstein T, Farnbacher M et al (2004) Extracorporeal shockwaver lithotripsy of gallstones in cystic duct remnants and Mirizzi syndrome. Gastrointest Endosc 60:454-459
45. Delcenserie R, Joly JP, Dupas JL (1992) Endoscopic diagnosis and treatment of Mirizzi syndrome. J Clin Gastroenterol 15:343-346
46. Binmoeller KF, Thonke F, Soehendra N (1993) Endoscopic treatment of Mirizzi's syndrome. Gastrointest Endosc 39:532-536
47. Oxtoby JW, Yeong CC, West DJ (1994) Mirizzi syndrome treated by percutaneous stone removal. Cardiovasc Intervent Radiol 17:207-209
48. Adam A, Roddie ME, Benjamin IS (1993) Mirizzi syndrome—treatment with metallic endoprosthesis (case report). Clin Radiol 48:198-200

Chapter 31

Biliary Lithiasis in Children

Ciro Esposito, Marianna De Marco, Claudia della Corte, Raffaele Iorio, Pietro Vayro, Alessandro Settimi

Introduction

Cholelithiasis is generally considered an uncommon disease in children. The frequency of pediatric gallstones, documented in studies conducted at the end of the eighties in which patients were selected according to initial symptoms, was reported to be between 0.13 and 0.22% [1, 2]. However, in recent years, following the extensive use of abdominal ultrasound scanning (AUS) in the pediatric population, an increasing number of children with cholelithiasis have been identified. In a population-based study, the prevalence of cholelithiasis retrospectively evaluated in 4,200 children submitted to AUS for different reasons, such as typical biliary symptoms, general abdominal symptoms or routinely check-ups, was 1.9% [1, 3]. Further, following the routine use of ultrasound examination during pregnancy, fetal gallstones are emerging as a new entity. The prognosis of fetuses with gallstones is very good and complete spontaneous resolution between 1 and 12 months after birth is generally observed [2].

Although cholelithiasis in children is idiopathic in the majority of cases, many risk factors for pediatric cholelithiasis have been identified, including hemolytic disorders, family history of gallstones, obesity, total parenteral nutrition (TPN), hepatobiliary chronic disease, cystic fibrosis (CF), therapy with ceftriaxone or cyclosporine, abdominal surgery, IgA deficiency, Gilbert's disease and Down's syndrome [3–5]. A greater prevalence of cholelithiasis, approximately 20 times more than normal children, is reported in Down's syndrome. In adolescents, obesity represents an important risk factor, above all in Western countries.

On the basis of gallstone composition, cholelithiasis in children can be distinguished as:

1. Cholesterol stones: radiotransparent, yellow or green, round or faceted, smooth or mamillated, multiple or solitary and variable in diameter. They are composed of between 70 and 100% cholesterol.
2. Black pigment stones: radio-opaque, dark brown or black, small, multiple and with an irregular surface; they are composed of calcium bilirubinate in a protein matrix and are associated with hemolysis and TPN.
3. Mixed cholesterol stones: besides cholesterol, they also contain protein, bilirubin and carbonate.
4. Brown pigment stones: they have a rough surface and contain large amounts of fatty acid and calcium bilirubinate; they are formed when bacterial enzymes deconjugate bilirubin from glucuronic acid and hydrolyze phospholipids, making excess bilirubin and free fatty acids precipitate with calcium. They are associated with bile duct dilatation, bile stasis and bacterial infection [3, 6, 7].

In prepuberal children black pigment stones tend to predominate, but from adolescence onwards, the majority of stones are cholesterol [1, 3].

Biliary sludge is a non-shadowing, echogenic sediment present in the gallbladder lumen; its frequency in children has recently increased, with a current prevalence of 1.46%. It is generally considered a dynamic condition not predisposing to the development of gallstones [2, 8].

In the pediatric population cholelithiasis is often asymptomatic; in fact, in almost 40% of cases gallstones are diagnosed accidentally on ultrasound examination for causes unrelated to cholelithiasis [9, 10]. Symptomatic children can show colicky pain and jaundice often associated with nausea and vomiting. Colicky pain is described as a suddenly developing pain, usually located in the right upper quadrant or in the epigastrium, which may radiate to the back or right shoulder [11, 12]. In other cases children complain of non-specific abdominal pain, right upper quadrant or epigastric pain, tenderness, nausea, vomiting and food intolerance. In rare cases cholelithiasis can begin with complications such as cholecystitis, acute pancreatitis and cholangitis [13, 14]. Spontaneous perforation of the gallbladder is an extremely rare event in children; it appears above all in immunodeficient children, and is characterized by an acute abdomen [3, 15].

Little is known about the natural history and therapy of cholelithiasis in children. So far, guidelines for management of this disorder in the pediatric age are lacking.

Diagnosis

The most accurate and useful diagnostic test for the diagnosis of cholelithiasis is abdominal ultrasound scanning; it allows the recognition of echogenic foci and acoustic shadows with mobility in the gallbladder and assessment of gallbladder size and wall thickness and the diameter of the common bile duct [1, 16]. AUS is accurate for the diagnosis of gallstones in the gallbladder in up to 96% of patients [2, 17, 18]. Ultrasonographic diagnosis of biliary sludge is based on the presence of a non-shadowing, echogenic, intraluminal sediment.

An X-ray of the abdomen plays a marginal role in the diagnosis of cholelithiasis, in rare cases showing radio-opaque images in the right hypocondrium. This finding would be only useful for the choice of treatment because oral bile acid therapy is effective only for radiolucent gallstones [19, 20].

Laboratory tests are usually normal but in some cases, particularly in the presence of an obstruction of the biliary outflow and cholecystitis, they show an increased rate of aspartate aminotransferase (AST), alanine aminotransferase (ALT), gamma glutamyl transpeptidase (GGT), alkaline phosphatase (ALP), conjugated bilirubin and leucocytosis [1, 4, 21].

The introduction of ultrasound in pediatric cases has made cholecystography obsolete.

Magnetic resonance cholangiopancreatography (MRCP) has emerged as an accurate, noninvasive diagnostic modality for investigating the biliary and pancreatic ducts. It provides excellent anatomic details of the biliary tree and has a sensitivity of 81–100% and a specificity of 92–100% for detecting choledocholithiasis [2, 3, 22].

Endoscopic retrograde cholangiopancreatography (ERCP) can also be a useful tool in preoperative diagnosis and in the management of choledocholithiasis [23]. When compared to other tests such as ultrasonography and MRCP, ERCP has the advantage of providing a therapeutic option when gallstones are identified. Complications associated with ERCP include pancreatitis, cholangitis, perforation of the duodenum or bile duct and bleeding. These individual complications occur in 5–8% of patients [4, 24, 25]. The usefulness of this procedure is limited in the pediatric age because of a deficiency of adequate sized instruments.

Management of Children with Cholelithiasis

Guidelines for the management of cholelithiasis in adults are available. Cholecystectomy is recommended for symptomatic patients and for the asymptomatic patients with a predisposition for malignancy (calcified gallbladder wall or family history of gallbladder cancer). For asymptomatic patients, an expectant management with periodical clinical and echographic controls is recommended [2, 3, 26]. On the contrary, little is known about natural history and management of cholelithiasis in childhood.

Children with gallstones should be divided into two groups based on their clinical presentation: symptomatic or asymptomatic [1, 27]. Considering the low rate of complications of asymptomatic gallstones and the favorable natural history described in adults, an expectant management with periodical clinical and ultrasonographic controls is recommended [4, 28]. On the other hand, considering the low rate of post-operative complications and post-cholecystectomy syndrome for symptomatic gallstones, a surgical approach with laparoscopic cholecystectomy seems to be appropriate. Ursodeoxycholic acid (UDCA) should not be used to treat pediatric gallstones, except in cases of symptomatic children with contraindications to surgery in order to reduce the clinical symptoms [2, 3, 29, 30].

Cholelithiasis can also be due to hemolytic diseases that can provoke an increase in the concentration of biliary salts. These patients should therefore be followed with ultrasound monitoring to discover possible gallbladder pathologies, beyond the treatment for the hematological disorder.

Acalculous cholecystitis (AC) is more commonly found in children than adults. Two-thirds of cases result as a complication of other illnesses: trauma, shock, burns, sepsis or operative procedures [31, 32]. Contributing causes are obstruction, congenital tortuosity or narrowing of the cystic duct, decreased blood flow to the gallbladder, and long-term parenteral nutrition. Males are more commonly affected than females.

Another type of emergent gallbladder pathology is represented by Ceftriaxone-associated biliary pseudolithiasis, which is a benign condition, usually asymptomatic, that resolves spontaneously. Cessation of drug therapy is unnecessary and patients can be managed conservatively by observation. Knowledge of this condition is important in order to prevent unnecessary treatment [3, 33].

Medical Treatment

The pharmacological approach to pediatric cholelithiasis is based on the use of UDCA: the rationale of bile acid therapy is to interfere with the supersaturation of bile, which is the major factor responsible for the formation of cholesterol gallstones [2, 3, 34]. Oral bile acid therapy enriches the bile acid pool, reducing cholesterol saturation in bile and progressively dissolving cholesterol gallstones. The treatment of cholesterol radiolucent gallstones with UDCA is well documented in adults and is recommended for a specific subset of symptomatic patients with radiolucent gallstones less than 5 mm of diameter [4, 35]; on the contrary, there are few data regarding the use of UDCA in children for treatment of gallstones and guidelines for the selection of patients to be treated are lacking [36]. On the basis of the available data, UDCA in children is ineffective for the dissolution of gallstones probably because cholesterol is not the main component of stones [1, 37]. However, UDCA has a positive effect on abdominal discomfort in the vast majority of the symptomatic patients treated [10].

Surgical Treatment

The indications for surgery in cases of cholelithiasis in children are the same as those adopted in the adult population. Therefore, cholecystectomy is indicated in all cases of symptomatic cholelithiasis and in the presence of complications. The treatment for accidentally discovered cholelithiasis has been strongly influenced by the development of minimally invasive surgery (MIS). Although there are no guidelines universally accepted in pediatrics, it seems advisable to perform a follow-up of approximately 6 months and a medical therapy if necessary in asymptomatic patients [38, 39].

In both pediatric patients and adults, laparoscopic cholecystectomy (LC) has become the procedure of choice for the removal of the gallbladder disease and the best standard procedure to treat children with cholelithiasis. The benefit of this procedure in children is obvious: it is safe, effective, well tolerated, it results in a short hospital stay, early return to activity and reduced hospital expenses.

Preoperative evaluation should include verification of gallstones by ultrasound, as well as liver function tests [40].

Children are placed in a supine decubitus position on the operating table in a reverse Trendelenburg position. A nasogastric tube is positioned before surgery.

As for operative set-up, the surgeon can stand between the patient's legs (French position) or lateral to the patient (American position).

Most surgeons prefer to use open laparoscopy to introduce the first trocar. A 0-degree optics (5 or 10 mm) is always positioned infra-umbilically to give a general exposition of the abdomen.

The other three ports (5 or 3 mm) are positioned as follows: the first is placed in the upper midline just below the xiphoid appendix for the second operative instrument; the other two ports are placed along the right costal margin for the first operative instrument and for the grasper, which is used to retract the gallbladder fundus. Pneumoperitoneum pressure is kept between 8 and 12 mmHg [37, 41].

The first step in the surgical technique is to gently elevate the liver. The gallbladder may be immediately visible, or may be surrounded by omental adhesions that must be dissected.

The traction on the gallbladder fundus allows clear identification of the cystic duct.

Throughout dissection, the direction of the traction by an infundibular grasper is critical to prevent errors in identification of the biliary structures in this area [42].

With the grasper, the infundibulum of the gallbladder is retracted to expose Calot's triangle. A careful search for congenital biliary tree abnormalities, which are sometimes found in children, is carried out. Dissection is begun directly adjacent to the gallbladder.

The cystic duct is identified and isolated with a blunt dissection. After having identified the cystic duct–common bile duct junction, the cystic artery is bluntly dissected. Two clips are placed side by side as close to the gallbladder as possible and two similar clips are placed on the cystic duct. Enough space is left between the set of the clips to divide the duct with scissors. Two clips are placed on the artery. The artery is sectioned between the clips. The dissection of the gallbladder from its bed is initiated, taking care to stay away from the porta hepatis and to avoid perforation onto the gallbladder. Most surgeons use a hooked cautery for this phase. The gallbladder is then removed from its bed using a coagulating hook or sometimes with the aid of a harmonic hook. The gallbladder is always removed through the umbilical orifice.

Cholangiography before any dissection of Calot's triangle is advised in adults to avoid iatrogenic common bile duct injuries during dissection due to anomalous anatomy, but it is rarely adopted in pediatric patients [7, 43].

Complications

Bleeding during LC can vary from inconsequential oozing to major hemorrhage.

Excluding trocar site bleeding, the most frequent source of bleeding is represented by Calot's triangle and the hepatic bed. A safe and effective use of dissection and coagulation can usually solve this problem.

Dissection can be difficult above all in cases of inflamed gallbladder. The gallbladder wall is thinner in pediatric patients and sometimes there can be gallbladder perforation during dissection. Postoperative bile leaks or collections may be the result of common duct or right hepatic duct injury, cystic duct stump leakage or injury to an accessory bile duct [15, 19].

An accurate and delicate dissection can reduce these complications, considering that sometimes pediatric patients present with a biliary anatomic variations.

It is absolutely forbidden to use coagulation near clips in order to avoid a secondary clip dislocation. Injury to the main bile duct usually occurs during the dissection of Calot's triangle, exposing the cystic duct. Cephalad traction often causes the cystic duct to lie in a straight line with the common bile duct, causing the common duct to be mistaken for the cystic duct [23].

These complications are rare but reported in the literature, above all in less experienced centers [44].

Conclusion

Gallbladder stones are a frequent pathology in adults and LC is one of the most largely employed procedures in general surgery units. On the contrary, cholelithiasis is rare in children; for this reason, it is difficult to evaluate the validity of this procedure in a large case series of pediatric patients.

The presence of gallbladder stones is generally idiopathic, and their discovery is sometimes accidental during a sonographic exam performed to search for other abdominal pathologies. However, there are well-known predisposing factors to the development of gallbladder stones in children. Among infants affected by hemolytic disease—hemolytic anemia, for instance—the incidence of gallbladder stones is much higher than in the normal population; its reported incidence ranges from 10 to 40% in various series [3, 42].

The management of children with cholelithiasis requires great caution; an accurate hematological study is always necessary in order to detect possible underlying hematological disease.

In cases of incidentally discovered gallstones, an accurate follow-up is suggested, since a spontaneous resolution of the pathology is possible.

Non-calcified gallbladder stones in children generally disappear within 3–6 months. By contrast, surgery is needed for calcified stones in both non-symptomatic and symptomatic children.

Based on our experience, LC is the treatment of choice for symptomatic gallbladder in pediatric patients.

It is important to remember that in pediatric patients, owing to the small size of the abdominal cavity, it is preferable to place the first trocar using the open laparoscopy technique [34].

Moreover, for the same reason, laparoscopy in infants should be performed using very small instruments (3 or 5 mm in diameter). Technically, this approach is similar to the one employed for adults, although careful consideration of a child's anatomical differences is essential in order to avoid complications.

An interesting finding is that the gallbladder wall of infants is thinner than in adults, therefore perforations of the gallbladder wall are more frequent in children.

It is important to keep in mind that pediatric patients may have biliary tree anomalies, such as gallbladder duplication, ductal abnormalities, accessory bile ducts, or accessory cystic arteries.

These findings do not represent a contraindication to the laparoscopic procedure if the surgeon is able to perform a delicate and accurate dissection of the elements at the level of Calot's triangle [17, 19].

Bile duct injuries, which are often reported in adults, are very rare in children.

We were also able to observe that the junction between the cystic duct and the common bile duct is much more visible in children, due to the scarcity of fatty tissue and adhesions at the level of Calot's triangle at this age. This improved visualization makes the dissection of the cystic duct easier and less dangerous than in adult patients.

The presence of common bile duct stones in children is an extremely rare event; indeed, we have not come across any such cases in our series. At any rate, the presence of jaundice, dilatation of the biliary tree at ultrasonography, alkaline phosphatase and total bilirubin > 5 mg/dl above the normal range, and/or a history of pancreatitis are indications for a cholangiography or an ERCP.

With respect to the ERCP, the sequential approach of endoscopic sphincterectomy and stone extraction followed by LC is a safe and effective method in children as well as in adults, although we have no experience with this procedure [25, 37].

One important advantage is that LC in children can be associated, if necessary, with other technical procedures, such as the closure of a peritoneal vaginal duct in case of inguinal hernia; thus, a second operation or another incision can be avoided. However, if another procedure is required, laparoscopic expertise on the part of the surgeon is fundamental to avoid additional morbidity.

The most important key points are that pediatric patients need a complete preoperative evaluation to search for the possible coexistence of hematological diseases, an open laparoscopic technique to introduce the first trocar to reduce risk of complications, and a more accurate biliary dissection due to possible anatomic variations or anomalies [2, 31].

LC was found to be superior to the open conventional procedure, reducing the operating time, length of stay, diet resumption, and use of pain medication. The child is more pleased with his cosmetic results and activities are more promptly established. We also found that common bile duct stones can be managed safely with simultaneous endoscopic papillotomy and costs of LC are further reduced by employing re-usable equipment and selective cholangiographic indications.

References

1. Wesdorp I, Bosman D, de Graaff A et al (2003) Clinical presentation and predisposing factors of cholelithiasis and sludge in children. J Pediatr Gastroenterol Nutr 31:411-417
2. Suma V, Marini A, Bucci N et al (1998) Fetal gallstones: sonographic and clinical observations. Ultrasound Obstet Gynecol 12:439-441
3. Stringer MD, Taylor DR, Soloway RD (2003) Gallstones composition: are children different? J Pediatr 142:435-440
4. Al-Salem AH, Nourallah H (1997) Sequential endoscopic/laparoscopic management of cholelithiasis and choledocholithiasis in children who have sickle cell disease. J Pediatr Surg 32:1432-1435
5. Palanduz A, Yalcin I, Tonguc E et al (2000) Sonographic assessment of Ceftriaxone-associated biliary pseudolithiasis in children. J Clin Ultrasound 28:166-168
6. Al-Salem AH, Qaisaruddin S, Al-Abkari H et al (1997) Laparoscopic versus open cholecystectomy in children. Pediatr Surg Int 12:587-590
7. Davidoff AM, Branum GD, Murray EA et al (1992) The technique of laparoscopic cholecystectomy in children. Ann Surg 215:186-191

8. Caprotti R, Franciosi C, Motta M et al (1999) Combined laparoscopic splenectomy and cholecystectomy for the treatment of hereditary spherocytosis: Is it safe and effective? Surg Laparosc Endosc Percutan Tech 9:203-206
9. Carney DE, Kosoka ER, Resercola FJ et al (2004) Predictors of successful outcome after cholecystectomy for biliary dyskinesia. J Ped Surg 39:813-816
10. Esposito C, Gonzales Sabin MA, Corcione F et al (2001) Results and complications of laparoscopic cholecystectomy in childhood. Surg Endosc 15:890-892
11. Iwai N, Goto Y, Kano M et al (1985) Cancer of gallbladder in a 9-year-old girl. Z Kinderchir 40:106-107
12. Farah RA, Rogers ZR, Thompson WR et al (1997) Comparison of laparoscopic and open splenectomy in children with hematologic disorders. J Pediatr 131:41-46
13. Holcomb GW, Naffis D (1993) Laparoscopic cholecystectomy in infants. Pediatr Ann 22:657-662
14. Jawad AJ, Al-Khudairy N, Al-Sanie A (1995) Laparoscopic cholelithiasis in infancy. Pediatr Surg Int 10:212-214
15. Holcomb GW, Morgan WM, Neblett WW et al (1999) Laparoscopic cholecystectomy in children: lesson learned from the first 100 patients. J Pediatr Surg 34:1236-1240
16. Kasirajan K, Obermeyer RJ, Kehris J et al (1998) Microinvasive laparoscopic cholecystectomy in pediatric patients. J Laparoendosc Adv Surg Tech 8:131-135
17. Kim PC, Wesson D, Superina R, Filler R (1995) Laparoscopic cholecystectomy versus open cholecystectomy in children: which is better? J Pediatr Surg 30:971-973
18. Miltenburg DM, Schaffer R, Breslin T, Brandt ML (2000) Changing indications for pediatric cholecystectomy. Pediatrics 105:1250-1253
19. Lobe TE (1999) Cholelitiasis and cholecystectomy in children. Semin Pediatr Surg 9:170-176
20. Lotan G, Efrati Y, Halevy A et al (1995) Laparoscopic cholecystectomy in early infancy. Pediatr Surg Int 10:215-217
21. Toscano E, Trivellini V, Andria G (2001) Cholelithiasis in Down's syndrome. Arch Dis Child 85:242-243
22. Lugo Vicente HL (1997) Trends in management of gallbladder disorders in children. Pediatr Surg Int 12:348-352
23. Mattioli FP, Jasonni V, Cagnazzo A et al (1993) Infantile laparoscopic cholecystectomy; 2 cases. Endosurgery 2:91-92
24. Vegunta RK, Raso M, Pearl RH et al (2005) Biliary dyskinesia: the most common indication for cholecystectomy in children. Surgery 138:726-731
25. Mucio M, Felemovicius J, De la Concha F (1994) The Mexican experience with laparoscopic cholecistectomy and common bile duct exploration: a multicentric trial. Surg Endosc 8:306-309
26. Newman KD, Marmon LM, Attorri R, Evans S (1991) Laparoscopic cholecystectomy in pediatric patients. J Pediatr Surg 26:1184-1185
27. Newman KD, Powel DM, Holcomb GW (1997) The management of choledocholithiasis in children in the era of laparoscopic cholecystectomy. J Pediatr Surg 32:1116-1119
28. Pasquale MD, Nauta R (1989) Selective vs routine use of intraoperative cholangiography. Arch Surg 124:1041-1042
29. Schwesinger WH, Diehl AK (1996) Changing indication for laparoscopic cholecystectomy. Stones without symptoms and symptoms without stones. Surg Clin North Am 76:493-504
30. Schoenfield LJ, Berci G, Chumley D et al (1990) The effect of ursodiol on the efficacy and safety of extracorporeal shock-wave lithotripsy of gallstones. The Dornier National Biliary Lithotripsy Study. N Engl J Med 323:1239-1245
31. Patton ML, Moss BE, Haith LR Jr et al (1997) Concomitant laparoscopic cholecystectomy and splenectomy surgical management of hereditary spherocytosis. Am Surg 63:536-539
32. Peters HJ, Gibbons GD, Innes JT et al (1991) Complications of laparoscopic cholecystectomy. Surgery 110:769-778
33. Radke M, Helms B, Czarnetzki HD et al (1994) Laparoscopic cholecystectomy in a young girl. Eur J Pediatr Surg 4:108-109
34. Rosser JC, Boeckman CR, Andrews D (1992) Laparoscopic cholecystectomy in an infant. Surg Laparosc Endosc 2:143–147
35. Sanada Y, Yamaguchi M, Chiba M et al (1998) Endoscopic sphincterotomy and laparoscopic cholecystectomy in an infant with cholecystocholedocholithiasis. J Pediatr Surg 33:1312-1314
36. Shea JA, Healey MJ, Berlin JA et al (1996) Mortality and complications associated with laparoscopic cholecystectomy: a meta-analysis. Ann Surg 5:609-620
37. Tagge EP, Othersen HB, Jackson SM et al (1994) Impact of laparoscopic cholecystectomy on the management of cholelithiasis in children with sickle cell disease. J Pediatr Surg 2:209-213
38. Sigman HH, Laberge JM, Croitoru D et al (1991) Laparoscopic cholecystectomy: a treatment option for gallbladder disease in children. J Pediatr Surg 26:1181-1183
39. Stringer MD (2004) Informed consent and choice in cholecystectomy. Pediatr Surg Int 20:741-743
40. Stringer MD, Taylor DR, Soloway RD (2003) Gallstones composition: are children different? J Pediatr 142:435-40
41. Villanova N, Bazzoli F, Festi D et al (1989) Gall-

stone recurrence after successful oral bile acid treatment. A 12 years follow-up study and evaluation of long-term postdissolution treatment. Gastroenterology 97:726-731
42. Vinograd I, Halevy A, Klin B et al (1993) Laparoscopic cholecystectomy: treatment of choice for cholelithiasis in children. World J Surg 17:263-266
43. Zani A, Pacilli M, Conforti A et al (2005) Adenomyomatosis of the gallbladder in childhood: report of a case and review of the literature. Pediatr Dev Pathol 8:577-580
44. Wolfe BM, Gardiner BN, Leary BF, Frey CF (1991) Endoscopic cholecystectomy: an analysis of complications. Arch Surg 126:1192-1198

Chapter 32

Biliary Lithiasis in Pregnancy

Paul Sungler, Horst Steiner

Specification of Problems Related to Biliary Lithiasis in Pregnancy

Surgery during pregnancy always has an emotional touch because it entails the obvious added risk of morbidity for two – mother and fetus. Laparoscopic surgery in pregnancy is a technically challenging procedure because of the limitations of positioning, low intra-abdominal pressure and hindrance due to the uterus enlargement in later pregnancy; many surgeons are therefore reluctant to perform such surgery. In Reddick and Olson's original article [1], pregnancy was stated to be a contraindication to laparoscopic cholecystectomy.

It is estimated that 1–3% of pregnant women undergo surgical procedures unrelated to their pregnancy [2].

Gallstones are present in 4.5–12% of all pregnancies [3–5] and are the most frequent cause of pancreatitis in pregnancy [6]. The majority of symptomatic patients are treated medically in an attempt to carry the patient until term or at least until the second trimester. However, medical treatment fails in more than one third of patients leading to endoscopic or surgical intervention for recurrent symptoms or recurrent attacks of biliary pancreatitis [4, 7–9].

Delay in definitive treatment of biliary disease during pregnancy increases repeated hospital admissions, emergency room visits and premature contractions, necessitating tocolytic and corticoid therapy [10]. Nonoperative management of symptomatic cholelithiasis increases the risk of complications of biliary lithiasis, such as cholecystitis and empyema, while obstructing common bile duct stones with or without cholangitis and biliary pancreatitis raise maternal mortality to 15–37% and fetal demise to 10–60% [4, 11–13].

Pregnancy-associated acute pancreatitis may be severe and poses a survival threat even in the youngest patients [14]. A spontaneous abortion rate of 12% is associated with nonoperative management of symptomatic cholelithiasis in the first trimester and premature labor in up to 40% of cases [15, 16].

Surgery during pregnancy always carries an increased risk of fetal loss, but there is sufficient data in the literature to indicate that laparoscopic surgery is safe and can be performed during all gestational ages [8, 17–26]. However, in the first trimester, conventional and laparoscopic surgery is associated with an increased risk of postoperative abortion and, in later pregnancy, a hindrance of operation due to the enlarged uterus [1, 27–29]. Premature labor occurs postoperatively in the third trimester in up to 40% of patients [16], meaning that surgery during pregnancy should be performed during the second trimester whenever possible. Laparoscopic cholecystectomy during pregnancy has advantages for the mother in that it speeds up her recovery, giving her less pain and decreasing the chance of incisional hernias from large incisions [2, 8]. Above all, it can facilitate natural birth without a Cesarean section, especially in patients requiring cholecystectomy later in their pregnancies [22].

Statements on Laparoscopic Surgery in the Literature

The Society of Gastrointestinal Endoscopic Surgeons (SAGES) guidelines state that despite the growing clinical experience suggesting laparoscopy is as safe as laparotomy in pregnancy, long-term clinical studies are lacking. For this reason, caution must be exercised. SAGES encourages future studies into methods that increase the safety of laparoscopy in the pregnant patient (e.g., alternative gases or abdominal lift devices) [30]. Unfortunately, there are almost no "scientific" data about laparoscopic surgery during pregnancy, but gynecologists seem to have no fear of the procedure for their patients [31]. The number of pregnant patients undergoing laparoscopic cholecystectomy has been increasing since the first publications in 1991 [25, 32]: a MEDLINE search using the keywords "cholecystectomy", "laparoscopy", "pregnancy" and "surgery" produces 126 papers, most of them case reports and small series. The reported rate of fetal death is very low, only two papers described fetal death following laparoscopic operation on a pregnant mother [6, 33]. Eichenberg et al. [34] reviewed the literature over the last 30 years and found no reported case of open or laparoscopic cholecystectomy in the third trimester of pregnancy that had not resulted in a viable birth. According to the literature, expert recommendations, and daily practice, there are no contraindications to laparoscopic cholecystectomy during pregnancy when surgery is required [31].

Technical Aspects of Laparoscopic Surgery in Pregnancy

Laparoscopy in pregnancy should mainly be performed in centers with special experience, interest and skills in laparoscopy in close collaboration with experienced gynecologists. All gravidas should be consulted by an obstetrician prior to surgery. Gestational age, fetal status and signs of premature labor should be checked. Premature contractions are evaluated mainly by cervical ultrasound. From 24 weeks on fetal heart rate and uterine activity should be monitored pre- and postoperatively by external cardiotocography in addition to measurements of cervical length and the depiction of cervical funneling by transvaginal ultrasound. In case of preterm contractions, pregnancy should be managed as in the absence of surgery. There is an increased risk of aspiration because of mechanically and hormonally decreased lower esophageal sphincter tonus during pregnancy in addition to possible nausea due to cholecystitis. Nasogastric tubes should be inserted liberally to decompress the stomach prior to anesthesia. A tilted position to the left should be adapted with gravidas in order to prevent supine hypotension syndrome due to aortocaval compression and to optimize uterine perfusion. Surgeons should be aware of the size of the uterus before inserting trocars and take into consideration the alterations in the uterine fundus. Especially in the end of the second or during the third trimester, triangulation may be hindered and alternative positions of trocar insertion points have to be chosen [14, 35]. If in doubt, ultrasound should be used in the operating room to avoid uterine lesions. For safe access, the open technique, as described by Hasson [36], is preferred.

Intra-abdominal pressure should be kept as low as possible (8–10 mmHg) [22, 29, 37], as increased intra-abdominal pressure may decrease maternal respiratory compliance, decrease uterine blood flow and lead to premature labor [8, 37]. Most of the concerns about the side effects of carbon dioxide, leading to increased fetal acidosis, fetal loss and other detrimental side effects are based on experimental studies only and need to be confirmed by randomized controlled studies [28]. Hypoxemia, hypotension, acidosis, hypoventilation and hyperventilation should be avoided. Teratogenic effects of drugs such as antibiotics have to be taken into consideration [38, 39]. There is no need for prophylactic administration of perioperative antibiotics or prophylactic tocolysis. If there is a high risk of preterm birth, antenatal glucocorticoid administration for fetal lung maturation should be initiated preoperatively.

Endoscopic Retrograde Cholangiopancreatography (ERCP)

Endoscopy represents the third treatment option for complicated biliary lithiasis during pregnancy. Unlike in former days, ERCP is no longer a diagnostic, but is now mainly a therapeutic pathway, since the introduction of magnetic resonance cholangiopancreatography (MRCP). Once diagnosis of choledocholithiasis is made, therapeutic ERCP should be performed by a highly experienced, high volume endoscopist. Therapeutic ERCP either replaces or precedes laparoscopic cholecystectomy. As shielding of the fetus is more difficult during surgery, laparoscopic common bile duct exploration does not seem to be a good alternative to ERCP.

As for the risk of X-rays in the second and third trimester, Sorensen et al [40] conclude that radiological studies, other diagnostic modalities, and operative intervention should not be delayed because of possible adverse effects on the fetus. They assert that the best way to achieve fetal survival is to assure maternal survival and avoid unnecessary maternal morbidity.

The first reports of therapeutic ERCP during pregnancy were in 1990 [41, 42]; Friedman and Friedman presented a pregnant patient with calculus biliary duct obstruction and cholecystitis, using ERCP, papillotomy, and stone extraction in combination with laparoscopic cholecystectomy [43].

ERCP during pregnancy seems to be a safe procedure for both the mother and the fetus, but should be restricted to therapeutic interventions.

Special Strategies for Endoscopic Interventions

Exposure of the fetus to radiation has to be minimized by shielding the pelvis and reducing fluoroscopy to the absolute minimum. Most radiation sources are underneath the patient, so the lead apron has to be positioned underneath the patient or wrapped around the lower abdomen and pelvis. Digital radiography reduces radiation exposure. Especially in later pregnancy, patients should be supported by cushions in the left lateral position.

Procedure time should be minimized, which can be achieved most realistically by a highly experienced endoscopist. Proper sedation is required and it may be safe and reasonable to have anesthesiological standby to administer conscious sedation with, for example, propofol and monitor oxygenation.

Conclusion and Management

There is consensus that endoscopic and/or surgical intervention is indicated for obstructive jaundice and gallstone pancreatitis, failed medical treatment for acute and symptomatic cholecystitis, or suspected peritonitis. In our Institution we continue to perform laparoscopic cholecystectomy safely in all trimesters whenever indicated, as laparoscopic surgery is safe, reduces the rate of preterm deliveries, and reduces fetal morbidity.

References

1. Reddick EJ, Olson DO (1989) Laparoscopic laser cholecystecomy: a comparison with minilap cholecystectomy. Surg Endosc 3:131-133
2. Steinberg ES, Santos AC (1990) Surgical anaesthesia during pregnancy. International Anaesthesiology Clinics 28:58-65
3. Basso L, McCollum P, Darling MRN et al (1992) A study of cholelithiasis during pregnancy and its relationship with age, parity, menarche, breast-feeding, dysmenorrheal, oral contraception and a maternal history of cholelithiasis. Surg Gynecol Obstet 175:41-46
4. Curet MJ (1997) Laparoscopic surgery in pregnant patients. SAGES Congress Syllabus, 19-22 March, San Diego, USA, pp 227-237
5. Williamson SL, Williamson MR (1984) Cholecystosonography in pregnancy. J Ultrasound Med 3:329-331
6. Amos JD, Schorr SJ, Norman PF et al (1996) Laparoscopic surgery during pregnancy. Am J Surg 171:435-437
7. Axelrat AM, Fleischer DE, Strack LL et al (1994) Performance of ERCP for symptomatic choledocholithiasis during pregnancy: techniques to increase safety and improve patient management. Am J Gastroenterology 89:109-112
8. Curet MJ, Allen D, Josloff RK et al (1996) Laparoscopy during pregnancy. Arch Surg 131:546-551
9. Glasgow RE, Visser BC, Harris HW et al (1998) Changing management of gallstone disease during pregnancy. Surg Endosc 12:241-246
10. Muench J, Albrink M, Serafini F et al (2001) Delay in treatment of biliary disease during pregnancy increases morbidity and can be avoided with safe laparoscopic cholecystectomy. Am Surg 67:539-542
11. Wilkinson EJ (1973) Acute pancreatitis in pregnancy: a review of 98 cases and a report of 8 new cases. Obstet Gynecol Surve 28:281-303
12. Scott L (1992) Gallstone disease and pancreatitis in pregnancy. Gastroenterol Clin North Am 21:803-815
13. Al-Fozan H, Tulandi T (2002) Safety and risk of laparoscopy in pregnancy. Curr Opin Obstet Gynecol 14:375-379
14. Robertson KW, Stewart IS, Imrie CW (2006) Severe acute pancreatitis and pregnancy. Pancreatology 6:309-315
15. Schwartzberg BS, Conyers JA, Moore JA (1997) First trimester of pregnancy laparoscopic procedures. Surg Endosc 11:1216-1217
16. McKellar DP, Anderson CT, Boynton CJ, Peoples JB (1992) Cholecystectomy during pregnancy without fetal loss. Surg Gynecol Obstet 174:465-468
17. Affleck DG, Handrahan DL, Egger MJ, Price RR (1999) The laparoscopic management of appendicitis and cholelithiasis during pregnancy. Am J Surg 178:523-529
18. Palanivelu C, Rangarajan M, Senthilkumaran S, Parathasarathi R (2007) Safety and efficacy of laparoscopic surgery in pregnancy: experience of a single institution. Laparoendosc Adv Surg Tech A 17:186-190
19. Shay DC, Bhavani-shankar K, Datta S (2001) Laparoscopic surgery during pregnancy. Anaesthesiol Clin North America 19:57-67
20. Halkic N, Tempia-Caliera AA, Ksontini R et al (2006) Laparoscopic management of appendicitis and symptomatic cholelithiasis during pregnancy. Langenbecks Arch Surg 391:467-471
21. Rollins MD, Chan KJ, Price RR (2004) Laparoscopy for appendicitis and cholelithiasis during pregnancy: a new standard of care. Surg Endosc 18:237-241
22. Sungler P, Heinerman PM, Steiner H et al (2000) Laparoscopic cholecystectomy and interventional endoscopy for gallstone complications during pregnancy. Surg Endosc 14:267-271
23. Elerding SC (1993) Laparoscopic cholecystectomy in pregnancy. Am J Surg 165:625
24. Lang RD, Thiele H (1995) Laparoskopische Cholecystektomie in der Schwangerschaft. Chirurg 66:1225-1229
25. Weber AM, Bloom GP, Allan TR, Curry SL (1991) Laparoscopic cholecystectomy during pregnancy. Obstet Gynecol 78:958-959
26. Lu EJ, Curet MJ, El-Sayed YY, Kirkwood KS (2004) Medical versus surgical management of biliary tract disease in pregnancy. Am J Surg 188:755-759
27. Martin IG, Dexter SPL, McMahon MJ (1996) Laparoscopic cholecystectomy in pregnancy. Surg Endosc 10:508-510
28. Society of American Gastrointestinal Endoscopic Surgeons (1998) Guidelines for laparoscopic surgery during pregnancy. Surg Endosc 12:189-190
29. Neudecker J, Sauerland S, Neugebauer E et al (2002) The European Association for Endoscopic Surgery clinical practice guideline on the pneumoperitoneum for laparoscopic surgery. Surg Endosc 16:1121-1143
30. SAGES guidelines for laparoscopic surgery during pregnancy. SAGES publication 0023 (2000) www.sages.org/sg_pub23.html. Cited 30 July 2007
31. Holthausen UH, Mettler L, Troidl H (1999) Pregnancy: a contraindication? World J Surg 23:856-862
32. Arvidson D, Gerdin E (1991) Laparoscopic cholecystectomy during pregnancy. Surg Laparosc Endosc 1:193

33. Jamal A, Gorski TF, Nguyen HQ, Davis R (1997) Laparoscopic cholecystectomy during pregnancy. Surg Rounds pp 408-415
34. Eichenberg BJ, Vanderlinden J, Miguel C et al (1996) Laparoscopic cholecystectomy in the third trimester of pregnancy. Am Surg 62:874-877
35. Lemaire BMD, Vanerp WFM (1997) Laparoscopic surgery during pregnancy. Surg Endosc 11:15-18
36. Hasson HM (1971) A modified instrument and method for laparoscopy. Am J Obstet Gynecol 110:886-870
37. Hunter JG, Svanstrom L, Thornburg K (1995) Carbon dioxide pneumoperitoneum induces fetal acidosis in the pregnant ewe model. Surg Endosc 9:272-279
38. Shay DC, Bhavani-shankar K, Datta S (2001) Laparoscopic surgery during pregnancy. Anaesthesiol Clin North America 19:57-67
39. Halkic N, Tempia-Caliera AA, Ksontini R et al (2006) Laparoscopic management of appendicitis and symptomatic cholelithiasis during pregnancy. Langenbecks Arch Surg 391:467-471
40. Sorensen VJ, Bivins BA, Obeid FM, Horst HM (1990) Management of general surgical emergencies in pregnancy. Am Surg 56:245-250
41. Baillie J, Cairns SR, Putnam WS, Cotton PB (1990) Endoscopic management of choledocholithiasis during pregnancy. Surg Gynecol Obset 171:1-4
42. Binmoeller KF, Katon RM (1990) Needle knife papillotomy for an impacted common bile duct stone during pregnancy. Gastrointest Endosc 36:607
43. Friedman RL, Friedman IH (1995) Acute cholecystitis with calculous biliary duct obstruction in the gravid patient. Surg Endosc 9:910-913

Chapter 33

Biliary Lithiasis and Obesity

Mario Rizzello, Giovanni Casella, Francesca Abbatini, Gianfranco Silecchia, Nicola Basso

Epidemiology of Gallstones

Gallbladder stones are a common clinical finding in the Western population: a prevalence rate of 10–15% in adult European and of 3–5% in African and Asian populations has been reported. In several Western countries 80% of gallstones are cholesterol stones in a matrix of bile pigments, calcium salts and glycoproteins [1–5]. Adult age, female gender, fecundity and family history of gallstone disease are strongly associated with the formation of cholesterol stones. Moreover, specific dietetic regimens, such as high cholesterol and high carbohydrate diets, are associated with an increased risk of gallstone formation [6]. Obesity (body mass index, BMI > 30 kg/m^2), and other factors contributing to the metabolic syndrome, such as dyslipidemia, hyperinsulinemia, insulin resistance or type 2 diabetes, are also well established risk factors. On the other hand, rapid active weight loss and weight cycling are also strongly associated with an increased risk [7–8].

In many studies obesity appears to be an independent factor without correlation with age and gender: 25–35% of obese patients present gallstones [9]. Prevalence of gallbladder disease in the obese population has been found to range as high as 87–97% when evaluated by gross and histological examination after routine cholecystectomy in bariatric procedures [10–14].

Pathogenesis of Gallstones

In Obese Patients

Three abnormalities are considered to be responsible for gallstone formation: cholesterol bile saturation, enhanced nucleation of cholesterol crystals and gallbladder hypomotility. In obese patients adipose tissue produces several peptides (adipokines). Recent data have shown that aberrant plasma levels of adipokines can play a crucial role in obesity-related diseases and it could be possible that adipokines (such as leptin and adiponectin) are also involved in gallstone disease [7, 8].

Leptin, discovered by Friedman in 1994, is mainly produced by adipose tissue in proportion to body fat mass [15, 16]. Bile is the main route for cholesterol clearance and leptin should regulate biliary lipid metabolism by promoting mobilization of the stored excess cholesterol. Increased serum leptin levels may enhance bile cholesterol secretion and induce cholesterol bile saturation [17–19]. In addition, in leptin-deficient and leptin-resistant mice a shortened time of cholesterol crystal formation is observed [20]. Furthermore, some authors have hypothesized that increasing leptin serum levels could decrease gallbladder response to cholecystokinin [21]. Adiponectin levels are lower than normal in obese patients with insulin resistance, and/or type 2 diabetes. Low serum adiponectin levels are significantly associated with gallstone disease [22]. Although the direct relationship between hypoadiponectinemia and gallstone development has not been established, hyperglycemia secondary to hypoadiponectinemia may play a key role [23].

In Weight-losing Obese Patients

The risk of gallstone formation during weight loss increases if the weight loss rate exceeds 1.5 kg/week or when there is an excess weight loss of more than 24% [24–26]. Rapid weight loss induces cholesterol gallstone formation and the pathogenesis has been studied extensively. In obese patients, cholesterol concentration is elevated at baseline and more so during weight loss when fat stores are mobilized. A dietary caloric restriction induces a reduction of bile acid secretion, and the relative excess of cholesterol results in "supersaturated bile". Reduction of dietary fat also decreases gallbladder emptying. Impaired gallbladder motility may result in stasis and in gallstone formation. Biliary mucin is also increased during weight loss and causes a shorter gallstone nucleating time.

In Operated Bariatric Patients

Morbidly obese patients are at high risk of gallstone development (22–71%), also after weight loss inducing surgery [27–30]. A study by Kiewiet et al. [31] reported 30% incidence of gallstones after adjustable gastric banding (AGB) procedures. Miller et al. [32] reported an incidence of 22% a year after vertical banded gastroplasty (VBG) or AGB, and of 30% 2 years after surgery. Shiffman et al. [33] described an incidence of gallstone formation of 38% within 6 months after Roux-en-Y gastric bypass (RYGBP). Scopinaro et al. reported a 40% incidence of gallstones 1 year after biliopancreatic diversion (BPD) [34, 35]. In a recent paper, Gagner et al. [36] reported the incidence of gallstones after laparoscopic BPD with duodenal switch (BPD-DS) as only 7% when associated with prophylactic medical therapy.

Restrictive procedures determine: cholesterol bile saturation due to mobilization of cholesterol from mobilized fat, diminished gallbladder emptying due to diminished food intake and accelerated cholesterol crystal nucleation from bile stasis. In addition, the division of the hepatic branch of the vagus nerve, which may occur during bariatric procedures, results in decreased gallbladder motility. Cholecystokinin secretion is also decreased because of loss of the intraluminal stimulus when the duodenum is bypassed (Fig. 33.1). After BPD, Scopinaro found no increase in fecal bile salt concentration and concluded that the increased incidence of gallstones was due to failure of the gallbladder to empty because of lack of stimulation from the bypassed duodenum. In 1988 Hess [37] introduced a modified BPD by performing a sleeve gastrectomy and a duodenal switch (BPD-DS). In this procedure, cholecystokinin secretion is not completely inhibited since the initial 2–3 cm of duodenum are not bypassed by the food; further, the hepatic branch of the vagus nerve is left untouched, preserving gallbladder motility. A longer common limb (100 cm vs. 50 cm) allows a better uptake of biliary salts and reduces the risk of bile cholesterol supersaturation.

Natural History and Management of Gallstones

In Obese Patients

Data on gallbladder disease in the obese population based on ultrasound and other imaging procedures seem to underestimate the overall prevalence of the disease. In obese patients the ultrasound mean sensitivity is 64% [10].

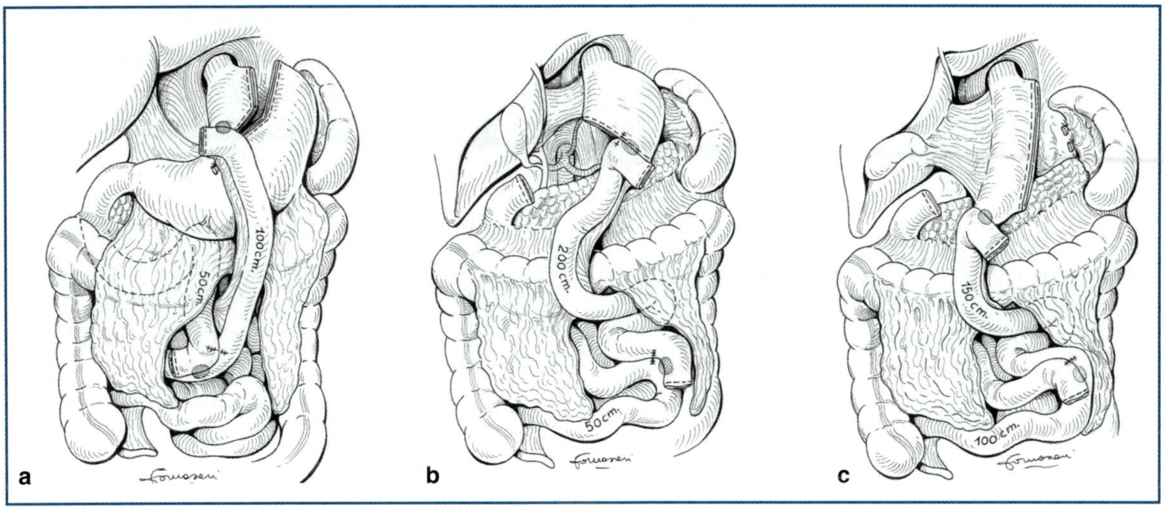

Fig. 33.1 Bariatric procedures with by-passed duodenum. **a** Roux-en-Y gastric bypass; **b** bilio-pancreatic diversion (Scopinaro's technique); **c** bilio-pancreatic diversion with duodenal switch

The natural history of gallbladder disease in the obese population is not known, but symptoms and complications are expected to be more frequent than in non-obese patients.

In the general population Friedman [38] found complications in 1–3% of patients with gallstones. Moreover, 6–8% of initially mildly symptomatic patients will ultimately require cholecystectomy [38]. Attili et al. [39] found that the probability of developing biliary colic was 12% at 2 years and 26% at 10 years in asymptomatic patients. The probability of developing gallbladder complications (cholecystitis, cholangitis and biliary pancreatitis) was 3% in asymptomatic patients and 7% in symptomatic patients after 10 years.

The standard treatment of symptomatic gallstones is laparoscopic cholecystectomy. In the "laparoscopic era", the early literature reports a conversion rate from laparoscopic to open cholecystectomy of 2–15% and obesity was considered one of the main causes of conversion [40]. Difficult trocar placement, "obscure" anatomy because of extensive abdominal fat, inability to retract the liver due to hepatomegaly and/or steatosis and difficult instrument manipulation were important factors leading to conversion and, then, a relative contraindication to the laparoscopic approach. With the development of laparoscopic technology and with the standardization of the laparoscopic approach, several reports have shown that, at present, obesity is no more associated with an increased rate of conversion, morbidity or prolonged hospital stay (Table 33.1) [41–42]. In these reports laparoscopic cholecystectomy seems to be a safe and effective treatment for gallbladder disease and represents the standard of care also in

Table 33.1 Laparoscopic cholecystectomy in obese vs. non-obese patients [41]

Group (BMI)	Conversion rate (%)*	Postoperative complication rate (%)*	Length of hospital stay*
≤ 25	4.1	1.6	1.08
25.1–30	10.1	0.7	1.11
≥ 30.1	6.5	0	1.01

* not statistically significant

the obese population (BMI > 30 kg/m^2). However, obese patients have a moderate risk of perioperative venous thromboembolism [43]. Prophylaxis with mechanical (sequential compression boots and early ambulation) and pharmacological (subcutaneous low molecular weight heparin) treatment is advised, prolonging the heparin treatment at least 7 days after hospital discharge. Parenteral antibiotic prophylaxis is standard. Positioning of the patient on the operating table must include considerations of prevention of pressure sores and neuropathy. Dedicated operative tables must be weight-rated appropriately. Long trocars and instruments and 30 degree laparoscopes may be useful. Placement of the "midline port" in the supraumbilical region and meticulous and careful dissection of the fat in the triangle of Calot are advised. In addition, the surgeon should not hesitate to place additional trocars when needed to retract the liver or to push down the omentum to achieve adequate exposure. Choledocolithiasis in obese patients can be managed by routine methods.

In Bariatric Surgery

In the "open bariatric surgery era", Amaral and Thompson [10] recommended a routine prophylactic concomitant cholecystectomy. Scopinaro advocated cholecystectomy as routine part of the standard BPD. The rational for this approach was the high prevalence of gallbladder disease in the obese population (87–97%), the low sensitivity of preoperative ultrasonography (64%) and the high risk of gallstones during weight loss. Nevertheless, other surgeons recommended cholecystectomy only when gallstones or cholesterolosis or chronic inflammation are present at the bariatric procedure. The potential increase of complication rate after routine cholecystectomy during "open" bariatric surgery, due to technical difficulties, and a relatively low incidence of gallstones complications has been described [44–46]. The gallbladder screening during "open" bariatric surgery using "palpation" or intraoperative ultrasonography (IOUS) has been proposed, but the use of IOUS requires a learning curve and increases the cost and time of the procedures. Moreover, in a study by Scott et al. [47], 10% of patients with negative IOUS developed symptomatic cholelithiasis and required cholecystectomy showing the accuracy of IOUS as 90% in the obese population.

In the "laparoscopic bariatric surgery era" routine prophylactic cholecystectomy has been abandoned. Postoperative prophylactic medical therapy with ursodeoxycholic acid is the standard treatment. Subsequently, if symptomatic gallstones are detected, a laparoscopic cholecystectomy can be easily performed after postoperative weight loss without increased risks compared to the general population.

In fact, a concomitant routine prophylactic cholecystectomy may add difficulty to the procedure with the potential for an increased incidence of complications: access ports are not placed in the "ideal" position for cholecystectomy and adequate access to the right upper quadrant can be difficult, requiring insertion of an additional port [48]. In these cases long instruments must span significant distances through a thick abdominal wall, creating torque and resistance and making precise movements a challenge (Fig. 33.2). In addition, visualization may be hindered by a large liver, especially in the case of an intrahepatic gallbladder, a fatty greater omentum or a fatty falciform ligament. Hamad et al. [14] report that the addition of cholecystectomy to laparoscopic bariatric procedures increases the operative time by nearly 50 minutes and hospital stay by 2 days. Thus, a concomitant cholecystectomy during laparoscopic bariatric procedures can be technically demanding and increase the risk of intraoperative complications.

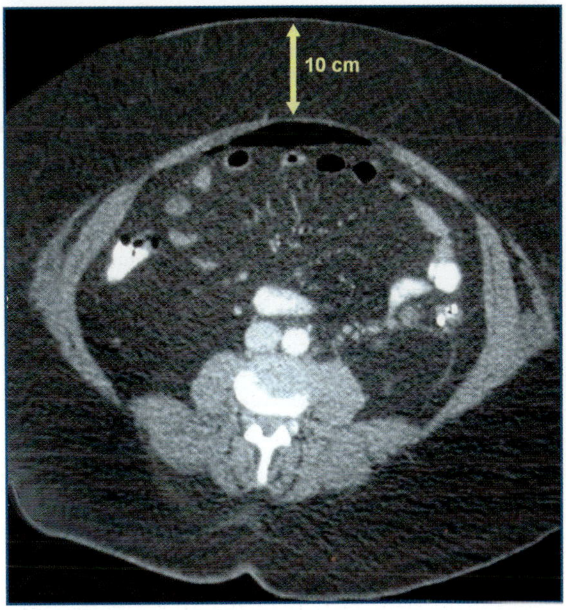

Fig. 33.2 CT scan: subcutaneous adipose tissue in an obese candidate for laparoscopic cholecystectomy

Moreover, Sugerman et al. [49] showed that the incidence of gallstones after bariatric surgery decreases from 32% (vs. placebo) to 2% when ursodeoxycolic acid prophylactic treatment (300 mg twice daily for six months) is undertaken. The same authors report that symptomatic gallstone disease after bariatric surgery was only 0.6% in the prophylactic group and 6–29% in the control group. Therefore the risk of concomitant cholecystectomy must be evaluated by looking at the real low risk of developing gallstones complications (acute cholecystitis, choledocholithiasis, cholangitis and pancreatitis) when postoperative prophylactic medical therapy is performed.

For the above reasons in the "laparoscopic era" the concomitant removal of the gallbladder is performed only in cases of preoperative or intraoperative gallstone diagnosis. When gallstones are not present, postoperative prophylactic medical therapy with ursodeoxycholic acid is the standard of care.

The effective and safe dose of ursodeoxycolic acid for gallstone prophylaxis is 600 mg/daily. A 6 month treatment appears to be adequate, since weight loss after bariatric surgery is most rapid during this period and gallstones formation is less common thereafter. However, the diarrheagenic effect of ursodeoxycolic acid, especially after malabsorptive procedures, reduces the compliance of the patients.

Choledocholitiasis and Bariatric Surgery

After bariatric procedures in which the duodenum is bypassed, endoscopic access to the bypassed structures becomes very difficult and, in most cases, impossible. If needed, endoscopic treatment of common bile duct stones may be problematic. For these reasons, before performing "duodenal bypass" bariatric procedures choledocholithiasis must be excluded. In these cases the limiting factor for an endoscopic approach is advancement of the scope along the afferent limb. Although anecdotic cases of choledocholitiasis are reported, the problem of the approaching bypassed duodenum is not new and different access techniques have been described to perform an endoscopic retrograde cholangiopancreatography (ERCP) and/or sphincterotomy.

The success rate reported using a retrograde approach is 65% in standard RYGBP (Fig. 33.3) [50]. After long limb RYGBP, traditional ERCP has been described as nearly impossible. Percutaneous computed tomography or ultrasound guided access to the gastric remnant is challenging because of the inability to distend the remnant stomach with air in order to place the endoscope percutaneously in the stomach remnant [51]. Fobi et al. [52] described routine placement of a gastrostomy tube with a radiopaque silastic ring around it at the initial bariatric surgery. However, the very low incidence of cholecocholithiasis does not justify routine use of gastrostomy tubes with their associated morbidity (postoperative pain and risks of leak and wound infection) as a prophylactic

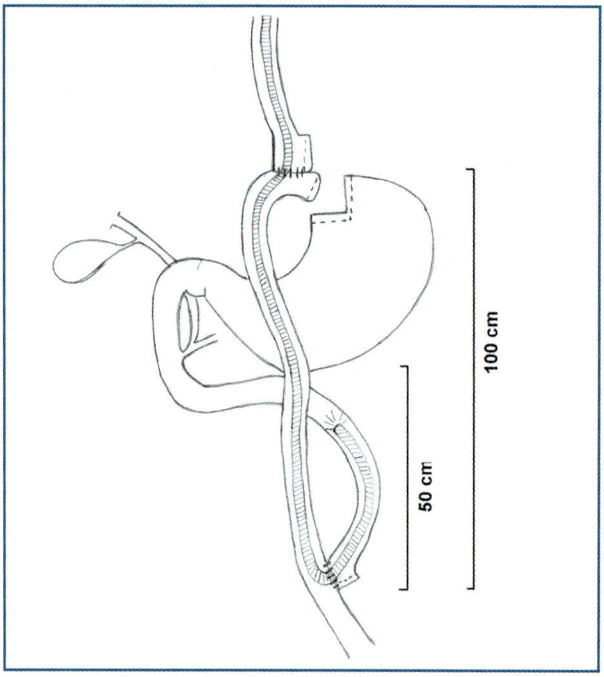

Fig. 33.3 Flexible upper gastro-intestinal endoscopy in standard Roux-en-Y gastric bypass

measure. Use of the double balloon enteroscopy to perform an endoscopic assisted placement of the trocar into the remnant stomach was recently reported (Fig. 33.4) [53]. Access to the residual stomach can be performed using an open procedure and creation of a gastrostomy. Recent studies described laparoscopic transgastric endoscopy to access the bypassed stomach after RYGBP. Once pneumoperitoneum is achieved, gastrostomy is performed using ultrasonic shears and a 15 mm trocar is placed in the stomach. The endoscope is then inserted through the trocar [54]. At the end of the procedure, the gastrostomy is closed with a running suture or linear stapler.

After BPD the possibility of reaching the papilla through a surgical gastrostomy or

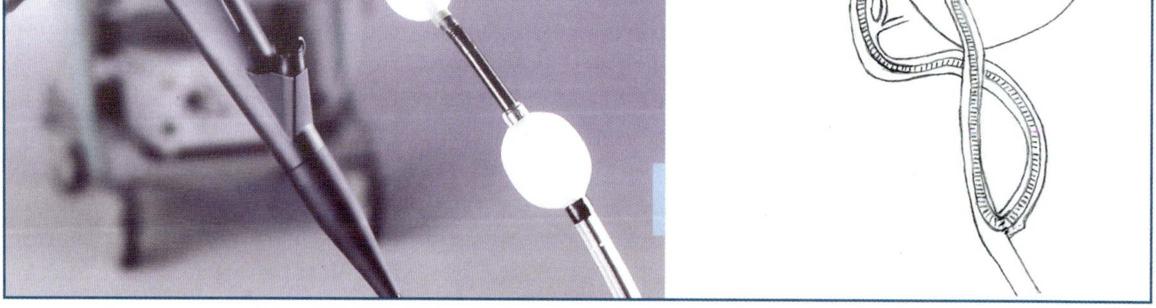

Fig. 33.4 Flexible upper gastro-intestinal endoscopy with double-balloon system (*left panel*); in Roux-en Y gastric bypass achieving the gastric lumen (*right panel*)

jejunostomy has been reported. Recently a case of laparoscopic assisted ERCP was reported by Mutignani et al. [55].

Conclusion

It is known that the prevalence of cholesterol gallstones is increased in the obese population (25–35% vs. 10–15% in the nonobese population). Laparoscopic cholecystectomy, when performed by expert laparoscopic surgeons, seems to be a safe and effective treatment for gallbladder disease in obese patients (Table 33.2). In candidates for bariatric surgery, gallstone disease should be routinely ruled out preoperatively or intraoperatively by ultrasonography. When gallstones are diagnosed cholecystectomy should be performed simultaneously. After bariatric surgery gallstone formation is related to the rapid weight loss. Our experience (Table 33.3) confirms that a daily dose of 600 mg of ursodeoxycolic acid for 6 months is an effective prophylaxis to reduce the incidence of gallstone formation. Routine postoperative ultrasonography surveillance is recommended during the weight-losing period (2 years postoperative). In operated bariatric patients, gallstones should be treated as in the general population: surgery is indicated when the disease is symptomatic (Fig. 33.5). In case of choledocolithiasis, safe and effective different access techniques have been described for diagnosis and treatment of the condition within the bypassed structures.

Table 33.2 Laparoscopic cholecystectomy in obese patients

Tips and tricks
1. Pneumoperitoneum induction with Veress needle
2. CO_2 pressure 14–16 mmHg
3. Long instruments and trocars in selective cases
4. 30 degree laparoscope
5. Placement of the "first midline port" in the supraumbilical region (do not consider the umbelicus a landmark)
6. Meticulous and careful dissection of the fat in the triangle of Calot
7. Placement of an additional trocar in case of hepatomegaly

Table 33.3 Personal experience in laparoscopic bariatric surgery using postoperative prophylactic medical therapy

Bariatric procedure	Previous cholecystectomy	Concomitant cholecystectomy (preoperative diagnosis of stones)	Postoperative laparoscopic cholecystectomy (%)
Lap AGB (n = 541)	20	27	2 (0.4) at 16 months
Lap RYGBP (n = 216)	14	22	3 (1.6) at 12 months
Lap sleeve gastrectomy (n = 94)	4	8	3 (3.6) at10 months

AGB, adjustable gastric banding; *RYGBP*, Roux-en-y gastric bypass

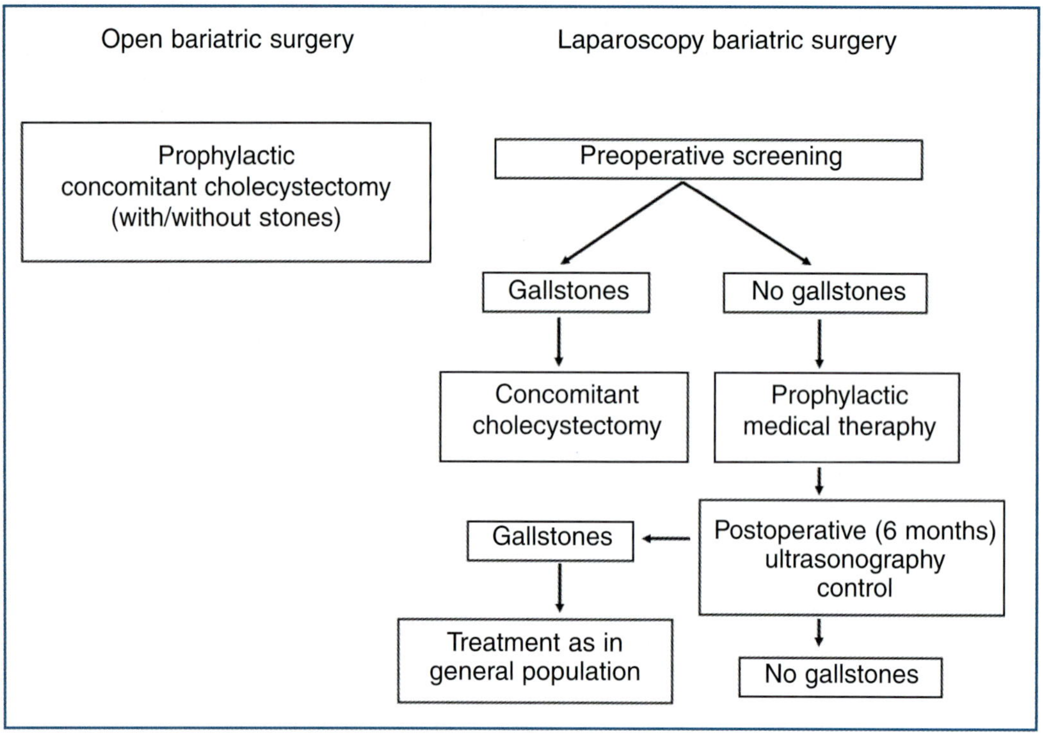

Fig. 33.5 Management of gallstones in bariatric surgery

References

1. Marschall HU, Einarsson C (2007) Gallstone disease. J Intern Med 261:529-542
2. Kratzer W, Mason RA, Kachele V (1999) Prevalence of gallstones in sonographic surveys worldwide. J Clin Ultrasound 27:1-7
3. Everhart JE, Khare M, Hill M et al (1999) Prevalence and ethnic differences in gallbladder disease in the United States. Gastroenterology 117:632-639
4. Sampliner RE, Bennett PH, Comess LJ et al (1970) Gallbladder disease in Pima Indians. Demonstration of high prevalence and early onset by cholecystography. N Engl J Med 283:1358-1364
5. Everhart JE, Yeh F, Lee ET et al (2002) Prevalence of gallbladder disease in American Indian populations: findings from the Strong Heart Study. Hepatology 35:1507-1512
6. EA Shaffer (2006) Epidemiology of gallbladder stone disease. Best Pract Res Clin Gastroenterol 20:981-996
7. Wang SN, Yeh YT, Yu ML et al (2006) Hyperleptinaemia and hypoadiponectinaemia are associated with gallstone disease. Eur J Clin Invest 36:176-180
8. Trayhurn P, Wood IS (2004) Adipokines: inflammation and the pleiotropic role of white adipose tissue. Br J Nutr 92:347-355
9. Friedman GD, Kamel WB, Dawber TR (1996) The epidemiology of gallbladder disease: observations in the Framingham study. J Chronic Dis 19:273-292
10. Amaral JF, Thompson WR (1985) Gallbladder disease in the morbidly obese. Am J Surg 149:551-557
11. Aidonopoulos AP, Papavramidis ST, Zaraboukas TG et al (1994) Gallbladder findings after cholecystectomy in morbidly obese patients. Obes Surg 4:8-12
12. Calhoun RC, Willbanks O (1987) Coexistence of gallbladder disease and morbid obesity. Am J Surg 154:665-658
13. Fobi M, Lee H, Igwe D et al (2002) Prophylactic cholecystectomy with gastric bypass operation: incidence of gallbladder disease. Obes Surg 12:350-353
14. Hamad GG, Ikramuddin S, Gourash WF et al (2003) Elective cholecystectomy during laparoscopic Roux-en-Y gastric bypass: is it worth the wait? Obes Surg 13:76-81
15. Zhang Y, Proenca R, Maffei M et al (1994) Positional cloning of the mouse obese gene and its human homologue. Nature 372:425-432

16. Friedman JM, Halaas JL (1998) Leptin and the regulation of body weight in mammals. Nature 395:763-770
17. VanPatten S, Ranginani N, Shefer S et al (2001) Impaired biliary lipid secretion in obese Zucker rats: leptin promotes hepatic cholesterol clearance. Am J Physiol Gastrointest Liver Physiol 281:393-404
18. Hyogo H, Roy S, Paigen B et al (2002) Leptin promotes biliary cholesterol elimination during weight loss in ob/ob mice by regulating the enterohepatic circulation of bile salts. J Biol Chem 277:117-124
19. Tran KQ, Swartz-Basile DA, Nakeeb A et al (2003) Gallbladder motility in agouti-yellow and leptin-resistant obese mice. J Surg Res 113:56-61
20. Graewin SJ, Kiely JM, Lee KH et al (2004) Nonobese diabetic mice have diminished gallbladder motility and shortened crystal observation time. J Gastrointest Surg 8:824-829
21. Graewin SJ, Lee KH, Kiely JM et al (2004) Gallbladder myocytes are short and cholecystokinin-resistant in obese diabetic mice. Surgery 136:431-436
22. Tsai CJ, Leitzmann MF, Willett WC et al (2005) Glycemic load, glycemic index, and carbohydrate intake in relation to risk of cholecystectomy in women. Gastroenterology 129:105-112
23. Sasazuki S, Kono S, Todoroki I et al (1999) Impaired glucose tolerance, diabetes mellitus, and gallstone disease: an extended study of male self-defense officials in Japan. Eur J Epidemio 15:245-251
24. Papavramidis S, Deligianidis N, Papavramidis T et al (2003) Laparoscopic cholecystectomy after bariatric surgery. Surg Endosc 17:1061-1064
25. Jiffry BO, Shaffer EA, Saccone GTP et al (2003) Changes in gallbladder motility and gallstone formation following laparoscopic gastric banding for morbid obesity. Can J Gastroenterol 17:169-174
26. Erlinger S (2000) Gallstones in obesity and weight loss. Eur J Gastroenterol Hepatol 12:1347-1352
27. Shiffman ML, Kaplan GD, Brinkman Kaplan V et al (1995) Prophylaxis against gallstone formation with ursodeoxycholic acid in patients participating in a very-low-calorie diet program. Ann Int Med 122:899-905
28. Shiffman ML, Sugerman HJ, Kellum JM et al (1991) Gallstone formation after rapid weight loss: a prospective study in patients undergoing gastric bypass surgery for treatment of morbid obesity. Am J Gastroenterol 86:1000-1005
29. Shiffman ML, Sugerman HJ, Kellum JM et al (1993) Gallstones in patients with morbid obesity: relationship to body weight, weight loss and gallbladder bile cholesterol solubility. Int J Obes 17:153-158
30. Worobetz LJ, Inglis FG, Shaffer EA (1993) The effect of ursodeoxycholic acid therapy on gallstone formation in the morbidly obese during rapid weight loss. Am J Gastroenterol 88:1705-1710
31. Kiewiet RM, Durian MF, van Leersum M et al (2006) Gallstone formation after weight loss following gastric banding in morbidly obese Dutch patients. Obes Surg 16(5):592-596
32. Miller K, Hell E, Lang B et al (2003) Gallstone formation prophylaxis after gastric restrictive procedures for weight loss. Ann Surg 238:697-702
33. Shiffman ML, Sugerman HJ, Kellum JM et al (1991) Gallstone formation after rapid weight loss: a prospective study in patients undergoing gastric bypass surgery for treatment of morbid obesity. Am J Gastroenterol 86:1000-1005
34. Scopinaro N, Gianetta E, Civalleri D (1979) Biliopancreatic bypass for obesity. II Initial experience in man. Br J Surg 66:618-620
35. Scopinaro N, Gianetta E, Civalleri D et al (1980) Two years experience with bilio-pancreatic bypass. Am J Clin Nutr 33:506-514
36. Bardaro SJ, Gagnér M, Consten E et al (2004) Is routine cholecystectomy during biliopancreatic diversion with duodenal switch really necessary? Abstract ASBS, San Diego
37. Hess DS, Hess DW (1998) Biliopancreatic diversion with a duodenal switch. Obes Surg 8:267-282
38. Friedman GD (1993) Natural history of asymptomatic and symptomatic gallstones. Am J Surg 165:399-404
39. Attili AF, De Santis A, Capri R et al (1995) The natural history of gallstones: the GREPCO experience. Hepatology 21:655-660
40. Alponat A, Kum CK, Koh BC (1997) Predictive factors for conversion of laparoscopic cholecystectomy. World J Surg 21:629-633
41. Sidhu RS, Raj PK, Treat RC (2007) Obesity as a factor in laparoscopic cholecystectomy. Surg Endosc 21:774-776
42. Simopoulos C, Polychronidis A, Botaitis S (2005) Laparoscopic cholecystectomy in obese patients. Obes Surg 15:243-246
43. Westling A, Bergqvist D et al (2002) Incidence of deep venous thrombosis in patients undergoing obesity surgery. World J Surg 26:470-473
44. Fakhry SM, Herbst CA, Buckwalter JA (1987) Cholecystectomy in morbidly obese patients. Am Surg 53:26-28
45. Jones KB Jr (1995) Simultaneous cholecystectomy: to be or not to be. Obes Surg 5:52-54
46. Mason E, Renquist KE (2002) Gallbladder management in obesity surgery obes surg 12:222-229
47. Scott DJ, Villegas L, Sims TL et al (2003) Intraoperative ultrasound and prophylactic ursodiol for gallstone prevention following laparoscopic gastric bypass. Surg Endosc 17:1796-802

48. Angrisani L, Lorenzo M, De Palma G et al (1995) Laparoscopic cholecystectomy in obese patients compared with nonobese patients. Surgical Laparosc Endosc 5:197-201
49. Sugerman HJ, Brewer WH, Shiffman ML et al (1995) A multicenter, placebo-controlled, randomized, double-blind, prospective trial of prophylactic ursodiol for the prevention of gallstone formation following gastric- bypass–induced rapid weight loss. Am J Surg 169:91-97
50. Martinez J, Guerrero L, Byers P et al (2006) Endoscopic retrograde cholangiopancreatography and gastroduodenoscopy after Roux-en-Y gastric bypass. Surg Endosc 20(10):1548-1550
51. Goitein D, Gagn DJ, Papasavas PK et al (2006) Percutaneous computed tomography-guided gastric remnant access after laparoscopic Roux-en-Y gastric bypass. Surg Obes Relat Dis 2(6):651-655
52. Fobi M, Lee H, Igwe D (2002) Prophylactic cholecystectomy with gastric bypass operation: incidence of gallbladder disease. Obes Surg 12(3):350-353
53. Ross AS, Semrad C, Alverdy J et al (2006) Use of double-balloon enteroscopy to perform PEG in the excluded stomach after Roux-en-Y gastric bypass. Gastrointest Endosc 64(5):797-800
54. Ceppa FA, Gagne DJ, Papasavas PK et al (2007) Laparoscopic transgastric endoscopy after Roux-en-Y gastric bypass. Surg Obes Relat Dis 3(1):21-24
55. Mutignani M, Marchese M, Tringali A et al (2007) Laparoscopy-assisted ERCP after biliopancreatic diversion. Obes Surg 17(2):251-254

Chapter 34

Biliary Lithiasis in Patients with Gastroesophageal Reflux (Acid and Alkaline)

Alberto del Genio, Gianluca Rossetti, Vincenzo Maffettone, Vincenzo Napolitano, Gianmattia del Genio, Luigi Brusciano, Francesco Pizza, Maria Di Martino, Salvatore Tolone

Gastroesophageal reflux (GERD) and cholelithiasis are both very common diseases. It is estimated that 15–20 million people in the United States have gallstones [1] and that 36% of the American population complains of at least one episode of heartburn per month. In Spain, 10% of the population has ultrasonographically demonstrated cholelithiasis [2] and 30% of the population suffers from reflux symptoms, 10% of these on a weekly basis [3]. The two diseases have been connected for years. Saint's triad [4], a well-known association of hiatal hernia with cholelithiasis and colon diverticula that was much in fashion during the 1980s, represented a paradigmatic expression of Westernization-induced gastrointestinal disturbances. However, this argument is very contentious, and we will try to analyze the controversy in this chapter.

Three questions have to be posed:

1. is there really an association between cholelithiasis and GERD?
2. Does cholecystectomy have an influence on the occurrence of GERD?
3. Is a combined surgical treatment of the two diseases safe?

The first matter of debate concerns the supposed association of cholelithiasis with GERD. As both are common conditions in Western countries, chances are high that a patient with one condition will have the other simply because of the frequency of the conditions; however, they are even higher when it is brought to our attention that being overweight is a risk factor for both.

What is the physiological and scientific basis for correlating cholelithiasis and GERD? It has been demonstrated that gallstone patients have impaired postprandial gallbladder motility [5–9] and increased cycle length of the migrating motor complex (the interdigestive motility pattern of the small intestine) with disruption of motilin release and decreased interdigestive gallbladder motility. In addition to impaired gallbladder motility, delayed intestinal transit time [10, 11] and frequent pathological gastroesophageal reflux have been reported in a significant number of gallstone patients. Two determining factors for the occurrence of GERD in these patients are probably the compromised competence of the lower esophageal sphincter [12] and delayed gastric emptying.

An interesting report on the argument has been published by Portincasa et al. [13]. Twenty patients with gallstones and 20 healthy subjects homogeneous for sex, age and body size were studied by ultrasonography to assess gallbladder and gastric emptying simultaneously in response to a standard liquid meal. The same subjects underwent ambulatory 24-hour gastroesophageal pH monitoring.

Both gallbladder and gastric motility were impaired in gallstone patients. Data concerning the motility of the stomach are given in Table 34.1 and Fig. 34.1. Although basal and maximal antral areas were similar between the patients and control subjects, gallstone patients had a larger minimal percentage antral area, less integrated emptying and a longer half-emptying time than control subjects ($p < 0.05$). The timing and the extent of antral emptying were similar

Table 34.1 Gastric emptying in gallstone patients and control subjects. From [13]

	Gallstones (*n*=20)	Control subjects (*n*=20)
Antral area		
Basal (cm^2)	4.7±0.3	5.1±1.7
Maximal post-prandial (cm^2)	12.7±0.6	11.7±0.7
Minimal post-prandial (cm^2)	10.2±4.2	4.9±0.5
Minimal post-prandial (%)†	20.8±5.3*	6.6±2.7
Integrated emptying (%120 min^{-1})	7716±383*	8828±251
Half-emptying time (min)	51±4**	36±3

Data are means ± SE. † Normalized to maximal area after substraction of basal area. **P*<0.05; vs. control subjects; **P<0.005 vs. control subjects

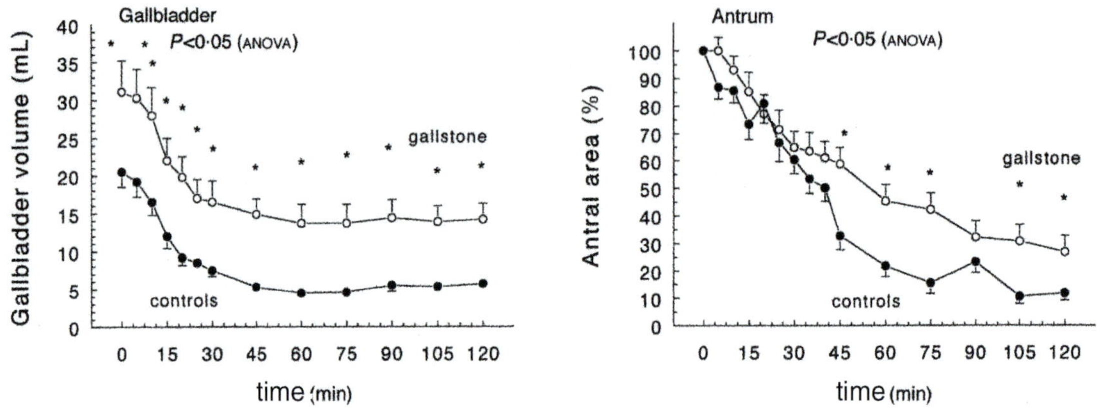

Fig. 34.1 Time course of gallbladder and gastric emptying in gallstone patients and healthy control subjects after ingestion of a standard liquid meal. From [13]

in patients with or without dyspeptic symptoms.

Concerning the acquisition data of esophageal and gastric pH monitoring, the percentage of interprandial pH in the acidic range was significantly higher, nearly sixfold, in gallstone patients that in control subjects ($p < 0.005$) (Fig. 34.2). Also in the postprandial period, gallstone patients had significantly more time spent at a pH of less than 4 and more episodes of prolonged refluxes than the control subjects ($p < 0.05$) (Table 34.2). Overall, pathological gastroesophageal reflux was present in 15 gallstone patients (75%) compared with three control subjects (15%) ($p < 0.00014$). Furthermore, there was a significant positive correlation between the duration of the longest episode of gastroesophageal reflux in the post-prandial period and the speed of antral emptying. Not only acid pathological gastroesophageal reflux but also, in the interpran-

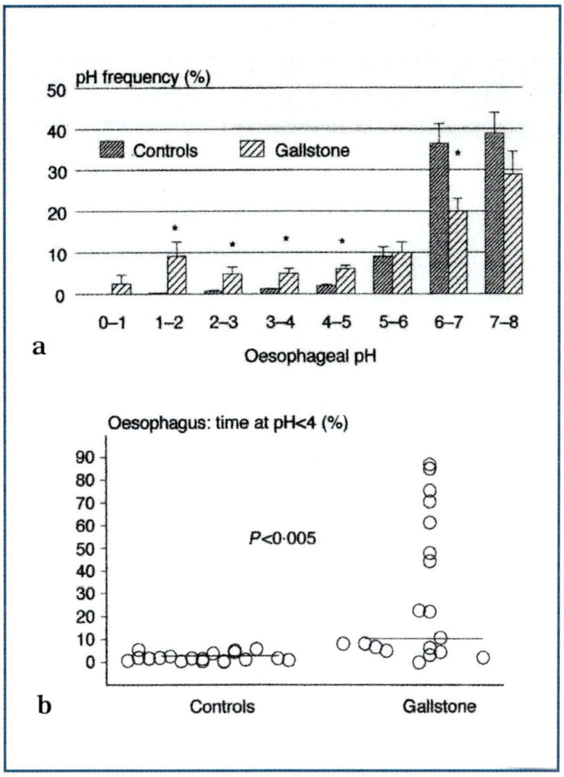

Fig 34.2 **a** Frequency distribution of esophageal pH in the interprandial period in 20 control subjects and 19 gallstone patients. **b** Individual values of percentage time spent at pH < 4 at the level of the esophagus in the interprandial period in 20 control subjects and 19 gallstone patients. From [13]

dial period, a prolonged alkaline shift in the antrum suggestive of duodeno-gastric reflux was seen in 20% of control subjects versus 35% of gallstone patients, even though the difference was not statistically significant. However, gallstone patients had significantly more and longer episodes of duodeno-gastric refluxes than control subjects ($p < 0.05$). In the opinion of the authors this explains how gallstone patients could be exposed to both acid and alkaline gastroesophageal reflux.

Another report confirming a delayed gastric emptying in gallstone patients was published by Ibrarullah et al. [14] who evaluated 43 patients with gallstones and 20 patients in a control group. The patients all underwent a scintigraphic gastric emptying study. The upper limit of the normal emptying time was set at 112 minutes. The mean gastric emptying time of the control group was 82 ± 15 minutes with all the patients in the normal range. On the other hand, delayed gastric emptying ($t_{1/2} > 112$ min) was observed in 18 gallstone patients (42%), as compared to the control group ($p < 0.002$).

The underlying mechanism explaining the supposed increased incidence of GERD

Table 34.2 Esophageal pH in gallstone patients and control subjects. From [13]

	Gallstones (n=20)	Control subjects (n=20)
Interprandial period		
Recording time	1139 (124-1387)	1083 (916-1259)
Time at pH<4 (min)	105.0 (0-1281)*	18.5 (2-79)
Percentage time at pH<4	10.7 (0-87)*\	1.8 (0.2-5.8)
No. GER episodes	19.0 (0-73)*	10.5 (0-24)
No. GER episodes >5 min	2 (0-18)*	1 (0-4)
Longest GER episode (min)	23 (0-723)*	5 (0-19)
Post-prandial period		
Recording time (min)	240 (58-570)	240 (120-430)
Time at pH<4 (min)	30.0 (0-153)*	5.5 (0-24)
Percentage time at pH<4	12.3 (0-84.9)*	2.9 (0.3-9.7)
No. GER episodes	8.0 (0-48)	3 (1-19)
No. GER episodes >5 min	1 (0-8)*	0 (0-1)
Longest GER episode (min)	12.0 (0-58)*	2 (0-12)

GER, gastroesophageal reflux. Data are medians (range). *$P<0.005$ vs. control subjects in gallstone patients remains to be elucidated. Disruption of one or more hormonal patterns might partly impair the function of several gastrointestinal target organs. The postprandial secretion of neurotensin seems significantly higher in gallstone patients than in control subjects [15]. Interestingly, neurotensin is able to inhibit gastric emptying [16] and reduce the pressure of the lower esophageal sphincter [17], thus affecting two pathogenetic factors of gastroesophageal reflux. Neurotensin might also inhibit gallbladder motility in man [15], and fasting levels are significantly higher in patients with duodeno-gastric reflux compared with control subjects [18].

Another hypothesis takes into consideration a reflex pyloroduodenal ileus resulting from inflammation in and around the gallbladder and/or a subclinical mechanical obstruction produced by recurrent cholecystitis leading to pericholecystic inflammatory adhesions involving the pyloroduodenum [14].

Another determining factor for the occurrence of GERD is the supposed frequency of association between cholelithiasis and hiatal hernia. Several studies have underlined this association [19–21]. Obviously, an increased occurrence of hiatal hernia in subjects with gallstones may suggest a greater susceptibility to the development of GERD. However, not all authors have reported the same results. Avidan et al. [22] observed 790 patients with various forms of GERD and 407 control subjects without GERD. Hiatus hernia was almost three times more common among case subjects with GERD than among control subjects without GERD. At the multivariate logistic regression analysis, the presence of hiatal hernia was found to be the most significant risk factor for the occurrence of GERD. On the other hand, the presence of gallstone disease was not found to exert any significant influence on the occurrence of GERD. Cholelithiasis alone was not associated with an increased occurrence of GERD or hiatal hernia. Moreover, it was not associated with more severe forms of reflux disease. Finally, the frequency of GERD among hiatus hernia patients with gallstones was similar to the frequency of GERD among hiatus hernia patients without gallstones (Table 34.3).

No conclusions can be definitively drawn at the moment on the frequency of correlation between cholelithiasis and GERD as data acquired from various reports are too contradictory. A determining contribution may be provided by pH inpedenzometry as it is able to detect both acid and nonacid gastroesophageal reflux, thus reducing the possible underestimation of duodenogastroesophageal reflux that could have a high incidence in these patients.

Another important question is the following: Is gastroesophageal reflux influenced by cholecystectomy?

It has long been hypothesized that a previous cholecystectomy could cause the occurrence of GERD: What are the determining factors?

Cholecystectomy has been claimed to affect the antropyloric barrier [23–25]; the loss of the reservoir function for bile after removal of the gallbladder leads to changes in the dynamics of bile flow. Instead of the intermittent meal-induced bile flow, a continuous flow ensues, which may affect antroduodenal motility and promote duodenogastric reflux [26–28], consequently favoring gastroesophageal reflux. Moreover, the alterations in bile flow dynamics result in post-prandial elevation of cholecystokinin [29, 30]. Elevated cholecystokinin levels have been shown to result in increased transient lower esophageal sphincter relaxation [30, 31], another possible determining mechanism of reflux in these patients.

Several studies have been conducted on this argument, confirming a delayed gastric emptying and an increased incidence of gastroesophageal reflux in these patients.

Lorusso et al. [32] followed up 15 patients who underwent cholecystectomy. All the examinations were carried out before and 6 months after cholecystectomy. Bile reflux and gastric acid secretion were evaluated by gastric drainage in all patients, who had been fasting since the previous day. Their findings revealed an increase in the duodenogastric reflux of bile after cholecystectomy, as shown in Figure 34.3.

Jazrawi et al. [33] evaluated 37 patients who underwent elective cholecystectomy. Patients were studied before operation and 3–4 months afterwards. A detailed questionnaire was completed on each patient, while esophageal function was evaluated by esophageal manometry and 24-hour esophageal pH recording with simultaneous gastric pH monitoring. Upper gastrointestinal endoscopy was performed and biopsies were taken from the lower esophagus and gastric antrum.

The results were the following: 13 (35%) of the 37 patients undergoing cholecystectomy had gastroesophageal reflux before operation, increasing to 27 (73%) after operation ($p < 0.002$). The mean DeMeester acid reflux score for the whole group increased from 15.2 to 34.2 after operation ($p < 0.001$). In the esophagus, eight (22%) preoperative biopsy reports were consistent with reflux esophagitis, increasing to 19 (51%) after operation. Gastric alkaline shift (proportion of time at gastric pH > 4) increased significantly in the supine position, from a mean of 9.2% to 17.7% after surgery ($p < 0.02$). All the above mentioned results are listed in Table 34.4.

However, manometric measurements in patients with abnormal pH profile after operation did not reveal a statistically significant modification in the lower esophageal sphincter pressure and in intra-abdominal sphincter length before and after operation; instead, the sphincter function index showed a significant reduction ($p < 0.01$) (Table 34.5).

Lujan-Mompean et al. [34] conducted a scintigraphic study comparing ten patients who had undergone cholecystectomy with ten control patients; their acquisitions also confirmed a significant increase in duodenogastric reflux in operated patients.

Rothwell et al. [35] evaluated 50 patients who had undergone an elective cholecystectomy (28 by open approach and 22 by laparoscopic approach). Preoperative 24-hour pH studies and manometry were performed. Studies were repeated 3 months after surgery. Pathological acid reflux was defined in terms of the DeMeester acid score.

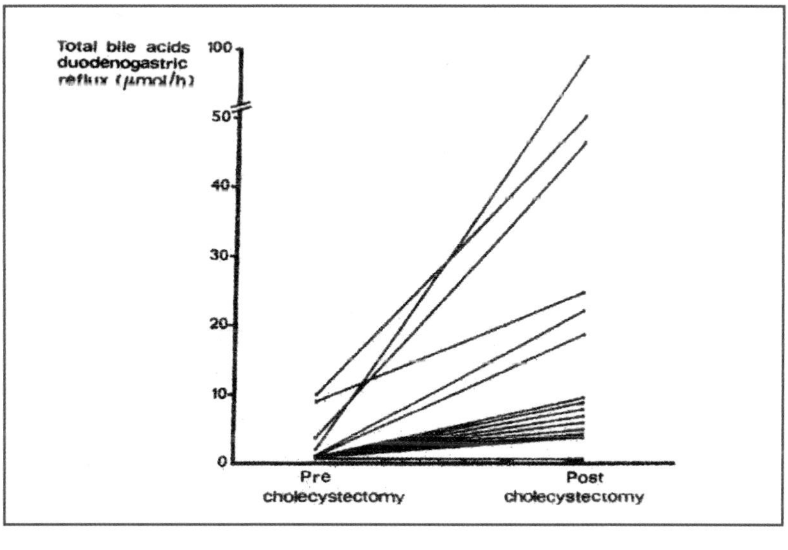

Fig. 34.3 Variation of the duodenogastric reflux in 15 patients before and after cholecystectomy. Reproduced from [13]

Table 34.3 Frequency of gallstones in patients with GERD and hiatal hernia. From [22]

Variable	No Gallstones (n=875)	Cholecystectomy (*n*=185)	Gallstones without surgery (*n*=137)	*p*
Presence of hiatal hernia				
No hiatal hernia	283(32%)	59(32%)	43(31%)	0.992
Hiatal hernia	592(68%)	126(68%)	94(69%)	
Presence of reflux disease				
No GERD	292(33%)	69(37%)	46(34%)	0.643
GERD	583(67%)	116(63%)	91(66%)	
Severity of reflux disease				
Nonerosive reflux disease	40(5%)	14(8%)	18(13%)	0.946
Erosive esophagitis (mild)	468(53%)	91(49%)	56(41%)	
Erosive esophagitis (moderate)	56(6%)	9(5%)	12(9%)	
Esophageal ulcers	19(2%)	2(1%)	5(4%)	

Table 34.4 Changes in duodenogastric and gastroesophageal reflux markers following cholecystectomy. From [12]

	Before operation	After operation	χ^2	s.n.d.	*P*
Reflux*	13 (35)	27 (73)	9.20	-	<0.002†
Mean (s.e.m.) acid reflux score	15.2 (2.1)	34.2 (5.2)	-	3.63	<0.001‡
Mean (s.e.m.) LES pressure (mmHg)	15.4 (0.7)	14.3 (0.9)	-	0.88	0.19‡
Mean (s.e.m.) percentage of supine time at gastric pH>4	9.2 (2.0)	17.7 (3.7)	-	2.27	0.017‡
Esophagitis*	8 (22)	19 (51)	5.83	-	0.016†
Gastritis*	8 (22)	23 (62)	10.88	-	<0.001†
Antral Helicobacter pylori*	8 (22)	19 (51)	5.83	-	.016†

*Values in parentheses are percentages. *s.n.d.*, Standardized normal deviate with continuity correction; † 1 d.f.; ‡ Wilcoxon's signed rank test

Table 34. 5 Manometric measurements in patients with abnormal pH profile after operation. From [12]

	Before operation	After operation	*P**
Lower esophageal sphincter pressure (mmHg)	11 (1)	10 (2)	0.06
Intra-abdominal sphincter length (mm)	24 (3)	23 (2)	0.48
Overall sphincter length (mm)	44 (2)	45 (2)	0.49
Sphincter function index	718 (98)	507 (115)	0.01

Values are mean (s.e.m.). *Wilcoxon's signed rank test

Mean DeMeester acid scores increased from 14.2 before surgery to 29.8 after surgery for the 50 patients studied ($p < 0.001$). For patients who had an open operation, the score increased from 14.8 to 34.0 ($p < 0.006$), and for patients who had laparoscopic surgery, from 13.9 to 28.9 ($p < 0.002$). Both groups were comparable, with no significant difference in the preoperative and postoperative DeMeester acid scores between the open and laparoscopic groups. Mean lower esophageal sphincter pressure fell from 14.5 mmHg before surgery to 13.5 mmHg after surgery ($p < 0.2$ NS), with no statistically significant difference between the open and laparoscopic group. All these result are summarized in Table 34.6. In conclusion, this study also seems to confirm that patients undergoing elective cholecystectomy have a significant increase in the incidence of gastroesophageal reflux.

In contrast to the above mentioned studies, other authors believe that cholecystectomy has no influence on the occurrence of duodenogastric or gastroesophageal reflux [36, 37].

Manifold et al. [37] compared 17 operated patients with 11 healthy controls and documented that cholecystectomy produced no significant change in acid gastroesophageal reflux or duodenogastric reflux; furthermore, no difference was detected between control subjects and operated patients (Fig. 34.4).

Also in this case, as a definitive conclusion on the argument at the moment cannot be drawn, pH impedenzometry studies could help to understand physiological modifications in this group of patients.

The last question that has to be posed is the following: When cholelithiasis and GERD coexist, is it advisable to perform a combined surgical treatment? In the presence of symptomatic cholelithiasis the choice is clear, as complications due to gallstones can be severe and range from acute cholecystitis and pancreatitis to occasional gallbladder cancer. It remains controversial whether asymptomatic patients should undergo elective cholecystectomy or take the wait-and-see approach, with surgical intervention reserved for

Table 34. 6 Pre- and postoperative results of pH and manometry studies. From [35]

	n	Preoperative Mean (SEM)	Postoperative Mean (SEM)	*P**
Group 1 (open surgery)				
Acid score				
All patients	28	14.8 (2.4)	34.0 (6.7)	0.0061
Patients with postoperative reflux symptoms	11	11.6 (2.2)	37.6 (7.1)	0.003
Manometry (LESP) mmHg				
All patients	28	16.4 (4.4)	15.6 (5.6)	0.575
Patients with postoperative reflux symptoms	11	13.8 (1.07)	15.4 (1.77)	0.296
Group 2 (laparoscopic surgery)				
Acid scores				
All patients	22	13.9 (2.5)	28.9 (4.3)	0.002
Patients with postoperative reflux symptoms	9	14.5 (3.8)	34.5 (7.1)	0.004
Manometry (LESP) mmHg				
All patients	22	12.0 (2.4)	10.8 (3.9)	0.163
Patients with postoperative reflux symptoms	8	8.78 (0.57)	9.67 (1.4)	0.389

*Wilcoxon signed rank test; *LESP*, Lower esophageal sphincter pressure

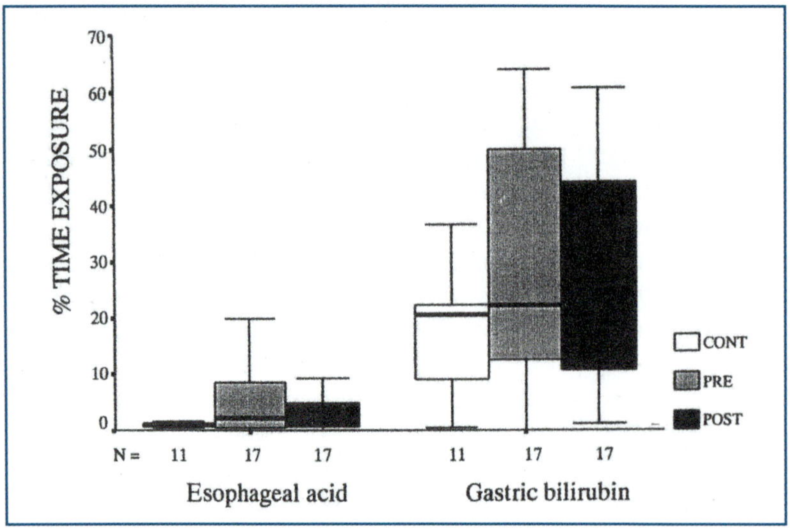

Fig. 34.4 Box-whisker plot of esophageal acid exposure (pH < 4) and gastric bilirubin exposure in control subjects before and after cholecystectomy in the patient group. From [37]

those who later develop symptoms or complications. The probability of ever needing a biliary operation for patients with asymptomatic cholelithiasis ranges from 15 to 40%, depending on the patient's age [38–41]. Nonbiliary surgery can result in complications from gallstones in some patients, and others may even develop acute cholecystitis in the postoperative period. This may become particularly important for elderly patients in whom the mortality of emergency surgery is 20 times higher than that of elective surgery. Furthermore, the wide diffusion of laparoscopic surgery has largely increased the indications to surgery for these patients because of reduced postoperative pain and faster recovery. Klaus et al. [42] compared the clinical outcome of 67 patients after laparoscopic fundoplication and incidental cholecystectomy for cholelithiasis with another 67 patients who underwent fundoplication alone. Surgical results including complications are summarized in Table 34.7. The addition of cholecystectomy did not prolong hospital stay and there were no

Table 34. 7 Laparoscopic fundoplication plus cholecystectomy vs. fundoplication alone – Perioperative results. From [42]

	ARS+CHOLE	ARS	*p* Value
Laparoscopic Nissen fundoplication	63	57	0.09
Laparoscopic Toupet fundoplication	4	10	0.09
Duration of GERD symptoms (months)	154.2	108.7	0.3
Hospital stay (days)	2.0	1.8	0.6
Blood loss (ml)	126.0	56.3	0.09
Duration of surgery (hours)	2.7	2.0	0.6
Complications			
Bleeding	3	1	0.31*
Pneumonia	0	2	1.0*

Mean is given for hospital stay, duration of symptoms, blood loss and duration of surgery; *Fisher's exact test used in lieu of chi-squared test; *ARS*, antireflux surgery; *CHOLE*, cholecystectomy statistically significant differences in blood loss and duration of surgery. In our experience, cholecystectomy was associated with laparoscopic fundoplication in 15 cases in a series of 487 patients operated upon for GERD (3.1%). We did not observe a significant increase in operative time, nor in morbidity or hospital stay in comparison with patients operated upon for laparoscopic fundoplication alone. Therefore, also in our opinion, it seems advisable to perform a combined intervention for cholelithiasis and GERD, as recommended by most authors.

In conclusion, no definitive answer can be given as to whether cholelithiasis and GERD are really associated, nor on the influence of cholecystectomy on the occurrence of GERD. We hope that future studies will be able to clarify this really interesting matter, elucidating the physiological modifications present in these patients and thus increasing therapeutic options.

References

1. Marshall JB (1994) Current opinions in gallstone management. What to do when symptoms are mild or absent. Postgrad Med 95:115-128
2. Martinez de Pancorbo C, Carballo F, Horcajo P et al (1997) Prevalence and associated factors for gallstone disease: results of a population survey in Spain. J Clin Epidemiol 50:1347-1355
3. Diaz-Rubio M, Moreno-Elola-Olaso C, Rey E et al (2004) Symptoms of gastroesophageal reflux: prevalence, severity duration and associated factors in a Spanish population. Aliment Pharmacol Ther 19:95-106
4. Burkitt DP, Walker ARP (1976) Saint's triad: confirmation and explanation. S Afr Med J 50:2136
5. Fisher RS, Stelzer F, Rock E, Malmud LS (1982) Abnormal gallbladder emptying in patients with gallstones. Dig Dis Sci 27:1019-1024
6. Portincasa P, Di Ciaula A, Baldassarre G et al (1994) Gallbladder motor function in gallstone patients: sonographic and in vitro studies on the role of gallstones, smooth muscle function and gallbladder wall inflammation. J Hepatol 21:430-440
7. Pomeranz IS, Shaffer EA (1985) Abnormal gallbladder emptying in a subgroup of patients with gallstones. Gastroenterology 88:787-791
8. Van Erpecum KJ, van Berge-Henegouwen GP, Stolk MFJ et al (1992) Fasting gallbladder volume, postprandial emptying and cholecystokinin release in gallstone patients and normal subjects. J Hepatol 14:194-202
9. Stolk MFJ, van Erpecum KJ, Renooij W et al (1995) Gallbladder emptying in vivo, bile composition and nucleation of cholesterol crystals in patients with cholesterol gallstones. Gastroenterology 108:1882-1888
10. Klapdor R, Hammer E (1983) Interdigestive motilin secretion and gallstone disease. Klin Wochenschr 61:251-253
11. Heaton KW, Emmett PM, Symes CL, Braddon FEM (1993) An explanation for gallstones in normal-weight women: slow intestinal transit. Lancet 341:8-10
12. Jazrawi S, Walsh TN, Byrne PJ et al (1993) Cholecystectomy and esophageal reflux: a prospective evaluation. Br J Surg 80:50-53
13. Portincasa P, Di Ciaula A, Palmieri V et al (1997) Impaired gallbladder and gastric motility and pathological gastroesophageal reflux in gallstone patients. Eur J Clin Invest 27:653-661
14. Ibrarullah M, Mittal BR, Agarwal DK et al (1994) Gastric emptying in patients with gallstone disease with or without dyspepsia: effect of cholecystectomy. Aust N Z J Surg 64:247-250
15. Walker JP, Khalil T, Wiener I et al (1985) The role of neurotensin in human gallbladder motility. Ann Surg 201:678-683
16. Blackburn AM, Bloom SR, Long RG (1980) Effect of neurotensin on gastric function in man. Lancet 1:987-989
17. Rosell S, Thor K, Nyquist O et al (1980) Plasma concentration of neurotensin-like immunoreactivity and lower esophageal sphincter pressure in man following infusion of (Gln4)-neurotensin. Acta Physiol Scand 109:369-375
18. Wilson P, Welch NT, Hinder RA et al (1993) Abnormal plasma gut hormones in pathologic duodenogastric reflux and their response to surgery. Am J Surg 165:169-176
19. Capron JP, Payenneville H, Dumont M et al (1978) Evidence for an association between cholelithiasis and hiatus hernia. Lancet 2:329-331
20. Baldwin JA (1978) Cholithiasis and hiatus hernia. Lancet 2:992
21. Honorf LH (1979) Cholelithiasis and hiatus hernia. Lancet 2:927-928
22. Avidan B, Sonnenberg A, Schnell TG, Sontag SJ (2001) No association between gallstones and gastroesophageal reflux disease. Am J Gastroenterol 96:2858-2862

23. Svensson JO, Gelin J, Svanvik J (1986) Gallstones, cholecystectomy and duodenogastric reflux of bile acid. Scand J Gastroenterol 21:181-187
24. Cabrol J, Navarro X, Simo-Deu J, Segura R (1990) Evaluation of duodenogastric reflux in gallstone disease before and after simple cholecystectomy. Am J Surg 160:283-286
25. Bates T, Ebbs SR, Harrison M, A'Hern RP (1991) Influence of cholecystectomy on symptoms. Br J Surg 78:964-967
26. Brough WA, Taylor TV, Torrance HB (1984) The surgical factors influencing duodenogastric reflux. Br J Surg 71:770-773
27. Lorusso D, Mangini V, Misciagna G et al (1986) Pre- and postcholecystectomy duodenogastric reflux. Dig Surg 3:305-310
28. Pedrikis G, Wilson P, Hinder R et al (1994) Altered antroduodenal motility after cholecystectomy. Am J Surg 168:609-615
29. Bailey I, Walsh TN, Hill AD et al (1992) Effect of cholecystectomy on plasma cholecystokinin. Br J Surg 79:456
30. McDonnell CO, Bailey I, Stumpf T et al (2002) The effect of cholecystectomy on plasma cholecystokinin. Am J Gastroenterol 97:2189-2192
31. Clavè P, Gonzalez A, Martin M et al (1996) Endogenous cholecystokinin enhances post-prandial gastroesophageal reflux in healthy volunteers. Gastroenterology 4:A649
32. Lorusso D, Misciagna G, Mangini V et al (1990) Duodenogastric reflux of bile acids, gastrin and parietal cells and gastric acid secretion before and 6 months after cholecystectomy. Am J Surg 159:575-578
33. Jazrawi S, Walsh TN, Byrne PJ et al (1993) Cholecystectomy and esophageal reflux: a prospective evaluation. Br J Surg 80:50-53
34. Lujan-Mompean JA, Robles-Campos R, Parrilla-Paricio P et al (1993) Duodenogastric reflux in patients with biliary lithiasis before and after cholecystecomy. Surg Gynecol Obstet 176:116-118
35. Rothwell JF, Lawlor P, Byrne PJ et al (1997) Cholecystectomy induced gastroesophageal reflux: is it reduced by the laparoscopic approach? Am J Gastroenterol 92:1351-1354
36. Maddern GJ, Baxter PS (1997) The effect of laparoscopic cholecystectomy on gastroduodenal reflux. Aust N Z J Surg 67:703-705
37. Manifold DK, Anggiansah B, Owen WJ (2000) Effect of cholecystectomy on gastroesophageal and duodenogastric reflux. Am J Gastroenterol 95:2746-2750
38. Ransohoff DF, Gracie WA (1993) Treatment of gallstones. Ann Intern Med 119:606-619
39. Peterson R (1995) Gallstones during the course of 1066 abdominal sections for pelvic disease. Surg Gynecol Obstet 20:284-291
40. Lund J (1960) Surgical indication in cholelithiasis: prophylactic cholecystectomy elucidated on the basis of long-term follow up on 526 non operated cases. Ann Surg 151:153-162
41. Wenckert A, Robertson B (1966) The natural course of gallstone disease: eleven-year review of 781 non operated cases. Gastroenterology 50:376-381
42. Klaus A, Hinder R, Swain J, Achem SR (2002) Incidental cholecystectomy during laparoscopic antireflux surgery. Am Surg 68:619-62

Chapter 35

Hepatic Cirrhosis and Biliary Stones

Patrick Pessaux, Emilie Lermite

Introduction

Different studies have suggested that the prevalence of gallstones is increased in patients with cirrhosis [1–3]. In the past, open cholecystectomy (OC) in cirrhotic patients was commonly accompanied by significant morbidity and mortality [4, 5]. Laparoscopic cholecystectomy (LC) has become the procedure of choice to treat symptomatic cholelithiasis in the general population. However, cirrhosis has been considered as a contraindication for LC due to the risk of bleeding and liver failure [6]. Currently, with the advances in laparoscopic technology, a range of increasingly complex procedures are performed, making traditional contraindications at best relative. Several studies have reported good results and suggested liberal use of LC in patients with early-stage cirrhosis and symptomatic cholelithiasis. The aim of this chapter is to review the results from the literature of LC in patients with cirrhosis.

Preoperative Workup

When a patient with cirrhosis needs surgery, the degree of hepatocellular insufficiency and portal hypertension are prognostic factors and must be well evaluated preoperatively. Clinical and radiological assessment is necessary in identifying patients with portal hypertension. The risk of portal hypertension should not be underestimated, and a preoperative upper gastrointestinal endoscopy is useful to evaluate the presence of esophageal varices.

Special individual measures should be taken to improve hepatic function. These include hepatic function protection and support, ascites control, nutrition support, improvement of coagulopathy disorders and reduction of portal vein pressure. Correction of coagulopathy with platelets or fresh frozen plasma before surgery is advisable, and intraoperative availability of these products is essential.

Technique

LC in cirrhotic patients should be considered advanced laparoscopic surgery and should not be attempted by surgeons with limited experience in laparoscopic surgery. Some modifications of the technique should be employed to avoid the risk of heavy bleeding. Particular care is necessary when the umbilical port is placed because a collateral venous circuit may be present. In such a case, it is best to avoid the periumbilical area in order to prevent injury to an umbilical vein. Additionally, major collateral veins may be identified by transillumination of the abdominal wall using the light of the laparoscope. A more laterally to the right placement of the subxifoid port is crucial to avoid injury to the falciform ligament. Sometimes cirrhosis can lead to atrophy-hypertrophy and displacement of liver lobes. This may cause inconvenient exposure of the operative field under laparoscopy. Tracker location is usually adjusted in this situation. Excessive traction is avoided in order to prevent avulsion of the gallbladder from the liver bed and, hence, bleeding from the gallbladder bed. In patients with important collateral veins around the gallbladder, some authors propose performing a subtotal cholecystectomy in order to prevent blood loss from the gallbladder bed [7].

Special care is recommended in the management of the liver with forceps.

All access ports must be checked internally just before completion of the procedure to detect possible bleeding.

Results

The first report on the use of LC in patients with cirrhosis was published by Yerdel et al. [8] in 1993. This report proved that LC was a safe procedure, with a short operative time and reduced hospital stay. These data were confirmed by different studies: more than 400 patients with Child-Pugh A and B cirrhosis who underwent LC have been reported to date with no mortality and with an overall morbidity rate of 20% (Table 35.1). The majority of these studies are too small to determine any statistically significant difference in outcomes.

Currently no prospective trial comparing LC to OC has been performed in cirrhotic patients. A meta-analysis summarised the results of the published studies [26]. This meta-analysis reported that cirrhotic patients had significantly increased blood loss compared with noncirrhotic patients during LC, but the mean blood loss was significantly lower for LC than for OC in the cirrhotic group. In addition, the operative time and length of hospitalisation in cirrhotic patients were significantly reduced

Table 35.1 Review of the literature

	Number of patients	Morbidity (%)	Mortality (%)	Operative time (min)	Hospital stay (days)
Yerdel et al., 1997 [9]	7	0	0	155	6
Angrisani et al., 1997 [10]	31	25	0	-	3
Jan et al., 1997 [11]	21	4.8	-	-	4.1
Sleeman et al., 1998 [12]	25	32	0	116	1.7
Poggio et al., 2000 [13]	26	19	0	116	2.3
Morino et al., 2000 [14]	33	0	0	114	2.8
Fernandes et al., 2000 [15]	48	12.5	0	-	6.5
Urban et al., 2001 [16]	15	0	0	105	3
Clark et al., 2001 [17]	25	52	4	107	4
Leone et al., 2001 [18]	24	20.8	0	89	4.7
Tuech et al., 2002 [19]	26	27	0	126	5
Yeh et al., 2002 [20]	226	6.6	0.88	-	4.7
Cucinotta et al., 2003 [21]	22	36	0	115	5
Wu Ji et al., 2004 [22]	38	13.2	0	-	-
Curro et al., 2004 [23]	42	35	4.76	128	7.3
Schiff et al., 2005 [24]	31	-	0	156	2
Flores Cortes et al., 2005 [25]	14	21.42	0	77	3
Palanivelu et al., 2006 [7]	265	25.6	0	65	4

for LC compared with OC. These data seem to be associated with several causes. Magnification of the surgical field in laparoscopy permits meticulous care during haemostasis, and pneumoperitoneum seems to play a role in determining haemostasis (barohaemostasis). Laparoscopy avoids the subcostal incision that would increase haemorrhage, particularly in patients with coagulopathy. Furthermore, LC reduces the risk of infections, dehiscences, postoperative hernias, and infiltration of ascites through the abdominal wound.

In the literature, the conversion rate is between 0 and 12%. In a difficult situation, it is better to convert the procedure. Conversion is not a complication, but should be considered a means of preventing more serious problems. The surgeon should convert the procedure immediately when there is uncertainly about the safety and efficiency of the operative procedure.

Another advantage of LC over laparotomy is a lower rate of postoperative adhesions in patients who may need liver transplantation in the future. Morino et al. [14] have also described the advantages to the staff of the use of LC in patients with viral cirrhosis, as the risk of contamination decreases from 9 to 4.7% [14].

Particular Situations: Acute Cholecystitis, Child-Pugh Class C

Patients with acute cholecystitis should be treated conservatively and reassessed later because emergency operative management has always been associated with high morbidity and mortality. Acute cholecystitis can induce deterioration of the liver reserve and change a Child-Pugh Class B to C.

For patients with Child-Pugh Class C cirrhosis, the benefits and risks of LC must be carefully evaluated, as mortality is extremely high. There is very little in the literature about Child-Pugh Class C patients undergoing LC [23]. A meta-analysis reported only six Child-Pugh C cirrhotic patients who underwent LC [26]. In these high risk patients, cholecystectomy should be avoided. Some authors have suggested endoscopic stenting of the cystic duct [27]. Alternatively, percutaneous cholecystostomy may reverse the progression of the inflammation in patients with cholecystitis and provide prompt symptomatic relief [28]. However, in the presence of portal hypertension, coagulopathy, and/or ascites, the use of this approach is also associated with haemorrhage and sepsis.

Conclusion

The overall incidence of complications and blood loss related to LC seems to be higher in cirrhotic patients compared to the general population. However, LC is a safe and effective alternative for treatment of symptomatic cholelithiasis in patients with well-compensated Child-Pugh class A or B cirrhosis. Postoperative morbidity/mortality and bleeding are low, and both operative time and hospital stay are short in comparison with OC. Nevertheless, because of the high risk of liver failure and heavy haemorrhage in patients with Child-Pugh class C, LC is not recommended.

References

1. Del Olmo JA, Garcia F, Serra MA et al (1997) Prevalence of gallstones in liver cirrhosis. Scand J Gastroenterol 32:1061-1065
2. Schwesinger WH, Kurtin WE, Levine BA, Page CP (1985) Cirrhosis and alcoholism as pathogenetic factors in pigment gallstone disease. Ann Surg 210:319-322
3. Conte D, Fraquelli M, Fornari F et al (1999) Close relationship between cirrhosis and gallstones: cross-sectional and longitudinal survey. Arch Intern Med 159:49-52
4. Aranha GV, Sontag SJ, Greenlee HB (1982) Chole-

cystectomy in cirrhotic patients: a formidable operation. Am J Surg 143:55-60
5. Schwartz SI (1981) Biliary tract surgery and cirrhosis: a critical combination. Surgery 90:577-583
6. NIH consensus conference statement on gallstones and laparoscopic cholecystectomy (1993) Am J Surg 165:390-398
7. Palanivelu C, Rajan PS, Jani K et al (2006) Laparoscopic cholecystectomy in cirrhotic patients: the role of subtotal cholecystectomy and its variants. J Am Coll Surg 203:145-151
8. Yerdel MA, Tsuge H, Mimura H (1993) Laparoscopic cholecystectomy in cirrhotic patients: expanding indications. Surg Laparoscoc Endosc 3:180-183
9. Yerdel MA, Koksoy C, Aras N, Orita K (1997) Laparoscopic versus open cholecystectomy in cirrhosis patients: a prospective study. Surg Laparosc Endosc 7:483-486
10. Angrisani L, Lorenzo M, Corcione F, Vincenti R (1997) Gallstones in cirrhotics revisited by a laparoscopic view. L Laparoendosc Adv Surg Tech A 7:213-220
11. Jan YY, Chen MF (1997) Laproscopic cholecystectomy in cirrhotic patients. Hepatogastroenterology 44:1584-1587
12. Sleeman D, Namias N, Levi D et al (1998) Laparoscopic cholecystectomy in cirrhosis patients. J Am Coll Surg 187:400-403
13. Poggio JL, Rowland CM, Gores GJ et al (2000) A comparison of laparoscopic and open cholecystectomy in patients with compensed cirrhosis and symptomatic gallstone disease. Surgery 127:405-411
14. Morino M, Cavuoti G, Miglietta C et al (2000) Laparoscopic cholecystectomy in cirrhosis: contraindication or privileged indication? Surg Laparosc Endosc Percutan Tech 10:360-363
15. Fernandes NF, Schwesinger WH, Hilsenbeck SG et al (2000) Laparoscopic cholecystectomy and cirrhosis: a case-control study of outcomes. Liver transpl 6:340-344
16. Urban L, Eason GA, ReMine S et al (2001) Laparoscopic cholecystectomy in patients with early cirrhosis. Curr Surg 58:312-315
17. Clark JR, Wills VL, Hunt DR (2001) Cirrhosis and laparoscopic cholecystectomy. Surg Laparosc Endosc Percutan Tech 11:165-169
18. Leone N, Garino M, De Paolis P (2001) Laparoscopic cholecystectomy in cirrhotic patients. Dig Surg 18:449-452
19. Tuech JJ, Pessaux P, Regenet N et al (2002) Laparoscopic cholecystectomy in cirrhotic patients. Surg Laparosc Endosc Percutan Tech 12:227-231
20. Yeh CN, Chen MF, Jan YY (2002) Laparoscopic cholecystectomy in 226 cirrhotic patients. Surg Endosc 16:1583-1587
21. Cucinotta E, Lazzara S, Melita G (2003) Laparoscopic cholecytectomy in cirrhotic patients. Surg Endosc 17:1958-1960
22. Wu JI, Ling-Tang Li, Xun-Ru Chen, Jie-Shou Li (2004) Application of laparoscopic cholecystectomy in patients with cirrhotic portal hypertension. Hepatobiliary Pancreat Dis Int 3:270-274
23. Curro G, Lapichino G, Melita G et al (2005) Laparoscopic cholecystectomy in Child-Pugh Class C cirrhotic patients. JSLS 9:311-315
24. Schiff J, Misra M, Rendon G et al (2005) Laparoscopic cholecystectomy in cirrhotic patients. Surg Endosc 19:1278-1281
25. Flores Cortes M, Obispo Entrenas A, Docobo Durantez F et al (2005) Laparoscopic treatment of cholelithiasis in cirrhotic patients. Rev Esp Enferm Dig 97:648-653
26. Puggioni A, Wong LL (2003) A metaanalysis of laparoscopic cholecystectomy in patients with cirrhosis. J Am Coll Surg 197:921-926
27. Feretis C, Apostolidis N, Mallas E et al (1993) Endoscopic drainage of acute obstructive cholecystitis in patients with increased operative risk. Endoscopy 25:392-395
28. Welschbilling-Meunier K, Pessaux P, Lebigot J et al (2005) Percutaneous cholecystostomy for high-risk patients with acute cholecystitis. Surg Endosc 19:1256-1259

Chapter 36

Biliary Stones and Gastrectomy

Giovanni De Manzoni, Simone Giacopuzzi, Giuseppe Borzellino, Claudio Cordiano

Epidemiology

A possible association of biliary stones and gastric surgery has been hypothesised since the clinical observations of Majoor in 1947 on a series of 147 gastric resections for peptic ulcer [1]. Although the pathophysiology of such an association was not completely understood, vagotomy and neuro-hormonal changes after gastric resections were advocated and an 18% prevalence of new gallstones was reported at 5 years follow up, 13.5% of which required a surgical treatment [2, 3].

Since the introduction of endoscopy and new pharmaceutical products, such indications for gastric surgery have dramatically decreased. However, gastrectomy with lymphadenectomy remains the most valuable option for gastric cancer, improvements in the surgical treatment of which in recent years have resulted in an increase in 5 year survival rates [4]. Epidemiological data and survival analysis therefore suggest that the question of new cases of gallstones after gastric surgery for gastric cancer needs to be considered. The question of a prophylactic cholecystectomy during gastrectomy is emphasised not only on the basis of the aforementioned data but also by the lower feasibility of a minimally invasive treatment for biliary lithiasis in patients with previous either total or partial gastrectomy. Upper abdominal previous surgery may be a contraindication for laparoscopic cholecystectomy due to parietal and visceral adhesions, most annoying at the duodenal closure; furthermore, Roux-en-Y loop digestive reconstruction may close the door to a common bile duct stone endoscopic approach.

Overall incidence of gastric cancer has decreased in the last decades but such a trend has not been registered for adenocarcinoma of the oesophago-gastric junction, which remains the fourth highest cause of tumours in general population and the second cause of tumour-related death. In 2000, 880,000 news cases were registered, with 650,000 related deaths worldwide [5]. Early diagnosis has, however, allowed a higher 5 year survival rate to be reached for such tumours. Data from the American Cancer Society, based on the National Cancer Data Base, revealed that in the year 2000, the 5 year overall survival rate after gastrectomy was 28%, and the survival rates for stage IA and IB were 78% and 58%, respectively [6]. In our experience, the 5 year survival rate is 54% after R0 surgery and up to 95% in the cases without nodal metastases (Fig. 36.1) [7].

The incidence of cholelithiasis after gastric surgery for gastric cancer has been reported to be higher than that of general population, with reported incidences varying from 10 to 47% [8–15]. Different extents of gastrectomy and/or lymphadenectomy and different digestive reconstruction modalities may explain the wide range of cholelithiasis incidence in different series. In a recent study on 749 either partial or total gastrectomies for gastric carcinoma, the prevalence of gallbladder stones was 13.6% and 22.1%, 5 years and 10 years after gastric surgery, respectively [8]. In a study

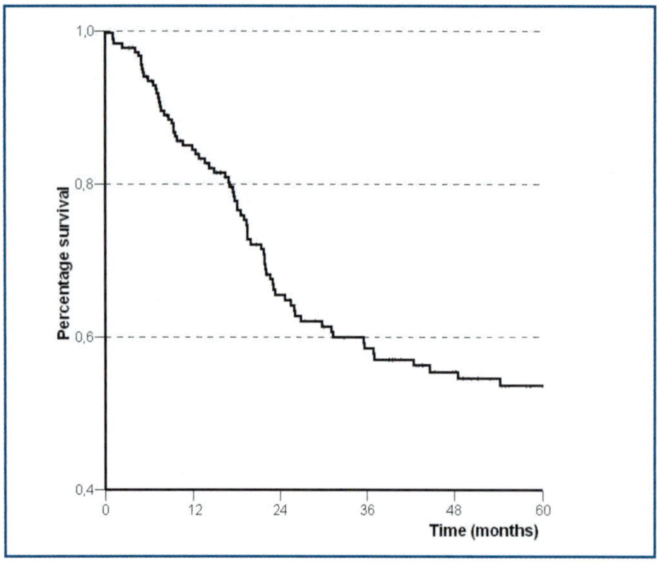

Fig. 36.1 Survival after R0 surgery. From [7]

of total gastrectomies, the prevalence of cholelithiasis was 47% within 2 years of gastric surgery [15], while a study with different extents of gastrectomy and lymphadenectomy reported a 12.7% prevalence of gallstone, 90.1% of which occurred within 5 years of gastric surgery [10].

Pathophysiology

The role of vagotomy and that of neuro-hormonal factors involved in gallstone formation after gastrectomy were reported in the era of gastrectomy for peptic ulcer [3]. More recent studies based on ultrasonographic examinations have confirmed gallbladder volume and gallbladder contractility alterations after gastrectomy for gastric cancer [11, 16], while a study on the surgical anatomy of innervation of the gallbladder has emphasised the role of the vagus in such a process [17].

However, sludge formation associated with a lower contractility of the gallbladder has been observed in a very high percentage of patients soon after gastrectomy. The sludge disappeared in most cases one year after the recovery of contractile function of the gallbladder, and the formation of stones occurred later and seemed independent of early sludge formation [11].

Two hepatic plexuses innervating the biliary tree and gallbladder, one anterior and one posterior, have been described, along with nerve offshoots arising from the phrenic nerves. The anterior plexus contains shepatic division of the anterior vagal trunk, parasympathetic and sympathetic fibres arising from celiac plexus, wounding around hepatic artery it sends branches to the peritoneum and bed of the gallbladder via the cystic artery; via the cystic duct as well the plexus sends also direct branches to the neck, body and fundus of gallbladder. The posterior plexus arises from the right side of the celiac plexus and runs along the dorsal sides of the portal vein, branches extend along the upper part of the common bile duct and join the liver and the gallbladder, while descending branches are sent to the proximal part of the descending duodenum and distal common bile duct. Bidirectional neural connection between the papilla and gallbladder is sustained by numerous communicating branches behind the common bile duct and portal vein [17, 18].

A general pathway may be recognised: sections of vagus directly alter gallbladder tone, while a lack of acid production due to vagus denervation and deviation of food from the jejuno-duodenal tract are responsible for impaired hormonal secretion of active peptides, such as cholecystokinin and secretin, acting on gallbladder motility and bile composition. The role of cholecystokinin in gallbladder contraction and sphincter of Oddi relaxation has been reported [3, 19], while impairment of secretin leads to a reduction in rich bicarbonate fluid secretion in the bile, therefore favouring crystal aggregation of cholesterol [20]. However, in a study on cholecystokinin response to oral fat after gastrectomy, an increase in hormone secretion was observed in gastrectomised patients with either Billroth I or Billroth II reconstruction when compared with normal subjects [21]. These observations indicate that a large amount of hormone can be released from the jejunum and may be increased by rapid gastric emptying. Although different molecular forms of the hormone may have different potencies in terms of action on the gallbladder contractility, such an elevated amount of jejunal cholecystokinin plays a role in the lithogenesis of the bile as a result.

The nutritional status of patients and total parenteral nutrition may also play a role in the increased risk of biliary lithiasis after gastrectomy [22, 23]. Tissutal mobilisation of cholesterol and post-operative fasting have been hypothesised [24, 25], but such a correlation is still controversial since a pattern of transient post-operative sludge formation rather than a real increase incidence of gallstone formation has been reported [11].

Gallstone formation after gastric surgery is therefore mainly due to complex interactions between different levels of vagus nerve sectioning and hormonal response in relation to the extent of gastrectomy and type of reconstruction. Furthermore, the level of vagus section depends on the extent of gastrectomy and that of lymphadenectomy, since with total gastrectomy the vagus is sectioned proximally, while in partial distal gastrectomy the section is more distal and may not influence biliary innervation. In the latter case, dissection of the hepato-duodenal ligament and celiac arteries for D2 lymphadenectomy may alter gallbladder innervation due to retroperitoneal destruction of sympathetic and parasympathetic fibers, gallbladder innervation remains only cholinergic with contractility dysfunction as a result. In both, exclusion of the duodenum adds a further predisposing factor due to impaired hormonal regulation. In proximal or pylorus-preserving gastrectomy, risk factors are limited to vagus damage since conserved passage of food through the duodenum does not alter hormonal regulation of gallbladder physiology.

The extent of gastrectomy, and the extent of lymphadenectomy in partial gastrectomy and digestive reconstruction have therefore to be taken into account when evaluating the risk of gallbladder stone occurrence after gastric surgery.

Risk Factors for Development of Gallstones

Extent of Gastric Resection

Two comparative studies have reported a significant increase in the prevalence of gallbladder stones after total gastrectomy, as compared to partial gastrectomy [8, 14], while two studies have reported no relationship between the extent of gastrectomy and incidence of post-operative gallstone disease [12, 26]. In the study of Koyabashi et al. [8], total gastrectomy with Roux en Y loop and near total gastrectomy with pylorus preservation were compared with partial gastrectomy comprising Billroth I, Billroth II and pylorus-preserving partial gastrectomy. A significantly higher proportion of patients developed gallstones after total gastrectomy, with a rate of 17.3% versus 8.4% ($p < 0.001$) after partial gastrectomy in the 10-years-follow-up. The results were rendered confusing by the fact that Billroth I was included in the partial gastrectomy group and therefore may have influenced the results by the way of a different hormonal response. However, based on the data reported by the author, re-calculation of the proportion of patients with gallstones after exclusion of the Billroth I patients in the partial gastrectomy group was only slightly higher (10.6 %), and therefore did not influence the comparison. The study of Nakamura et al. [14] in which post-operative symptomatic gallbladder stones were considered confirm these data, with gallstones in 38.5% of patients after total gastrectomy versus 6.2% after proximal and 1% after distal partial gastrectomy ($p < 0.001$), although no details on digestive reconstruction were provided.

The confounding nature of the comparative study's lack of subgroup analysis that would take into account extent of lymphadenectomy and digestive reconstruction should be kept in mind.

Extent of Lymphadenectomy

Four studies report a higher proportion of gallstone disease after extended lymphadenectomy [8, 10, 12, 26]. One of these compared D3 versus D1-2 and another one compared radical versus simple gastrectomy. Again, possible confusion related to a lack of subgroup analysis has to be taken into account. In one study [10], the incidence of gallstones was compared after a D1 and D2 lymphadenectomy. In this study the extent of gastrectomy and type of reconstruction did not differ in the two groups, but early stages were more likely to be treated with a D1 lymphadenectomy. At a 70.5 month follow up, the incidence of gallbladder stones was higher in the D2 group than in the D1 group, with an incidence of 17.8% versus 9.4% ($p = 0.001$) respectively, and occurred earlier, at 18.8 months versus 29.4 months ($p = 0.002$). In the study of Kobayashi et al. [8], a more accurate analysis of lymph node dissection was reported. Stations along the common hepatic artery, around the celiac artery, and in the hepatoduodenal ligament (stations 8, 9 and 12 of the Japanese Classification of Gastric Carcinoma, respectively) correlated statistically with a higher incidence of gallstone disease but only station 12 of the hepatoduodenal ligament was identified as a significant risk factor in a multivariate analysis of different extents of gastrectomy and types of reconstruction, with an Odds Ratio of 3.66 (95% CI: 2.16–6.22). One study has reported that the extent of lymphadenectomy does not influence the incidence of symptomatic post-operative cholelithiasis [14].

Digestive Reconstruction

Contradictory results are reported: in two studies no differences in the incidence of symptomatic and asymptomatic gallstone disease were found among different reconstructions after gastrectomy [12, 14], while a significantly higher incidence of gallstones were retrieved in the study of Kobayashi et al. [8]. Pylorus preservation and influence of passage of food were evaluated by comparison of incidence of gallstones after reconstructions in which the duodenum was excluded (Roux-en-Y loop and Billroth II) and those with a maintained duodenal food passage (Billroth I and pylorus-preserving gastrectomy). In these studies, the incidence of gallstones was 17% in the duodenal exclusion group versus 8% in the duodenal conservation group ($p < 0.001$).

Digestive reconstruction strongly depends, however, on the extent of gastrectomy and results may be biased since the duodenum is excluded in the most common and valuable reconstruction after total gastrectomy in which the truncal vagus is of course sectioned. Only partial proximal gastrectomy allows a pylorus-preserving procedure, while for distal gastrectomy Billroth I is rarely feasible with an oncologic purpose.

Treatment of Biliary Lithiasis in Previous Gastric Surgery

Laparoscopic cholecystectomy is the treatment of choice for symptomatic cholelithiasis; however, previous abdominal surgery was considered a contra-indication since high conversion rates were reported rising up to 50% of cases in patients with previous gastrectomy [27–29]. With increased experience, laparoscopy has proven to be feasible even in patients with previous abdominal surgery, although difficulties are encountered due to the problem of post-operative adhesion. In post-gastrectomy patients, significant difficulties with viscera-visceral adhesions at the site of cholecystectomy are added to the general problems of the viscera-parietal adhesion. The former, generated by a previous dissection of the hepatoduodenal ligament and duodenal stump closure, make it more difficult to recognise biliary structures that have to be freed from adhesion, while the latter have to be considered in the pneumoperitoneum creation and extent of adhesiolysis necessary to complete cholecystectomy [30, 31]. In a recent study, among 449 patients with previous abdominal surgery, 29 had a gastrectomy with a conversion rate of 10%, much higher than the 0.9% conversion rate reported in patients with other previous abdominal interventions [9]. In all cases the cause of laparoscopic failure was adhesions, and the complication rate of laparoscopic cholecystectomy was 14%. In a case control study no significant differences were found in patients with previous gastrectomy for peptic ulcer and patients without previous abdominal surgery, although only 15 patients were included in each group [31].

When extensive viscera-parietal adhesions secondary to previous gastrectomy are suspected, an open laparoscopy is recommended rather than blind needle puncture for the creation of pneumoperitoneum. In our experience, a pre-operative parietal ultrasonography has proven a valuable approach, with a 100% sensitivity reached and none of the complications reported in the literature even with open laparoscopy [32, 33]. The presence of viscera-visceral adhesions has to be managed according to personal experience, the duration of the intervention and risks of complication have to be considered when deciding whether or not to convert.

Acute cholecystitis adds further difficulties, since management occurs in an urgent setting and dissection of anatomical structures may be more difficult due to inflammation of the gallbladder, leading to an increased conversion rate [30, 31].

The type of reconstruction of gastric surgery is of major concern for the treatment of common bile duct stones. The exclusion of duodenum makes it impossible to achieve an endoscopic approach. An endoscopic sphincterotomy via a percutaneous transhepatic cholangioscopy has been reported in three patients [34]. However, this innovative technique needs to be validated by further studies. This approach may be indicated in cholecystectomised patients or in those unfit for surgery, otherwise comparative studies with the surgical approach are necessary. Laparoscopic surgical approach has been also reported in two patients with previous Billroth II operation [9], by choledocotomy with primary closure and T-tube closure of the main bile duct. Here again, only isolated cases are reported in the literature and the technique cannot be routinely recommended. The last solution is an open surgical approach to the main bile duct. We have attempted a Rendez-vous technique in two cases with previous gastrectomy with a Roux-en-Y reconstruction, one by laparoscopy and one by laparotomy. A guide wire was introduced via the cystic duct in the duodenal stump and under radioscopic guidance carried to the termino-lateral anastomosis of the Roux-en-Y loop. Here the wire was recovered by endoscopy and pulled out of the mouth in order to guide the further positioning of the endoscope to the level of the papilla in the duodenal stump. In the case of attempted laparoscopy, although the papilla was reached, cannulation was not possible due to difficulties in positioning the endoscope in the correct position in front of the papilla and conversion was necessary, while in the case approached by open surgery, the manoeuvre was feasible and endoscopic sphincterotomy was achieved.

A combined laparoscopic and endoscopic approach may be attempted, but if it does not prove to be feasible, conversion to open cholecystectomy in order to facilitate the Rendez-vous technique by handling the endoscope through the intestinal loop seems the most valuable and less invasive approach.

Prophylactic Cholecystectomy during Gastric Surgery

Since previous gastric surgery may impair minimally invasive treatment of biliary lithiasis and cholelithiasis is more frequent after gastrectomy, indications for prophylactic cholecystectomy during gastric surgery may be questionable. Literature data are scarce and controversial opinions have been expressed [8, 14, 26]. Arguments in favour arise from epidemiological observations, while arguments against include the possible complications of cholecystectomy in the course of gastric surgery and post-cholecystectomy syndrome in gastrectomised patients.

Although there is no specific data, morbidity for non complicated cholecystectomy is very low and may be considered to have no influence in the setting of gastric surgery. Post-cholecystectomy syndromes are mainly due to persistence of the symptoms that erroneously led to cholecystectomy, to duodeno-gastric bile reflux, to alteration of intestinal motility due to the action of non emulsioned fat or biliary dyskinesia due to sphincter of Oddi dysfunction [35, 36]. If cholecystectomy is just prophylactic and a Roux-en-Y reconstruction is performed, only symptoms related to intestinal motility and biliary dyskinesia may play a role. No specific studies on such a topic have been found, and it is not known to what extent the interaction between pathophysiology of gastric surgery and cholecystectomy may play a role. Incidence of symptoms due to biliary dyskinesia have been reported to be less than 1% [37] and up to 3% over a 10 year period of time [36]; however, survival after gastric cancer is not reported for such a long term. Furthermore, after gastrectomy a possible synergic effect of rapid passage of food through the jejunum and that of non emulsioned fat on increased jejunal cholecystokinin secretion with altered intestinal motility may be hypothesised, as well as sphincter of Oddi dyskinesia secondary to an impaired cholecysto-biliary reflex.

Among epidemiological data, those that may influence the question of a prophylactic cholecystectomy are the prevalence of symptomatic cholelithiasis, the only type that requires treatment, and their time of appearance. Since the most common indication for gastric surgery is actually gastric cancer, a careful consideration of incidence and time of appearance cannot be carried out without a survival analysis of gastric cancer.

Although incidence of post-gastrectomy cholelithiasis has been found to be higher than in the general population, the rate that becomes symptomatic and therefore needs surgical treatment seems to be much lower; it has been reported to vary from 3.5 to 15.9% of new cases of cholelithiasis and therefore from 0.4 to 2.3% of all patients operated upon for a gastric cancer, with a median time period for symptomatic gallstone detection from 40–48 months [8, 10, 14].

Overall rates of survival after gastric cancer surgery have been reported by the American Cancer Society to be 34% at 3 years and 28% at 5 years [6]. However, the pathological stage of the cancer and possibility of reaching R0 surgical excision influence survival rate. In our experience [7], overall survival is 54% at 5 years in R0 patients. With N2 nodal metastases, survival is 48% at 3 years, but it decreases to 14% when N3 nodal station metastases are retrieved (Fig. 36. 2), while for a T3/T4 TMN stage tumour the survival rate is 35% at 5 years, independent of nodal status (Fig. 36.3). In early gastric cancer (stage T1), a survival rate of 95% without nodal metastases and 73% with nodal involvement have been retrieved. However, pre- and peri-operative staging are not always predictive of the pathological findings: only the T parameter may be evaluated during surgery by the way of an ultrasound examination of the gastric wall with 91% accuracy [38], while nodal assessment requires an extended lymphadenectomy. Peri-operative staging is therefore not reliable for prognostic determination of gastric cancer. Extension of gastric resection also has to be taken into account, since total gastrectomy with Roux-en-Y reconstruction leads to a higher incidence of post-operative cholelithiasis and since D2 lymphadenectomy is associated with a significantly higher rate of symptomatic cholelithiasis than D1 lymphadenectomy, with 19.5% of cases requiring surgical treatment in the former versus 4.3% in the latter (p = 0.033) [10].

It could therefore be estimated that in about one-third to one-half of patients with radical gastric surgery the risk of requiring a cholecystectomy is no more than 2.5%.

Conclusion

Gallbladder lithiasis is a relevant physiopathological event after gastric surgery, but epidemiological data do not support the indication for a prophylactic cholecystectomy during gastric surgery for cancer, despite the reported lower feasibility of minimally invasive treatment of biliary lithiasis in patients with previous gastrectomy. However, due to a longer survival time in early gastric cancer and a higher incidence of cholelithiasis after total gastrectomy with Roux-en-Y reconstruction and extended lymphadenectomy, an indication restricted to

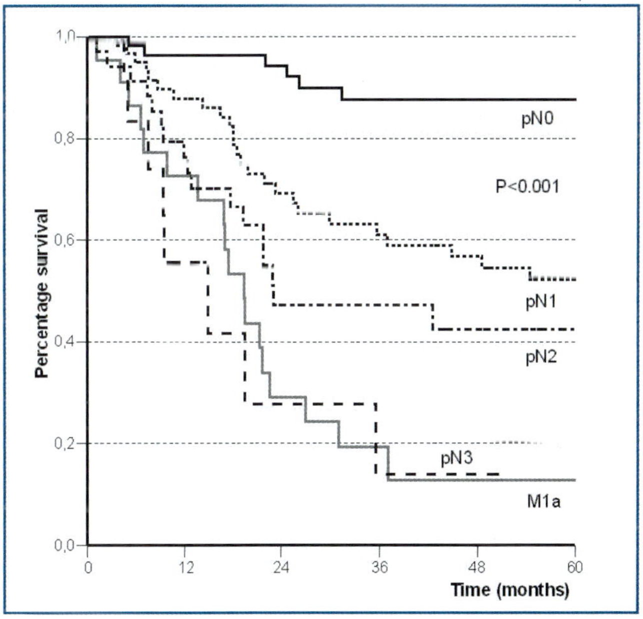

Fig. 36.2 N subgroup 5 year survival after R0 surgery. From [7]

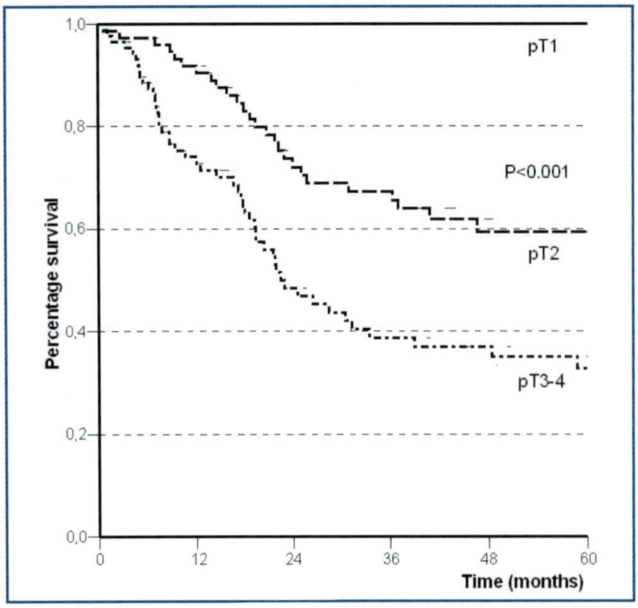

Fig. 36.3 T subgroup 5 year survival after R0 surgery. From [7]

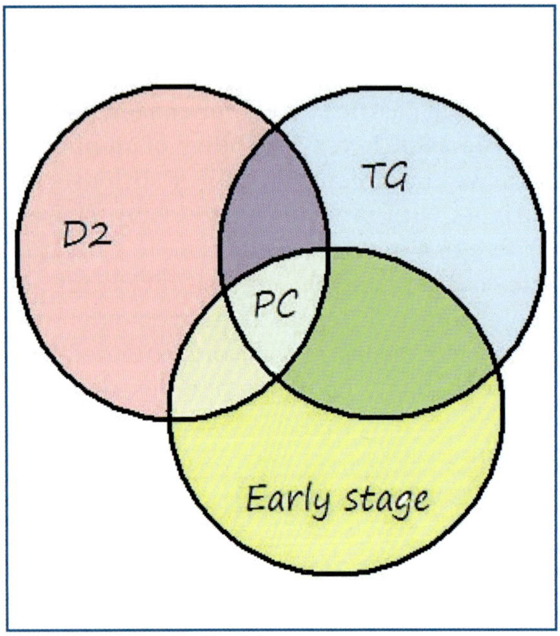

Fig. 36.4 Prophylactic cholecystectomy (*PC*) based on lymphadenectomy (*D2*), early stage of gastric cancer and extent of gastrectomy (*TG*, total gastrectomy)

this group of patients (Fig. 36.4) may be contemplated, although staging uncertainties have to be taken into account. A better understanding of gastrectomy with associated cholecystectomy pathophysiology and more precise epidemiological data on such patients are therefore needed.

References

1. Majoor CLH, Suren TJJ (1947) Gallbladder complications following resection of stomach for peptic ulcer. BMJ ii:8-11
2. Rehnberg O, Haglund U (1985) Gallstone disease following antrectomy and gastroduodenostomy with or without vagotomy. Ann Surg 201:315-318
3. Bouchier IA (1970) The vagus, the bile, and gallstones. Gut 11:799-803
4. Folli S, Morgagni P, Roviello F et al; Italian Research Group for Gastric Cancer (IRGGC) (2001) Risk factors for lymph node metastases and their prognostic significance in early gastric cancer (EGC) for the Italian Research Group for Gastric Cancer (IRGGC). Jpn J Clin Oncol 31:495-499
5. Crew KD, Neugut AI (2006) Epidemiology of gastric cancer. World J Gastroenterol 21:354-362
6. Hundahl SA, Phillips JL, Menck HR (2000) The National Cancer Data Base Report on poor survival of U.S. gastric carcinoma patients treated with gastrectomy: Fifth Edition American Joint Committee on Cancer staging, proximal disease, and the "different disease" hypothesis. Cancer 88:921-932
7. Roviello F, Marrelli D, Morgagni P et al; Italian Research Group for Gastric Cancer (2002) Survival benefit of extended D2 lymphadenectomy in gastric cancer with involvement of second level lymph nodes: a longitudinal multicenter study. Ann Surg Oncol 9:894-900
8. Kobayashi T, Hisanaga M, Kanehiro H et al (2005) Analysis of risk factors for the development of gallstones after gastrectomy. Br J Surg 92:1399-1403

9. Kwon AH, Inui H, Imamura A et al (2001) Laparoscopic cholecystectomy and choledocholithotomy in patients with a previous gastrectomy. J Am Coll Surg 193:614-619
10. Akatsu T, Yoshida M, Kubota T et al (2005) Gallstone disease after extended (D2) lymph node dissection for gastric cancer. World J Surg 29:182-186
11. Inoue K, Fuchigami A, Higashide S et al (1992) Gallbladder sludge and stone formation in relation to contractile function after gastrectomy. A prospective study. Ann Surg 215:19-26
12. Kodama I, Yoshida C, Kofuji K et al (1996) Gallstones and gallbladder disorder after gastrectomy for gastric cancer. Int Surg 81:36-39
13. Hara S, Ogoshi K, Mitomi T (1993) Ultrasonic findings of the cholecyst and biliary tract after gastrectomy. J Jpn Surg Soc 94:352-358
14. Nakamura K, Ogoshi K, Makuuchi H (2005) Clinicopathological study of cholelithiasis following gastric cancer surgery. Eur Surg Res 37:29-35
15. Hauters P, de Neve de Roden A, Pourbaix A et al (1988) Cholelithiasis: a serious complication after total gastrectomy. Br J Surg 75:899-900
16. Takahashi T, Yamamura T, Utsunomiya J (1990) Pathogenesis of acute cholecystitis after gastrectomy. Br J Surg 77:536-539
17. Yi SQ, Ohta T, Tsuchida A et al (2007) Surgical anatomy of innervation of the gallbladder in humans and Suncus murinus with special reference to morphological understanding of gallstone formation after gastrectomy. World J Gastroenterol 13:2066-2071
18. Yi SQ, Ohta T, Miwa K et al (2005) Surgical anatomy of the innervation of the major duodenal papilla in human and Suncus murinus, from the perspective of preserving innervation in organ-saving procedures. Pancreas 30:211-217
19. Waitman AM, Dyck WP, Janowitz HD (1969) Effect of secretin and acetazolamide on the volume and electrolyte composition of hepatic bile in man. Gastroenterology 56:286-294
20. Magee DF (1965) Physiology of gallbladder emptying. In: Taylor W (ed) The biliary system. Oxford, Blackwell, pp 233-247
21. Hopman WP, Jansen JB, Lamers CB (1984) Plasma cholecystokinin response to a liquid fat meal in vagotomized patients. Ann Surg 200:693-697
22. Messing B, Bories C, Kunstlinger F, Bernier JJ (1983) Does total parenteral nutrition induce gallbladder sludge formation and lithiasis? Gastroenterology 84:1012-1019
23. Bolondi L, Gaiani S, Testa S, Labo G (1985) Gallbladder sludge formation during prolonged fasting after gastrointestinal tract surgery. Gut 26:734-738
24. Liddle RA, Goldstein RB, Saxton J (1989) Gallstone formation during weight-reduction dieting. Arch Intern Med 149:1750-1753
25. Roslyn JJ, Pitt HA, Mann LL et al (1983) Gallbladder disease in patients on long-term parenteral nutrition. Gastroenterology 84:148-154
26. Wu CC, Chen CY, Wu TC et al (1995) Cholelithiasis and cholecystitis after gastrectomy for gastric carcinoma: a comparison of lymphadenectomy of varying extent. Hepatogastroenterology 42:867-872
27. Yu SC, Chen SC, Wang SM, Wei TC (1994) Is previous abdominal surgery a contraindication to laparoscopic cholecystectomy. J Laparoendosc Surg 4:31-35
28. Jorgensen JO, Hunt DR (1993) Laparoscopic cholecystectomy. A prospective analysis of the potential causes of failure. Surg Laparosc Endosc 3:49-53
29. Miller K, Holbling N, Hutter J et al (1993) Laparoscopic cholecystectomy for patients who have had previous abdominal surgery. Surg Endosc 7:400-403
30. Karayiannakis AJ, Polychronidis A, Perente S et al (2004) Laparoscopic cholecystectomy in patients with previous upper or lower abdominal surgery. Surg Endosc 18:97-101
31. Pezzolla F, Lorusso D (1998) Does previous gastric resection increase the risks of laparoscopic cholecystectomy? A case-control study. Minerva Chir 53:603-607
32. Borzellino G, de Manzoni G, Ricci F et al (1996) Mappa ecografica delle aderenze peritoneali. Radiol Med 92:390-393
33. Borzellino G, De Manzoni G, Ricci F (1998) Detection of abdominal adhesions in laparoscopic surgery. A controlled study of 130 cases. Surg Laparosc Endosc 8:273-276
34. Itoi T, Shinohara Y, Takeda K et al (2004) A novel technique for endoscopic sphincterotomy when using a percutaneous transhepatic cholangioscope in patients with an endoscopically inaccessible papilla. Gastrointest Endosc 59:708-711
35. Evans PR, Bak YT, Dowsett JF et al (1997) Small bowel dysmotility in patients with postcholecystectomy sphincter of Oddi dysfunction. Dig Dis Sci 42:1507-1512
36. Konsten J, Gouma DJ, von Meyenfeldt MF, Menheere P (1993) Long-term follow-up after open cholecystectomy. Br J Surg 80:100-102
37. Bar-Meir S, Halpern Z, Bardan E, Gilat T (1984) Frequency of papillary dysfunction among cholecystectomized patients. Hepatology 4:328-330
38. Manzoni G, Di Leo A, Pedrazzani C et al (2001) Intraoperative US staging of T in gastric cancer: final results of a blind prospective study. J Surg Oncol 78:158-61

Chapter 37

Biliary Ileus

Benoit Navez, Hwai-Ding Lam, Jean-François Gigot

Introduction

Gallstone ileus (also known as biliary ileus), a rare complication of cholelithiasis, is defined as a mechanical intestinal obstruction due to a gallstone lodging in the intestinal lumen. This entity was first described by the Danish physician Thomas Bartholin in 1654 during an autopsy [1]. The average age of occurrence is about 70 years old. The youngest case reported was a 13 year old patient and the eldest patient was 97 years old [2]. About 85% of patients are women. Gallstone ileus accounts for 1–2% of all causes of mechanical intestinal obstruction but should be always considered whenever small bowel obstruction is encountered in an elderly patient [3].

The overall perioperative mortality from gallstone ileus was 18% in the second half of the nineteenth century. It has decreased in recent years, but remains high, at up to 11–17% [4]. This is mainly attributed to the fact that such a complication is often seen in the eldery, who are often tolerant of pain, and that more than half of the patients are known to have concurrent cardiorespiratory diseases, diabetes mellitus and obesity. On the other hand, the decision to operate on these patients is often delayed because of the so-called "tumbling" phenomenon, whereby the obstructing stone continues on its migration more distally into the bowel with symptoms of intestinal obstruction that appears to improve.

Etiology and Pathophysiology

The disease starts with recurrent episodes of acute cholecystitis due to the impaction of a gallstone in the gallbladder neck. This inflammation causes adhesions between the gallbladder and the adjacent viscera. The resultant phlegmon is composed of omentum and nearby bowel, commonly the duodenum. If the inflammatory process is of sufficient intensity and duration, then the diseased gallbladder can form a fistulous communication with adjacent hollow organs. In most cases the fistula is between the gallbladder and the duodenum (in more than 60% of the cases), but cholecystocolic, cholecystojejunal, cholecystogastric and choledochoduodenal fistula have been described [4–7]. Having entered the alimentary tract, the gallstone, which is usually single, may be vomited or passed spontaneously via the rectum. The gallstone can also grow "in situ" after migration to the bowel, especially after papillotomy. This could explain the reported cases of biliary ileus in which the gallbladder was removed several years prior to intestinal obstruction [7–10].

Most stones are asymptomatic as their size is smaller than 2 cm in diameter and they normally pass down the alimentary tract without causing obstruction. Stones larger than 2.5 cm can impact in the bowel, causing a mechanical obstruction. The site of impaction is usually the terminal ileum

(60% of the cases), as it is the narrowest part of the alimentary tract. Other levels of obstructions are the jejunum in 16% of the cases and the colon in 4%. Impaction in the stomach (14%) or in the duodenum (3.5%) [4] causes gastric outlet obstruction known as Bouveret's syndrome, a subgroup of gallstone ileus first described in 1896 [11]. Up to approximately 300 cases of Bouveret's syndrome have been described in the medical literature [12–17].

As the gallstone moves down the small intestine, it may temporarily block the lumen and create obstructive symptoms; then it can dislodge, pass further along and impact again, recreating obstructive symptoms. This intermittent phenomenon of gallstone lodging and dislodging along the alimentary tract is known as "tumbling" and is reflected clinically by the intermittent character of symptoms. Complete obstruction develops when a segment of intestine is reached where further passage is impossible.

Clinical and Radiological Findings

The usual clinical presentation is distal small bowel obstruction with non specific signs such as abdominal pain, nausea and vomiting, which can resolve spontaneously and reappear later intermittently. As previously mentioned, the symptoms may be episodic, leading the physician to optimistically predict a spontaneous resolution of the problem and delay operation. This "tumbling" effect is characteristic of biliary ileus, which can easily be mistaken for gastroenteritis and explains why its diagnosis is often missed.

A past history suggestive of chronic gallbladder disease is present in 50–75% of cases [18–20]. Symptoms of acute cholecystitis immediately preceding the onset of obstruction occur in one-quarter to one-third of cases. Occasionally, there may be an initial episode of biliary colic, but major pain is usually not experienced until intestinal colic occurs. Classical symptoms of intestinal obstruction can be encountered, including nausea, vomiting, abdominal cramps and distension. Bouveret's syndrome can present with haematemesis due to the mucosal ulceration caused by the impacted stone [21, 22], but mostly it presents with gastric outlet obstruction symptoms (repeated projectile vomiting and epigastric pain).

In most patients, the findings on physical examination are typical of distal small bowel obstruction, except in cases of Bouveret's syndrome, in which abdominal distension is absent. Right upper quadrant tenderness and a mass may sometimes be present. Occasionally the stone can be palpated within the ileum. Laboratory tests show a lower intestinal obstruction pattern with hypokalemia, hyponatremia, hypochloremia and sometimes elevated cholestatic parameters [23, 24].

The classical radiological signs seen in biliary ileus on plain abdominal radiograph as described by Rigler et al. [25] include presence of gas in the bile ducts (40% of cases) (Fig 37.1), visualisation of the stone in the intestine if radio-opaque (less than 20% of cases), radiological evidence of partial or complete bowel obstruction and change in position of a previously observed stone. Two small air-liquid levels in the gallbladder and in the duodenal bulb have been added as a frequent finding in biliary ileus by Bathalzar et al. [26]. Due to the intermittent character and sometimes to incomplete obstruction, the sensitivity for gallstone ileus on plain abdominal radiograph remains low (40–70%). The biliary-enteric fistula can sometimes also be demonstrated on a gastrointestinal series and ultrasonography can be useful. A recent study has shown that a computed tomography (CT) scan can improve the sensitivity to 93% with a specificity of 100% [27] (Fig. 37.2).

It is therefore important to put biliary ileus on the top of the diagnostic list in a

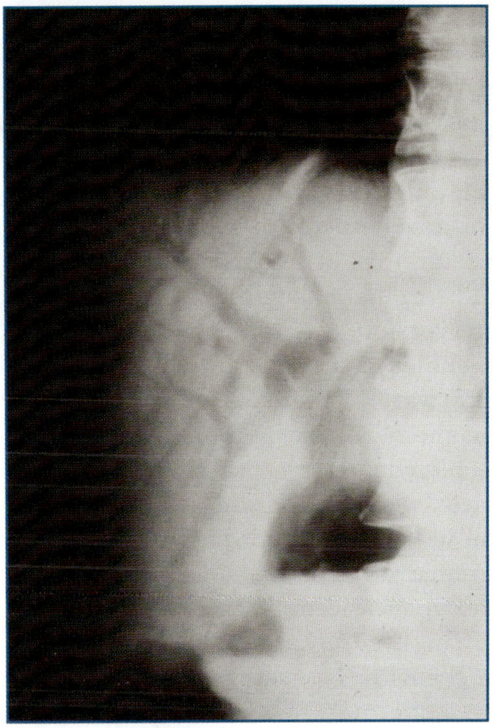

Fig. 37.1 Aerobilia

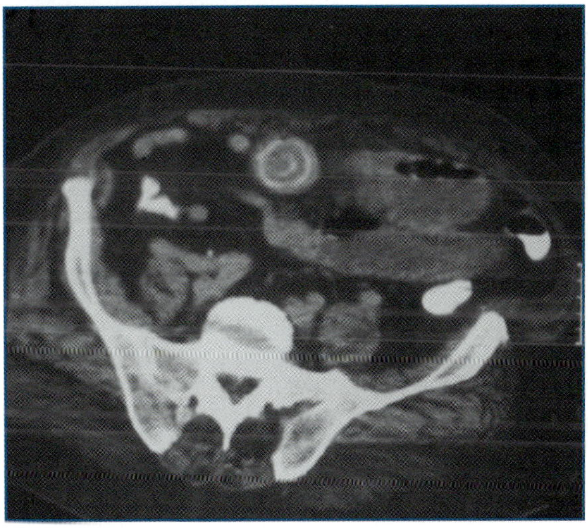

Fig. 37.2 Obstructing stone on a CT scan

geriatric patient with mechanical bowel obstruction and no previous abdominal surgery after exclusion of an incarcerated hernia. The work-up should include laboratory tests, plain films and a CT scan to diagnose and exactly localise the gallstone. The knowledge of remaining cholelithiasis may have an impact on the further surgical strategy.

Treatment

Biliary ileus remains a surgical emergency and the proper treatment is relief of the mechanical obstruction. Classically, this is done by a standard midline incision. The removal of the obstructive gallstone is performed through a small longitudinal enterotomy at the antimesenteric border just proximal to the impacted segment in order to avoid suture on the fragile bowel wall (Fig. 37.3). The gallstone is milked proximally and extracted. The enterotomy is then closed transversely in order to avoid stenosis and the proximal bowel is carefully inspected for the presence of any additional stones (Fig. 37.4). Recurrence rate due to overlooked stones can be as high as 10% and multiple stones can be expected in 3–16% of cases. This is especially the case when the obstructive stone is faceted.

Concomitant definitive correction of the internal fistula remains debatable. Many authors agree that cholecystectomy and closure of the fistula should not be performed

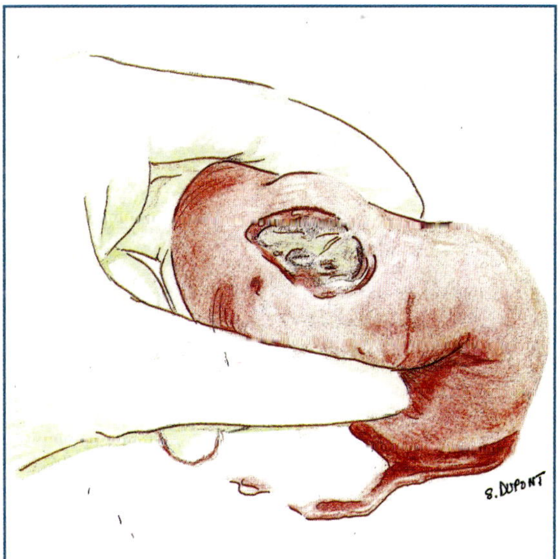

Fig. 37.3 Longitudinal enterotomy proximal to the impacted bowel segment. Reproduced with permission of Stéfanie Dupont

during the emergency procedure. This would transform a simple operation into a long and difficult procedure that may last several hours and have no immediate benefit for a fragile geriatric patient. Besides, it increases the short-term postoperative morbidity and mortality [28]. Furthermore, the fistula will close spontaneously in up to 50% of cases, especially if there is no evidence of cholelithiasis with a patent cystic duct. An elective cholecystectomy can also be performed later on if the patient has persistant biliary symptoms; this seems to be the case in 15–30% of cases [4, 23].

With improvement in preoperative resuscitation, some authors believe that a more definitive operation should be undertaken. Advocates for the one-stage procedure with concomitant cholecystectomy and fistula closure argue that leaving the fistula and gallbladder in situ places the patient at risk of further biliary complications. The ascending cholangitis rate due to open fistula can be as high as 11%, gallbladder carcinoma can develop in up to 15% in patients with persistent fistula. Recurrent cholecystitis and recurrence of gallstone ileus have also been reported. However, the mortality rate might be higher than in enterotomy alone, although no statistical significance (12 vs. 17%) has yet been proven [4, 6, 8, 29].

It seems to be wise to handle only highly selected patients with few comorbid conditions in a one-stage procedure. The fragile geriatric patient with high degree cholecystitis and serious concomitant diseases should undergo simple enterolithotomy and interval cholecystectomy should be performed afterwards if there is evidence of symptomatic cholelithiasis or cholecystitis.

The high mortality and morbidity rates associated with open surgical treatment justify the use of videoendoscopic techniques to minimise surgical trauma to the patient. Laparoscopic procedures have been described in small case series [30–34]. This approach seems to be useful and a safe alternative technique for treating gallstone ileus.

There are several advantages of laparoscopic surgery over the open approach:

1. complete abdominal exploration to rule out other associated pathologic conditions;

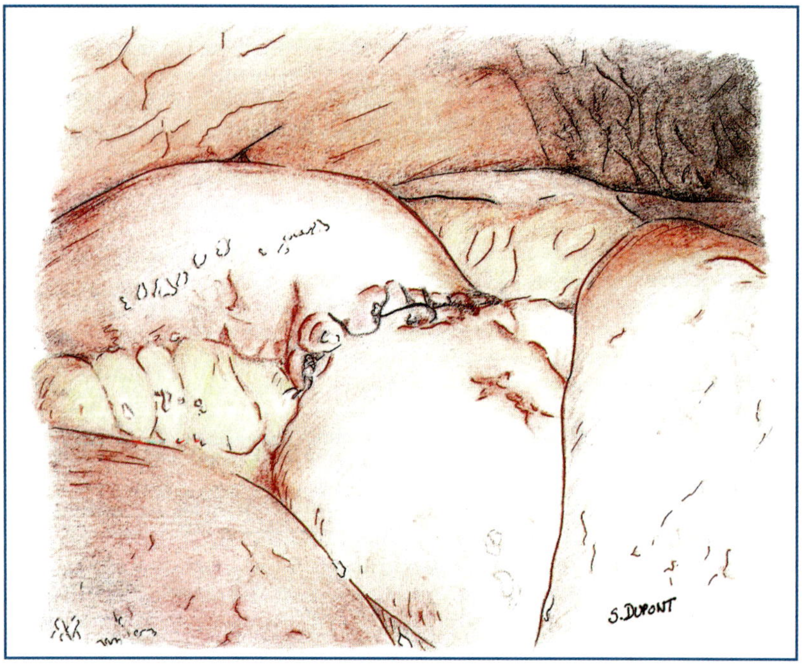

Fig. 37.4 Transversal suture of the small bowel. Reproduced with permission of Stéfanie Dupont

2. avoidance of unnecessary laparotomy;
3. in case of video-assisted laparoscopy, proper location and minimal size of incision (minilaparrotomy);
4. reduced associated morbidity: such as wound infection, dehiscence and incisional hernia.

The open Hasson technique must be used to achieve pneumoperitoneum and a 10 mm blunt balloon trocar is introduced in the left hypochondrium. Two additional 5 mm ports are inserted usually in the left flank and the epigastric area. The non-distended small bowel is carefully run back from the ileocaecal valve using atraumatic forceps until the obstructing stone is detected. Care must be taken when manipulating the dilated bowel loops to avoid injury. By using careful inspection and soft palpation, it is essential to rule out the presence of intraluminal additional stones in the proximal intestine that could be the cause of a recurrent gallstone ileus [30–34].

The segment of small intestine containing the obstructing stone is brought out through a minilaparotomy in the midline usually around or below the umbilicus. After placement of a bowel clamp proximally, a longitudinal enterotomy is performed and the stone is removed as described in the open procedure. The bowel is closed transversely using a single layer suture. Then it is reintegrated into the abdomen and a last check of the abdominal cavity is performed. In the vast majority of cases, the gallbladder is left in place.

Limitations to the laparoscopic procedure are the inadequate exploration of the abdominal cavity in case of massive ileus (distal obstruction) and the difficulties that can occur in searching for additional stones, what is mandatory if the extracted stone is faceted. Laparoscopy should therefore only be performed by skilled surgeons with experience in laparoscopic approach for small bowel obstruction. In a retrospective comparison of laparoscopically assisted and open enterolithotomy for gallstone ileus, the overall morbidity rate was low with predominantly minor complications in the laparoscopic group and major complications after an open procedure; the results were similar in terms of operating time and hospital stay [34].

References

1. Martin F (1912) Intestinal obstruction due to gallstones. Ann Surg 55:725
2. Kasahara Y, Umemura H, Shiraha S et al (1980) Gallstone ileus. Review of 112 patients in the Japanese literature. Am J Surg 140:437-440
3. Jones PF (1987) Emergency abdominal surgery, 2nd edn. Blackwell scientific publications
4. Reisner RM, Cohen JR (1994) Gallstone ileus: a review of 1001 reported cases. Am Surg 60:44-446
5. Abou-Saif A, Al-Kawas FH (2002) Complications of gallstone disease: Mirrizzi syndrome, cholecystocholedochal fistula, and gallstone ileus. Am J Gastroenterol 97:249-254
6. Clavien PA, Richon J, Burgan S et al (1990) Gallstone ileus. Br J Surg 77:737-742
7. Atli AO, Coskun T, Ozenc A et al (1997) Biliary enteric fistulas. Int Surg 82:280-283
8. Day EA, Marks C (1975) Gallstone ileus. Review of the literature and presentation of thirty-four new cases. Am J Surg 129:552-558
9. Cushieri, Steele, Moosa (2002) Essential surgical practise, 4th edn AJ2
10. Lobo DN, Jobling JC, Balfour TW (2000) Gallstone ileus: diagnostic pitfalls and therapeutic successes. J Clin Gastroenerol 30:72-76
11. Bouveret L (1896) Stenose du pylore adherent à la vesicule. Rev Med (Paris) 16:1-16
12. Halaz NA (1964) Gallstone obstruction of the duodenal bulb (Bouveret's syndrome). Am J Dig Dis 9:856-861
13. Togeron SA, Greening GK, Juniper K et al (1979) Gallstone obstruction of duodenal cap (Bouveret's syndrome) diagnosed by endoscopy. Am J Gastroenterol 72:165-167
14. Murphy GD (1995) Bouveret's syndrome. Am J Gastroenterol 90:638-639
15. Ariche A, Czeiger D, Gortzak Y et al (2000) Gastric outlet obstruction by gallstone: Bouveret syndrome. Scand J Gastroenterol. 35:781-783
16. Masannat Y, Caplin S, Brown T (2006) A rare complication of a common disease: Bouveret syndrome, a report of a case. World J Gastroenterol 12:2620-2621
17. Sica GS, Sileri P, Gaspari AL (2005) Laparoscopic treatment of Bouveret's syndrome presenting as acute pancreatititis. JSLS 9:472-475

18. Masannat Y, Masannat Y, Shatnawei A (2006) Gallstone ileus: a review. Mt Sinai J Med 73:1132-1134
19. Courvosier LT (1890) Zasurstich-Statistische Beiträge zur pathologie und chirurgie der gallenwege. Leipzig, FCW Vogel
20. Cooperman AM, Dickson RE, ReMine WH (1968) Changing concepts in the surgical treatment of gallstone ileus: a review of 15 cases with emphasis on diagnosis and treatment. Ann Surg 167:377-383
21. Salah-Eldin AA, Ibrahim MA, Alapati R et al (1990) The Bouveret syndrome: an unusual cause of hematemesis. Henry Ford Hosp Med J 38:52-54
22. Heinrich D, Meier J, Wehrli H et al (1993) Upper gastrointestinal hemorrhage preceding development of Bouveret's syndrome. Am J Gastroenterol 88:777-780
23. Mulholland MW, Lillemoe KD, Doherty GM et al (2006) Greenfield's surgery scientific principles and practise, 4th edn. Philadelphia, Lippincot Williams & Wilkins
24. Galloway AC, Shires GT, Daly JM et al (1999) Principles of surgery by Schwartz, 7th edn. New York, McGraw Hill
25. Rigler LG, Borman CN, Noble JF (1941) Gallstone obstruction: pathogenesis and roentgen manifestations. JAMA 117:1753-1759
26. Balthazar EJ, Schrechter LS (1978) Air in gallbladder: a frequent finding in gallstone ileus. AJR Am J Roentgenol 131:219-222
27. Yu CY, Lin CC, Shyu RY et al (2005) Value of CT in the diagnosis and management of gallstone ileus. World J Gastroenterol 11:2142-2147
28. Doko M, Zovak M, Kopljar M et al (2003) Comparison of surgical treatment of gallstone ileus: preliminary report. World J Surg 27:400-404
29. Kirchmayr W, Muhlmann G, Zitt M et al (2005) Galstone ileus: rare and still controversial. ANZ J Surg 75:234-238
30. Soto DJ, Evan SJ, Kavic MS (2001) Laparoscopic management of gallstone ileus. JLJS 5:279-285
31. Sarli L, Costi R, Gobbi S (1998) Gallstone ileus: laparoscopic assisted enterolithotomy. J Am Coll Surg 186:370-371
32. Moberg AC, Montgomery A (2007) Laparoscopically assisted or open enterolithotomy for gallstone ileus. Br J Surg 94:53-57
33. Ferraina P, Gancedo MC, Elli F et al (2003) Video-assisted laparoscopic enterolithotomy: new technique in the surgical management of gallstone ileus. Surg Laparosc Endosc Percutan Tech 13:83-87
34. Montgomery A (1993) Laparoscope-guided enterolithotomy for gallstone ileus. Surg Laparosc Endosc 3:310-314

Chapter 38

Clinical Pictures of Intrahepatic Lithiasis

Andrea Ruzzenente, Chiara Zugni, Alfredo Guglielmi

Intrahepatic stone disease, or hepatolithiasis, is a disease with distinctive epidemiological, pathogenetic and therapeutic features. This disease is rare in Western countries, whereas it is endemic in some Asian countries. It is defined as presence of gallstones in intrahepatic the bile ducts, proximal to bile duct bifurcation [1]. Hepatolithiasis is primary when stones are formed de novo in the intrahepatic bile ducts, whereas it is secondary when extrahepatic gallstones migrate into the intrahepatic bile ducts [2–4]. The disease is associated with biliary stricture, primary disease of bile ducts (primitive sclerosing cholangitis, Caroli's disease, choledochal cysts), neoplasm or parasitic infestation.

Epidemiology

Intrahepatic stone disease was originally described as oriental cholangiohepatitis according to its high prevalence in Asian countries and in some geographical areas where it is an endemic disease (Fig. 38.1) [1].

The disease is more frequent from fifth to the seventh decades of life and the male/female proportion is 1 to 1.2 [5–7].

In Western countries intrahepatic lithiasis is rare, with a prevalence lower than 1% among all patients suffering from stone diseases (the prevalence varies between 0.6 and 1.3% in different studies) [8, 9]. Most patients with hepatolithiasis suffer from secondary

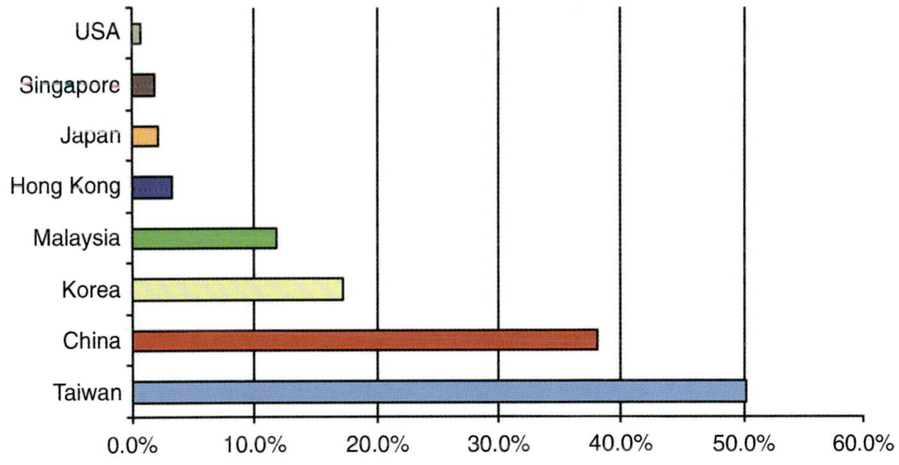

Fig. 38.1 Prevalence of hepatolithiasis in relation to gallstone disease in Western and Asian Countries

hepatolithiasis, associated with gallbladder or common bile duct stones. The incidence of intrahepatic lithiasis in Western countries has increased in the last decades due to immigration from countries with a higher prevalence: a significant proportion of patients with hepatolithiasis are immigrants [10].

Primary bile duct stones without concomitant gallbladder stones are quite common in Asian countries due to differences in the pathogenesis of the disease and are frequently associated with parasite infestation. The prevalence of intrahepatic stones is higher in countries with poor sanitary and nutritional conditions suggesting that socio-economic conditions are implicated in the pathogenesis of the disease. The variation in economic conditions and in lifestyle recently observed in Japan may have contributed to a decrease in the incidence of intrahepatic stones and to an increase in gallbladder stones [11]. Also in Taiwan and Korea the decreased incidence of intrahepatic stones has also been related to an improvement in economic conditions [12, 13]. The prevalence of intrahepatic stones in relation to gallstone disease is 1.7% in Singapore, 2% in Japan (where the frequency has decreased since the seventies when the reported frequency was 4%), 3.1% in Hong Kong, 11.7% in Malaysia, 17% in Korea, 38% in China and 47.3 % in Taiwan [1, 14]. Hepatolithiasis is a health-care problem in Japan where several nationwide survey have been conducted. The relative proportion of hepatolithiasis in relation to gallbladder stones was 4.1% between 1970 and 1977, 3% in the years 1975–1984, 2.3% in the years 1985–1988, 2.2% in the years 1989–1992 and 1.7% in the years 1993–1995 [5–7, 11]. In Latin America the relative proportion of hepatolithiasis varies from 2 to 7% [15].

Pathogenesis

Pathogenesis of intrahepatic stones is complex and has not been completely clarified yet. The steps of stone formation probably involve a combination of different factors: bile stasis, bile infection, malnutrition and parasitic infestation [16]. Frequent causes of the disease are summarized in Table 38.1.

Biliary strictures lead to bile stasis and to bacterial colonization due to translocation from the gut. Bacterial infection is strictly related with hepatolithiasis and bacteria have been detected in the bile of more than the 90% of people affected by intrahepatic stones [17]. Intrahepatic stones increase biliary stasis, favoring bacterial proliferation and creating a vicious cycle.

Bacteria reach the biliary system by the hematogenous (portal) route, the lymphatic route and the ascending route through the common papilla of Vater (thought to be the most frequent pattern). The bacteria most frequently isolated from the bile are aerobes such as *Escherichia coli* and *Enterobacter* species (*Klebsiella* and *Pseudomonas*) or anaerobes such as *Bacteroides* and *Clostridium* [17]. β-glucuronidase and other enzymes produced by bacteria cause the hydrolysis of bilirubin diglucuronide to unconjugated bilirubin, which can precipitate as calcium

Table 38.1 Pathogenesis and causes of hepatolithiasis

Pathogenesis	Causes
Primary hepatolithiasis	
Biliary strictures	Postoperative or iatrogenic Primary sclerosing cholangitis Caroli's disease Cholangiocarcinoma
Infection	Biliary parasites Recurrent bacterial cholangitis
Genetic disorders	Hemolytic diseases
Secondary hepatolithiasis	
Stone migration	Gallbladder or common bile duct stones

bilirubinate [18]. The breakdown of biliary lecithin caused by bacterial phospholipase produces free fatty acids and lysophospholipids such as calcium palmitate that may precipitate [16, 18]. Recently, it has been suggested that lipopolysaccharide produced by bacteria can upregulate the expression of mucins such as MUC2 and MUC5AC, both directly and indirectly through the stimulation of tumor necrosis factor-alpha (TNF-α). The mucin overexpression increases the formation of bile brown pigment stones [19].

Biliary mucin secretion is regulated by multiple factors, including cystic fibrosis transmembrane conductance regulator (CFTR), which has an important role in the pathogenesis of hepatolithiasis. The CFTR is a membrane chloride channel receptor expressed by epithelial cells of the biliary tract. In patients affected by cystic fibrosis the CFTR mutation induces the production of dense mucus that obstructs the biliary ducts. Some authors hypothesize that CFTR is overexpressed in patients affected by hepatolithiasis; in particular, they identified that the increased expression of CFTR is related with the active inflammation of bile ducts with cholangitis. This CFTR expression pattern indicates that the active inflammatory phase of chronic proliferative cholangitis can increase mucin hypersecretion and intrahepatic stone formation [20].

Parasite infestation by *Clonorchis sinensis* and *Ascaris lumbricoides* (which are quite common in East Asia) can cause chronic inflammation, enhance mucin secretion and provide the nidus for stone formation; fragments of parasites and their eggs can be the starting point for calcium bilirubinate precipitation and stone formation.

Bile stasis can also be caused by anatomical abnormalities (congenital or acquired) and genetic disorders. Congenital causes of biliary strictures or dilatation are Caroli's disease, choledochal cysts, primary sclerosing cholangitis and anomalous pancreaticobiliary ductal union. The acquired biliary strictures can be benign, malignant or iatrogenic due to surgical and endoscopic procedures (i.e., iatrogenic strictures of the biliary duct, stenosis of bilio-enteric anastomosis or stenosis of bile duct following endoscopic retrograde cholangiopancreatography [ERCP]).

The genetic disorders with increased risk of intrahepatic lithiasis include hemolytic diseases due to the increased formation of bilirubin, which increase the risk of stone formation in all parts of biliary tree.

Environmental and socio-economic factors have proven to be important in the pathogenesis of intrahepatic stones. In particular, the disease is more frequent in rural areas with low economical status. A diet low of saturated fatty acids may increase biliary stasis. A low protein diet is also responsible for a decreased level of β-glucuronidase inhibitors that leads to increased deconjugating reactions and to the formation of calcium bilirubinate stones [21].

Stone Type and Location

Gallstones found in hepatolithiasis can be divided into two different types: brown pigment stones (calcium bilirubinate stones) and cholesterol stones.

Calcium biliriubinate stones are more frequently observed (in more than 90% of patients); they have a color that varies from brown to orange, a rough surface, an ovoid or faceted shape, and a soft and friable consistency. They are made up of more than 60% calcium bilirubinate, fatty acids and less than 20% cholesterol; their matrix consists of glycoproteins. On the cut surface a lamellar structure can be observed. This type of stone is frequently associated with bacterial colonization and bacterial cholangitis.

Cholesterol stones, which are more frequently found in the gallbladder and in the common bile duct, are quite uncommon in the intrahepatic biliary tree. They are

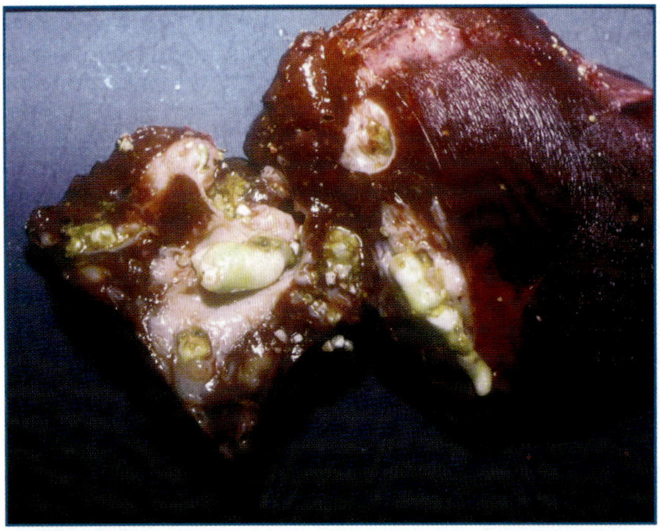

Fig. 38.2 Surgical specimen of hepatolithiasis of the left hepatic lobe

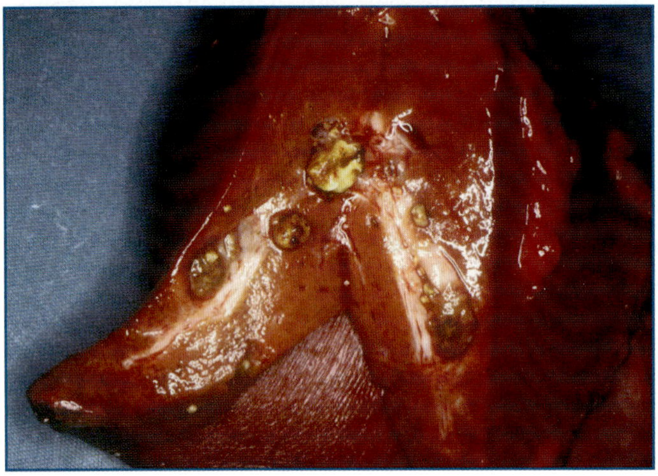

Fig. 38.3 Surgical specimen of hepatolithiasis of the right hepatic lobe

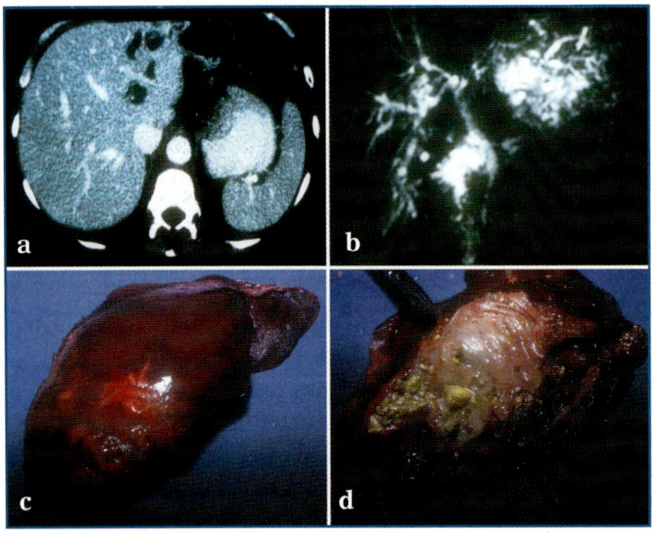

Fig. 38.4 Hepatolithiasis of the left hepatic lobe. **a** CT shows dilated left bile ducts. **b** MRCP shows dilated left hepatic ducts with intrahepatic stones. **c** Surgical specimen after left lobectomy showing alteration of the surface of the liver. **d** Surgical specimen with evidence of hepatolithiasis

whitish yellow, small hard stones. It is possible to observe on the cut surface radial or crystalloid structures [18].

The distribution of stones within the intrahepatic biliary system has specific features; in particular, the left biliary system is more frequently involved (Figs. 38.2-38.4). The stones are identified in the left lobe in 45.5–55% of patients, in the right lobe in 11.5–26.1% of patients and in both the left and right lobe in 26.3–31.3% of patients. Stones are identified in the caudate lobe bile ducts in 6.6% of patients [22].

Pathology

Macroscopically, the liver appears enlarged and scarred, with frequent capsular adhesions. In patients with recurrent cholangitis it is possible to observe segmental liver atrophy due to segmental portal vein thrombosis.

The primary pathological sign of hepatolithiasis is bile duct dilatation, usually with stones, detritus, mud or frank pus. Histological signs of cholangitis can be usually found, including bile duct proliferation; inflammatory cells, mostly polymorphonuclear leukocytes; and focal hepatocellular necrosis can be frequently demonstrated in the portal space [23, 24]. The chronic inflammation leads to an increase in fibrous tissue in the portal space around the bile ducts. Bile duct epithelium can show several alterations due to chronic cholangitis. Atypical epithelial changes in bile ducts are frequently observed, and cholangiocarcinoma can be identified in about 5% of patients.

Clinical Manifestations

The clinical history of hepatolithiasis is characterized by recurrent abdominal pain and fever. Intrahepatic lithiasis-induced abdominal pain is located in the epigastrium and in the right upper quadrant of the abdomen, and may last for hours or days before spontaneously resolving. Transient jaundice may follow the pain episode. Biliary obstruction favours bacterial colonization and the occurrence of cholangitis, which is characterized by the typical Charcot's triad: fever with chills, jaundice and pain. The distribution of symptoms among Asian and Western patients is reported in Table 38.2. About 16% of patients are asymptomatic, with the alterations only identifiable in liver blood tests. In particular frequent alterations involve increases in alkaline phosphates (ALP), gamma-glutamyltranspeptidase (GGT) and bilirubin levels.

Hepatolithiasis causes chronic obstruction of the biliary tree with chronic segmental cholestasis that can induce the formation of liver abscesses. Frequently, chronic segmental cholangitis induces portal thrombophlebitis with segmental portal vein thrombosis. An unusual complication of liver abscesses is fistulization with portal vein and occurrence of hemobilia.

From a clinical point of view the Hepatolithiasis Research Group in Japan has classified four grades of clinical severity in intrahepatic stone disease: grade 1 with no symptoms; grade 2 with abdominal pain; grade 3 with transient jaundice or cholangitis; grade 4 with continuous jaundice, sepsis or cholangiocarcinoma [26].

In a Japanese survey of 473 patients with hepatolithiasis, 20% presented with grade 1 symptoms, 25% with grade 2 and 55 % with grade 3 and 4 [14].

Table 38.2 Common symptoms observed in patients with hepatolithiasis

Symptoms	East [25]	West [10]
	N=96	N=54
Abdominal pain	30%	63%
Cholangitis	59%	67%
Jaundice	10%	39%

Chronic cholestasis with recurrent cholangitis can lead to biliary strictures and secondary biliary cirrhosis. Portal hypertension and esophageal varices characterize the last stages of chronic liver disease.

Hepatolithiasis and Caroli's Disease

Caroli's disease is a rare congenital condition characterized by non-obstructive saccular or fusiform multifocal segmental dilatation of the intrahepatic bile ducts [27]. The mode of inheritance is not clear yet but it seems to be usually inherited by autosomal recessive fashion. Caroli's disease may occur in the pure form, characterized by dilatations of intrahepatic bile ducts without any other histological alteration; the so-called Caroli's syndrome is defined when it is associated with congenital periportal fibrosis and renal cystic disease (from renal tubular ectasia to polycystic kidney disease).

The clinical history of these patients starts from childhood and is characterized by hepatomegaly and recurrence of abdominal pain, recurrent cholangitis (sometimes with biliary abscess), lithiasis and the onset of cirrhosis; cholangiocarcinoma may occur in 7% of cases. Intrahepatic stones are common in Caroli's disease due to bile stasis and bacterial infection. The presence of hepatolithiasis worsens the clinical picture of Caroli's disease and makes treatment more complicated. At pathology, the saccular dilatation of peripheral bile ducts are filled with detritus and stones, and histological signs of cholangitis are also frequently observed.

Hepatolithiasis and Parasites

Ascaris lumbricodes is a large nematode responsible for most of the helminthic infestations in the world; the prevalence of ascariasis is high in countries with low economical and sanitary conditions; in particular, it is endemic in South East Asia. After ingestion of food contaminated by *Ascaris* eggs, *Ascaris* larvae unfold in the upper bowel and migrate through the jejunal mucosa towards lymphatic and portal circulation thus reaching the liver and the lung. From the lung larvae are coughed up and they are swallowed into the digestive system where they develop as the adult worm. Adult *Ascaris* remain alive in the gut and tend to slip into Vater's ampulla thus causing biliary or pancreatic obstruction.

Ascaris infestation is often asymptomatic or slightly symptomatic. When *Ascaris* infests the biliary duct, it can cause a range of symptoms, from biliary colic (56%) to acute cholangitis (25%), acute alithiasic cholecystitis (13%), liver abscess (less than 1%) and acute pancreatitis (6%) [28].

Clonorchis sinensis is a small trematode; its intermediate host is a particular species of snail, moreover some type of fish can also act as a host. When people eat contaminated food such as freshwater fish, *Clonorchis* larvae hatch in the duodenum and go upstream the biliary tract to the peripheral ducts; their oral and ventral suckers allow the parasites to move into the biliary duct, thus causing epithelial chronic damage leading to hyperplasia, fibrosis and then cirrhosis. The fluke can survive in the human biliary system for up to 30 years. Clinical manifestations due to *Clonorchis* can be acute or chronic. Acute symptoms are characterized by fever, abdominal pain, diarrhea, hepatomegaly and jaundice that can be confused with acute hepatitis. Upon blood testing, eosinophilia may be present, which can help in the differential diagnosis. Otherwise, chronic infestation is characterized by abdominal pain, nausea, anorexia and slight fever. The chronic pattern of infestation may be sometimes worsened by recurrent episodes of cholecystitis and cholangitis (sometimes with liver abscess). Chronic infestation can cause progressive biliary cirrhosis and cholangiocarcinoma.

Opistorchis viverrini, *Opistorchis felineus* and *Dicrocoelium dendriticum* are closely related to *Clonorchis* and can also infest the biliary tree with similar clinical signs and complications. *Opistorchis viverrini* is considered a strong risk factor for cholangiocarcinoma. *Fasciola hepatica* and *Fasciola gigantica* can also be involved in biliary disease [29].

Hepatolithiasis and Primary Sclerosing Cholangitis

Primary sclerosing cholangitis (PSC) is a rare chronic cholestatic liver disease characterized by a generalized and beading and stenosis of the biliary tree. It mainly affects young male people and its pathogenesis is a quite complex and mostly unknown multistep process including autoimmune mechanisms, immunogenetic susceptibility (related to HLA-B8 and HLA-DR3 haplotype) and disorders of biliary epithelia. It is a progressive disease characterized by inflammation and fibrosis of the biliary tree resulting in diffuse stenosis. In the advanced stages of the disease PSC causes liver dysfunction and cirrhosis up to liver failure; it is also associated with a high risk of cholangiocarcinoma. PSC often coexists with inflammatory bowel disease such as ulcerative colitis.

The increased incidence of hepatolithiasis in patients affected by PSC can be explained by an increased lithogenicity of the bile and the concomitance of biliary stasis due to diffuse intrahepatic biliary strictures.

Patients with PSC have a significantly higher incidence of gallstones compared with patients without PSC, 57% versus 10-20%, respectively. Also hepatolithiasis has an higher incidence in PSC with a prevalence of 8% [30].

Recent studies hypothesized defects on ABCB4 gene, which codes for a glycoprotein involved as a transmembrane carrier in biliary phosphatidylcholine excretion; since phospholipids act as carrier and solvent of cholesterol and rule a protective effect against bile-salt induced biliary mucosa injury, mutations of this gene may explain increased lithogenicity of bile and damage to biliary epithelial cells. Mutations of ABCB4 have been reported in some patients with a history of intrahepatic cholestasis [31].

People affected by PSC and intrahepatic stones are more prone to recurrent ascending cholangitis than those affected by PSC without calculi.

The presence of hepatolithiasis worsens the clinical picture, with increased episodes of cholangithis. Moreover, the presence of hepatolithiasis complicates the medical management of the disease.

Hepatolithiasis and Cholangiocarcinoma

Hepatolithiasis is considered as a risk factor for intrahepatic cholangiocarcinoma; its incidence is up to 10% among people affected by intrahepatic stone disease in Japan [32]. Hepatolithiasis precedes cholangiocarcinoma by at least 10 years; this temporal relationship suggests that hepatolithiasis worsens a chronic inflammatory process (chronic proliferative cholangitis) and then causes epithelial degeneration (atypical epithelial hyperplasia) that can result in neoplastic trasformation [33].

Many genetic alterations in the biliary mucosa can be demonstrated in patients with hepatolithiasis; these can be part of the multi-step carcinogenesis pathway that leads to the formation of cholangiocarcinoma [34, 35].

Recent studies have shown the presence of bile-resistant *Helicobacter pylori* species in the bile and biliary epithelium of some people affected by hepatolithiasis; the studies on the proliferative index of biliary cells suggest that *H. pylori* infection may stimulate the proliferative cycle of bile duct cells, thus promoting neoplastic transformation.

Intrahepatic cholangiocarcinoma should be suspected in people with a long history of hepatolithiasis (at least 10 years), age around 40 years or older, with weight-loss and increased level of serum alkaline phosphatase, increased level of serum albumin, and carcinoembryonic antigen (CEA) higher than 4.2 ng/ml; if hepatolithiasis involves both the liver lobes, the risk of cholangiocarcinoma is significantly higher [36].

However, the association rate of cancer appears to be significantly higher in people with cholesterol intrahepatic stones (up to 30% of cancers) than in people affected by brown pigment stones (about 3%) [37].

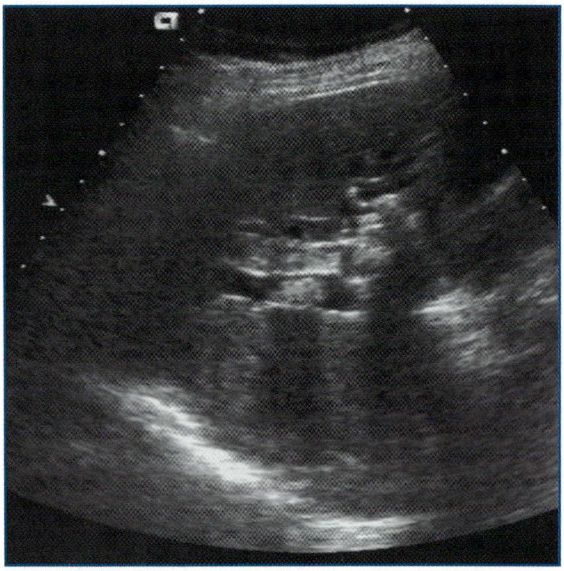

Fig. 38.5 Ultrasonography showing dilated bile ducts with stones

Diagnosis

Noninvasive diagnostic imaging of hepatolithiasis is based on ultrasonography (US), computed tomography (CT) and magnetic resonance imaging (MRI). These diagnostic tools have both advantages and limits, but the three methods together can provide precise information not only about the presence of intrahepatic stones, but also about their localization and the presence of abnormalities of the biliary tree [1]. The severity of involvement of the biliary tree observed in hepatolithiasis can be classified into four different types according to the classification proposed by Tsunoda [25]: Type I has no marked dilatation or strictures of intrahepatic ducts; Type II has diffuse dilatation of the intrahepatic biliary tree without strictures; Type III has unilateral solitary or multiple cystic intrahepatic dilatation of intrahepatic ducts accompanied by stenosis; and Type IV has the same as III but with bilateral involvement of hepatic lobes.

Ultrasonography

US is the first step in diagnosis of hepatolithiasis; it has the advantage of being easy to perform without any preparation of the patient (Fig. 38.5). US describes the anatomy of the bile ducts, and it defines and describes the presence of biliary ducts dilatation. In most patients (85–90%) with hepatolithiasis US can identify the presence of stones in dilated bile ducts [38]. The stones at US appear as echogenic spots with an acoustic shadow behind them; stones with a higher calcium content appear with a high echo rim on the front surface. Cholesterol stones with lower calcium content can be better visualized. The presence of pneumobilia can be difficult to distinguish from stones but postural variation of the patients can help for differential diagnosis. US can therefore identify cystic dilatation of intrahepatic bile ducts and liver abscesses.

Computed Tomography

CT is a helpful diagnostic tool in hepatolithiasis. It precisely describes the anatomy of dilated bile ducts and the site of stricture. The direct visualization of biliary strictures can rarely be directly identified with CT. The detection rate of intrahepatic stones is not as good as for US because the visualization of stones depends on the calcium content. The stones rich of calcium appear as a high-density intrahepatic formation in the dilated bile ducts, whereas the stones with low calcium content are difficult to differentiate from bile, due to a similar density. Moreover, CT describes signs of chronic liver disease and the presence of complications such as liver abscesses. This diagnostic tool is useful for the identification vascular complications such as segmental portal vein thrombosis.

Magnetic Resonance Imaging

Magnetic resonance cholangiopancreatography (MRCP) has become the gold standard among noninvasive diagnostic tools for the study of the biliary tree (Fig. 38.6). MRCP identifies biliary anatomy, the presence of dilatation and the presence of intrahepatic stones. It has completely replaced invasive investigations such as ERCP and percutaneous transhepatic cholangiography (PTC), which nowadays have only therapeutic aims. The sensitivity and specificity of MRCP in detecting right and left intrahepatic duct stones is greater than 90% [39]. Stones appear as low-intensity areas and the alterations of the biliary tree are accurately depicted. MRCP identifies the presence of primary sclerosing cholangitis or the presence of other types of biliary strictures. Gadolinium-enhanced MR identifies the vascular structures and the presence of vascular complications.

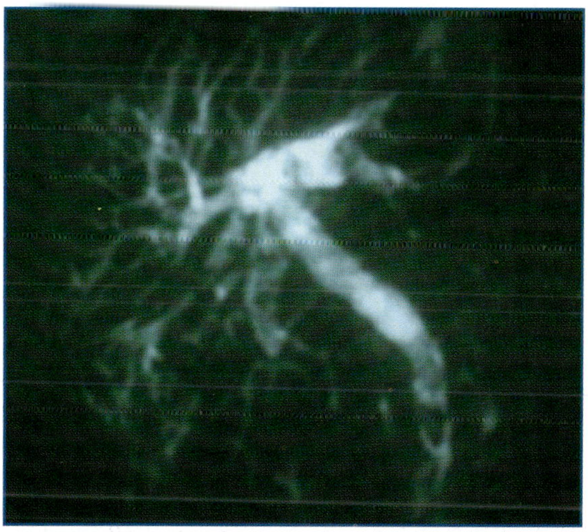

Fig. 38.6 MRCP showing hepatolithiasis of the left hepatic ducts

ERCP and PTC

Direct cholangiography techniques reveal optimal definition of bile duct anatomy and have the best sensitivity in identifying biliary strictures (Fig. 38.7). Direct cholangiography has now been replaced by noninvasive imaging techniques. The sensibility and specificity of ERCP seem to be lower than MRCP in detecting intrahepatic stones because the visualization of bile ducts peripheral to strictures is not always possible, or requires forced injection of contrast medium that may increase the risk of cholangitis. Moreover, ERCP is related to

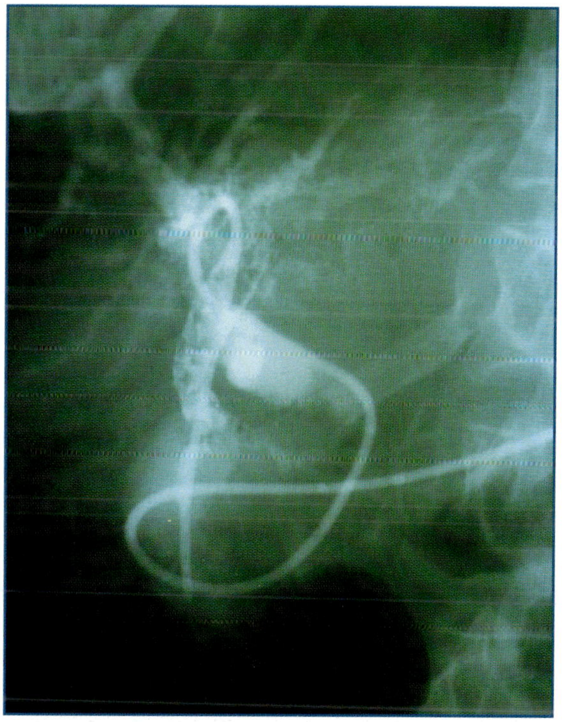

Fig. 38.7 ERCP showing dilated left hepatic ducts with hepatolithiasis of the hepatic segment 4

complications such as cholangitis, pancreatitis, hemorrhage and perforation. PTC is a highly sensitive investigation for detecting peripheral bile ducts but it is invasive, with significant morbidity. PTC is limited to those patients in whom therapeutic procedures such as stone extraction, intraductal lesion biopsy and biliary drainage positioning are indicated.

Conclusion

Hepatolithiasis is a disease with a variable geographical distribution related to socioeconomic conditions. It has different causes and can result in life-threatening complications such as severe cholangitis and chronic liver disease. The recent advances in non-invasive diagnostic tools have improved diagnosis of hepatolithiasis and can precisely identify the presence of bile ducts dilatation or strictures. These tools are useful in defining the correct type of therapeutic approach.

References

1. Mori T, Sugiyama M, Atomi Y (2006) Gallstone disease: management of intrahepatic stones. Best Pract Res Clin Gastroenterol 20:1117-1137
2. Leung JW, Yu AS (1997) Hepatolithiasis and biliary parasites. Baillieres Clin Gastroenterol 11:681-706
3. Pridgen JE Jr, Aust JB, McInnis WD (1977) Primary intrahepatic gallstones. Arch Surg 112:1037-1043
4. Saunders KD, Cates JA, Roslyn JJ (1990) Pathogenesis of gallstones. Surg Clin North Am 70:1197-1216
5. Nakayama F, Keida Y et al (1987) The survey of hepatolithiasis. Annual reports of the Japanese Ministry of Health and Welfare, Tokyo, Japan. Japanese Government p 37
6. Ozawa K, Takabayashi Y et al (1992) The survey of hepatolithiasis. Annual reports of the Japanese Ministry of Health and Welfare, Tokyo, Japan. Japanese Government (37):11
7. Tanimura H (1997) The survey of hepatolithiasis. Annual reports of the Japanese Ministry of Health and Welfare, Tokyo, Japan. Japanese Government, 1997: p 8
8. Lindstrom CG (1977) Frequency of gallstone disease in a well-defined Swedish population. A prospective necropsy study in Malmo. Scand J Gastroenterol 12: 341-346
9. Simi M, Loriga P, Basoli A (1979) Intrahepatic lithiasis. Study of thirty-six cases and review of the literature. Am J Surg 137:317-322
10. Pitt HA, Vebrux AC, Coleman J (1994) Intrahepatic stones. The transhepatic team approach. Ann Surg 219:527-535; discussion 535-537
11. Nakayama F, Furusawa T, Nakama T (1980) Hepatolithiasis in Japan. Am J Surg 139:216-219
12. Su CH, Lui WY, P'Eng FK (1992) Relative prevalence of gallstone diseases in Taiwan. A nationwide cooperative study. Dig Dis Sci 37:764-768
13. Kwon OJ, PY, Kim JP (1982) A clinical study of cholelithiasis in Korea. J Korea Surg Soc 24:1052-1057
14. Tanimura H, Uchiyama K (1998) Epidemiological status of hepatolithiasis. J Biliary Tract Pancreas 19:5
15. Nakayama (1997) The survey of hepatolithiasis. Cause and treatment. Tokyo, New York, Igaku-Shoin Ltd, p 12
16. Tazuma S (2006) Gallstone disease: epidemiology, pathogenesis, and classification of biliary stones (common bile duct and intrahepatic). Best Pract Res Clin Gastroenterol 20:1075-1083
17. Tabata M, Nakayama F (1984) Bacteriology of hepatolithiasis. Prog Clin Biol Res 152:163-174
18. Leung JW, Sung JY, Costerton JW (1989) Bacteriological and electron microscopy examination of brown pigment stones. J Clin Microbiol 27:915-921
19. Zen Y, Harada K, Sasaki M (2002) Lipopolysaccharide induces overexpression of MUC2 and MUC5AC in cultured biliary epithelial cells: possible key phenomenon of hepatolithiasis. Am J Pathol 161:1475-1484
20. Kim HJ, Lee SK, Kim MH (2002) Cystic fibrosis transmembrane conductance regulators (CFTR) in biliary epithelium of patients with hepatolithiasis. Dig Dis Sci 47:1758-1765
21. Matsushiro T, Suzuki N, Sato T, Maki T (1977) Effects of diet on glucaric acid concentration in bile and the formation of calcium bilirubinate gallstones. Gastroenterology 72(4 Pt 1):630-633
22. Kamiya J, Nimura Y (2007) Intrahepatic Stones. Surgery of the Liver, Biliary Tract and Pancreas, Saunders Elsevier, Philadelphia (USA). Vol 1:586-596
23. Cook J, How PC, HO HC, Mcfadzean AJ (1954) Recurrent pyogenic cholangeitis. Br J Surg 42:188-203

24. Chou ST, Chan CW (1980) Recurrent pyogenic cholangitis: a necropsy study. Pathology 12(3):415-428
25. Tsunoda T, Tsuchiya R, Harada N et al (1985) Long-term results of surgical treatment for intrahepatic stones. Jpn J Surg 15:455-462
26. Nimura Y, MM, Yamada T et al (2001) Annual reports of the Japanese Ministry of Health and Welfare. Tokyo, Japan, p 6
27. Gupta AK, Gupta A, Bhardwa VK, Chansoria M (2006) Caroli's disease. Indian J Pediatr 73:233-235
28. Khuroo MS, Zargar SA, Mahajan R (1990) Hepatobiliary and pancreatic ascariasis in India. Lancet 335:1503-1506
29. Rana SS, Bhasin DK, Nanda M, Singh K (2007) Parasitic infestations of the biliary tract. Curr Gastroenterol Rep 9:156-164
30. Dodd GD 3rd, Niedzwiecki GA, Campbell WL, Baron RL (1997) Bile duct calculi in patients with primary sclerosing cholangitis. Radiology 203:443-447
31. Rosmorduc O, Hermelin B, Boelle P-Y et al (2004) ABCB4 Gene Mutations and Primary Sclerosing Cholangitis. Gastroenterology 126:1220-1222
32. Chijiiwa K, Ichimya H, Kuroki S et al (1993) Late development of cholangiocarcinoma after the treatment of hepatolithiasis. Surg Gynecol Obstet 177:279-282
33. Holzinger F, Z'Graggen K, Buchler MW (1999) Mechanisms of biliary carcinogenesis: a pathogenetic multi-stage cascade towards cholangiocarcinoma. Ann Oncol 10(Suppl 4):122-126
34. Kuroki T, Tajima Y, Kanematsu T (2005) Hepatolithiasis and intrahepatic cholangiocarcinoma: carcinogenesis based on molecular mechanisms. J Hepatobiliary Pancreat Surg 12:463-436
35. Ishikawa A, Sasaki M, Sato Y et al (2004) Frequent p16ink4a inactivation is an early and frequent event of intraductal papillary neoplasm of the liver arising in hepatolithiasis. Hum Pathol 35:1505-1514
36. Kim YT, Byun JS, Kim J et al (2003) Factors predicting concurrent cholangiocarcinomas associated with hepatolithiasis. Hepatogastroenterology 50:8-12
37. Chijiiwa K, Ohtani K, Noshiro H et al (2002) Cholangiocellular carcinoma depending on the kind of intrahepatic calculi in patients with hepatolithiasis. Hepatogastroenterology 49:96-99
38. Lim JH (1991) Oriental cholangiohepatitis: pathologic, clinical, and radiologic features. AJR Am J Roentgenol 157:1-8
39. Kim TK, Kim BS, Kim JH et al (2002) Diagnosis of intrahepatic stones: superiority of MR cholangiopancreatography over endoscopic retrograde cholangiopancreatography. AJR Am J Roentgenol 179:429-434

Chapter 39

Treatment of Intrahepatic Lithiasis

Yuji Nimura

Percutaneous Approach

The percutaneous approach for the non-surgical treatment of intrahepatic stones was developed with flexible cholangioscopy via a T-tube sinus tract to remove retained intrahepatic stones after intraoperative choledochohepaticolithotomy through choledochotomy [1, 2]. Another route of percutaneous cholangioscopic lithotomy was established through choledochojejunostomy with subcutaneous jejunostomy after intraoperative choledochohepaticolithotomy [3]. Further development of interventional techniques and fiber optic flexible cholangioscopes enabled percutaneous transhepatic cholangioscopy (PTCS) via dilated sinus tract of percutaneous transhepatic biliary drainage (PTBD) (Fig. 39.1) [4–8].

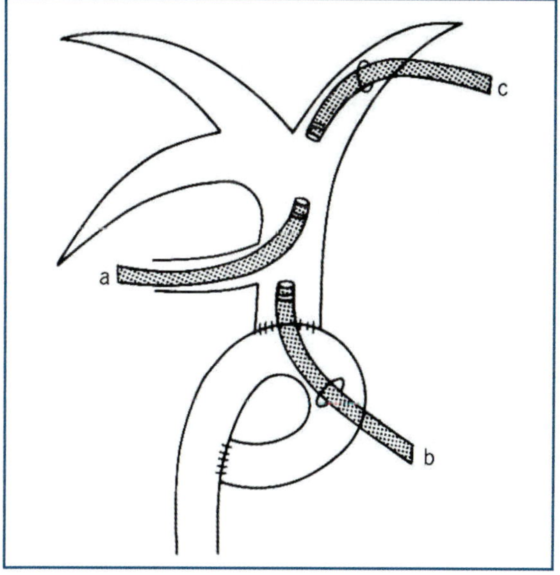

Fig. 39.1 Cholangioscopic lithotomy. Postoperative cholangioscopy via T-tube sinus tract (T-POC) (*a*). Postoperative cholangioscopy via jejunostomy (J-POC) (*b*). Percutaneous transhepatic cholangioscopy (PTCS) (*c*)

Postoperative Cholangioscopy via T-tube Sinus Tract (T-POC)

The time of intraoperative cholangioscopic lithotomy through choledochotomy should not be prolonged. Especially in cases of difficult intrahepatic stones, postoperative cholangioscopy (POC) with the help of fluoroscopy is more effective in removing the numerous impacted stones in the bilateral lobe of the liver. The T-tube sinus tract can be established 2–3 weeks after T-tube drainage. Location of the intrahepatic stones with possible biliary stenosis and/or dilation should be diagnosed by T-tube cholangiography prior to POC. In case of impacted stones in the intrahepatic segmental duct, the operator should be careful not to overlook the possible non-pictured segmental duct at T-tube cholangiography (Fig. 39.2a). After removing the impacted stones at the confluence of the involved segmental ducts, selective cholangiography should be employed to clarify the segmental anatomy of the involved intrahepatic ducts and possible retained stones with or without biliary stenosis in the further peripheral branches (Fig. 39.2b, c). A thin cholangioscope is used to remove small stones in the peripheral small branches with or without biliary stenosis and to confirm the absence of residual stones (Fig. 39.2d).

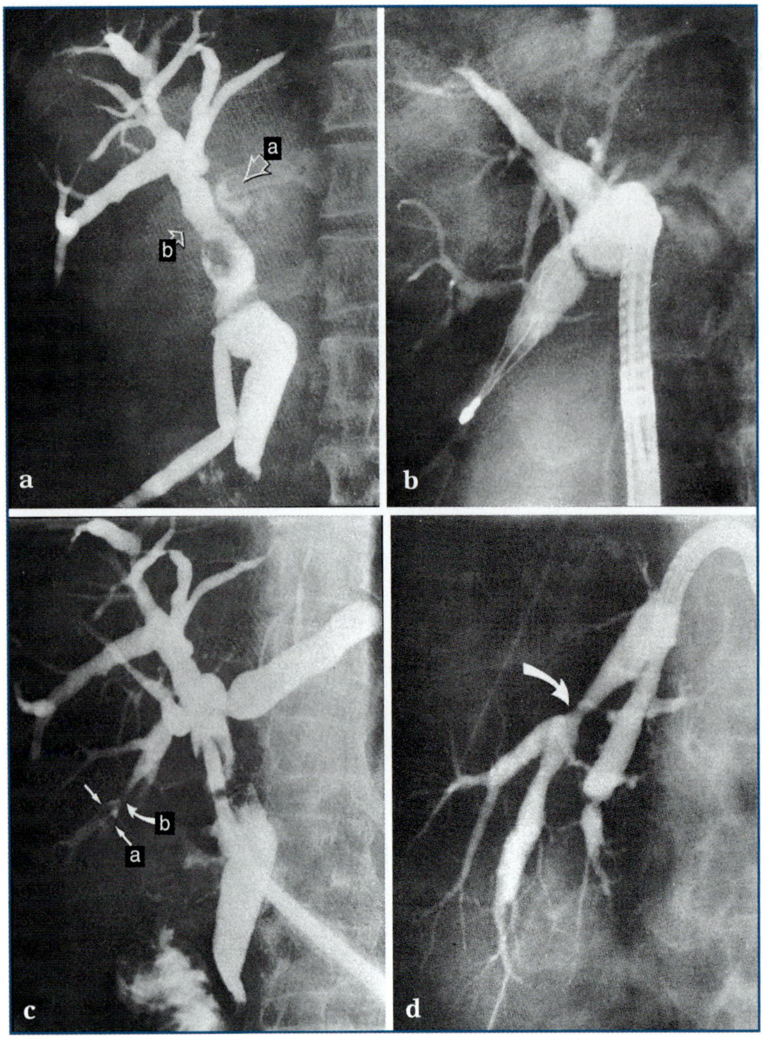

Fig. 39.2 a T-tube cholangiography only visualizes the right anterior sectional ducts. The left hepatic duct (*arrow a*) and the right posterior sectional duct (*arrow b*) are not demonstrated because of impacted stones. **b** Cholangioscopic lithotomy with a basket catheter in the right posterior sectional duct. **c** T-tube cholangiography after cholangioscopic lithotomy clearly shows the left hepatic duct and biliary stenosis (*b*) with small impacted stones in the peripheral branches (*a*) of the right posterior sectional duct. **d** Cholangioscopic selective cholangiography demonstrates improved biliary stenosis (*arrow*) without residual stones

Postoperative Cholangioscopy via Jejunal Limb (J-POC)

A cholangioscope is introduced through a jejunostomy made proximal to choledochojejunostomy in case of a retained intrahepatic stone. Involved segmental ducts are also confirmed by cholangioscopic selective cholangiography under fluoroscopy (Fig. 39.3a). Retained stones with or without biliary strictures can be demonstrated by cholangioscopic selective cholangiography (Fig. 39.3b, c). After completing cholangioscopic lithotripsy, a drainage catheter placed through the jejunostomy is removed to close the jejunostomy [9].

Percutaneous Transhepatic Cholangioscopy (PTCS)

PTCS is applied for primary or retained intrahepatic stones that cannot be treated by T-POC, J-POC or peroral transpapillary cholangioscopy because of peripheral stones with biliary stenosis or more difficult intrahepatic stones complicated with biliary sepsis and/or liver cirrhosis [6, 9].

Firstly, PTBD is performed through the left hepatic duct under a direct anterior approach. The PTBD sinus tract is dilated by replacing a 6Fr drainage catheter with a 10Fr or 11Fr PTCS catheter (Fig. 39.4). PTBD tube cholangiography is more useful

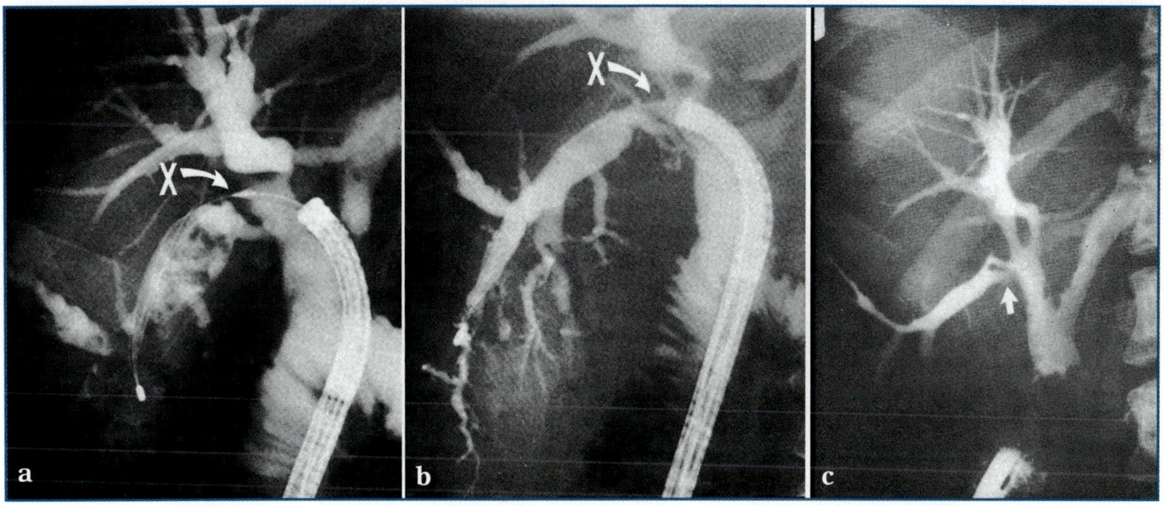

Fig. 39.3 a Postoperative transjejunal cholangioscopy reveals retained intrahepatic stones in the right posterior sectional duct with biliary stenosis (*X*). **b** A basket catheter is introduced through the stenotic segment (*X*) to remove the impacted stones. **c** The biliary stenosis (*arrow*) is recovered after cholangioscopic lithotomy

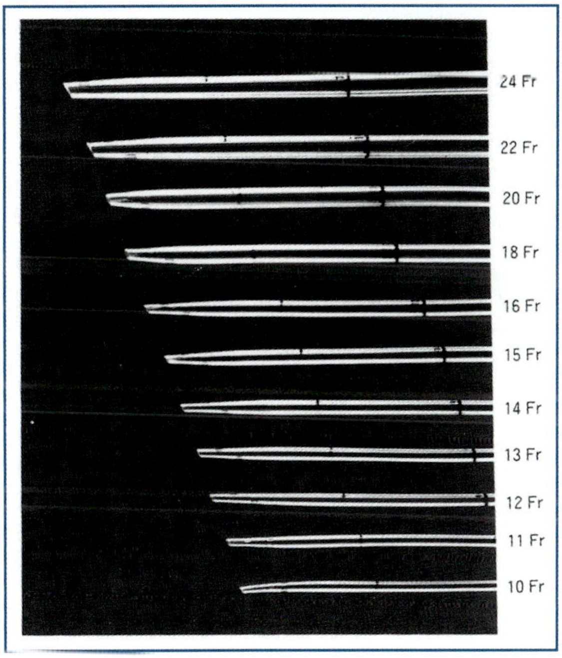

Fig. 39.4 PTCS catheters. Eleven kinds of catheters from 10 Fr to 24 Fr have two side holes at the tapered tip of the catheter

than ERCP for demonstrating intrahepatic stones and/or common bile duct stones with or without biliary strictures and/or anomalous anatomy of the intrahepatic segmental ducts (Fig. 39.5a). The PTBD sinus tract is further dilated by exchanging the catheter for a bigger one step-by-step, until a 16Fr catheter can be introduced approximately 2 weeks after the initial PTBD. Then PTCS can be carried out with a commercially available cholangiofiberscope. Distal bile duct stones are easily removed by PTCS lithotomy with a basket catheter (Fig. 39.5b). Selective cholangioscopy under PTCS gives more detailed information about biliary anatomy and impacted stones proximal to a biliary stenosis (Fig. 39.5c). In case of the above abnormality with severe stenosis, a basket catheter cannot be introduced through the biliary stenosis into the dilated segmental ducts filled with stones (Fig. 39.5d). In this situation, another PTBD should directly be performed through the affected segmental duct (Fig. 39.5e), and PTCS lithotomy should be carried out under direct cholangioscopic control (Fig. 39.5f). Complete clearance of intrahepatic stones is confirmed by cholangioscopic observation together with selective cholangiography (Fig. 39.5g).

If an ill patient with intrahepatic stones develops septic cholangitis with or without liver cirrhosis, urgent PTBD is indicated. The most advantageous site for PTBD is the left

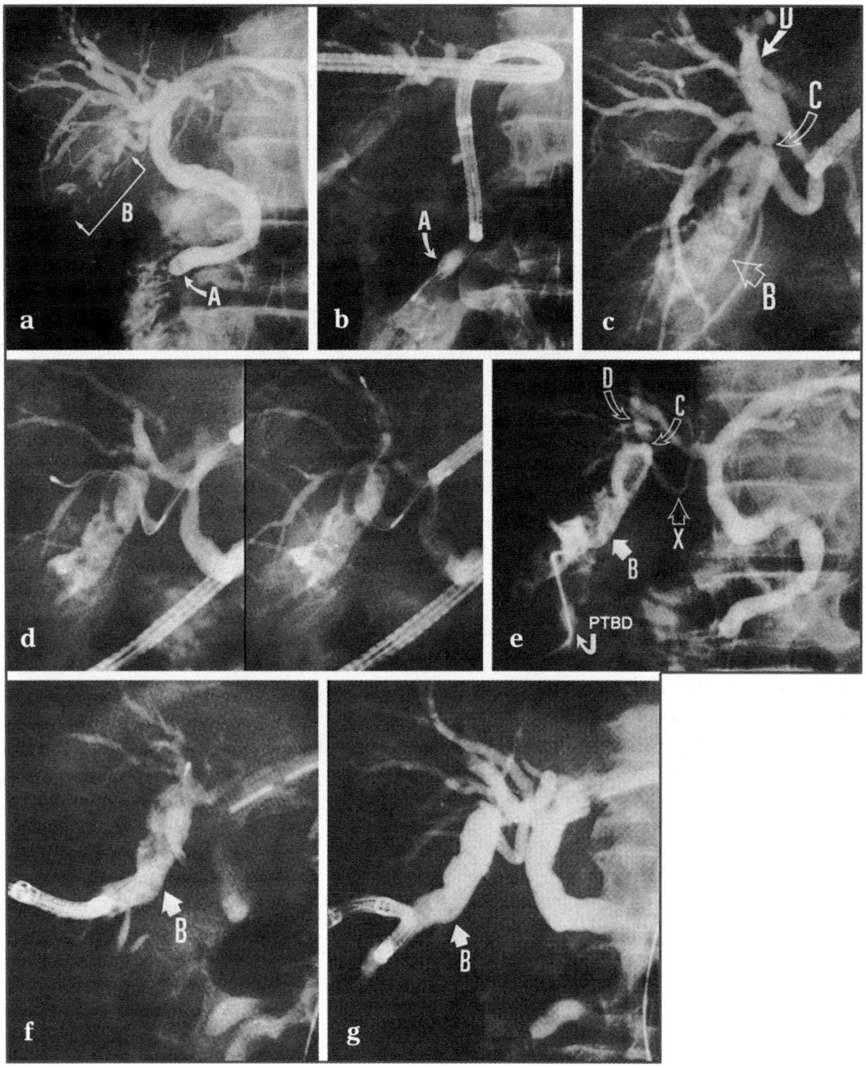

Fig. 39.5 **a** PTBD tube cholangiography shows a distal bile ducts stone (*A*) and possible intrahepatic stone in the right posterior inferior segmental duct (*B*). **b** A distal bile duct stone (*A*) is easily removed with a basket catheter. **c** Cholangioscopic selective cholangiography demonstrates biliary stenosis (*C*) at the confluence of the involved posterior inferior branch (*B*) and posterior superior branch (*D*). **d** Selective introduction of a basket catheter was applied but failed to remove the stones because of the biliary stenosis distal to the impacted stone. **e** Selective PTBD was performed directly to the involved right posterior inferior segmental duct (*B*). *C*, biliary stenosis; *D*, posterior superior duct; *X*, right posterior duct. **f** PTCS lithotomy was carried out through the right posterior inferior segmental duct (*B*). **g** Cholangioscopic cholangiography clearly shows no residual stone after PTCS lithotomy (*B*, posterior inferior duct)

hepatic duct through the anterior approach, providing easy access for a cholangioscope not only to the right anterior and posterior sectional ducts, but also into the left medial and lateral sectional ducts. The PTBD catheter should be exchanged for a larger one when the cholangitis has subsided. PTCS lithotomy is conducted in the usual manner. Even in case of possible biliary stenosis at the initial cholangiography (Fig. 39.6a), cholangiographic biliary stenosis often disappears after PTCS lithotomy and a cholangioscope can be further introduced peripherally through the stenotic segment to remove the peripheral stones (Fig. 39.6b, c). Initially, undemonstrated segmental ducts are also

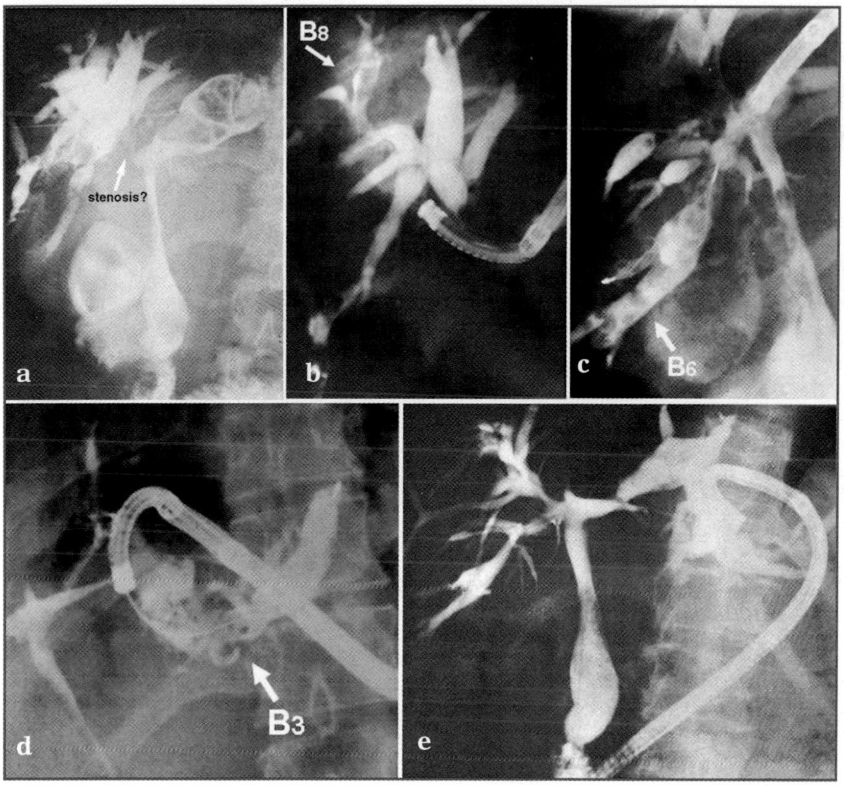

Fig. 39.6 a Urgent PTC for a septic patient with cholangitis shows bilateral intrahepatic stones, biliary stenosis and dilation. **b** PTCS lithotomy in the right anterior superior segmental duct (*B8*). **c** PTCS lithotomy in the right posterior inferior segmental duct (*B6*). **d** PTCS lithotomy in the left lateral inferior segmental duct (*B3*). **e** Cholangioscopic cholangiography after complete removal of intrahepatic stones shows multiple deformities of the intrahepatic segmental ducts, which look stenotic or dilated

revealed after removing impacted stones at the confluence of the segmental ducts (Fig. 39.6d). Cholangioscopic cholangiography after removing all the peripheral stones clearly shows the absence of residual stones and the presence of deformities of the intrahepatic segmental ducts that look stenotic or dilated (Fig. 39.6e).

Recent progress in diagnostic procedures has allowed early detection of small lesions localized in the intrahepatic segmental ducts. Ultrasonography (US) detects a high echoic lesion in the slightly dilated intrahepatic segmental duct in a patient complaining of abdominal pain and fever (Fig. 39.7a). ERCP reveals the absence of the intrahepatic segmental duct that is involved by a high echoic lesion in US (Fig. 39.7b). US guided percutaneous transhepatic cholangiography (PTC) clearly demonstrates segmental stenosis with proximal dilation of the posterior branch of the left lateral section (B2) (Fig. 39.7c). Subsequently, PTBD followed by PTCS is performed through this dilated duct and an impacted cholesterol stone is detected in the proximal site of this duct (Fig. 39.7 d, e). The cholesterol stone is easily removed with a basket catheter. Precise investigation of the affected duct is carried out by cholangioscopic observation and selective cholangiography (Fig. 39.7f). In case of severe biliary stenosis, the stenotic portion should be carefully observed by PTCS with biopsy to exclude possible association of cholangiocarcinoma. If a negative biopsy is obtained, non-surgical treatment should be applied as the first treatment of choice. A guide wire is inserted into the stenotic segment under cholangioscopic and fluoroscopic control (Fig. 39.7g), and a PTCS catheter is introduced over the guide wire to dilate the stenosis (Fig. 39.7h). This dilation procedure is repeated in the same manner to dilate the PTBD sinus tract. Complete dilation of the biliary stenosis makes it possible to pass a cholangioscope through the dilated stenotic segment and to observe the entirety of the intrahepatic segmental ducts in order not to

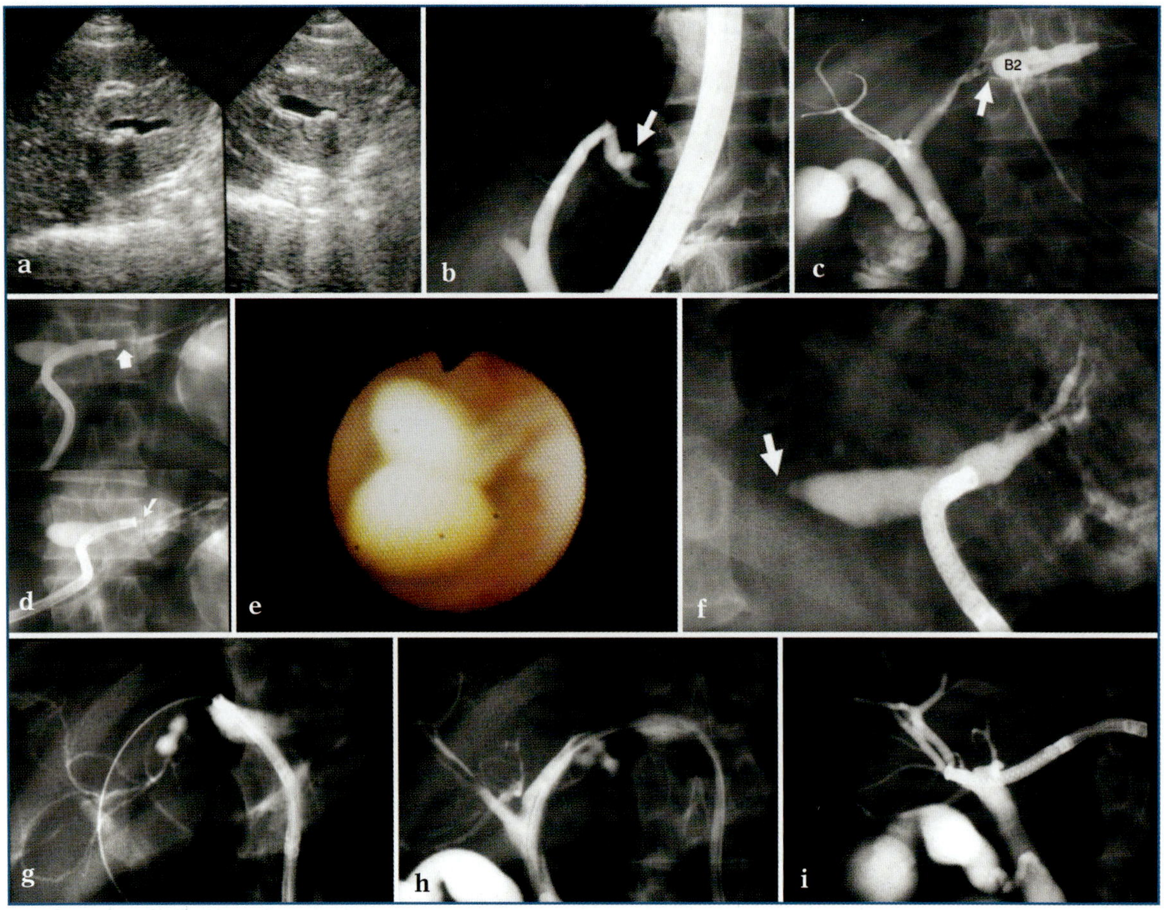

Fig. 39.7 a A high echoic lesion with acoustic shadow is detected in a slightly dilated intrahepatic duct by US. **b** ERCP dose not reveal the affected segmental duct (*arrow*) detected by US. **c** PTBD is performed through the slightly dilated left lateral superior segmental duct (*B2*). Biliary stenosis (*arrow*) is also revealed. **d** Cholangioscopic cholangiography demonstrates a shadow defect (*arrow*) in the proximal site of the B2. **e** Cholangioscopic inspection revealed impacted cholesterol stones that were easily removed with a basket catheter. **f** Cholangioscopic selective cholangiography shows no residual stone in the B2. However, the marked stenosis (*arrow*) remains unchanged. **g** A guide wire is inserted through the stenotic segment under cholangioscopic and fluoroscopic control. **h** A PTCS catheter is introduced over the guide wire to dilate the biliary stenosis. **i** A cholangioscope passes through the dilated stenotic segment to observe the entire biliary tract and not to overlook residual stones

overlook residual intrahepatic stones (Fig. 39.7i).

With the help of recent progress in computed tomography (CT), the composition of intrahepatic stones can be estimated at the time of diagnosis. If calculi less dense than water (a characteristic finding of cholesterol stones in CT) are detected in a symptomatic patient, a non-surgical approach is recommended as the first treatment of choice [10]. Contrary to calcium bilirubinate intrahepatic stones, inflammatory changes and degree of dilatation of the affected segmental duct are minimal. Therefore, endoscopic lithotomy followed by dissolution therapy is useful to prevent recurrent intrahepatic cholesterol stones [11].

Conservative Surgery

As a conservative surgery, hepaticojejunostomy followed by choledocholithotomy has been performed for choledochohepaticolithiasis to prompt postoperative spontaneous discharge of the intrahepatic stones into the jejunum. However, this surgical strategy conveyed septic cholangitis to the ill patients with retained intrahepatic stones, one of the strong prognostic factors of this disease. The risk of cholangitis in retained intrahepatic stones is higher in patients with hepaticojejunostomy than in those without bilioenteric anastomosis. Therefore, if hepaticojejunostomy (end-to-side anastomosis is preferable) is indicated for patients with retained intrahepatic stones, percutaneous jejunostomy should be made proximal to the anastomosis and postoperative cholangioscopic lithotomy must be carried out to remove the all residual stones. Hepaticojejunostomy in patients with residual intrahepatic stones will lead to ascending cholangitis with or without sepsis, which is a strong factor in the formation of new intrahepatic stones and the development of biliary cirrhosis with or without intrahepatic cholangiocarcinoma [12]. Complete removal of the residual stones is the most important factor to improve the quality of life of the treated patients [3].

Hepaticojejunostomy is indicated for patients with bilateral intrahepatic stones associated with proximal biliary stenosis. In such a difficult case, PTCS should first be performed to remove some stones, to treat cholangitis and to clarify the local anatomy of the biliary system and extent of biliary stenosis (Fig. 39.8a). After improving the general condition of the ill patient, the stenotic segment of the proximal bile duct is resected and hepaticojejunostomy is carried out at the hepatic confluence above the biliary stricture. Postoperative PTCS should be performed to remove possible residual stones and to confirm complete stone clearance and biliary passage (Fig. 39.8b).

Resective Surgery

Hepatic resection is an established treatment strategy for intrahepatic stones localized in the atrophic unilateral lobe of the liver [13]. Chronic segmental or sectional biliary dilation with impacted intrahepatic stones associated with chronic cholangitis develops aggressive periductal fibrosis and periphlebitis, inducing chronic portal stenosis followed by segmental or sectional atro-

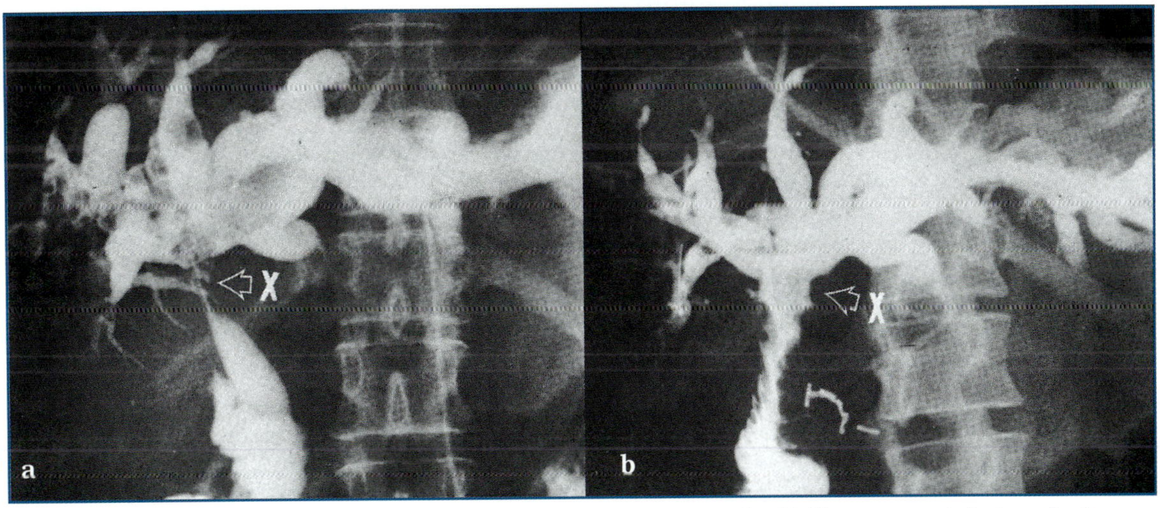

Fig. 39.8 a PTBD tube cholangiography clearly demonstrates marked biliary stenosis below the hepatic confluence (*X*), atrophy of the right liver and multiple stones in bilateral intrahepatic ducts. **b** Postoperative PTBD tube cholangiography shows no residual stone and reconstructed biliary tract at the hepatic hilus (*X*)

phy of the liver. The location of an intrahepatic stone with liver atrophy is predominantly in the left liver rather than in the right or bilateral lobe, therefore left lateral sectionectomy or left hepatectomy with or without hepaticojejunostomy are often used with a low long-term stone recurrence rate [12, 14]. In case of a bilateral intrahepatic stone, a definitive surgical procedure cannot be designed at the initial presentation because the evidence of impacted stones hinders detection of a causative lesion is in such cases difficult before removing the stones either by US, CT, ERCP and TCP.

In the case we present, ERCP showed a dilated left hepatic duct filled with stones, and an intrahepatic stone was suspected also in a part of the right hepatic duct (Fig.39.9a). PTBD was performed through the affected left hepatic duct and PTBD tube cholangiography clearly demonstrated impacted stones in the left hepatic duct and the right posterior sectional duct. However, the hepatic confluence could not be demonstrated clearly in order to understand whether or not a causative lesion involved the hepatic confluence (Fig. 39.9b). When PTCS lithotomy was progressed, the undemonstrated right intrahepatic ducts B6 and B7, and the caudate lobe branches B1r and B1l were clearly visualized (Fig. 39.9c).

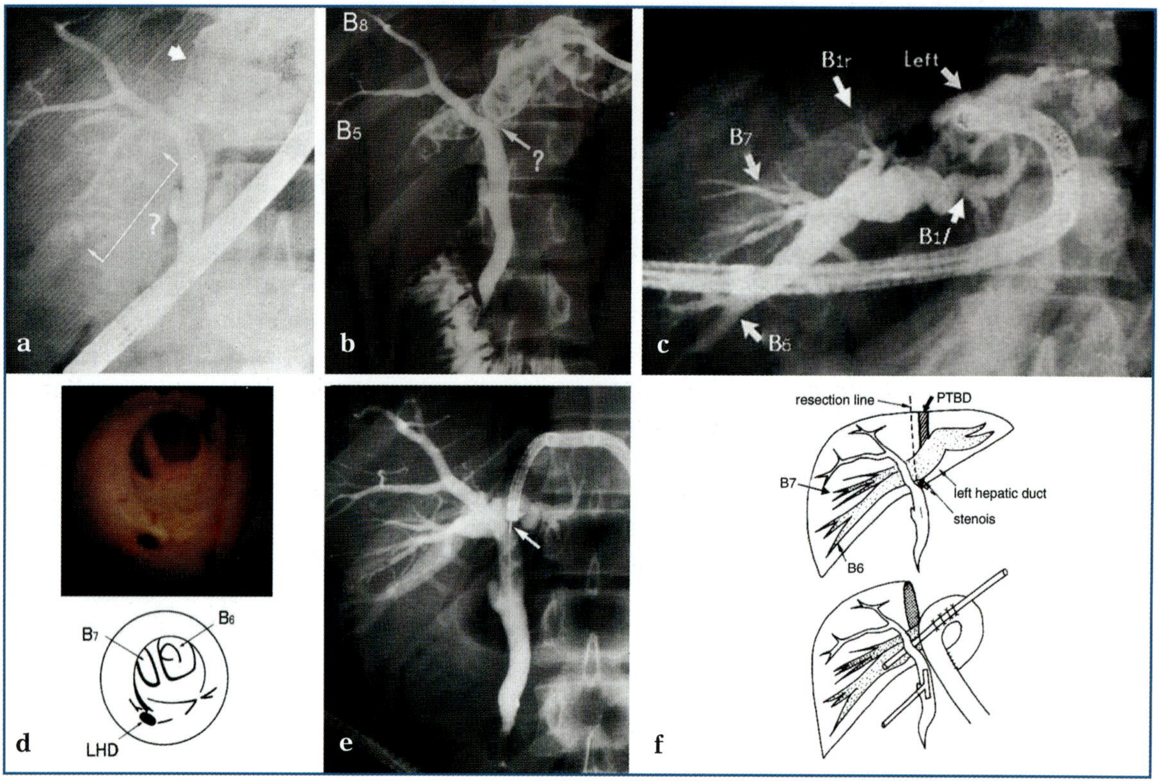

Fig. 39.9 a ERCP shows a dilated left hepatic duct filled with stones (*arrow*) and an irregular shadow is faintly witnessed in the right liver (*?*). **b** PTBD cholangiography clearly demonstrates intrahepatic stones filled in the left hepatic duct in continuity with the right hepatic duct. The anterior sectional ducts (*B5, B8*) and extrahepatic duct are normal. The hepatic confluence (*?*) is not clearly visualized. **c** The right posterior sectional ducts (*B6, B7*) and the right and left caudate lobe branches (*B1r, B1l*) are clearly demonstrated during PTCS lithotomy. **d** Cholangioscopic finding after PTCS lithotomy. The right posterior sectional duct (*B6, B7*) are slightly dilated, and a narrow duct was diagnosed as the left hepatic duct confluence (*LHD*). **e** Cholangioscopic cannulation with cholangiography reveals that the stenotic segment is the left hepatic duct at the hepatic confluence (*arrow*). **f** Left hepatectomy, hepaticojejunostomy and T-tube drainage were performed to remove the causative lesion and to provide access routes for postoperative cholangioscopy

A severe stricture of the left hepatic duct was detected by cholangioscopic inspection of the hepatic confluence (Fig. 39.9d). Cholangioscopic selective introduction of a catheter into the stenotic duct demonstrated the passage to the common bile duct (Fig. 39.9e). According to the above findings, the causative lesion of an intrahepatic stone was defined as the stenotic left hepatic duct proximal to the hepatic confluence and distal to the confluence of the left hepatic duct and the right posterior sectional duct. Therefore, left hepatectomy, hepaticojejunostomy and T-tube drainage were performed to remove the causative lesion (Fig. 39.9f). Postoperative cholangioscopy via the T-tube sinus tract and through a performed percutaneous jejunostomy should be carried out to confirm the absence of residual stone.

Another patient with a past history of cholecystectomy and transduodenal papilloplasty for cholecystocholedocholithiasis, complained of epigastric pain. CT demonstrated atrophy of the left lateral section, hypertrophy of the caudate lobe and high density lesions in the left lateral section and the right posterior section (Fig. 39.10a). Balloon ERCP showed slight dilation of the common bile duct and absence of the left lateral and right anterior sectional ducts, and multiple intrahepatic stones were shown in the right posterior sectional duct. Long biliary branches of the left medial section and the caudate lobe were also demonstrated (Fig. 39.10b). PTBD was performed through the affected right posterior sectional duct, and selective cholangiography after PTCS lithotomy clearly showed marked stenosis of the right anterior sectional duct. Small retained stones were shown in the branches of the right posterior inferior segment (Fig. 39.10c). Further selective cholangioscopic cholangiography demonstrated impacted stones in the atrophic right anterior sectional duct (Fig. 39.10d) and left lateral sectional duct (Fig. 39.10e). Selective cannulation in the left medial sectional duct made it possible to demonstrate an elongated sectional duct without stones that indicated hypertrophy of segment 4 (Fig. 39.10f). Selective hepatic arteriography and portography showed the atrophic left lateral and right anterior sections and portal obstruction of the left lateral branch, a small right anterior branch and big left medial branch and caudate lobe branches (Fig. 39.10g). Composition of the retrieved intrahepatic stones was variable as shown in Table 39.1, and the pathogenesis of each intrahepatic stone was also suspected as variable. According to the final diagnosis of this case (Fig. 39.10h), transduodenal papilloplasty was suspected as a main cause of lithogenecity of the intrahepatic stone, and left lateral sectionectomy, right anterior sectionectomy and hepaticojejunostomy were indicated to prevent postoperative ascending cholangitis followed by intrahepatic stone recurrence. Intraoperatively, marked atrophy of the left lateral (L) and right anterior sections, and hypertrophy of the left medial section (M) and the caudate lobe (S1) were observed (Fig. 39.10i). Postoperative PTBD tube cholangiography showed resected margins of the left lateral and right anterior sectional ducts and good passage of contrast into the jejunal limb (Fig. 39.10j).

Table 39.1 Composition of gallstones removed from different hepatic sections

Location	Calcium bilirubinate	Fatty acid calcium	Cholesterol
Left lateral section	10%	6%	84%
Right anterior section	49%	28%	23%
Right posterior section	60%	25%	15%

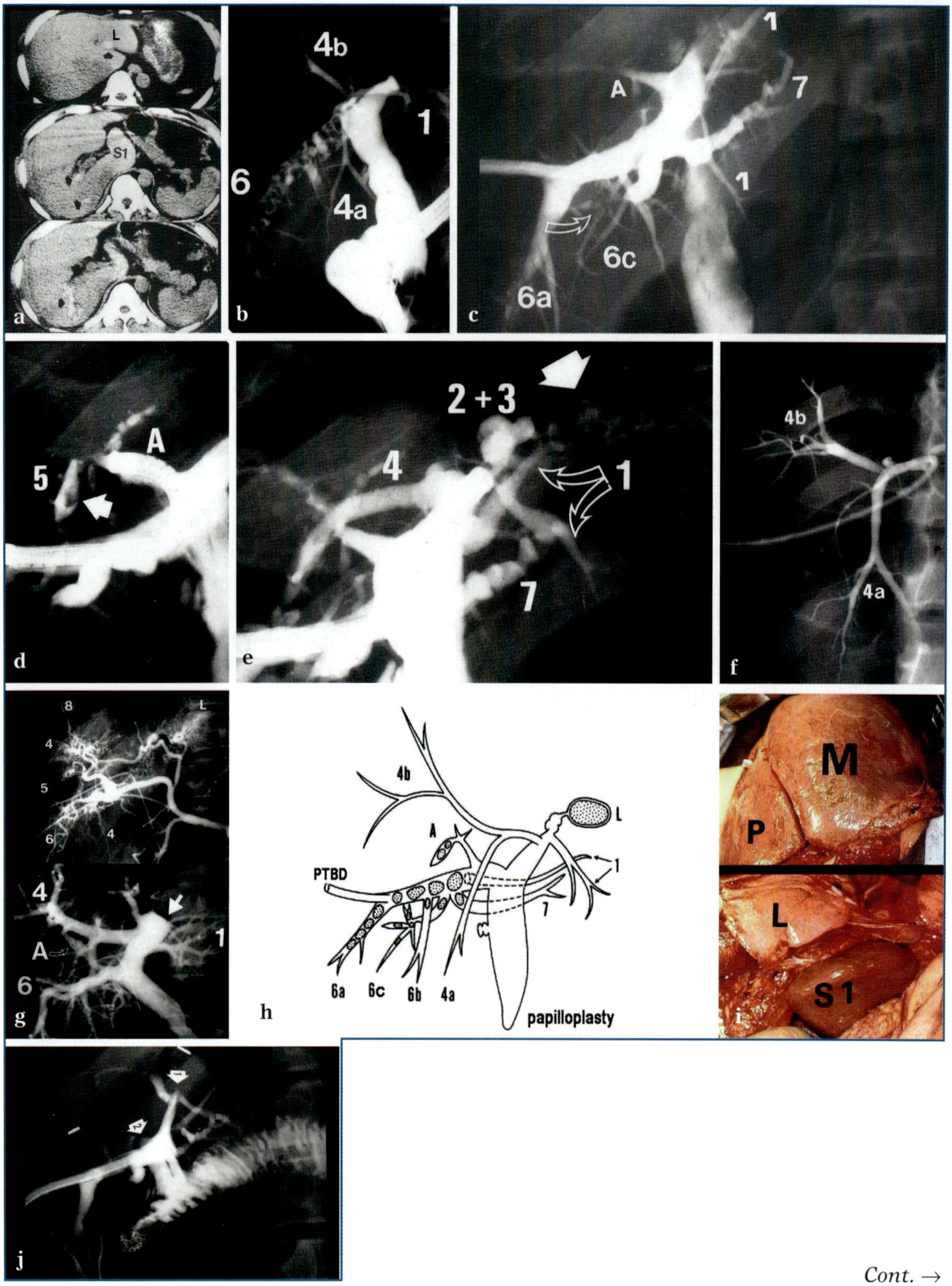
L
S1
4b
1
6
4a
A
7
1
6c
6a
5
2+3
4
1
7
4b
4a
8
L
4
5
6
4
4
A
1
6
4b
A
L
PTBD
1
7
6a
6c
6b
4a
papilloplasty
M
P
L
S1
a
b
c
d
e
f
g
h
i
j

Cont. →

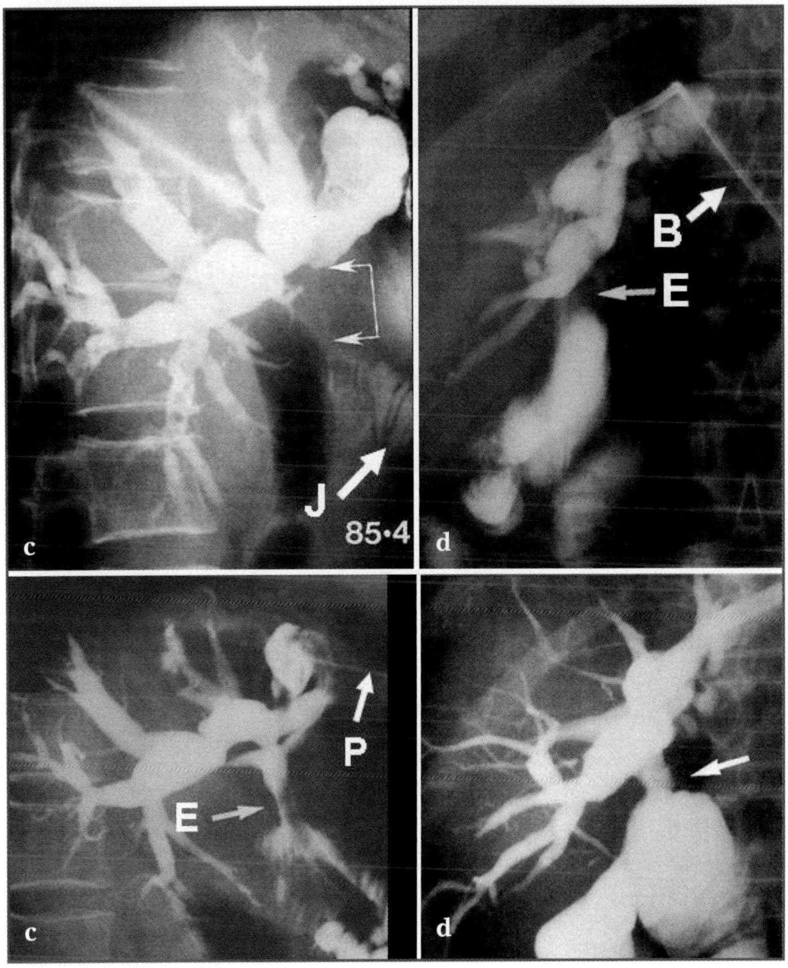

Fig. 39.11 a PTC in a left lateral position. PTC shows dilation of the bilateral intrahepatic bile ducts with multiple stones. Although hepaticojejunal anastomosis is not demonstrated, the jejunum is faintly seen (*J*). **b** PTBD tube (*B*) cholangiography shows clear passage of the contrast medium through an endoprosthesis (*E*) placed across the hepaticojejunal anastomosis. **c** PTC (*P*) demonstrates clear passage of the contrast medium over the obstructed endoprosthesis (*E*). **d** Cholangioscopic cholangiography shows clear passage of the contrast medium through the dilated hepaticojejunostomy (*arrow*)

Cont. **Fig. 39.10 a** CT demonstrates atrophy of the left lateral section (*L*), hypertrophy of the caudate lobe (*S1*) and high density lesions in the left lateral and right posterior sections (*arrows*). **b** Balloon ERCP shows dilated common bile duct, the right posterior sectional duct filled with stones (*6*), absence of the left lateral and right anterior sectional ducts and elongation of the biliary branches of the left medial inferior (*4a*) and medial superior (*4b*) segments and the caudate lobe (*1*). **c** PTBD tube cholangiography after PTCS lithotomy shows marked stenosis of the right anterior sectional duct (*A*) and small retained stones in the peripheral branches of the segment 6 (*arrow*). Numerals indicate the number of Couinand's segments – 6a: ventral branch; 6c: lateral branch. **d** Cholangioscopic selective cholangiography demonstrates marked stenosis of the right anterior sectional duct (*A*) with stones in the atrophic anterior inferior segmental duct (*5, arrow*). **e** Cholangioscopic selective cholangiography also shows marked stenosis with proximal dilation of the left lateral sectional duct (*2+3*) filled with stones (*white arrow*). Numerals indicate the number of Couinand's segments. **f** Selective cholangiography of the left medial section clearly demonstrates hypertrophy of this section without an intrahepatic stone. *a*: inferior branch, *b*: superior branch. **g** Hepatic arteriography and portography show atrophy of the left lateral (*L*) and right anterior sections (*5, 8*) and portal obstruction of the left lateral sectional branch (*white arrow*), a small right anterior branch (*A*) and big left medial branch (*4*) and caudate lobe branches (*1*). Numerals indicate the number of Couinand's segments. **h** Preoperative diagnosis of this case. *L*, left lateral section; *A*, right anterior section. Numbers indicate the number of Couinand's segments: 4a, inferior branch; 4b, superior branch; 6a, ventral branch; 6b, dorsal branch; 6c, lateral branch. **i** Intraoperative finding. The left medial section (*M*) and the caudate lobe (*S1*) are hypertrophic and left lateral section (*L*) is atrophic. The right anterior section forms a sulcus between the left medial section (*M*) and the right posterior section (*P*) due to marked atrophy. **j** Postoperative PTBD tube cholangiography shows resected margins of the left lateral (*arrow 1*) and right anterior (*arrow 2*) sectional ducts

Relapsing Bile Duct Stones in Patients with Previous Hepatico-juno-anastomosis

Some patients with difficult intrahepatic stones have a past history of biliary surgery. The cause of lithogenesis is variable. A cause may be inadequate hepaticojejunostomy because of intrahepatic biliary stenosis with or without proximal dilation [12]. Another cause of relapsing symptoms may be increasing number of residual stones [9]. The first choice of precise diagnosis and treatment is PTBD tube cholangiography followed by PTCS lithotomy. Most of the cases have bilateral intrahepatic stones proximal to the stricture of hepaticojejunostomy (Fig. 39.11a). Precise diagnosis should be made after PTCS lithotomy. If anastomotic stenosis is diagnosed as a main cause of relapsing intrahepatic stones after hepaticojejunostomy, nonsurgical techniques, preferably PTCS, should be selected as the treatment of choice. In the case shown (Fig. 39.11b), the stenotic portion was dilated by cholangioscopic balloon dilation or cholangioscopic incision with electric cautery and a silicon endoprosthesis was placed across the anastomosis to prevent restenosis. Three years later, PTC clearly demonstrated good passage of the contrast medium over the obstructed endoprosthesis (Fig. 39.11c), which was removed by PTCS. Clear passage of the contrast medium through the hepaticojejunostomy was demonstrated by PTCS cholangiography after removing the endoprosthesis (Fig. 39.11d).

References

1. Yamakawa T, Komaki F, Shikata J (1978) Experience with routine postoperative choledochoscopy via the T-tube sinus tract. World J Surg 2:379-385
2. Chen MF, Jan YY, Chou FF et al (1983) Use of fiberoptic choledochoscope in common bile duct and intrahepatic duct exploration. Gastrointest Endosc 29:276-278
3. Ker CG, Kuo KK, Tsai CC et al (1994) Evaluation of choledochojejunostomy with subcutaneous jejunostomy for treatment of intrahepatic stones. Int Surg 79:110-113
4. Nimura Y, Hayakawa N, Toyoda S et al (1981) Percutaneous transhepatic cholangioscopy. Stomach Intestine (Japanese with English abstract) 16:681-689
5. Nimura Y (1984) Percutaneous transhepatic cholangioscopy (PTCS) in the treatment of intrahepatic stones. In: Sheen PC, Ker CG (eds) Gallstone and Choledochoscope. Kaohsiung, Mei Yue, pp 71-85
6. Nimura Y, Shionoya S, Hayakawa N et al (1988) Value of percutaneous transhepatic cholangioscopy (PTCS). Surg Endosc 2:213-219
7. Chen MF, Jan YY (1986) Percutaneous transhepatic removal of common bile duct and intrahepatic duct stones with a fiberoptic choledochoscope. Gastrointest Endosc 32:347-349
8. Chen MF, Jan YY, Lee TY (1987) Percutaneous transhepatic cholangioscopy. Br J Surg 74:728-730
9. Yeh YH, Huang MH, Yang JC et al (1995) Percutaneous trans-hepatic cholangioscopy and lithotripsy in the treatment of intrahepatic stones: a study with 5 year follow-up. Gastrointest Endosc 42:13-18
10. Kondo S, Nimura Y, Hayakawa N et al (1995) A clinicopathologic study of primary cholesterol hepatolithiasis. Hepatogastroenterology 42:478-486
11. Strichartz SD, Abedin MZ, Ippoliti AF et al (1991) Intrahepatic cholesterol stones: a rationale for dissolution therapy. Gastroenterology 100:228-232
12. Jan YY, Chen MF, Wang CS et al (1996) Surgical treatment of hepatolithiasis: long-term results. Surgery 120:509-514
13. Chen MF, Jan YY, Wang CS et al (1997) Role of hepatic resection in surgery for bilateral intrahepatic stones. Br J Surg 84:1229-1232
14. Chen DW, Poon RTP, Liu CL et al (2004) Immediate and long-term outcomes of hepatectomy for hepatolithiasis. Surgery 135:386-393

Chapter 40

Extracorporeal Shock Wave Treatment of Gallbladder Stones

Luís Carrilho-Ribeiro, Miguel Carneiro de Moura

Introduction

Extracorporeal shock wave lithotripsy (ESWL) is a treatment option for selected patients with gallbladder stone disease. The word 'lithotripsy' stems from the Greek word for stones (*litos*) and the Latin word for crushing (*tritura*). Accordingly, ESWL consists in the generation of special acoustic waves, referred to as shock waves, which can penetrate and pass through body tissues. These waves can be targeted at and focused on the stones. This method was developed in Germany in the 1970s. Its first clinical application, for the treatment of urinary stones, was reported in 1980 [1].

Shock waves are high-pressure waves that follow acoustic laws and are generated when a pressure front moves faster than sound [2], as after an explosion or when an airplane breaks the speed of sound. They differ from sound waves in their higher frequency (in the range of ultrasound) and higher amplitude (high energy) and, mainly, in not presenting the sinusoidal positive and negative deflections of acoustic waves. These waves have a saw-toothed shape, with almost no negative component (Fig. 40.1). They may in fact be considered distorted ultrasound waves.

Not unexpectedly, shock waves exhibit some different properties from ultrasound waves, such as: (1) they are mainly pressure waves, and their power is measured in units denominated as 'bar' or 'pascal' (1 bar=10^5 pascal); (2) they are freely transmitted in aqueous media, such as the human body, with little loss of energy; (3) like light waves, they suffer changes when the characteristics of the conductive media change (acoustic impedance), being partially

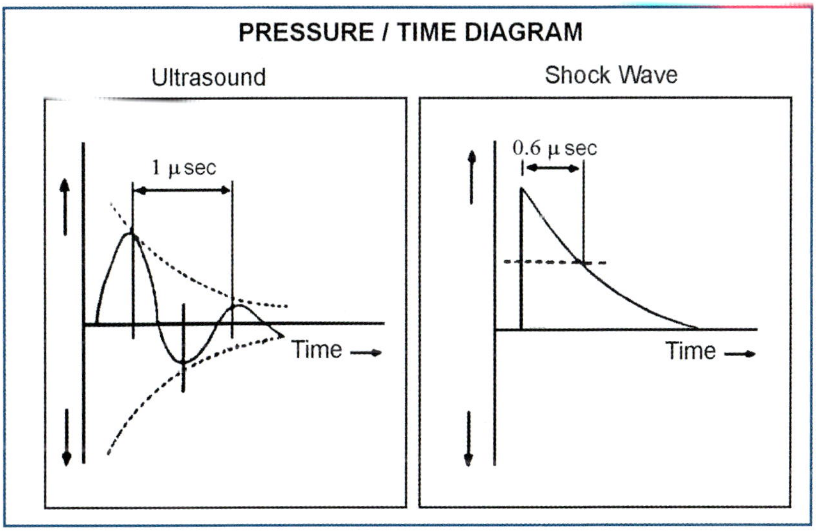

Fig. 40.1 Difference between ultrasound waves and shock waves

reflected or refracted, modifying their original trajectory; and (4) they can be made to converge on a focal space of maximal intensity (denominated F2) by means of reflectors or acoustic lenses.

There are three main types of extracorporeal shock wave generators: electrohydraulic (“spark-gap”), electromagnetic, and piezoelectric types. The main difference in the shock waves generated by these different devices is the size of the focal space, F2, which is much smaller in piezoelectric lithotripters, being measured in millimeters. In the other two types of machines, F2 is a few centimeters wide. There seem to be other slight differences in the characteristics of the shock waves generated by these three different devices [3], but all of them are capable of delivering over 500 bar in F2, and it is accepted that a pressure over 200 bar is necessary for fragmenting urinary stones [4] and pressure of over 300 bar for biliary stones [5]. Both the power and the frequency of the shock wave generation can be adjusted on the command console of the lithotripters.

Procedure

Patients are usually positioned lying prone with the abdomen over the shock wave generator. In this position the gallbladder is closer to the anterior abdominal wall, without intestinal gas interposition. This is the case with the Dornier MPL-9000, a machine with an electrohydraulic generator, which has been used throughout in our unit (Fig. 40.2).

In the machines that are equipped with an ‘overhead generator’ treatment is performed with the patient lying supine or, preferably, in left lateral decubitus, because this usually immobilizes the stones in the gallbladder fundus [6].

The positioning of the gallstones in the F2 focal space is sonographically oriented, usually by an inline transducer mounted inside the generator, coaxially oriented, so as to guarantee maximal precision.

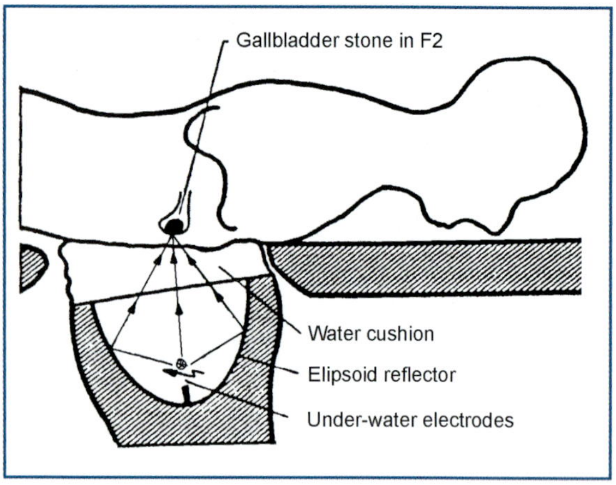

Fig. 40.2 Positioning of a gallbladder stone patient in the Dornier MPL 9000 lithotripter

The stretcher is mobilized by remote control until the stones are correctly positioned in the F2 focus, and as shock wave administration begins the effects are monitored sonographically in real time. It is usually necessary to start with high-energy shock waves to fragment large stones [7], and since those generated by electrohydraulic machines frequently cause pain, the treatments are frequently done under i.v. analgesia. Piezoelectric machines usually do not cause pain and do not therefore necessitate analgesia, but a larger number of shock waves per session and larger number of sessions are needed to achieve the same results [2]. Electromagnetic devices are associated with an intermediate need for analgesia [8].

Clinical Use

There is a double rationale for fragmenting gallbladder stones: (1) to facilitate the expulsion of the residual debris to the duodenum; and (2) to increase the surface-to-volume ratio of the stone burden so as to enhance the effect of oral dissolution with bile acids [9]. Usually, ursodeoxycholic acid (UDCA) is used, alone or, less commonly, with chenodeoxycholic acid (CDCA).

The first objective is hampered by an anatomical barrier, the cystic channel spiral valves of Heister [10]. Nevertheless, it has been demonstrated that small (2–3 mm) fragments are easily passed without causing biliary pain [11]. The advantage of achieving the second objective is amplified by the fact that stone volume is proportional to the third power of stone diameter and stone surface, only to the second power. Figure 40.3 shows an example of a successful treatment of a gallstone patient in our unit.

Candidate patients for gallbladder stone lithotripsy should be symptomatic (biliary pain) but without past or present complications such as cholecystitis, choledocal stones, or pancreatitis. They must have a functioning gallbladder with a permeable cystic duct. This can be checked by opacification of the organ on oral cholecystography or by measuring gallbladder contraction after a liquid fatty meal. Preferably the stones should be: (1) single and small, more amenable to fine (≤3 mm) fragmentation; and (2) radiolucent (cholesterol rich, no calcifications), so that the post-ESWL fragments respond better to adjuvant oral dissolution with bile acids.

The initial gallbladder ESWL protocols, in the 1980s, consisted in one or two low-energy sessions, which frequently did not achieve fine fragmentation of the stones [12,13]; this meant that its efficacy relied heavily on the effect of adjuvant oral dissolution. Indeed, the use of oral bile acids has proved to be essential in this context [14]. In the early 1990s there was an evolution towards the use of high-energy shock waves [15] and/or more repeat ESWL sessions [16], leading to better results in the quality of stone fragmentation and subsequent faster dissolution and clearance of the gallbladder debris.

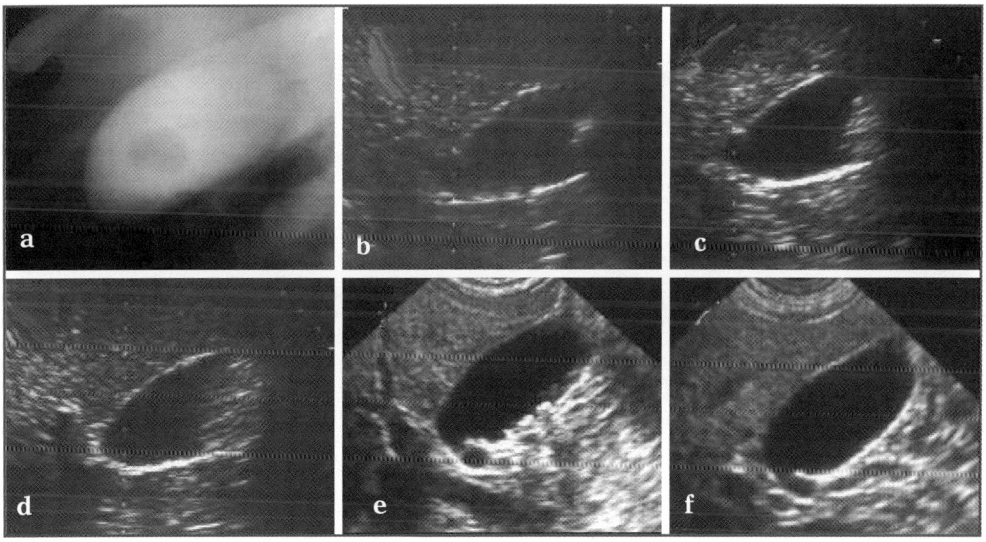

Fig. 40.3 Successful treatment with ESWL plus oral dissolution: 52-year-old male patient with a single 18-mm radiolucent gallbladder stone. **a** Oral cholecystography prior to ESWL. **b** Sonographic image in the initial stage of the ESWL session; some "clouds of dust" can be seen at the surface of the stone. **c** In the middle of the session there is clear fragmentation but the fragments are still coarse. **d** At the end of the session (40 min) fragmentation is finer and more homogeneous. **e** On the sonographic control after 6 weeks there still are some small (≤4 mm) fragments in the gallbladder. **f** On the next sonography, 4 months after ESWL, the gallbladder is completely free of stones and sludge

Later, some groups proposed the so-called pulverization strategy [17–19]. This consisted in greater numbers of ESWL sessions with a larger total number of shock waves until ultrafine fragments that were not measurable by sonography, or biliary sludge, resulted. This modality relies mainly on expulsion of the debris through the cystic duct, the effect of oral dissolution being less important [19, 20]. The new strategy achieved stone-free status of the gallbladder in a shorter period of time, and it was even claimed that good results could be obtained with multiple and calcified stones [18]. However, a Munich-led multicenter study published in 1997 did not confirm this assertion about multiple stones [20]. The following year saw publication of another German study, which also did not confirm this claim for calcified stones [21].

Therefore, the pulverization strategy leads to better and faster results, but does not solve the problem of the lower efficacy of ESWL in the case of multiple and/or calcified stones. The need for adjuvant oral bile acid therapy in this context is still an open question owing to the small number of patients and short follow-up in the two randomized trials that have addressed this issue [19, 20], and it is unlikely that larger studies will be available in the near future, in these times of widespread availability of laparoscopic cholecystectomy.

Efficacy

A single radiolucent stone up to 2 cm in diameter is the ideal candidate for ESWL, irrespective of the type of protocol adopted. Table 40.1 shows the results obtained in some of the series reported on by different groups: stone-free status was obtained in 68–84% of the patients after 12 months of adjuvant oral dissolution [15, 16, 19, 20, 22–24].

Larger stones, multiple stones, and stones with slight calcifications are associated with worse ESWL results. In the case of single radiolucent stones between 2 and 3 cm in diameter stone-free status was achieved in 13–50% of patients after 12 months of oral dissolution (Table 40.2) [15, 16, 19, 20, 22–24]. With this type of stone, the benefit of adjuvant bile acids seems to be greatest when pulverization protocols are used [19, 20].

Table 40.1 Results of gallbladder ESWL in patients with single radiolucent stones up to 2 cm in diameter (*M*, months)

Authors [ref.]	Year	No. of patients	Sessions Mean (range)	Percentage stone free after 6 M	12 M	18 M
Sackmann et al. [15]	1991	316	1.1 (1–2)	55%	71%	78%
Pelletier et al. [22]	1991	147	1.6 (1–5)	46%	69%	–
McSherry et al. [23]	1991	175	1.9 (1–3)	47%	68%	–
Elewaut et al. [16]	1993	169	2.5 (1–5)	61%	84%	91%
Tsuchiya et al. [19]	1995	49	4.2 (1–19)	63%	–	–
		44[a]		66%	–	–
Sauter et al. [20]	1997	34	4.3 (1–6)	76%	–	–
		27[a]		63%	–	–
Carrilho-Ribeiro et al. [24]	1998	138	2.6 (1–6)	49%	71%	80%

[a]Without adjuvant oral dissolution

Table 40.2 Results of gallbladder ESWL in patients with single radiolucent stones 2–3 cm in diameter (*M*, months)

Authors [ref.]	Year	No. of patients	Sessions Mean (range)	Percentage stone free after 6 M	12 M	18 M
Sackmann et al. [15]	1991	257	1.2 (1–2)	38%	50%	61%
Pelletier et al. [22]	1991	50	1.6 (1–5)	10%	25%	–
McSherry et al. [23]	1991	60	1.9 (1–3)	13%	13%	–
Elewaut et al. [16]	1993	56	3.4 (1–5)	41%	50%	–
Tsuchiya et al. [19]	1995	16	4.2 (1–19)	56%	–	–
		14[a]		29%	–	–
Sauter et al. [20]	1997	12	4.3 (1–6)	58%	–	–
		8[a]		12%	–	–
Carrilho-Ribeiro et al. [24]	1998	43	2.6 (1–6)	23%	38%	57%

[a]Without adjuvant oral dissolution

Patients with multiple stones, usually two or three, seem to need longer dissolution times after ESWL (Table 40.3) [15, 16, 19, 20, 22–24]. The three studies with longer follow-up showed that 51–68% patients had achieved stone-free status after 18 months.

Stones with slight calcification, usually defined as less than 3 mm thick, whether rim-like or in the core, take even longer to clear from the gallbladder, probably because they are less responsive to oral dissolution and passage of the insoluble debris through the cystic duct can be a lengthy process. Our experience has shown that it takes 24 months to achieve stone-free status in 51% of patients (Table 40.4) [15, 16, 24].

Sonography and oral cholecystography used to be the mainstay for selection of patients for ESWL. It might still be possible to improve results further by selecting

Table 40.3 Results of gallbladder ESWL in patients with multiple (usually two or three) radiolucent stones (*M*, months)

Authors [ref.]	Year	No. of patients	Sessions Mean (range)	Percentage stone free after 6 M	12 M	18 M
Sackmann et al. [15]	1991	138	1.4 (1–2)	12%	27%	51%
Pelletier et al. [22]	1991	163	1.6 (1–5)	17%	37%	–
McSherry et al. [23]	1991	115	1.9 (1–3)	31%	43%	–
Elewaut et al. [16]	1993	360	3.4 (1–5)	31%	57%	68%
Tsuchiya et al. [19]	1995	11	4.2 (1–19)	36%	–	–
		9[a]		22%	–	–
Sauter et al. [20]	1997	31	4.3 (1–6)	30%	–	–
		41[a]		30%	–	–
Carrilho-Ribeiro et al. [24]	1998	60	2.6 (1–6)	9%	40%	52%

[a]Without adjuvant oral dissolution

Table 40.4 Results of gallbladder ESWL plus oral dissolution in patients with single or multiple slightly calcified stones (*M*, months)

Authors [ref.]	Year	No. of patients	Sessions Mean (range)	Percentage stone free after 12 M	18 M	24 M
Sackmann et al. [25]	1992	86	1.5 (1–2)	36%	55%	–
Elewaut et al. [16]	1993	360	3.6 (1–5)	43%	–	–
Carrilho-Ribeiro et al. [24]	1998	60	2.6 (1–6)	21%	32%	51%

patients whose stones show low attenuation on computed tomography [26] or particular sonographic patterns [27] or in whom good gallbladder emptying is observed [28]. These possibilities have never been fully tested because of the general availability of laparoscopic cholecystectomy.

Complications

Gallbladder ESWL is a safe treatment: in all published results, involving thousands of patients, no deaths related to the procedure have been reported.

The most important complication is acute biliary pancreatitis, which is due to the migration of stone fragments in the first few weeks after the treatment and is reported to occur in 2–4% of patients [15, 29]. Nevertheless, most cases are mild, with fast recovery. In our experience, half of such patients eventually achieve a stone-free gallbladder by continuing treatment with UDCA [24].

Transient cholestasis occurs in about 1% of the patients and seldom needs endoscopic retrograde cholangiopancreatography and sphincterotomy [15]. Acute cholecystitis is a complication only in about 1% of patients [16], and is an indication for cholecystectomy.

Biliary pain is reported by about one third of patients [15, 16] while they are still harboring gallbladder stone fragments. These episodes are usually mild to moderate and can be managed with analgesic drugs, which are prescribed on an as-needed basis for the ambulatory setting.

About 4% of patients report transient hematuria a few hours after gallbladder ESWL when electrohydraulic devices are used. This is due to the effect of shock waves on the right kidney and seldom (1%) occurs with piezoelectric machines [30], whose F2 focal space is smaller.

Stone Recurrence

The risk of stone recurrence is common to all treatments that do not include removal of the gallbladder. Therefore, patients who achieve a stone-free gallbladder with medical treatments are usually enrolled in surveillance protocols and undergo gallbladder sonography once a year to detect any stone recurrence.

In the case of oral dissolution, long-term follow-up studies have shown recurrence rates of around 40% at 5 years, the recurrence curves flattening thereafter to reach 50–60% at 6–8 years, with little or no further increase up to 11–12 years of follow-up [31, 32]

Two large and long-term (more than 10 years) follow-up studies after ESWL [33, 34] have shown similar recurrence rates to those observed after oral dissolution. These studies, however, did not confirm that there was a plateau in the recurrence curves after 6–8 years. Instead, the cumulative recurrence rates continued to rise, albeit less steeply, meaning that new recurrences are only less likely after that time. The Janssen et al. study [33] followed up 120 stone-free patients and showed 30%, 40% and 60% risks of recurrence at 3, 5, and 10 years, respectively. Our own study [34] followed up 192 stone-free patients and showed 27%, 41% and 54% risks of recurrence after the same time intervals (Fig. 40.4).

When patients are followed up in this way, most gallstone recurrences are diagnosed before biliary pain is reported and most patients are good candidates for repeat nonsurgical therapy, harboring few and/or small stones [34]. In our experience most patients opt for repeat UDCA, with or without ESWL, depending on the size of the recurrent stone(s). After 1 year, 70% are again stone free. Unfortunately, the patients so treated show significantly higher rates of second and third recurrences after stopping UDCA [35]. Therefore, until measures are available to prevent gallstone recurrence, repeating nonsurgical treatments should not be encouraged.

In fact, no effective and acceptable strategy for preventing recurrence is available. Low-dose Aspirin fails to prevent it [36].

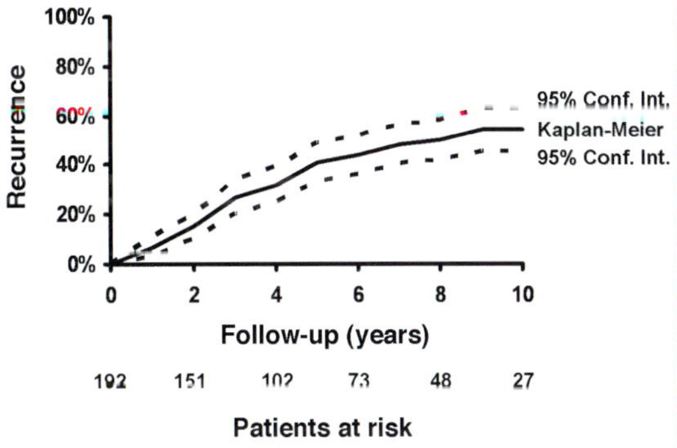

Fig. 40.4 Recurrence rates of our own prospective study [34] on recurrence after successful ESWL. Patients were followed up with yearly sonography without UDCA or any other prophylactic treatment. Recurrence rates were 41% and 54% at 5 and 10 years, respectively

With repeated courses of UDCA, about 80% of patients may remain gallstone free for 4–5 years after complete stone dissolution [37]. However, the prospect of life-long medication with bile acids does not seem appropriate for the great majority of patients.

Conclusion

In the laparoscopic era, cholecystectomy has widley been confirmed as the treatment of choice for gallbladder stones, however ESWL could be an effective treatment for some carefully selected patients. It is safe and noninvasive, and it does not require hospital admission. As a gallbladder-conserving treatment, it preserves the biliary anatomy and physiology and may thus be associated with less dyspepsia than cholecystectomy. In fact, a matched-pairs comparison study performed in our unit suggests that patients who had undergone cholecystectomy reported more frequent dyspeptic symptoms than post-ESWL stone-free patients [38].

Nevertheless, the long-term risk of stone recurrence seems unacceptably high. Until we learn to prevent their recurrence, nonsurgical treatments of gallbladder stones should be offered only in special cases, such as when patients refuse or are unfit to undergo laparoscopic cholecystectomy.

References

1. Chaussy C, Brendel W, Schmiedt E (1980) Extracorporeally induced destruction of kidney stones by shock waves. Lancet 12:1265-1268
2. Ferruci JT(1989) Biliary lithotripsy. AJR Am J Roentgenol 153:15-22
3. Sauerbruch T, Holl J, Sackmann M, Paumgartner G (1988) The role of extracorporeal lithotripsy (ESWL) in the treatment of gallstones. Endoscopy 20:305-308
4. Sass W, Steffen K, Matura E et al (1992) Experiences with lithotripters: measurements of standardized fragmentation. J Stone Dis 4:129-140

5. Esquivel MU, Sánchez JM, Méndez-Sánchez N, Villota SM (1996) Litotripsia biliar con ondas de choque extracorpóreas. Fundamentos físicos y aplicación clínica. In: Uribe M, Méndez N, Morán S (eds) Litiasis biliar: actualización para el estudio y tratamiento. Editorial Medica Panamericana, Mexico
6. Classen M, Cremer M, Faustini S et al (1990) Electromagnetic shock-wave lithotripsy of gallbladder calculi. Multicentered preliminary report on experience with 276 patients. Hepatogastroenterology 37:425-427
7. Paumgartner G (1998) Nonsurgical management of gallstone disease. In: Feldman M, Scharschmidt BF, Sleisenger MH (eds) Sleisenger & Fordtran's Gastrointestinal and liver disease, 6th edn. WB Saunders, Philadelphia
8. Staritz M (1989) Is extracorporeal biliary lithotripsy painless? My experience with three shockwave sources (letter to the editor). N Engl J Med 320:811
9. Senior JR, Johnson MF, DeTurck DM et al (1990) In vivo kinetics of radiolucent gallstone dissolution by oral dihydroxy bile acids. Gastroenterology 99:243-251
10. Ferrucci JT (1989) Biliary lithotripsy—a preview. J Lithotr Stone Dis 1:3-15
11. Greiner L, Munks C, Heil W, Jakobeit C (1990) Gallbladder stone fragments in feces after biliary extracorporeal shock-wave lithotripsy. Gastroenterology 98:1620-1624
12. Sauerbruch T, Delius M, Paumgartner G et al (1986) Fragmentation of gallstones by extracorporeal shock waves. N Engl J Med 314:818-822
13. Sackmann M, Delius M, Sauerbruch T et al (1988) Shock-wave lithotripsy of gallbladder stones: the first 175 patients. N Engl J Med 318:393-397
14. Schoenfield LJ, Berci G, Carnovale RL et al (1990) The effect of ursodiol on the efficacy and safety of extra-corporeal shock wave lithotripsy of gallbladder stones: The Dornier National Biliary Lithotripsy Study. N Engl J Med 323: 1239-1245
15. Sackmann M, Pauletzki J, Sauerbruch T et al (1991) The Munich gallbladder lithotripsy study: results of the first 5 years with 711 patients. Ann Intern Med 114:290-296
16. Elewaut A, Crape A, Afschrift M et al (1993) Results of extracorporeal shock wave lithotripsy of gallbladder stones in 693 patients: a plea for restriction to solitary radiolucent stones. Gut 34:274-278
17. Boscaini M, Piccinni-Leopardi M, Andreotti F, Montori A (1994) Gallstone pulverization strategy in patients treated with extracorporeal lithotripsy and follow-up results of maintenance therapy with ursodeoxycholic acid. Gut 35:117-121
18. Sohendra N, Nam VC, Binmoeller KF et al (1994) Pulverization of calcified and non-calcified gallbladder stones: extracorporeal shock wave lithotripsy used alone. Gut 35:417-422
19. Tsuchiya Y, Ishihara F, Kajiyama G et al (1995) Repeated piezoelectric lithotripsy for gallstones with and without ursodeoxycholic acid dissolution: a multicenter trial. J Gastroenterol 30:768-774
20. Sauter G, Kullak-Ublick GA, Schumacher R et al (1997) Safety and efficacy of repeated shockwave lithotripsy of gallstones with and without adjuvant bile acid therapy. Gastroenterology 112:1603-1609
21. Brand B, Groth J, Lerche L, Stange EF (1998) Intensified ESWL of gallstones: dissociation of pulverization, pain relief and stone-clearance. Hepatogastroenterology 45:70-76
22. Pelletier G, Delmont J, Capdeville R et al (1991) Treatment of gallstones with piezoelectric lithotripsy and oral bile acids: a multicenter study. J Hepatol 12:327-331
23. McSherry CK, the EDAP Investigators Group (1991) The results of the EDAP multicenter trial of biliary lithotripsy in the United States. Surgery 173:461-464
24. Carrilho-Ribeiro L (1998) A litotrícia extra-corporal da litíase vesicular: influência na história natural. PhD thesis, Lisbon
25. Sackmann M, Pauletzki J, Delius M et al (1992) Noninvasive therapy of gallbladder calculi with a radiopaque rim. Gastroenterology 102:988-993
26. Ell C, Schneider HT, Benninger J et al (1991) Significance of computed tomography for shockwave therapy of radiolucent gallbladder stones. Gastroenterology 101:1409-1416
27. Tsuchiya Y, Saito H, Saito N et al (1995) Sonographic patterns of radiolucent gallbladder stones for predicting successful shock-wave lithotripsy. J Gastroenterol Hepatol 10:426-431
28. Pauletzki J, Sailer C, Klüppelberg U et al (1994) Gallbladder emptying determines early gallstone clearance after shock-wave lithotripsy. Gastroenterology 107:1496-1502
29. Carrilho-Ribeiro L, Pinto Correia A, Contente LF, Carneiro de Moura M (1995) An aggressive protocol of ESWL and dissolution therapy of gallbladder stones. Hepatogastroenterology 42:259-264
30. Han JK, Choi BI, Yoon YB et al (1993) Piezoelectric lithotripsy of radiopaque gallstones. Results and six-month follow-up. J Stone Dis 5:89-95
31. O'Donnell LDJ, Heaton KW (1988) Recurrence and re-recurrence of gallstones after medical dissolution: a long-term follow-up. Gut 29:655-658
32. Villanova N, Bazzoli F, Taroni F et al (1989) Gallstone recurrence after successful oral bile acid treatment. Gastroenterology 97:726-731
33. Janssen J, Johanns W, Weickert U, Rahmatian M,

Greiner L (2001) Long-term results after successful extracorporeal gallstone lithotripsy: outcome of the first 120 patients. Scand J Gastroenterol 36:314-317
34. Carrilho-Ribeiro L, Pinto-Correia A, Velosa J, Carneiro de Moura M (2006) A ten-year prospective study on gallbladder stone recurrence after successful shock-wave lithotripsy. Scand J Gastroenterol 41:338-342
35. Carrilho-Ribeiro L, Pinto-Correia A, Velosa J, Carneiro de Moura M (2006) Recurrence, retreatment and subsequent recurrences after initially successful gallbladder stone extra-corporeal shock-wave lithotripsy (ESWL) (abstract). J Hepatol 44 (Suppl 2):S119
36. Adamek HE, Buttmann A, Weber J, Riemann JF (1994) Can Aspirin prevent gallstone recurrence after successful extracorporeal shockwave lithotripsy? Scand J Gastroenterol 29:355-359
37. Petroni ML, Jazrawi RP, Lanzini A et al (1996) Repeated bile acid therapy for the long-term management of cholesterol gallstones. J Hepatol 25:719-724
38. Carrilho-Ribeiro L, Serra D, Pinto-Correia A et al (2002) Quality of life after cholecystectomy and after successful lithotripsy: a matched-pairs comparison. Eur J Gastroenterol Hepatol 14:741-744

Chapter 41

Shock Wave for Main Bile Duct Stones

Stefano Amplatz, Fausto Chilovi

Introduction

The introduction of endoscopic sphincterotomy by Demling and Kawai in 1974 [1, 2] with or without mechanical lithotripsy followed by stone extraction with a Dormia basket or with a Fogarty-type balloon has gained wide acceptance as a standard nonoperative modality for the removal of common bile duct (CBD) stones [3-5]. The rate of successful stone removal has been reported to be more than 92% [5-9]. The most frequent causes that can hinder the endoscopic extraction of bile duct stones are the presence of impacted or large stones, bile duct strictures, unusual anatomy, or the presence of intrahepatic stones.

The relatively high morbidity of bile duct surgery [10] has driven the search for less invasive techniques to remove these refractory stones; besides extracorporeal shock wave lithotripsy (ESWL), these have included percutaneous transhepatic removal, chemical dissolution, laser lithotripsy and electrohydraulic lithotripsy.

Chemical dissolution does not play a significant role in the management of CBD stones because of the associated side effects, and the success rates are often reported at less than 50% [11-13]. The use of methyl tert-butyl ether, especially when combined with mechanical lithotripsy, may be more promising [14].

Electrohydraulic lithotripsy requires continuous visual control of the fragmentation procedure under duodenoscopic and choledochoscopic control to avoid potential bile duct injuries caused by high-pulse energies [15-17]. Electrohydraulic lithotripsy is seldom used, mainly because of the high potential for tissue damage.

Laser lithotripsy with pulsed dye laser (crushing effect) can be performed under choledochoscopic control in CDB stones.

The effect of laser stone fragmentation is similar to that of electrohydraulic lithotripsy and has demonstrated some advantages when compared to ESWL [18-20], but the high cost of the apparatus continues to be a major drawback of laser lithotripsy.

There are some CBD stones that are difficult to remove even by any of the abovementioned endoscopic methods and also by ESWL. In this case, to prevent acute cholangitis, immediate endoscopic drainage can also be achieved by the insertion of an endoprosthesis, which, in older patients, can be considered definitive treatment [21, 22].

ESWL

Extracorporeal shock-wave lithotripsy is a treatment option for patients with "refractory" bile duct stones. Since the first successful shock wave treatments of patients with biliary calculi by Sauerbruch et al. [23] in 1985 with a modified kidney electrohydraulic waterbath generator (Dornier HM3, Germany), a great number of different lithotripter devices have come into clinical use throughout the world.

Improved second-generation electrohydraulic lithotripters available today are complemented by piezoelectric and electromagnetic systems.

The first generation of lithotripters required the patient's immersion in water, and the treatment was done under general or epidural anesthesia. With second and third generation machines, the treatment is carried out without immersion and only under sedation and analgesia.

Principles of ESWL

Lithotripters are composed of four essential parts, which differ significantly among the devices: a shock wave generator, a localization system, and shock wave coupling and auxiliary equipment. The shock wave generator is based on electrohydraulic, electromagnetic or piezoelectric sources.

In the electrohydraulic generator, an underwater electrode is discharged, resulting in evaporation of water with a high-pressure wave. This is focused by an ellipsoid to generate a shock wave within the focal point. The disintegrative capacity of this system is high but causes pain, and deep analgesia or anesthesia is necessary for highly effective stone disintegration.

In electromagnetic generators, high-energy acoustic waves are focused using an acoustic lens or a paraboloid reflector. The shock wave is constant, and the energy is focused to a smaller focal point with higher peak energy.

Piezoelectric generators consist of multiple spherically-aligned piezo-elements inducing a very high peak pressure within a very small focal point. This induces less pain and can be used without analgosedation. The disadvantages are the large diameter of the source and the limited total energy in the focus.

A localization system identifies the stones and guides the positioning of the stone within the focal point: fluoroscopy or ultrasonography can be used for this.

When the shock wave reaches the stone, energy is liberated leading to a change in acoustic impedance and to cavitation phenomena on the surface of the stone causing stone destruction [24].

Shock Wave Therapy

The evaluation is based on published studies with more than 50 patients and our own experience with 376 patients published in 2006 (Table 41.1) [25].

Selection of Patients and Entry Criteria

Patients selected for treatment were those in whom bile duct stones could not be removed by the usual endoscopic manipulation.

Most centers observe the following selection criteria: 1) endoscopic papillotomy already performed; 2) successful positioning of the calculi into the focal area of the lithotriptor (with radiological or sonographical targeting; 3) no severe coagulative disorders, and 4) focal axis of the shock waves avoiding lung, aneurysm, calcified vessel and bone tissue.

The mean age of patients with stones in the biliary tree is in the range of 70 to 80 years with a high percentage of comorbidity factors and a relatively high risk for surgery.

Technique

Most patients have been treated by electrohydraulic or electromagnetic lithotripter machines with X-ray capability. Radiological monitoring and positioning of stones seems to be considerably more reliable than ultrasound. The targeting is done under biplanar fluoroscopy control after

Table 41.1 Studies of extracorporeal shock wave lithotripsy of bile duct stones (> 50 patients)

Author	Year	No. of patients	Device	Pain relief	Mean Ø of largest stone (range)	Method of targeting	Fragmentation rate	Clearance rate
Amplatz et al. [25]	2006	376	EM Lithostar	A, S	21 mm (7-80)	X-ray	97%	90%
Sackmann et al. [26]	2001	313	EH Dornier HM3 EH Dornier HM4 EM Dornier	GA PA A, S	20 mm (8-60)	X-ray	-	90%
Sauerbruch et al. (multicenter) [23]	1989	113	EH Dornier HM3	GA, PA	24 mm (7-70)	X-ray	91%	86%
van der Hul et al. [32]	1994	90	EM Lithostar EH Dornier HM3	A, S GA	25mm (10-50)	X-ray	85%	69%
Ellis et al. [27]	2000	83	EM Storz Modulith	A, S	15 mm	X-ray	-	83%
Conigliaro et al. [28]	2006	82	EM Storz Modulith	A, S	20 mm (7-45)	X-ray	-	85%
Hinz et al. [33]	1990	80	EM Lithostar	A, S	-	X-ray	-	72%
Lee et al. [34]	1990	70	EM Lithostar EH Dornier HM3	A, S GA	20 mm	X-ray	-	61%
Adamek et al. [35]	1993	64	Piezolith 2300	A, S	25 mm (10-50)	Sonography	86%	77%
Moody et al. (multicenter) [30]	1989	56	EH Dornier HM3	A, S	20 mm (10-50)	X-ray	91%	79%
Wenzel et al. [29]	1989	55	EH Dornier HM3 EM MPL 9000	GA A, S	23 mm (9-35)	X-ray Sonography	- -	92%
Nicholson et al. [31]	1992	54	EM Lithostar	A, S	16mm (8-36)	X-ray	81%	70

EH, electrohydraulic; *EM*, electromagnetic; *GA*, general anaesthesia; *A, S*, intravenous analgesia/sedation; *PA*, peridural anaesthesia

the injection of contrast. This is achieved by nasobiliary tubes, or following surgical placement of T-tubes, or transhepatically placed catheters.

During treatment the following parameters must be monitored: 1) pulse oximetry; 2) arterial pressure; and 3) continuous electrocardiography.

Endoscopic retrograde cholangiography is usually performed after ESWL to extract the residual fragments. In rare cases there is a spontaneous passage through the papilla.

Efficacy

Studies have reported success in treating retained bile duct stones with ESWL. Complete stone clearance is achieved in 70-90% of the patients treated (Table 41.2).

First generation electrohydraulic lithotripters (Dornier HM3) delivered higher shock wave energy and achieved higher clearance rates than second and third electromagnetic machines but required the patient to be

Table 41.2 Clearance rate of main bile duct after ESWL: comparison between the different devices

Lithotripter	No. patients treated	No. studies	Clearance rate (range)
Electrohydraulic (Dornier HM3, HM4)	552	5	83% (69-92%)
Electromagnetic (Lithostar Siemens, Storz, Dornier)	820	7	78% (61-90%)
Piezoelectric (Piezolith)	64	1	77%

Table 41.3 Distribution of number of sessions and shocks per session reported in various studies

Author	No. of patients	Device	Mean no. of sessions (range)	Shocks per session (range)
Amplatz et al. [25]	376	EM Lithostar	3.7 (1-12)	3470 (1500-5400)
Sackmann et al. [26]	313	EH Dornier HM3 EH Dornier HM4 EM Dornier	1 (62%) 2 (29%)	1960 (333-3000)
Sauerbruch et al. (multicenter) [23]	113	EH Dornier HM3	1 (84%) 2 (14%)	1502 (350-2400)
van der Hul et al. [32]	90	EM Lithostar EH Dornier HM3	1.8	4360
Ellis et al. [27]	83	EM Storz Modulith	1.3	3913
Conigliaro et al. [28]	82	EM Storz Modulith	1	3550 (800-7100)
Hinz et al. [33]	80	EM Lithostar	1.4	- (1000-5000)
Lee et al. [34]	70	EM Lithostar EH Dornier HM3	2.26 (1-7)	7254
Adamek et al. [35]	64	Piezolith 2300	2.3 (1-8)	7595 (1000-30800)
Moody et al. (multicenter) [30]	56	EH Dornier HM	2	1914 (600-2400)
Wenzel et al. [29]	55	EH Dornier HM3 EM MPL 9000	1-4	1793 (430-3000) 684 (420-2000)
Nicholson et al. [31]	54	EM Lithostar	1-2	5270 (4000-6000)

immersed in a waterbath, and also required either general or spinal anesthesia.

In our study - one of the largest case studies published to the present - using the electromagnetic lithotripter Lithostar Plus (Siemens, Erlangen, Germany) the fragmentation was obtained in 97% of the patients treated and stone clearance was achieved in 90.2% of patients with retained bile duct stones. These results are comparable to those obtained in previous studies [23, 26-29].

There are certainly differences in clearance rate between the various lithotripters: these need to be considered when interpreting the results. In our study, the high fragmentation and clearance rate, similar to that obtained with the more powerful electrohydraulic devices, was achieved after a mean of 3.7 ESWL sessions, higher than other published studies, with a mean number of discharges of 3470 per session (Table 41.3).

The application of high discharge energy and the repetition of ESWL sessions until stone fragmentation is sufficient (Figs. 41.1, 41.2) may contribute to the high percentage of bile duct clearance obtained in our study.

Described factors limiting the successful treatment with ESWL can be the presence of bile duct stenosis [25] and the size of the stone [28, 30, 31]. Reported neural network analysis indicates a better stone clearance rate in younger patients [27]. In other studies there were no significant differences between patients in whom ESWL was successful versus those in whom it was unsuccessful [23, 26].

No data on the recurrence rate of bile duct stone after ESWL are available today.

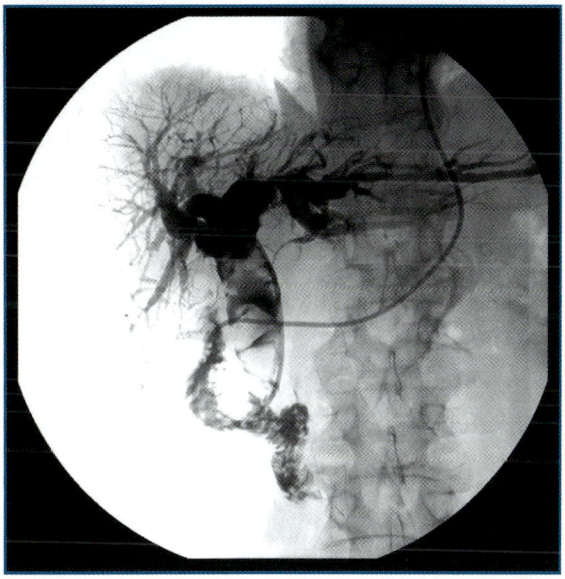

Fig. 41.1 Digital fluoroscopic image of bile duct stones before ESWL treatment

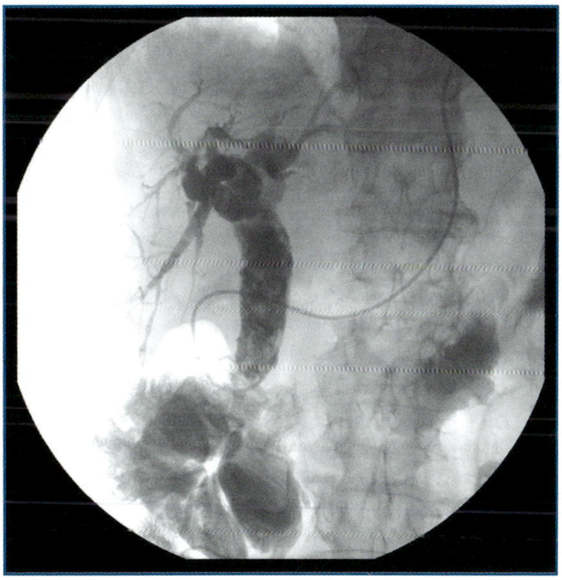

Fig. 41.2 After three ESWL treatments the nasobiliary cholangiogram reveals multiple stone fragments

Adverse Effects

Serious adverse effects are rare, considering the age and the associated comorbidity factors in such patients. The most important complication during or after ESWL is cholangitis. This complication occurred in 0.5-7% of the patients in larger series. Hemobilia and macrohematuria, while being directly attributable to shock wave-induced damage, are of no clinical relevance in most patients.

Ventricular premature complexes are often observed predominantly in elderly patients during ESWL treatment but they rarely result in the termination of the lithotripsy session.

Conclusion

Different studies have shown the efficacy of ESWL for the treatment of large or impacted biliary calculi "refractory" to endoscopic extraction. In this chapter, we reviewed twelve studies including more than 50 patients, published since 1989.

After the failure of conventional endoscopic procedures, 1436 patients were treated for bile duct stones. Most of the patients who presented with multiple bile duct stones were elderly patients at increased operative risk.

Stone clearance rate was about 80 to 90% in series of up to 376 patients, achieved with a mean of 1-3 sessions per patient. The main complication observed was cholangitis. However, we believe this complication can partly be avoided by prophylactic application of antibiotics.

We conclude that ESWL of stones in the common bile duct is a noninvasive and effective treatment with minimal discomfort to the patient. If endoscopic removal of the stone proves impossible, ESWL should be tried before an operation is undertaken, particularly in elderly or high-risk patients.

References

1. Demling L, Koch H, Classen M et al (1974) Endoscopic papillotomy and removal of gallstones: animal experiments and first clinical result. Dtsch Med Wochenschr 99:2255-2257
2. Kawai K, Akasaka Y, Murakami K et al (1974) Endoscopic sphincterotomy of the ampulla of Vater. Gastrointest Endosc 20:148-151
3. Cotton PB (1984) Endoscopic management of bile duct stones; (apples and oranges). Gut 25:587-597
4. Ikeda S, Tanaka M, Yoshimoto H, Matsumoto S (1984) Endoscopic sphincterotomy: 9 years experience using a long-tipped sphincterotome. In: Okabe H, Honda T, Oshiba S (eds) Endoscopic surgery. Amsterdam, Elsevier Science, pp 47-55
5. Tanaka M (2000) Problems inherent to balloon dilatation for the treatment of common bile duct stones in comparison with endoscopic sphincterectomy. Dig Endosc 12:112-115
6. Binmoeller KF, Schafer TW (2001) Endoscopic management of bile duct stones. J Clin Gastroenterol 32:106-118
7. NIH state of the science statement on endoscopic retrograde cholangiopancreatography (ERCP) for diagnosis and therapy (2002) NIH Consens State Sci Statements 19(1):1-26
8. Disario JA, Freeman ML, Bjorkman DJ et al (2004) Endoscopic balloon dilatation compared with sphincterotomy for extraction of bile duct stones. Gastroenterology 127 (5):1291-129
9. Baron TH, Harewood GC (2004) Endoscopic balloon dilation of the biliary sphincter compared endoscopic biliary sphincterotomy for removal of common bile duct stones during ERCP: a meta-analysis of randomized, controlled trials. Am J Gastroenterol 99(8):1455-1460
10. Vellacott KD, Powell PH (1979) Exploration of the common bile duct: a comparative study. Br J Surg 66:389-391
11. Neoptolemos JP, Hall C, O'Connor HJ et al (1990) Methyl-tert-butyl-ether for treating bile duct stones. The British experience. Br J Surg 77:32-35
12. Leuschner U, Baumgartel H (1984) Chemical dissolution of common bile duct stones. Prog Clin Biol Res 152:193-225
13. Binmoeller KF, Schafer TW (2001) Endoscopic management of bile duct stones. J Clin Gastroenterol 32:106-18
14. Diaz D (1992) Methyl-tert-butyl-ether in the endoscopic treatment of common bile duct radiolucent stones in elderly patients with nasobiliary tube. Dig Dis Sci 37:97-100
15. Tanaka M, Yoshimoto H, Ikeda S, Itho H (1982) Endoscopic electrohydraulic lithotripsy for choledocholithiasis; dog experiments and preliminary clinical experience. Gastroenterol Endosc 24:1544-1551
16. Binmoeller KF, Bruckner M, Thonke F, Soehendra N (1993) Treatment of difficult bile duct stones using mechanical electrohydraulic and extracorporeal shock wave lithotripsy. Endoscopy 25:201-206
17. Hochberger J, Tex S, Maiss J, Hahn EG (2003) Management of difficult common bile duct stones. Gastrointest Endoscopy Clin N Am 13:623-634
18. Jakobs R, Adamek HE, Maier M et al (1997) Fluoroscopically guided laser lithotripsy versus extracorporeal shock wave lithotripsy for retained bile duct stones: a prospect randomised study. Gut 40:678-682
19. Neuhaus H, Zillinger C, Born P et al (1998) Randomized study of intracorporeal laser lithotripsy versus extracorporeal shock-wave lithotripsy for difficult bile duct stones. Gastrointest Endoscop 47(5):327-334
20. Hochberger J, Bayer J,May A et al (1998) Laser lithotripsy of difficult bile duct stones: results in 60 patients using a rhodamine 6G dye laser with optical stone tissue detection system. Gut 43:823-829
21. De Palma GD, Galloro G, Siciliano S (2002) Endoscopic stenting for treatment of irretrievable common bile duct calculi. A long-term follow-up study of 49 patients. Hepatogastroenterology 48:56-58
22. Jain SK, Stein R, Bhuva M (2000) Pigtail stents: an alternative in the treatment of difficult bile duct stones. Gastrointest Endosc 52:490-449
23. Sauerbruch T, Stern M, and the Study Group for shock-wave lithotripsy of bile duct stones (1989) Fragmentation of bile duct stones by extracorporeal shockwaves: a new approach to biliary calculi after failure of routine endoscopic measures. Gastroenterology 96:146-152

24. Delius M, Miller M, Vogel A, Brendel W (1989) Extracorporeal shock waves: properties and principles of generation. In: Ferrucci T, Delius M, Burhenne HJ (eds) Biliary lithotripsy. Year Book Medical Publisher, Chicago, pp 9-16
25. Amplatz S, Piazzi L, Felder M et al (2006) Extracorporeal shock wave lithotripsy for clearance of refractory bile duct stones. Dig Liver Dis 39:267-272
26. Sackmann M, Holl J, Sauter GH et al (2001) Extracorporeal shock wave lithotripsy for clearance of bile duct stones resistant to endoscopic extraction. Gastrointest Endosc 53:27-32
27. Ellis RD, Jenkins AP, Thompson PH, Ede RJ (2000) Clearance of refractory bile duct stones with extracorporeal shockwave lithotripsy. Gut 47:728-731
28. Conigliaro R, Camellini L, Zuliani CG et al (2006) Clearance of irretrievable bile duct and pancreatic duct stones by extracorporeal shockwave lithotripsy, using a transportable device. J Clin Gastroenterol 40:213-219
29. Wenzel H, Greiner L, Jakobeit C et al (1989) Extrakorporale Stosswellenlithotripsie von Gallengangssteinen. Dtsch Med Wschr 114:738-743
30. Moody FG, Amerson JR, Berci G et al (1989) Lithotripsy for bile duct stones. Am J Surg 158:241-247
31. Nicholson DA, Martin DF, Tweedle DE, Rao PN (1992) Management of common bile duct stones using a second-generation extracorporeal shockwave lithotriptor. Br J Surg 79: 811-814
32. Van der Hul RL, Plaisier PW, Van Blankenstein M et al (1994) Extracorporeal shock wave lithotripsy of common bile duct stones in patients with increased operative risk. Eur J Surg 160:31-35
33. Hinz K, Schulz HJ, Natho W, Brien G (1990) Extracorporeal shockwave lithotripsy (ESWL) a new procedure for treating choledocholithiasis. Gastroenterol J 50:175-178
34. Lee SH, Fache JS, Burhenne HJ (1990) The value of extracorporeal shock-wave lithotripsy in the management of bile duct stones. AJR 155:775-779
35. Adamek HE, Buttmann A, Hartmann CM et al (1993) Extrakorporale piezoelektrische Lithotripsie von intra- und extrahepatische Gallengangssteinen. Dtsch Med Wochenschr 118:1053-1059

Chapter 42

Acute Gallstone Cholangitis: Clinical Pictures, Diagnosis and Treatment

Luigi Roncoroni, Leopoldo Sarli, Gabriele Regina

Introduction

Acute cholangitis is an infectious disease of the biliary tract with a wide spectrum of presentations, ranging in severity from a mild form, characterised mainly by fever and jaundice, to a severe form with septic shock. Reported mortality rates vary from 13 to 88% [1].

Cholangitis occurs in 6–9% of patients admitted with gallstone disease [2]. This type of cholangitis is typically found in Europe and USA and is different from oriental cholangiohepatitis, which is endemic in Eastern Asia.

Only a small number of patients with bile duct stones suffer from acute suppurative cholangitis. There are some factors predisposing patients with bile duct stones to acute cholangitis [3]. Risk factors for acute suppurative cholangitis secondary to gallstone disease are the following [4]: (1) age ≥ 70 years; (2) comorbid medical problems; (3) dysfunction of Oddi's sphincter by peripapillary diverticulum; and (4) decreased gallbladder motility in prolonged bed rest due to neurological disease.

Although bile duct stones are the most frequent cause of acute cholangitis in the Western world, other causes of cholangitis should be kept in mind if stones are absent (Table 42.1).

Experimental and clinical models strongly suggest that cholangitis is produced by biliary stasis in association with biliary infection. In fact, patients with partial bile duct obstruction are at increased risk compared to those with complete obstruction. Cholangitis is generally thought to be the result of ascending infection from the duodenum superimposed on a biliary system obstructed by gallstones. Haematogenous spread through the portal venous system could be another route. The rate of biliary infection correlates with the severity of gallstone disease.

Table 42.1 Causes of acute bacterial cholangitis

Gallstones within the biliary tree, sludge
Benign or malignant biliary strictures
Choledochal cyst, choledochocele, Caroli's disease
Stenosis papilla of Vater
Parasitic infections
Iatrogenic: Post-endoscopic retrograde cholangiopancreatography Postoperative: "sump" syndrome post-choledochoduodenostomy choledochojejunostomy

The term "bactobilia" refers to the presence of bacteria within bile; bactobilia without biliary stasis generally does not result in cholangitis. Acute bacterial cholangitis develops when bacterial infection complicates obstruction within the biliary tract. Conditions predisposing to bactobilia are the increased colonisation of the proximal small intestine by coliforms, and achlorhydria in the elderly. Bactobilia without symptoms in gallstone patients may be more common than previously thought.

The infecting organism is usually a gram-negative bacillus (most commonly coliforms), but *Staphylococcus* and *Streptococcus* are also reported.

In patients with bile duct stones associated cholangitis, there is a significantly higher pressure in the common bile duct [5]. When bile duct pressure (normally 7–14 cmH_2O) exceeds 20 cmH_2O, reflux of bacteria from the obstructed bile duct into the systemic circulation occurs; in severe cholangitis, biliary pressure exceeds 30 cmH_2O.

Clinical Features

Acute gallstone cholangitis may present as anything from a mild, self-limiting, intermittent disease to a fulminant and life-threatening one, depending on the presence of ascending cholangitis, acute suppurative cholangitis, the presence of frank pus within the biliary tree or the formation of multiple intrahepatic abscesses and septicaemia.

Fever, right upper quadrant abdominal pain and jaundice constitute the triad described by Charcot in 1877 that is a generally accepted clinical finding of acute cholangitis.

About 50–70% of patients with acute cholangitis develop all three symptoms; milder disease may not exhibit all three features, and, particularly in the elderly, abdominal pain may be absent; this might lead to misdiagnosis or delayed diagnosis.

In severe disease, which Reynolds and Dargan [6] in 1959 defined as acute obstructive cholangitis, shock and a decreased level of consciousness are also observed in up to 30% of patients. Authors have described this pentad as a well-characterised syndrome indicating the need for urgent decompression of the biliary tree.

Despite these cases, up to 80–90% of cholangitis patients will respond to initial conservative therapy including broad-spectrum antibiotics.

Laboratory Investigation

Laboratory investigation for the diagnosis of acute cholangitis is characterised by:

1. aspecific indicators of infection and flogosis such as leucocytosis, increased C-reactive protein and high erithrocyte sedimentation rates;
2. specific indicators of cholestasis such as increased bilirubin, alkaline phosphatase and gamma glutamyl tranferase (GGT);
3. indicators of hepatocellular disease with a pronounced and disproportionate increase in aspartate aminotransferase (AST) or alanine aminotransferase (ALT) that may cause confusion with viral hepatitis.

Laboratory investigations for the assessment of the illness include platelet count, blood urea nitrogen, creatinine, and prothrombin time (PT).

Positive blood cultures and severe hyperamylasaemia are also helpful parameters for severity assessment and for the identification of complications of choledocholithiasis such as biliary pancreatitis.

Imaging Findings

It is usually impossible to identify evidence of bile infection itself by imaging modalities. The role of diagnostic imaging in acute cholangitis is to determine the presence/absence of biliary obstruction, the level of the obstruction, and the cause of the obstruction, such as gallstones and/or biliary strictures.

Ultrasound Scanning

Transabdominal ultrasound is the first step in detecting bile duct (as well as associated gallbladder) stones. Ultrasound examination has satisfactory diagnostic capability when performed both by specialists and by emergency physicians. However, the distal bile duct in particular may be difficult to visualise because of air-containing intestinal loops in front of it. Therefore, the sensitivity of ultrasound in detecting bile duct stones is rather low (depending on the experience of investigators and stone size: 27–49%) [7]. In contrast, the specificity of ultrasonographic bile duct stone detection is extremely high (99–100%) [7]. Also, the finding of bile duct dilation during ultrasonographic exam is very valuable, since it indicates the presence of posthepatic biliary obstruction.

Normal bile duct diameter is considered to be less than 7 mm. Nevertheless, the upper limit of normal for bile duct diameter may increase with age (approximately 1 mm for each decade above 50 years of age) and after cholecystectomy. One should also realise that normal-sized bile ducts do not exclude the presence of bile duct stones.

Endoscopic Ultrasonography

With this procedure, ultrasonographic pictures may be obtained with the aid of a small ultrasound transducer at the tip of a side-viewing endoscope. When the endoscope is introduced into the descending duodenum at the level of the papilla, excellent visualisation of the bile duct is possible, including the distal part, which may be too difficult to examine with transabdominal ultrasound. In expert hands, this technique has a high sensitivity for the detection of bile duct stones [8].

Magnetic Resonance Cholangiopancreatography (MRCP)

MRCP has recently been introduced as a one-step noninvasive investigation providing additional important information. MRCP allows the visualisation of bile ducts as well as pancreatic ducts. The advantage of this technique compared to transabdominal ultrasound is its increased sensitivity (overall > 90%) in detecting bile duct stones. Sensitivity may be lower in the case of small stones in strongly dilated bile ducts. MRCP has also proved to be superior to ultrasound and direct cholangiography since it allows to assess both the presence of hepatolithiasis and associated pyogenic abscesses.

Endoscopic Retrograde Cholangiopancreatography (ERCP)

ERCP is commonly considered the gold standard for diagnosing bile duct stones. Although widely regarded as a safe procedure, ERCP carries a small but significant number of serious complications [9]. Recent studies have shown a morbidity of 3% for diagnostic ERCP, particularly post-ERCP pancreatitis, and a mortality of 0.2% [10]. In expert hands, success rates to cannulate the bile ducts are at least 90–95%. A considerable advantage of the procedure is the possibility to proceed to therapeutic ERCP with papillotomy, stone extraction and/or nasobiliary drainage or stenting.

Diagnostic Criteria for Acute Cholangitis

An International Consensus Meeting took place in Tokyo in 2006, to establish practical guidelines for the management of cholangitis. The diagnostic criteria for acute cholangitis adopted by the Tokyo Consensus Meeting are reported in Table 42.2. The basic concepts of the criteria are as follows: (1) Charcot's triad is a definite diagnostic criterion for acute cholangitis; and (2) if a patient does not have all the components of Charcot's

Table 42.2 Diagnostic criteria for acute cholangitis

A. Clinical context and clinical manifestations	1. History of biliary disease 2. Fever and/or chills 3. Jaundice 4. Adominal pain
B. Laboratory data	5. Evidence of inflammatory response (a) 6. Abnormal liver function tests (b)
C. Imaging findings	7. Biliary dilatation, or evidence of an aetiology (stricture, stone, stent, etc.)
Suspected diagnosis	Two or more items in A
Definite diagnosis	(1) Charcot's triad (2+3+4) (2) Two or more items in A + both items in B and item C

(a) Abnormal WBC count, increase of serum CRP level, and other changes indicating inflammation
(b) Increased serum ALP, GGT, AST, and ALT levels
WBC, white blood cells; *CRP*, C-reactive protein; *ALP*, alkaline phosphatase; *GGT*, Gamma Glutamyl Transferase; *AST*, Asparate Aminotransferase; *ALT*, Alanine Aminotransferase

triad, then definite diagnosis can be achieved if both an "inflammatory response" and "biliary obstruction" are demonstrated by the laboratory data and imaging findings.

Differential Diagnosis

Diseases that should be differentiated from acute cholangitis are acute cholecystitis, gastric and duodenal ulcer, acute pancreatitis, acute hepatitis, and septicaemia of other origins.

Severity Assessment

Patients with acute cholangitis may present with anything from a mild, self-limited illness to a severe, potentially life-threatening illness. Table 42.3 summarises the risk factors for poor outcome reported in the literature in patients with acute cholangitis [11].

Severity of acute cholangitis should be divided into three grades: mild (Grade I), moderate (Grade II), and severe (Grade III). To stratify acute cholangitis into the three grades, two different criteria should be utilised.

Organ dysfunction is the most common predictor of a poor outcome. On the other hand, based on the pathophysiology, "severe" acute cholangitis can also be defined as that which accompanies organ dysfunction caused by sepsis. Thus, "the onset of organ dysfunction" is an important factor in the definition of severe (Grade III) acute cholangitis.

The other factor for the severity assessment of acute cholangitis is "response to medical treatment", consisting of general supportive care and antibiotics. Patients with gallstone acute cholangitis that is not complicated by organ dysfunction, who did not respond to medical treatment and who continue to have systemic inflammatory response syndrome and/or sepsis, are classified as having moderate (Grade II) disease. Patients who respond to medical treatment and whose clinical manifestation and laboratory data improve are classified as having mild (Grade I) disease. Criteria for severity assessment of acute cholangitis are reported in Table 42.4.

Table 42.3 Prognostic factors in gallstone acute cholangitis

Prognostic factor	Value
Related to organ dysfunction	
Mental confusion	
Elevated serum creatinine	> 1.5 mg/dl
Elevated BUN	> 20 mg/dl
Prolonged prothrombin time	> 1.5 s
Hyperbilirubinaemia	> 2.2 mg/dl
Reduced platelet count	< 10x10 ^{4}/mm^{3}
Hypoalbuminaemia	< 3.0 mg/dl
Liver abscess	Number and size
Pre-existing cirrhosis	(Child Score)
Unrelated to organ dysfunction	
Advanced age	> 75 years old
Female sex	
Shock	
Hyperpyrexia	> 39°C
Leukocytosis	> 20,000/mm^{3}
Bacteriaemia	
Endotoxaemia	
Medical comorbidity	(ASA status)

BUN, blood urea nitrogen; *ASA*, American Society of Anestesiologists

Table 42.4 Criteria for severity assessment of acute cholangitis

	Severity of acute gallstone cholangitis		
Criterion	Mild (Grade I)	Moderate (Grade II)	Severe (Grade III)
Onset of organ dysfunction	No	No	Yes
Response to medical treatment *	Yes	No	No

* Consisting of general supportive care and antibiotics

Treatment

There are a number of factors to be considered when planning treatment strategies for acute gallstone cholangitis. These include the severity of cholangitis, the presence of concurrent medical illnesses, the underlying cause, and the available treatment options at each institution.

Except for mild (Grade I) disease, patients with cholangitis are best treated in hospitals where a management protocol exists, including resuscitation, antibiotic therapy, and the possibility of performing an effective, also endoscopic, biliary drainage. Identifying high-risk patients (Table 42.3) is also important, because they require urgent admission to an intensive or high-care unit.

Biliary drainage and antibiotics are the two milestones in the treatment of acute cholangitis.

Initial management of all patients with acute cholangitis should include intravenous fluid resuscitation, parenteral vitamin K to counteract any coagulopathy due to hepatic dysfunction, nutritional parenteral support and intravenous antibiotics.

Oxygen, intravenous colloids and inotropic support, together with invasive monitoring in intensive care unit, may be required in severe cases.

Antibiotics

One of the main goals of antibiotics is to control bacteraemia and sepsis.

Septicaemia may occur in up to 50% of patients, and because the underlying microbiology is usually unknown, it is essential to obtain blood samples for cultures before initiating empirical antibiotic therapy. The yield of positive blood cultures is usually 20–30%, but may be higher in elderly patients. In patients with choledocholithiasis, the most frequent organisms are gram-negative (*Escherichia coli*, *Klebsiella*, *Proteus* and *Pseudomonas aeruginosa*), while gram-positive anaerobes and fungi are less common, at least initially.

Theoretically, one should aim to achieve adequate biliary excretion of the antibiotic. In this respect, it is important to remember that in the case of biliary obstruction many antibiotics have little – or no – biliary excretion (e.g., imipenem, gentamycin, ampicillin), whereas quinolones exhibit a high degree of biliary excretion, even in the case of obstruction.

In practice, the primary aim is to reach adequate levels of antibiotic in the blood and in the liver around the biliary tract, rather than in the bile. Given the wide range of possible infecting organisms and the common finding of a mixed infection, a broad-spectrum antibiotic regimen is required.

The choice of antibiotics is also influenced by patient characteristics (e.g., antibiotic hypersensitivity, renal function), and by antibiotic sensitivity patterns in the structure.

Suitable regimens include the combination of an aminoglycoside with amoxycillin-clavulanic acid, benzylpenicillin with aminoglycoside and metronidazole, a second- or third-generation cephalosporin with metronidazole, a synthetic ureidopenicillin such as mezlocillin, or one of the newer generations of antibiotics, such as imipenem or ciprofloxacin.

The choice of the antibiotic and the modalities of its administration will depend on the severity score of the cholangitis and the positivity (or not) of blood cultures; the duration of therapy will be a function of the clinical course and the outcome of the biliary drainage.

Biliary Decompression

Biliary drainage is essential in the treatment of acute cholangitis, and its importance has been recognised for nearly the last 100 years [12]. Urgent biliary decompression is required by 10–20% of patients, based on their clinical condition at presentation. Biliary decompression may be achieved through open surgery, however, it is associated with high levels of morbidity and reported mortality rates up to 40% [13]. In recent years these figures have been improved by the use of less invasive techniques for biliary decompression. Non-operative biliary drainage (endoscopic or transhepatic) has revolutionised the treatment of acute cholangitis and is now preferred to emergency surgical decompression.

Between 80% and 90% of cholangitis patients will respond satisfactorily to initial conservative therapy with broad-spectrum antibiotics. The timing and choice of biliary decompression will depend on the response to antibiotic therapy, the presence of comorbid disease, and, to a certain extent, the underlying cause.

In patients with stones in the common bile duct, it appears wise to perform decompression as early as possible in all cases, even if theoretically almost all these patients could receive elective biliary decompression and stone removal after the resolution of cholangitis. Both morbidity and mortality increase with increasing delay from the onset of cholangitis to the time of biliary drainage; therefore, patients with severe acute cholangitis or those who have shown a poor response to conservative measures require urgent endoscopic biliary decompression [14].

Endoscopic Drainage

ERCP is now considered the treatment of choice in the case of acute gallstone cholangitis. The aim of ERCP with endoscopic sphincterotomy (ES) in patients affected by acute cholangitis due to choledocholithiasis is to quickly decompress the biliary tree to resolve the biliary stasis, which is responsible for sepsis. In 1977, good results were already being obtained in employing endoscopic decompression for the management of acute cholangitis [1]. This choice allows for the extraction of stones via the duodenum or, if this is not possible, for the placement of an internal stent or nasobiliary tube to drain the biliary tree obstructed by stones.

It has been shown that endoscopic drainage effectively relieves the endotoxaemia associated with acute cholangitis [15] and can be performed with a much lower mortality rate and fewer complications than open surgical drainage [16].

An aggressive management with early endoscopic biliary drainage has been shown to be associated with a very low mortality rate [17]. On the other hand, delay in ERCP for patients with severe cholangitis has resulted in increased mortality and morbidity [14]. Even those authors who maintain that surgical treatment of patients with common bile duct stones should be preferred to endoscopic management followed by cholecystectomy agree that urgent endoscopic management of bile duct stones should be preferred in patients with severe cholangitis [18].

An advanced level of endoscopic skill is required to perform therapeutic ERCP. In the hands of an experienced endoscopist, cannulation rates should exceed 90%, as should the rate of successful common bile duct clearance [19, 20].

Cautious sedation is advised during ERCP, especially in septic patients. Injection of contrast medium under pressure should be avoided, as this may lead to cholangio-venous reflux and exacerbation of cholangitis and septicaemia. Therefore, it is wise to aspirate bile after bile duct cannulation and before contrast injection, in order to avoid increased bile duct pressure and bacteraemia. Aspirated bile should be sent for culture. In patients with mild to moderate cholangitis, papillotomy with stone extraction can be performed during the initial procedure. In severe cholangitis, prolonged procedures with excessive manipulation in order to remove large or multiple impacted stones should be avoided, and the definitive treatment should be delayed after the improvement or resolution of cholangitis.

In fact, endoscopic biliary decompression in acute cholangitis can be obtained not only by ES with clearance of bile duct stones, but also by nasobiliary drainage with or without ES [19], or by stent placement [21]. Some authors consider endoscopic nasobiliary drainage or stent placement to be safer than ES in acute cholangitis as an initial step [22], while others believe that elderly patients should undergo endoscopic biliary drainage without sphincterotomy [23]. In accordance with other authors [17], we prefer to carry out ES in all cases, since it allows for the control of sepsis as well as biliary drainage, and also for the removal of the endoscopic bile duct stone, which constitutes the cause of the disease [24]. Only for patients with unstable haemodynamic status or expected difficulty of stone removal is ES postponed to a later date, initial drainage being obtained by nasobiliary tube or by the insertion of an endoprosthesis to control the sepsis.

Cannulation of the bile duct and the placement of a nasobiliary tube or stent is usually easy and can be performed without papillotomy, thus avoiding the risk of bleeding in patients who have an associated coagulopathy. Under these circumstances, a nasobiliary drain and an endoprosthesis are equally effective [25].

The placement of a nasobiliary tube has the advantage of allowing for regular irrigation, which prevents its obstruction, and for radiographic controls, although it carries the risk of dislocation. Stents, on the other hand, may obstruct or become displaced without being recognised. Removal of residual stones is deferred until the cholangitic process has subsided. Indefinite stenting, although associated with a higher incidence of recurrent cholangitis, may be the best option for high-risk patients in whom stone removal is endoscopically impossible.

Following biliary decompression, it is advisable to continue antibiotics up to full resolution of symptoms, since it has been noted that after ES around 5% of patients with cholangitis develop empyema of the gallbladder [26]. Apart from this, if full clearance of the biliary tree is achieved, the risks of further problems are minimal.

Patients who do not respond to endoscopic drainage and appropriate antibiotics should be investigated for the following:

1. malfunction of the biliary drainage system;
2. presence of associated empyema of the gallbladder;
3. associated cholangitic abscesses;
4. undrained segments of the liver, as seen with intrahepatic stones.

A repeat ultrasound or computed tomography (CT) or MRCP or ERCP are helpful in identifying the underlying cause of failure. If non-operative measures fail or are not possible, surgery may be life-saving.

Percutaneous Transhepatic Drainage

Percutaneous transhepatic drainage is reserved for patients in whom endoscopic drainage fails for either technical or anatomical reasons. Percutaneous transhepatic cholangiography can be used for biliary drainage by passing a catheter into a dilated intrahepatic duct, and this route may also be used to retrieve stones via a Dormia basket [27]. Studies, however, have shown rates of stone retention or recurrence of up to 40% [28], which may be associated with further attacks of cholangitis [29]. The passage of cannulas of sufficient diameter to retrieve stones through the liver can also cause significant bleeding.

Patients with intrahepatic stones associated with segmental hepatic duct strictures are best managed by percutaneous transhepatic drainage [30].

Surgical Drainage

Surgery represents a second option if instrumental techniques have failed. Its aim is to resolve the biliary stasis and, as a consequence, the cholangitis, and to treat gallbladder and common bile duct lithiasis. Since it is necessary to perform general anaesthesia, in the rare cases in which a severe cholangitis is complicated by sepsis and acute renal failure, haemodialysis may be required before the surgical intervention. In these conditions, after performing cholecystectomy and intraoperative cholangiogram (if a previous study of the biliary tree with a MR-cholangiogram was not possible), stone removal and drainage of the common bile duct with a Kehr tube constitutes the treatment of choice and the only life-saving option. In the case of mild to moderate cholangitis, if instrumental techniques have failed, the definitive surgical treatment of the cholelithiasis can be reasonably performed through cholecystectomy and bile duct stone treatment, as in an elective setting.

The surgical options are choledocolithotomy, bilioenteric anastomosis and papillosphincterotomy. It is also possible to perform an endoscopic-surgical Rendez-vous, in order to treat the bile duct lithiasis in a combined fashion and to allow for easier endoscopic cannulation of the common bile duct, which previously failed [31]. This combined access may also be useful when further endoscopic manoeuvres are indicated for the definitive treatment of bile tract stones. When repeated endoscopic procedures are needed in patients with previous hepaticojejunostomy, and biliary tree is not endoscopically accessible, the externalization of the afferent jejunal loop (jejunostomy) of hepaticojejunostomy opens a route to the biliary tract, through which appropriate instruments can be passed [32].

The results of the multicentric study reported by Cuschieri et al. [33] suggest that laparoscopy is the best option for the treatment of bile duct stones. When a laparoscopic approach for bile duct exploration is elected, the best method to be used is still controversial. The first laparoscopic explorations were done using the transcystic approach, which for some is still the best option [34, 35]. Choledochotomy has the advantage of allowing the surgeon to perform more complete and direct visual exploration of the bile ducts [36]. Urgent laparoscopic common bile duct exploration for cholangitis has been reported [37], as has elective laparoscopic bile duct exploration in selected cholangitis patients with failed endoscopic stone clearance [17]. At the few centres with the expertise and technology required, laparoscopic bile duct exploration can be carried out. Although laparoscopy appears promising, it is not readily available and its use is not standardised, particularly in choledocholithiasis complicated with cholangitis.

Definitive Treatment

The treatment of gallstone acute cholangitis, of choledocholithiasis and of biliary stasis, responsible for sepsis, is usually an endoscopic treatment that does not allow for the treatment of gallbladder stones. Patients with gallstone cholangitis, in fact, are usually affected by gallbladder stones, and definitive treatment should include cholecystectomy.

In the laparoscopic era many surgeons, including ourselves [24], consider preoperative endoscopy followed by laparoscopy to be the best two-step approach to cholecystocholedocholithiasis [39].

If the stones are successfully cleared endoscopically, the patient simply proceeds to laparoscopic cholecystectomy (LC), and the need for surgical exploration of the common bile duct is avoided. In this way, patients suffering from a possibly serious illness such as acute cholangitis can also benefit from the advantages that are now offered by mini-invasive treatments.

Only patients in whom ERCP or endoscopic stone clearance failed are managed by emergency open common bile duct exploration.

Although relatively high compared with LC for uncomplicated gallstone disease, the conversion rate is acceptable [17]. The main reason for conversion is dense adhesion around Calot's triangle as a result of previous cholangitis. The morbidity observed

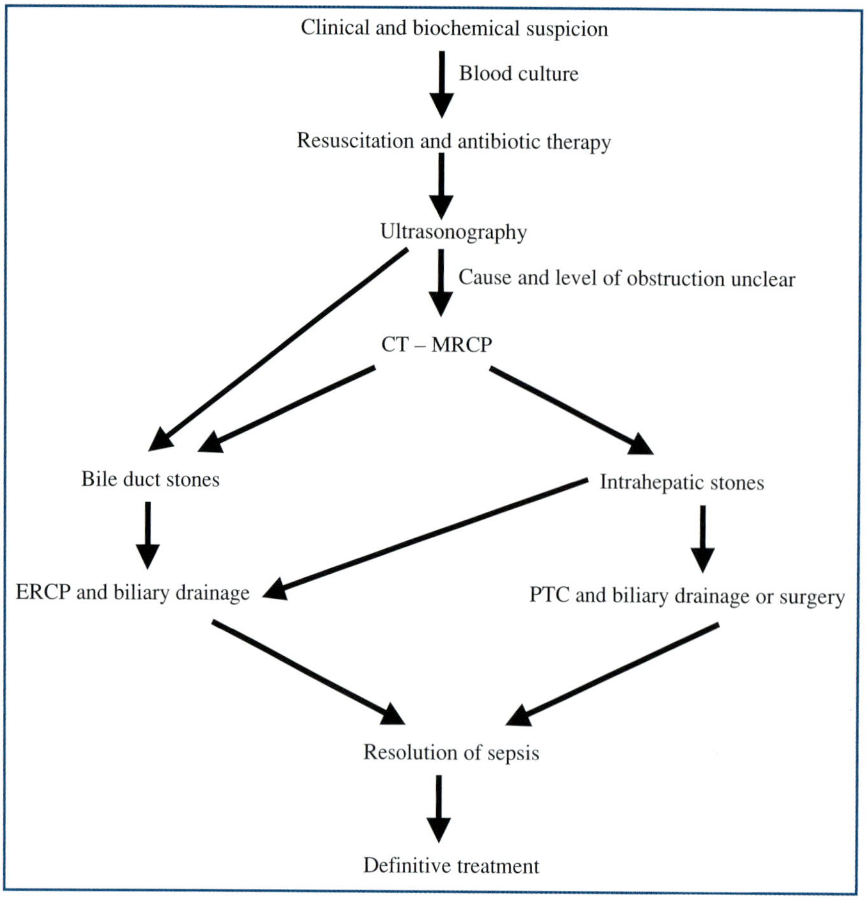

Fig. 42.1 Gallstone cholangitis: management algorithm [38]. *MRCP*, magnetic resonance cholangiopancreatography; *ERCP*, endoscopic retrograde cholangiopancreatography; *PTC*, percutaneous transhepatic drainage

after interval LC is low and not significantly different from that observed after standard LC.

For the treatment of cholecystocholedocholithiasis, a growing number of reports propose the combination of ES and LC, with ES performed under general anaesthesia immediately prior to or immediately after cholecystectomy, for a single-session performance of the two techniques [40, 42]. However, none of these reports specifically involved cases of acute cholangitis, and thus it is not possible to evaluate whether this approach is useful in these particular conditions.

Long-term findings in our recent experience [43] suggest that ES alone is insufficient for the treatment of patients with gallstone cholangitis. Patients managed with ES alone had a significantly higher risk of recurrent biliary symptoms than those with cholecystectomy. Mortality due to causes unrelated to cholangitis were also higher in the group of patients managed with ES alone, probably because this group included above all high operative risk or elderly patients and those with severe comorbid illnesses. A diagnostic-therapeutic algorithm for acute gallstone cholangitis [39] is proposed in Figure 42.1.

Follow-up

Patients who have undergone previous treatment of gallstone cholangitis may have recurrent bile tree obstruction, presenting as ascending cholangitis. Frequent recurrences of gallstone cholangitis may cause biliary cirrhosis which, as well known, can eventually lead to liver transplantation.

Periodic instrumental surveillance with stone removal decreases the incidence of recurrent episodes of ascending cholangitis as well as its associated morbidity and mortality [44].

References

1. Leese T, Neoptolemus JP, Baker AR, Carr-Locke DL (1986) Management of acute cholangitis and the impact of endoscopic sphincterotomy. Br J Surg 73:988
2. Saik RP, Greenburg AG, Farris JM, Peskin GW (1975) Spectrum of cholangitis. Am J Surg 130:143
3. Tsujino T, Sugita R, Yoshida H et al (2007) Risk factors for acute suppurative cholangitis caused by bile duct stones. Eur J Gastroenterol Hepatol 19:585-588
4. van Erpecum KJ (2006) Complications of bile duct stones: acute cholangitis and pancreatitis. Best Pract Res Clin Gastroenterol 20:1139-1152
5. Csendes A, Sepulveda A, Burdiles P et al (1988) Common bile duct pressure in patients with common bile duct stones with or without acute suppurative cholangitis. Arch Surg 123:697-699
6. Reynolds BM, Dargan EL (1959) Acute obstructive cholangitis; a distinct clinical syndrome. Ann Surg 150:299-303
7. Abboud PA, Malet PF, Berlin JA et al (1996) Predictors of common bile duct stones prior to cholecystectomy: a meta-analysis. Gastrointest Endosc 44:450-455
8. Palazzo L (1997) Which test for common bile duct stones? Endoscopic and intraductal ultrasonography. Endoscopy 29:655-665
9. Trap R, Adamsen S, Hart-Hansen O, Henriksen M (1999) Severe and fatal complications after diagnostic and therapeutic ERCP: a prospective series of claims to insurance covering public hospitals. Endoscopy 31:125-130
10. Loperfido S, Angelini G, Benedetti G et al (1998) Major early complications from diagnostic and therapeutic ERCP: a prospective multicenter study. Gastrointest Endosc 48:1-10
11. Wada K, Takada T, Kawarada Y et al (2007) Diagnostic criteria and severity assessment of acute cholangitis: Tokio Guidelines. J Hepatobiliary Pancreat Surg 14:52-58
12. Rogers L (1903) Biliary abscess of the liver with operation. BMJ 2:706-710
13. Neoptolemos JP, Carr-Locke DL (1980) ERCP in acute cholangitis and pancreatitis. In: Jacobson IM (ed.) ERCP: Techniques Application. New York, Elsevier, pp 91-126
14. Boender J, Nix GAJJ, de Ridder MAJ et al (1995) Endoscopic sphincterotomy and biliary drainage in patients with cholangitis due to common bile duct stones. Am J Gastroenterol 90:233-238
15. Lau JYW, Ip SM, Chung SCS et al (1996) Endoscopic drainage aborts endotoxemia in acute cholangitis. Br J Surg 83:181-187
16. Lai ECS, Mok FPT, Tan ESY et al (1992) Endoscopic biliary drainage for severe acute cholangitis. N Engl J Med 326:1582-1592
17. Poon RT, Liu CL, Lo CM et al (2001) Management of gallstone cholangitis in the era of laparoscopic cholecystectomy. Arch Surg 136:11-16
18. Suc B, Escat J, Cherqui D et al (1998) Surgery vs endoscopy as primary treatment in symptomatic patients with suspected common bile duct stones: a multicenter randomized trial. French Association for Surgical Research. Arch Surg 133:702-708
19. Cotton PB (1993) Endoscopic retrograde cholangiopancreatography and laparoscopic cholecystectomy. Am J Surg 165:474-478
20. Chan ACW, Chung SC, Wyman A et al (1996) Selective use of pre-operative endoscopic retrograde cholangiopancreatography in laparoscopic cholecystectomy. Gastrointest Endosc 43:212-215
21. Misra SP, Dwivedi M (1996) Biliary endoprosthesis as an alternative to endoscopic nasobiliary drainage in patients with acute cholangitis. Endoscopy 28:746-749
22. Sharma BC, Agarwal DK, Baijal SS et al (1997) Endoscopic management of acute calculous cholangitis. J Gastroenterol Hepatol 12:874-876
23. Sugiyama M, Atomi Y (1997) Treatment of acute cholangitis due to choledocholithiasis in elderly and younger patients. Arch Surg 132:1129-1133
24. Sarli L, Pietra N, Franzè A et al (1999) Routine intravenous cholangiography, selective ERCP, and endoscopic treatment of bile duct stones before laparoscopic cholecystectomy. Gastrointest Endosc 50:200-208
25. Sharma BC, Kumar R, Agarwal N et al (2005) Endoscopic biliary drainage by nasobiliary drain or by stent placement in patients with acute cholangitis. Endoscopy 37:439-443
26. Davidson BR, Neoptolemos JP, Carr-Locke DL (1988) Endoscopic sphincterotomy for common bile duct calculi in patients with gallbladder in situ considered unfit for surgery. Gut 29:114-118
27. Günter RW, Vorwerk D (1994) Percutaneous therapy of gallstones. Chirurg 65:430-437
28. Curtois CS, Picus DD, Hicks ME et al (1996) Percutaneous gallstone removal: long-term follow-up. J Vasc Intervent Radiol 7:229-234
29. Jan YY, Chen MF (1995) Percutaneous trans-hepatic cholangioscopic lithotomy for hepatolithiasis: long-term results. Gastrointest Endosc 42:1-5

30. Lee DWH, Chung SCS (1997) Biliary infection. Baillière's Clin Gastroenterol 11:707-724
31. Calvo MM, Bujanda L, Heras I et al (2001) The Rendez-vous technique for the treatment of choledocholithiasis. Gastrointest Endosc 54:511-513
32. Takada T, Yasuda H, Uchiyama K et al (1989) The relationship between a subcutaneously placed afferent jejunal loop in a hepaticojejunostomy and postoperative cholangitis. Int Surg 74:167-170
33. Cuschieri A., Croce E, Faggioni A et al (1996) EAES ductal stone study: preliminary findings of multicenter prospective randomized trial comparing two-stage management. Surg Endosc 10:1130-1135
34. Phillips E, Carroll BJ, Pearlstein AR et al (1993) Laparoscopic choledochoscopy and extraction of common bile duct stones. World J Surg 17:22-25
35. DePaula AL, Hashiba K, Bafutto M (1994) Laparoscopic management of choledocholithiasis. Surg Endosc 8:1399-1403
36. Carroll B, Phillips B, Daykhorsky L et al (1992) Laparoscopic choledochoscopy: an effective approach to the common bile duct. J Laparoendosc Surg 2:15-17
37. Lo CM, Liu CL, Fan ST, Lai ECS, Wong J (1998) Prospective randomized study of early versus delayed laparoscopic cholecystectomy for acute cholecystitis. Ann Surg 227:461-467
38. Borman OC, van Nelion JI, Krige JEJ (2003) Management of cholangitis. J Hepatobiliary Pancreat Surg 10:406-414
39. Dorenbusch NJ, Maglinte DDT, Micon LT et al (1995) Intravenous cholangiography and the management of choledocholithiasis prior to laparoscopic cholecystectomy. Surg Laparosc Endosc 5:188-192
40. Sarli L, Sabadini G, Pietra N et al (1995) Laparoscopic cholecystectomy and endoscopic sphincterotomy under a single anaesthetic: a case report. Surg Laparosc Endosc 5:68-71
41. De Palma GD, Angrisani L, Lorenzo M et al (1996) Laparoscopic Cholecystectomy, intraoperative ES and CBDS extraction for management of patients with cholecystocholedocholithiasis. Surg Endosc 10:646-652
42. Deslander E, Gagner M, Pomp A et al (1993) Intraoperative endoscopic sphincterotomy for common bile duct stones during laparoscopic cholecystectomy. Gastrointest Endosc 39:45-58
43. Sarli L, Iusco D, Sgobba G, Roncoroni L (2002) Gallstone cholangitis: a 10-year experience of combined endoscopic and laparoscopic treatment. Surg Endosc 16:975-980
44. Bowser L, Schutz SM (2000) The role of surveillance endoscopic retrograde cholangiopancreatography in preventing episodic cholangitis in patients with recurrent common bile duct stones. Gastrointest Endosc 51:247-248

SUBJECT INDEX

D

Printed in June 2008